Introductory nutrition

Introductory nutrition

Helen Andrews Guthrie, B.A., M.S.

Foods and Nutrition Department,
The Pennsylvania State University,
University Park, Pennsylvania

Illustrated

The C. V. Mosby Company

Saint Louis   1967

Preface

This presentation of the fundamentals of nutrition has been prepared for the new kind of student entering college, one who has graduated from high school well prepared for the serious study of elementary nutrition. Although the approach in this book does not presuppose formal training in physiology or biochemistry, it does take into account the experience most students have had dealing with the concepts of the biological and physical sciences. It is assumed that students using this book have the capacity and the desire to achieve a considerable understanding of nutritional processes. To help make this understanding possible, basic concepts and terms from related sciences are presented in the first chapter. In addition, a glossary of terms and a list of meanings of prefixes and suffixes are included.

I hope that in mastering the material presented the student will become a discerning consumer of nutrition information with a comprehension of the basic principles adequate to enable him to discriminate the scientific from the pseudoscientific and fact from fallacy in the vast literature which is appearing in both the lay and the scientific press. In addition to developing his own understanding of nutrition, the student should be adequately prepared to interpret fundamental knowledge about nutrition to the general public. One of the prime purposes of this text is to motivate the student to apply his knowledge to himself, for his own benefit. I also hope that I will achieve in some cases a different order of personal application of this information. Nutrition is an exciting, rapidly changing, vital area of science with challenging career opportunities and broad social implications. Nutritionists have a wide range of opportunities for research and service in the social and behavioral sciences as well as medical and biological fields. It would be gratifying if some of the readers of this book became sufficiently stimulated and challenged by the subject matter and limitless possibilities which the study of nutrition presents to continue with advanced work in the field.

The tremendous rate of development of research techniques and findings not only in nutrition but also in related fields means that certain aspects of the study of nutrition presented in this book may be open to question, outdated, or even disproved before the ink is dry. For instance, many of the relatively new theories of metabolism and the interrelationship of nutrients have been included with the full knowledge that they may not be substantiated by further research.

The social implications of this science must not be overlooked. It is known that physical growth, within the limits imposed by heredity, is to a large extent a reflection of the adequacy of nutrition of the individual. Recent evidence suggesting that severe nutritional inadequacy in early infancy may cause irreversible damage to the central nervous system places even more responsibility and a greater challenge in the hands of world nutrition authorities. Through its influence on the productivity, behavior, health, and emotional stability of the individual, nutrition plays a crucial role in world politics, with implications for the future of a nation as well as an individual.

The illustrations used in the text have been developed for the most part from current data and relatively recent publications. This should not be interpreted as a rejection of the historical aspects of the field and the tremendous contributions and impetus which early workers provided. Rather it is an attempt to reflect the current status of the field and to focus attention on the present rather than on the past.

Like most books this one was not produced single-handedly. It was possible only through the encouragement and cooperation of a great many individuals, including my colleagues in the Foods and Nutrition Department at the Pennsylvania State University, the scientists who generously consented to have their work reproduced or quoted, the many secretaries involved in the preparation of the manuscript, and my husband and three children whose encouragement and patience throughout the whole process went well beyond all reasonable expectations.

Helen A. Guthrie
University Park, Pennsylvania
January, 1967

Contents

Appendices

Part I

Basic principles
of
nutrition

1

Introduction

The science of nutrition has been defined in many ways. Most simply it has been expressed as the science of nourishing the body properly. Others have chosen to define it as a science devoted to ascertaining the requirements of the body for food constituents both qualitatively and quantitatively and to the selection of food in kinds and in quantity to meet these requirements. The Council of Foods and Nutrition of the American Medical Association elaborates still further in declaring nutrition as "the science of food, the nutrients and other substances therein, their action, interaction, and balance in relation to health and disease and the processes by which the organism ingests, digests, absorbs, transports, utilizes and excretes food substances." In addition, nutrition must be concerned with certain social, economic, cultural, and psychological implications of food and eating. Regardless of the basic definition, persons studying nutrition agree that they are concerned with the changes that occur in food and the way in which the body uses food from the time it is ingested until it is even-

tually incorporated into the body tissues, participates in biological reactions, or is excreted from the body. This includes the study of digestion, absorption, and transportation of nutrients to the cells and their metabolism within the many types of body cells.

The nutrients in food are those chemical components of the food that perform one of three roles in the body: to supply energy, to regulate body processes, or to promote the growth and repair of body tissue.

The science of nutrition is a relative youngster in the scientific community, having been recognized as a distinct discipline only in 1934 with the organization of the American Institute of Nutrition. By its very nature, a science relying on the techniques of the chemist and biologist, nutrition had to await the development of scientific techniques of these other branches of science. Nutrition, like other sciences, does not stand alone. It draws heavily on the basic findings of chemistry, biochemistry, microbiology, physiology, medicine, and, most recently, cellular biology. In turn, it also

3

contributes to these fields of scientific investigation.

HISTORICAL BACKGROUND

Although the organized study of nutrition has been confined to the twentieth century, there is evidence of a long-standing curiosity about the subject. A few well-conceived nutritional experiments were performed earlier, but these stimulated little interest. Schneider has very aptly divided the history of nutrition into three eras: the *naturalistic era* (400 B.C.-1750 A.D.), the *chemical-analytical era* (1750-1900), and the *biological era* (1900 to present). Running concurrently with the latter from 1955 to the present could be added the *cellular* or *molecular* era, in which emphasis has been directed to the study of metabolism within the highly organized individual cells. While no attempt will be made to discuss all the findings of each era, we will mention a few highlights to give some picture of the extent of the knowledge of nutrition in each stage.

Naturalistic era. During the naturalistic era people had many vague ideas about the quality of food, most of which revolved around taboos, magical powers, or the medicinal value of food. In Biblical times Daniel observed that men who ate pulses and drank water thrived better than those who ate the king's food and drank wine. Hippocrates, the father of medicine, in his discussion of food in health and disease in 400 B.C. considered food one universal nutrient. He felt that weight loss during starvation was caused by insensible perspiration. In the early seventeenth century an Italian physician, Sanctorius, curious about the fate of food in the body, weighed himself before and after each meal. His only explanation of his failure to gain weight commensurate with the amount of food taken in was that there must be weight loss in insensible perspiration. It was during this period that such men as Harvey and Spallanzani, with their interest in circulation

and digestion, made observations that eventually facilitated the study of nutrition. At the end of this era the first controlled nutrition experiment was carried out in 1747 by a British physician, Lind, who attempted to find a cure for scurvy by treating twelve sailors ill with the disease with six different substances. He determined that either lemon or lime juice was effective while the others, such as oil of vitriol, sea water, or vinegar, were ineffective in curing this scorbutic condition.

Chemical-analytical era. The chemical-analytical era in the study of nutrition was initiated by Lavoisier, who became known as the father of nutrition. He worked with guinea pigs on the rate of uptake of oxygen with and without food and during work—the first investigation of the question of energy. Black and Priestley also contributed to the growing knowledge of respiration and energy metabolism. All of these men worked in the eighteenth century.

Early in the nineteenth century methods for determining the carbon, hydrogen, and nitrogen in organic compounds were developed. Analyses of foods for these elements led Liebig to suggest that the nutritive value of foods was a function of its nitrogen content. He also postulated that an adequate diet must provide plastic foods (protein) and fuel foods (carbohydrate and fat). Dumas, a French chemist, tested this hypothesis during a siege of Paris in 1871. His efforts to produce a synthetic milk of carbohydrate, fat, and protein in the proportions believed to be found in cow's milk proved unsuccessful, and the infants to whom he fed it died. Dumas logically concluded that milk must contain some unknown nutritive substance.

A similar conclusion was reached in 1881 by Lunin, who found that mice fed a diet of purified casein (a protein), milk sugar (a carbohydrate), milk fat, and the inorganic ash from milk died, while those who were fed milk thrived. Between then and 1906 there were reports of twelve experiments in the use of purified diets in the feeding of animals. All led to essentially the same conclusion that the addition of "astonishingly" small amounts of natural foods was necessary to promote growth and maintain health in the animals. Obviously food contained more than carbohydrate, fat, protein, and mineral ash, but the nature of the other substances remained a mystery. In spite of these findings the United States Department of Agriculture steadfastly maintained until 1910 that carbohydrate, fat, and protein were the only nutrients essential in the human diet.

By 1912 it had been well established that there was an additional dietary essential besides carbohydrate, fat, protein, and mineral ash. Funk, recognizing that this dietary component was essential to life *(vita)* and believing it to be *amine-* or nitrogen-containing, introduced the term *vitamine* to describe this elusive dietary factor. Mc-Collum's work at the University of Wisconsin showing that some fats, such as butter, contained this essential growth factor whereas others, such as lard, did not and Eijkman's observations that a water-soluble substance in rice bran prevented beriberi, a disease common in the Orient, made it clear that at least two vitamins, fat-soluble A and water-soluble B, were essential. By 1920 it was established that all vitamins did not contain nitrogen and the final "e" was dropped to obtain the term *vitamin,* which is still used.

In spite of the relatively slow communication in this period scientists in Europe, Asia, and America made rapid progress in identifying essential dietary components. Many times discoveries were made almost simultaneously by scientists working independently and in widely separated laboratories. The concept that diseases such as beriberi, scurvy, rickets, and pellagra, previously considered to be caused by toxic substances or to be infectious in nature, were in reality the result of an absence of nutrients needed in very small amounts did

much to stimulate the attempts to identify the nature of these dietary essentials.

Biological era. The early part of the biological era was characterized by the discovery of many factors with vitamin-like properties. It soon became clear that there were several components of both fat-soluble A and water-soluble B. By 1940 four fat-soluble and eight water-soluble vitamins had been identified as essential elements of the human diet and several others had been identified for various species of animals. The chemical structure of each had been established, many had been synthesized, and knowledge of their biological roles was accumulating rapidly. Since 1940 only two essential vitamins, folic acid and vitamin B_{12}, have been identified. The emphasis in nutrition research has changed from a search for essential dietary components to a study of the interrelationship between nutrients, their precise biological roles, and the determination of human dietary requirements.

During this same period the noncombustible component or mineral ash of the diet was being studied, and it too proved to be a complex mixture of mineral elements—approximately fifteen of which have been established as dietary essentials for human beings. The essentiality of several others is still uncertain. Here again there was evidence of involved interrelationships among mineral elements; some were capable of replacing others while a high intake of one could cause the excretion of another.

Cellular or molecular era. Since 1955 and the discovery of the electron microscope and the ultracentrifuge, the development of microchemical techniques, and the use of radioactive isotopes, it has been possible to study the nutritional needs and metabolism of the individual cells and even the subcellular components or organelles of the cell, the smallest known units of body structure. At the present time a vast body of information is accumulating, which is leading to a more complete understanding

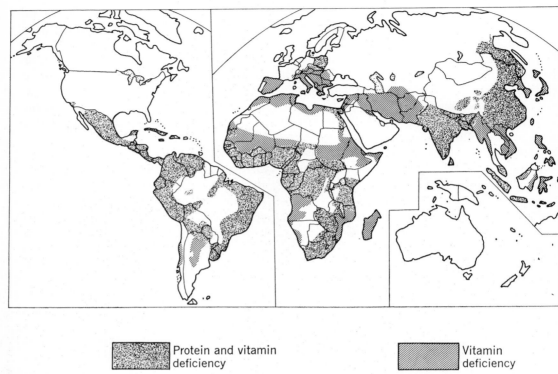

Fig. 1-1

Distribution of vitamin- and protein-deficiency diseases in the world.

of the intricacies of cell structure and the complex and vital role that nutrients play in the growth, development, and maintenance of the cell. Nourishment of the cell is basic to the nourishment of the collection of cells known as tissue, and this in turn is basic to the nourishment of organs of the body and ultimately of the whole complex body. Thus, a defect in nutrition at the cellular level can adversely affect the health of the whole body. The study of the cell has stimulated interest in the role that genetics may play in influencing the nutritional needs of the organism.

Present status. We now find ourselves, less than one hundred years after the first studies that showed that more than carbohydrate, fat, and protein were necessary for normal growth and development, with a vast, complex, and rapidly expanding knowledge of at least thirty-five nutritional principles that must be supplied by food for normal body functioning. The absence of any one of these, regardless of the amount needed, can have a profound effect on the functioning of the whole body.

Although it is now fourteen years since the discovery of the last vitamin, nutrition is a vital, exciting field in which new information is being accumulated at a phenomenal pace. The contributions of the nutritionist alone have been many and significant, but when one integrates with these the related findings of the biochemist, the physiologist, the biologist, and the physicist, one realizes that understanding the complexity of the process of nourishing the body is a challenging frontier of science that is only beginning to be explored.

The rate at which the time, effort, and

money expended on nutrition research increased after the concept of vitamins was first postulated can be judged by the number of scientific publications in the field. In 1913 there were four publications, all by Casimir Funk; by 1920 the number had risen to 73; and in 1930, 724 articles appeared. In 1962 a review of current literature on one of the vitamins, vitamin B_{12}, listed over 1300 references on this one topic. At least ten scientific journals are devoted entirely to reporting findings of nutrition research. The large number of investigators who consider nutrition their major interest is obvious from the large number of members in scientific organizations devoted to nutrition and from attendance at professional meetings. The Institute of Nutrition, whose membership is restricted to scientists who have made an outstanding contribution to the field, numbers over one thousand.

The importance that political leaders attach to nutrition is best illustrated by the fact that the first agency authorized within the United Nations was the Food and Agricultural Organization, commonly known as FAO. In 1944 it was charged with the responsibility of devising ways to improve the nutritional status of the world's population as one of the major pathways to peace. Since then interest in international nutrition problems has increased rapidly. Numerous conferences are devoted to discussion of efforts to improve the nutritional status of the expanding populations of developing countries. The necessity of making maximum use of indigenous food products to provide a level of nutrition capable of supporting the health and promoting individual productivity is an ever-present challenge to nutritionists. The worldwide incidence of nutritional deficiency diseases indicates the scope of the problem (Fig. 1-1).

IMPORTANCE OF GOOD NUTRITION

Before launching an intensive study of the individual nutrients, the student of nu-trition might legitimately ask, "What evidence is there that nutrition makes a difference?"

The available evidence is of two types. One points out the differences between poor and adequate nutrition and the other between adequate and enriched nutrition. A comprehensive review of studies in these areas is well beyond the scope of this text, but a few examples may serve to illustrate the point.

Difference between poor and adequate nutrition. A change from the use of poorly refined brown rice to more highly refined white rice with its improved keeping qualities occurred in the Philippines and other rice-eating countries around the turn of the century. With this change there was a marked increase in the incidence of the disease beriberi, which first was believed to be caused by a toxic substance in rice and later was attributed to unsanitary milling conditions. By 1935, however, an antiberiberi factor in rice bran had been identified, establishing that beriberi was the result of a lack of a nutrient that was apparently removed in the milling process. It became known as thiamine. Once this vitamin had been synthesized and was available commercially, the Philippine government and the Williams Waterman Fund backed a study of rice enrichment to determine the effect of adding thiamine back to the rice. People on one half of the island of Bataan ate rice enriched with thiamine while those on the other half ate the unenriched milled white rice. After nine months of rice enrichment 90% of the population that had previously shown mild or definite signs of the disease were improved and the death rate had dropped by two thirds. At the end of the second year there were no deaths at all from beriberi, indicating fairly clearly that the addition of a nutrient brought about a general improvement in the health and marked decrease in beriberi.

In 1946 Burke, working with patients at the Boston Lying-In Hospital at Harvard, studied the relationship between the quality of the diet of the mother during pregnancy and the health of the infant at the time of birth. Of the infants born to mothers whose diet was rated good or excellent, 94% were judged in superior physical condition at the time of birth, and only 6% were rated in poor condition. Conversely, when the diet was assessed as fair or poor, only 9% of the infants received a superior or good rating, while 67% were judged in poor condition. Since people change food habits slowly even under conditions of high motivation such as pregnancy, the dietary ratings undoubtedly reflected long-standing patterns of eating rather than those that prevailed during pregnancy. Failure of subsequent studies to show such a clearcut relationship may reflect an overall improvement of the diet of mothers.

The reduction in the incidence of simple goiter experienced in Michigan following an intensive educational campaign on the use of iodized salt is further evidence of the differences between poor and adequate nutrition in respect to one nutrient. In a thirty-year period there was a drop from 47.2% to 1.4% in the reported cases of endemic goiter. Similarly, the addition of fluoride to drinking water has resulted in a 50% to 70% reduction in the incidence of tooth decay.

Difference between adequate and enriched nutrition. In Newfoundland a nutritional survey in 1945 revealed a high incidence of subclinical evidence of nutritional deficiency, such as rough dry skin, cracks in the corner of the lips, and soft bleeding gums. This was attributed to suboptimal intakes of the B vitamins, vitamin A, and ascorbic acid. A program of enriching flour with thiamine, riboflavin, niacin, and iron and enriching margarine with vitamin A resulted in a marked reduction in these conditions.

The change in stature of children in the United States that has occurred in the past few decades has often been attributed to improved nutrition. There is ample evidence that children are heavier and taller than their parents. For instance, Philadelphia schoolchildren in first through fifth grades in all socioeconomic groups averaged 3 inches taller and 3 pounds heavier in 1951 than in 1925. In 1880 5% of male college freshmen were over 6 feet tall, whereas in 1955 30% reached this stature. Nutrition has undoubtedly contributed to this gain, but one must also keep in mind advances in other areas of medicine that have reduced the incidence of infection and other deterrents to maximum growth. The question is now being raised as to whether these large increases in growth rate are necessarily desirable. Evidence from animal studies indicates a decrease in life-span among animals fed at a level to stimulate early and rapid growth. On the other hand women over 5 feet 4 inches tall, possibly the better nourished members of the population, were found to have fewer complications during pregnancy and easier deliveries than those under 5 feet tall.

A study on a group of boys in an English boarding school to evaluate the effect of food supplements on a presumably adequate diet showed that those whose diets were enriched with an additional one pint of milk gained 7 pounds and grew 2.6 inches, while those on a regular diet gained only 3.9 pounds and grew 1.8 inches. Other supplements, such as casein, sugar, margarine, cress, and butter, also led to some increase in growth but not as much as the milk supplement.

HOW THE BODY USES FOOD

Food plays many roles for the individual. Its psychological value, its social significance, its satiety value, and the sheer pleasure it provides many people are constant determinants of when, how much, and what foods are consumed.

The role of food to which our interests will be directed primarily, however, is that of nourishing the body. In this role food chosen wisely provides all the nutrients essential for the normal functioning of the body. If food is not properly chosen there will be a deficiency of one or more of the essential nutrients. An essential nutrient is considered one that must be provided to the organism by food since it cannot be synthesized by the body. Nutrients essential for one species may not be essential for another.

Although we have a rapidly expanding body of information on the biological role and the need for specific nutrients, the long-established broad classification of the function of nutrients in the body is still valid. The major functions are to supply energy, to promote growth and repair of body tissues, and to regulate body processes.

The nutrients that perform these functions may be divided into six main categories: carbohydrate, lipid, protein, minerals, vitamins, and water. Following is a classification of the nutrients in each of these broad groupings that must be provided in the diet.

The nutrients listed are absolutely essential to body growth and functioning. Those classified as body regulators have an especially vital role since the body cannot release the energy from the energy-providing nutrients nor can it utilize those designated as needed for growth and maintenance without these nutrients. Indirectly, then, practically all nutrients can be considered as growth factors. Some nutrients are present in a wide variety of foods in nature and there is little likelihood of deficiency occurring in most diets. On the other hand, some are distributed in a very limited number of foods and will be present in less than optimal amounts if the variety of foods in the diet is limited.

It is clear from the following classification of nutrients according to functions that some, such as protein, perform all three functions, whereas some of the minerals are involved in two functions and vitamins, directly, only in one. A nutrient that performs only one function is equally as essential as one involved in all three functions.

Carbohydrate
  Glucose

Fat or lipid
  Linoleic acid

Protein
  Amino acids
    Leucine
    Isoleucine
    Lysine
    Methionine
    Phenylalanine
    Threonine
    Trytophan
    Valine
  Nonessential nitrogen

Minerals
  Calcium
  Phosphorus
  Sodium
  Potassium
  Sulphur
  Chlorine
  Magnesium
  Iron

Selenium
Zinc
Manganese
Copper
Cobalt
Molybdenum
Iodine

Vitamins
  Fat-soluble vitamins
    A
    D
    E
    K
  Water-soluble vitamins
    Thiamine
    Riboflavin
    Niacin
    Biotin
    Folacin
    Pyridoxine
    Cobalamin
    Pantothenic acid
    Ascorbic acid

Water

Source of energy
  Carbohydrate
  Lipid
  Protein
  Minerals*
  Vitamins*

Growth and maintenance of tissue
  Protein
  Mineral elements
  Vitamins*
  Water*

Regulation of body processes
  Protein
  Mineral elements
  Vitamins
  Water

The amount of each of the essential nutrients needed for normal body functions bears no relationship to its importance in

---

*These play an indirect role since they are necessary to catalyze the use of the nutrients directly involved.

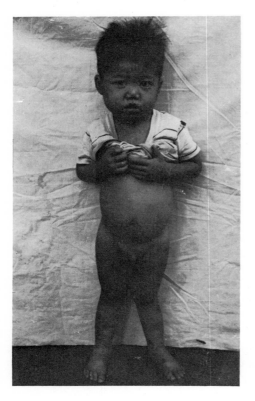

Fig. 1-2

Hidden hunger. This child, aged 4 years, looks plump enough. Closer inspection shows pitting edema of the legs caused by dietary protein deficiency and low serum albumin level. This is kwashiorkor (without dermatosis). The child is also dull, apathetic, potbellied, and has ophthalmic xerosis and Bitot's spots on the conjunctiva of both eyes. (Courtesy WHO Regional Office, Manila.)

the diet. In the adult male needs vary from $3 \mu g. \left(\dfrac{3}{28,000,000} \text{ oz.} \right)$ of cobalamin (vitamin B_{12}) to 70 gm. (2½ oz.) of protein to as much as three fourths of a pound of carbohydrate, depending on his energy needs. A deficiency of a nutrient needed in extremely small amounts may precipitate more severe symptoms more rapidly than a deficiency of one needed in much larger amounts. Figs. 1-2 and 1-3 show effects a severe and prolonged lack of a nutrient may have on an individual. It was the

search for a cause and cure of diseases such as these that stimulated much of the early research in nutrition.

One factor that influenced the ease with which nutritional factors were identified was the rapidity with which body reserves were depleted in times of dietary deficiency. Table 1-1 shows that the time varies from a few hours in the case of labile amino acids, which the body has virtually no capacity to store, to about sixty days for many water-soluble vitamins, to seven years for calcium. The major site of storage differs with the nutrient—liver for iron, vitamin A, and carbohydrate, the adrenal gland for vitamin C, and bone for calcium. For some nutrients there is no storage site. In these cases deficiency symptoms will become evident once the individual cells have become depleted of the nutrient.

The elucidation of the role of individual nutrients was further complicated by the interrelationship and interdependence that exists among the nutrients. For instance, the need for thiamine (vitamin B_1) is a function of the amount and kind of carbohydrate in the diet, the absorption of calcium is dependent on a supply of vitamin D, vitamin E protects vitamin A, and the nature and the amount of fat in the diet affects the vitamin E requirement. Current research is bringing forth even more evidence of the complexity of these interrelationships. Manipulation of one dietary component may lead to changes in the utilization or need of many others. Hence, the evaluation of the results of manipulating one dietary factor depends on knowledge of the existing status of all other dietary factors.

BASIC CONCEPTS FROM RELATED SCIENTIFIC FIELDS

Although this treatment of introductory material basic to the understanding of nutrition does not presuppose any previous training in the related fields of biochemistry, physiology, and cellular biology,

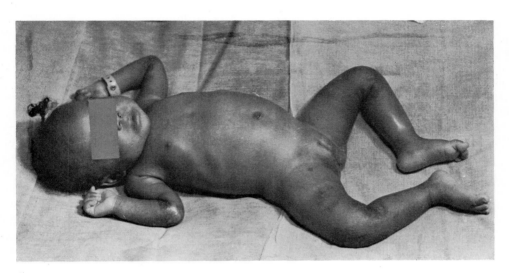

Fig. 1-3

Case of infantile scurvy caused by a lack of ascorbic acid (vitamin C). Note typical frog position, swelling of right thigh, and hyperpigmentation of skin. (From Ossofsky, H. J.: Infantile scurvy, Am. J. Dis. Child. **109**:173, 1965.)

Table 1-1. Extent of body reserves of nutrients

Nutrient	Time required to deplete reserves
Amino acids	Few hours
Carbohydrate	13 hours
Sodium	2-3 days
Water	4 days
Fat	20-40 days
Thiamine	30-60 days
Ascorbic acid	60-120 days
Niacin	60-180 days
Riboflavin	60-180 days
Vitamin A	90-365 days
Iron	125 days (women)
	750 days (men)
Iodine	1000 days
Calcium	2500 days

there are certain concepts from these fields that will facilitate the understanding of the processes involved in nourishing the body. They are well within the grasp of any college student and will be presented here as an elementary review for those with previous instruction in these fields and as the bare fundamentals for those unfamiliar with the subject matter.

Physiology. Before the cells, the smallest structural units of the body, can receive nourishment, the food taken into the body in a complex state must undergo many changes to reduce it to a form in which it can be transported to and used by the cells. These changes occur primarily in the digestive tract of the body (Fig. 1-4). The digestive tract is essentially a tube passing through the center of the body and until

food passes through the walls of this tube it is, from a physiologic standpoint, still outside the body. The walls of the intestines regulate not only the form in which nutrients enter the body but also the amounts.

The process of digestion is accomplished by mechanical and chemical processes. Mechanically, food is broken down into small pieces by the action of chewing in the mouth. This increases the surface area on which the enzymes of the digestive juices can act. As the food mass passes down the digestive tract, peristalsis, the churning action resulting from the contraction and relaxation of the very muscular wall of the tract, reduces the size of food particles still further and mixes them thoroughly with digestive juices.

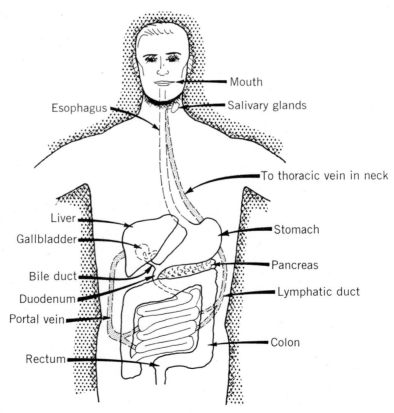

Fig. 1-4

Essential features of the human digestive system.

Chemically, the character of ingested food is changed by the action of digestive enzymes secreted in the salivary juice in the mouth, the gastric juice in the stomach, and by the pancreatic juice, the intestinal juices, and bile secreted into the small intestine. In addition it now appears that some digestion occurs within the wall of the small intestine. Together these digestive juices provide all the enzymes necessary to prepare food for use by the body.

Once the food has been changed chemically so that it is in the form in which the body can use it, it passes through the wall of the intestinal tract into the blood or lymph by which it is carried to the body cells. Most absorption occurs through walls of the small intestine, but some also occurs in the stomach and large intestine, and a very little in the mouth. For some nutrients the passage through the intestinal wall is by diffusion, for others by osmosis, and for many by *active transport*, a process that requires energy. In any case, the nature and amount of food that enters the body from the digestive tract is regulated by the intestinal wall.

After the digested food has passed through the wall of the digestive tract, it is picked up by one of two circulatory systems of the body, the arteriovenous or blood system or the lymphatic system. The relationship of these two systems is illustrated in Fig. 1-5. Nutrients that enter the arteriovenous system are carried by the portal vein to the liver, where they are released into the general circulatory system. In the circulatory system they are distributed through the arteries and very small blood vessels, the capillaries, and finally to the extracellular fluid bathing each individual cell of the body. Nutrients, primarily fats and fat-soluble nutrients that enter the lymphatic system, an auxiliary circulatory system that serves primarily to collect body fluids, bypass the liver and enter the general arteriovenous circulation at a point in the neck just before the blood flows through the heart. From this point, they are distributed to the cells in the same way as nutrients that passed through the liver. It is from the extracellular fluids bathing the cells that the cell obtains the nutrients it needs. In this case the cell membrane acts as a selective barrier to the entrance of material into the cell.

The waste products of cellular metabolism are released into the extracellular fluid, picked up by the bloodstream, and eventually excreted from the body, primarily through the lungs and kidneys.

The lungs serve as the main excretory organ for carbon dioxide and for much of the water. The kidney acts as a very efficient and selective filtering system for the bloodstream. It is capable of concentrating waste products of metabolism, such as creatinine and urea, in the urine and excreting them. It will also allow excesses of such nutrients as water-soluble vitamins to leave the body. However, for nutrients such as glucose, which the body needs to conserve, it will reabsorb practically all that is present in the blood filtered through the kidney. In the case of some other nutrients, it will reabsorb the amounts needed to maintain normal blood and tissue levels and release the rest. It is very sensitive to the demands of the body and will regulate the nature and amount of the metabolites excreted in response to the many regulatory forces that influence it. Some nutrients are also lost from the body through the skin—either in perspiration or in the sloughing of epithelial cells or the loss of hair and nails. Cells lining the intestinal tract are completely replaced every three to four days, the old ones falling off to be excreted in the feces. Fecal secretions may also contain nutrients that are part of the digestive juices, which are not reabsorbed. A determination of the kinds and amounts of nutrients lost from the body through any or all of these pathways sheds much light on the need for various nutrients and the way in which they are changed in the body.

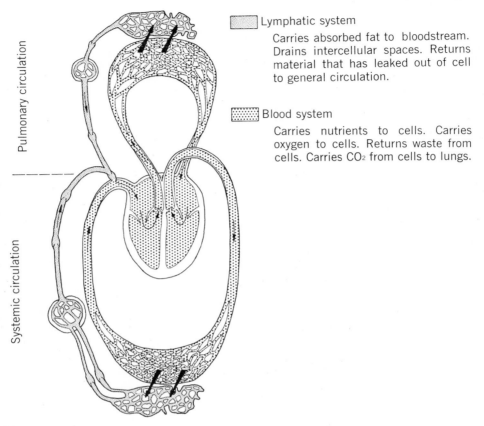

Lymphatic system

Carries absorbed fat to bloodstream. Drains intercellular spaces. Returns material that has leaked out of cell to general circulation.

Blood system

Carries nutrients to cells. Carries oxygen to cells. Returns waste from cells. Carries CO_2 from cells to lungs.

Pulmonary circulation

Systemic circulation

Fig. 1-5

Two circulatory systems, the blood and the lymphatic, are related in this schematic diagram. Oxygenated blood is pumped by the heart through a network of capillaries, bringing oxygen and nutrients to the tissue cells. Venous blood returns to the heart and is oxygenated in the course of the pulmonary (lung) circulation. Fluid and other substances seep out of the blood capillaries into the tissue spaces and are returned to the bloodstream by the lymph capillaries and larger lymphatic vessels. (From Mayerson, H. S.: The lymphatic system, Scient. Am. **208**:80 [June], 1963.)

Biochemistry. The nature of the nutrients and the chemical changes that occur in them from the time they are taken into the body until they are built into body tissue, used, or excreted is part of the subject matter of biochemistry—the chemistry of living material. All biological compounds contain the elements carbon and hydrogen, practically all contain oxygen, and they may have nitrogen, sulphur, or other inorganic elements.

Basic to any understanding of biochemistry is knowledge of the chemistry of carbon compounds. Carbon, an element capable of reacting with both positively and negatively charged elements, *always* has a valence of four, which means that there are four places on a carbon atom to which some other element is attached $\left(1 - \overset{\overset{\displaystyle 4}{|}}{\underset{\underset{\displaystyle 2}{|}}{C}} - 3\right)$.

If two adjacent carbon atoms are unsaturated or do not have anything to attach to their carbon bonds, they will join together, forming what is known as a double bond $(1-\overset{4}{C}=\overset{4}{C}-3)$. This is a relatively unstable bond that is easily broken to two single bonds if some elements become available to attach to the bonds. Compounds that contain double carbon bonds are quite active chemically since they are receptive to the addition of other elements. In general, however, carbon compounds are relatively inert, reacting very slowly with each other, with water, and with oxygen.

About 99% of the body is made up of biological material whose basic chemical structure involves carbon compounds. These range from simple two-carbon compounds such as acetic acid to the extremely large molecules of hormones and enzymes containing several hundred carbon atoms linked together in a straight chain, in a branched arrangement, or a three-dimensional molecule. Some compounds are biologically active, undergoing constant and sometimes very rapid change while others are relatively inert, changing slowly. A portion of the study of nutrition involves studying the nature and extent of the changes and the way in which various nutrients are involved in these changes. The biological material enters the body as carbohydrate, fat, protein, or vitamins and eventually is excreted through the lungs as carbon dioxide and water and in the urine as a variety of substances. The time elapsing between these two extremes may be a matter of seconds or a matter of years. In the interval they may be subjected to a few minor biochemical changes or a series of very complex biochemical actions and interactions, all of which involve the metabolism of carbon-containing compounds. Thus, when we refer to changes involving a single carbon unit such as a methyl group (CH_3), we are speaking of one small molecule or a small portion of a molecule; when we talk of a long-chain carbon unit such as a peptide chain or a fatty acid, we may be referring to a large portion of a biological compound.

Biochemical compounds are subject to the same fundamental reactions that inorganic compounds undergo. Thus, biochemical substances such as carbohydrate may unite with oxygen in a process called *oxidation* or combustion. The removal of a hydrogen atom has the same effect and is another way in which oxidation can occur. On the other hand, if hydrogen is incorporated, the substance is said to have been reduced or to have undergone hydrogenation. The removal of oxygen is also a reducing reaction. A compound that has been either reduced or oxidized will have physical, chemical, or biological properties that differ from the original compound. Nutritionally, the value of a nutrient may be completely destroyed or reduced by either oxidation or hydrogenation; in some cases the biological value of a nutrient is unaffected and in others it is enhanced.

In biochemical compounds the presence of an OH or hydroxyl group in a terminal position identifies the compound as an alcohol (comparable to hydroxide in inorganic compounds). When this is oxidized, it forms an aldehyde, —CHO, which can be further oxidized to an acid in which the terminal group is —COOH. This conversion of alcohol to aldehyde to acid by oxidation may be reversed by reduction reactions.

Other biochemical reactions to which a student of nutrition may be exposed are deamination, the removal of the amino group (NH_2) from a compound; transamination, the transfer of NH_2 from one compound to another; and transmethylation, the transfer of a methyl (CH_3) group.

Cellular biology. The smallest unit of body structure is the cell, which occurs in many sizes and shapes in the body. Fig. 1-6 shows various types of cells that have very specific characteristics, depending on the particular tissues of which they are a part. Recent discovery of the electron microscope has allowed scientists to determine a very definite structure within individual cells, indicating a high degree of organization of subcellular particles or organelles. The use of the ultracentrifuge and various microchemical techniques has made possible the determination of the bio-

chemical makeup of these organelles and has indicated definite biochemical specialization in these small subcellular units. Even the cell membrane has been determined as a highly structured, complex, and functional unit of the cell. Since many of the advances in nutrition are the result of the study of cellular nutrition and since popu-

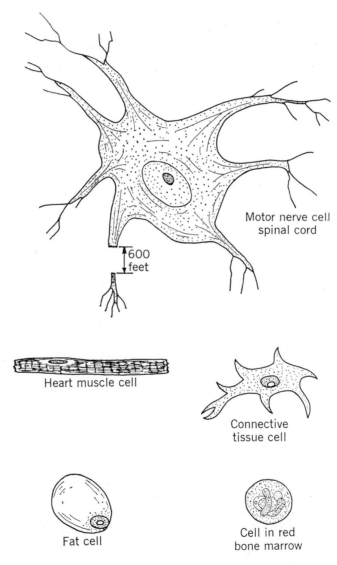

Fig. 1-6

Some typical mammalian cells (magnified two hundred times).

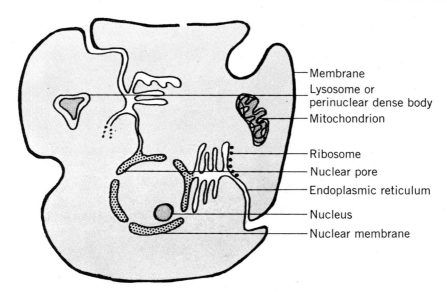

Membrane
Lysosome or
perinuclear dense body
Mitochondrion

Ribosome
Nuclear pore
Endoplasmic reticulum

Nucleus
Nuclear membrane

Fig. 1-7

Diagrammatic representation of a typical cell.

lar publications are using these findings with increasing frequency, a familiarity with cell structure seems desirable for a student of nutrition. Just as there is no typical human, there is no typical cell. Each varies according to its function. Fig. 1-7, however, is a representation of the essential features of most cells.

Among the main organelles or functional units of the cell is the cell membrane, composed of two layers of protein with a "filling" of fat, which regulates the uptake of material from the external environment of the cell, the extracellular fluid. It also governs the release of material, either newly synthesized material or waste products from the cell. In a sense, it is the "doorkeeper" of the cell. Within the cell is a mass of material, the cytoplasmic matrix, within which are several highly organized areas.

The mitochondrion, another double-membraned structure within the cell, contains upwards of five hundred enzymes involved in the release of energy from energy-yielding nutrients. Its vital role in energy metabolism has led to its designation as the powerhouse of the cell. The number of mitochondria within a cell var-

ies, depending on the function of the cell, but in very active cells, such as those of liver or heart muscle, there may be as many as one thousand.

Lysosomes or perinuclear dense bodies contain the digestive enzymes of the cell and serve to digest particles that may enter the cell in a form that must be changed before it can be used. Lysosomes are capable of digesting complex substances in the cytoplasm of the cell and releasing them as their simple components into the cytoplasm again. If released from their membranes, the enzymes of the lysosomes are capable of digesting the cell itself. This occurs at the death of the cell.

Throughout the cytoplasm is a network of canals, some of which are lined with small granules. The canals are known as endoplasmic reticulum and serve as communication channels within the cell and between cells. The small granules are microsomes or ribosomes in which the synthesis of protein within the cell occurs.

In the center of the cell, separated from the cytoplasm by a membrane, is the nucleus. The nucleus contains the genetic information that allows the cell to reproduce in the pattern of the parent cell. The code contained in the genetic material DNA, deoxyribonucleic acid, is transmitted through pores in the nuclear membrane to the ribosomes by another nucleic acid, RNA (ribonucleic acid), produced in the nucleolus of the nucleus.

SELECTED REFERENCES

Goldblith, S. A., and Joslyn, M. A. (editors): Milestones in nutrition, Westport, Conn., 1964, AVI Publishing Co.

Goldsmith, G. A.: Clinical nutritional problems in the United States today, Nutr. Rev. **23**:1, 1965.

Griffith, W. H.: Food as a regulator of metabolism, Am. J. Clin. Nutrition **17**:391, 1965.

McCollum, E. V.: A history of nutrition, Boston, 1957, Houghton Mifflin Company.

Todhunter, E. N.: Development of knowledge in nutrition. I. Animal experiments. II. Human experiments, J. Am. Dietet. A. **41**:328, 335, 1962.

Todhunter, E. N.: Some classics of nutrition and dietetics, J. Am. Dietet. A. **44**:100, 1964.

Williams, R. R.: The classical deficiency diseases, Fed. Proc. (No. 1, Supp. 7) **20**:323, 1961.

Youmans, J. B.: Changing face of nutritional diseases in America, J.A.M.A. **189**:672, 1964.

2

Carbohydrate

Carbohydrate, an energy-yielding nutrient, is the largest single component, aside from water, of most diets, about two thirds of a pound of carbohydrate being present in a 2400-calorie diet. It was one of the first nutrients to be chemically identified, yet only now is evidence appearing to indicate that it is essential in human nutrition. It is a compound composed of the three elements carbon, hydrogen, and oxygen. The ratio of hydrogen to oxygen in all carbohydrates is two to one, the same ratio found in water—hence the term *carbohydrate*. In simple carbohydrates there are equal numbers of carbon and oxygen atoms ($C_nH_{2n}O_n$); for complexes of two or more simple carbohydrates there is one less oxygen atom than carbon atoms ($C_n[H_2O]_{n-1}$). Carbohydrate foods are generally recognized as starches and sugars. It is in this form that plants store the energy they derive from the sun.

SYNTHESIS

Plants with green leaves are able to trap the energy of the sun through a process known as photosynthesis. As shown in Fig. 2-1, the carbon dioxide of the atmosphere and water from the soil are picked up by the plant and combined in the presence of chlorophyll, the magnesium-containing pigment of plants, to form the energy-rich carbohydrate—either starch or sugar.

In some plants, such as potatoes, wheat, and rice, the carbohydrate is in the form of starch; in others, such as sweet peas, bananas, cherries, and sugar beets, it is in the form of sugar.

In peas and corn carbohydrate is stored initially as sugar and changed to starch as the seed matures. The sweetness of carrots also declines as the sugar in the root is converted to starch with aging. Frequently we find the stored starch in fruits such as bananas, apples, and pears being converted to sugar during the ripening process. Regardless of the form in which it is stored or whether it is stored in the root, leaf, seed, or fruit of the plant, carbohydrate represents the reserve of energy for the plant.

CLASSIFICATION

Monosaccharides. The simplest structural unit of carbohydrates is a monosaccharide. This is the chemical building block from which all more complex carbohydrates **19**

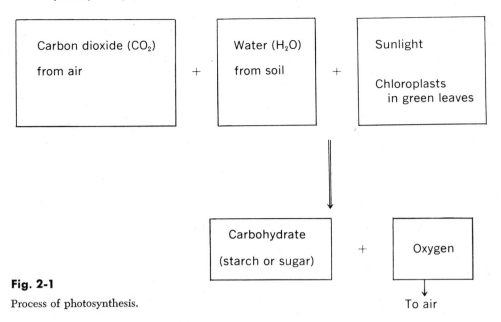

Fig. 2-1

Process of photosynthesis.

To air

are built. Most of the monosaccharides are also known as hexoses since they are composed of a six-carbon chain to which hydrogen and oxygen atoms are attached as hydrogen or hydroxyl (OH) groups. There are three monosaccharides of importance in nutrition—*glucose, fructose,* and *galactose.* A fourth, mannose, has limited significance in human nutrition since it is found free to a limited extent and only in poorly digested complexes. It has been used, however, in

intravenous feedings. They all contain the same number and kinds of atoms—six carbon atoms, twelve hydrogen atoms, and six oxygen atoms $(C_6H_{12}O_6)$. They differ from one another only in the way in which the hydrogen and oxygen atoms are arranged around the chain of carbon atoms. The combination of a hydrogen and oxygen atom (OH) is called a hydroxyl group. The differences in monosaccharides can be observed from the following formulas:

Glucose   **Fructose**   **Galactose**   **Mannose**

(Boxed areas are where structure differs from glucose.)

These different arrangements of atoms within the carbohydrate molecule account for the variation in sweetening power, solubility, and other properties of the different monosaccharides. One method of identifying sugars involves passing a beam of polarized light through a solution of the sugar. On the basis of its effect on polarized light, glucose, which causes the light to rotate to the right, has been named dextrose. A fructose solution, on the other hand, causes polarized light to rotate to the left. Hence, fructose is known as levulose.

Monosaccharides seldom occur free in foods. Some glucose is found in grapes, both glucose and fructose are found in honey, and fructose is found in the Jerusalem artichoke. Fructose is present in many syrups. So far no food has been found that contains galactose. It does occur as a component of the more complex carbohydrates in milk and the seed coat of legumes. Monosaccharides are usually derived from the digestion or breakdown of more complex carbohydrates.

Glucose is sometimes referred to as blood sugar since it is the only carbohydrate found in the general circulation of the body, where it occurs in both the blood plasma and the red blood cells. The total amount of glucose in blood and extracellular tissue is estimated at 17 gm. in an adult male. Normal fasting blood glucose levels are about 100 mg. per 100 ml. of blood. The level usually rises following a meal and falls gradually until it hits the fasting level, which is usually associated with hunger. When levels rise above 160 mg. per 100 ml., the condition is known as hyperglycemia; when they fall below 80 mg., hypoglycemia results. If blood glucose levels get so high that the kidney, which normally prevents the loss of sugar from the body, cannot reabsorb it, sugar appears in the urine. This occurs in diabetes mellitus.

Glucose can be reduced to an alcohol sugar, sorbitol. Sorbitol, with a sweetening power equivalent to glucose, has been used in some weight-reducing aids on the theory that the body cannot utilize it. It now appears the body can use it, but because of the slow rate at which it is absorbed it helps keep blood sugar levels high following a meal and delays the onset of hunger sensations. It has been found in many fruits and vegetables.

Mannitol, another alcohol sugar used as a drying agent in some foods, has a sweetening power similar to glucose, but because it is only partially absorbed yields only half as many calories per gram as other carbohydrates. It is found in pineapple, olives, asparagus, carrots, and sweet potatoes.

Some five-carbon sugars, pentoses, are found occasionally in plants but do not represent an appreciable source of dietary carbohydrate. Ribose, arabinose, and xylose are the most common. In the body ribose is part of some very vital body compounds, such as the riboflavin-containing enzymes and nucleic acids in the nucleus and cytoplasm of the cell. The body can produce ribose from glucose and so does not depend on a dietary source of five-carbon sugars to form the essential nucleic acids.

Disaccharides. More common in foods are the disaccharides, which are each composed of two monosaccharide units. When two monosaccharides are joined to form a disaccharide, one molecule of water is split off. Conversely, when a disaccharide is broken into its two component monosaccharide units, as occurs in digestion, a molecule of water must be added in a process known as hydrolysis. Thus we have a reversible reaction:

$$C_6H_{12}O_6 \quad + \quad C_6H_{12}O_6$$

Monosaccharides + Monosaccharides
(1) Hydrolysis
(2) Synthesis

$$\underset{(2)}{\overset{(1)}{\rightleftarrows}} \quad C_{12}H_{22}O_{11} \; + \; H_2O$$

Disaccharide + Water

The most common disaccharide, *sucrose,* a combination of glucose and fructose, is a familiar item in the diet. Granulated sugar is 100% sucrose. Brown sugar, the slightly less refined, more flavorful product of either beet or cane sugar, is 97% sucrose. Sucrose accounts for the sweetness of most fruits and vegetables. The world consumes 30 million tons of sucrose a year with two thirds of it coming from sugar cane and one third from beet sugar. Both cane and beet sugars yield far more calories per acre of land than any other crop. The consumption of sucrose in the American diet continues to increase and is felt to be a contributing factor to the high incidence of tooth decay.

Lactose, a combination of glucose and galactose, is found only in milk, where it accounts for half the total solids. Sometimes known as milk sugar, it was first identified in 1633 and is the only source of the monosaccharide galactose. In the intestine certain microorganisms cause the production of lactic acid from any unabsorbed lactose. This increased acidity in the lower intestinal tract creates a medium in which the organism *bifidus* grows to produce the *bifidus factor* believed to be beneficial to very young infants in preventing the growth of the less desirable bacteria that cause intestinal putrefaction. This factor is found primarily in the intestines of breast-fed infants, and its presence has been identified as one of the advantages of breast-feeding infants over bottle-feeding. The acid medium created by the formation of lactic acid from lactose has been suggested as an explanation of the favorable effect of lactose in the absorption of calcium and other alkaline metals. Recent evidence suggests that a relatively soluble calcium-lactose complex forms, increasing the extent to which calcium is absorbed. Others suggest that lactose increases the permeability of the intestinal membrane to cations. Whatever the mechanism, it is interesting to note that the best source of lactose and

of calcium in the diet is the same food—milk.

Maltose, the third disaccharide, is found in germinating cereals. It is composed of two molecules of glucose.

All members of the monosaccharide group and disaccharide group are considered sugars as indicated by the suffix *-ose.*

Sugars differ in their sweetening power, as shown in Table 2-1. The sweetening power of sugar parallels its solubility. Fructose, with the greatest sweetening power, is most soluble and therefore difficult to crystallize from a solution and obtain in crystalline form. This makes it useful in syrups but also means that the small amount of fructose available in crystalline form is very expensive. Lactose, which is relatively insoluble, is very difficult to incorporate in a solution and hence not practical as a sweetening agent for liquids.

Polysaccharides. The third group of carbohydrates, the polysaccharides, are much more complex and are considered starches rather than sugars. They represent about half of the dietary carbohydrates. They are composed solely of glucose units linked together in long chains. A polysaccharide may contain as many as two thousand glucose units, which may be in one long chain (an amylose) or in a branched arrangement (an amylopectin), as illustrated:

$$G-G-G-G-G-G-G-G---G_n$$

Amylose

$$G-G-G-G-G--------_n$$

Amylopectin

The number of glucose units and their arrangement within the molecule determine the characteristics of the starch. Each plant deposits a starch characteristic of its spe-

Table 2-1. Comparison of physical properties of carbohydrates

Monosaccharides	*Sweetening power*	*Soluble*	*Rate of absorption*
Hexoses			
Glucose	74	Yes	100
Fructose	173	Yes	30
Galactose	32	Yes	110
Mannose			10
Alcohol sugars			
Sorbitol	54	Yes	
Mannitol		Slightly	
Pentoses			
Ribose	—	Yes	
Xylose	40	Yes	15
Arabinose	—	Yes	9
Sorbose			30
Disaccharides			
Sucrose	100	Yes	
Lactose	16	Yes	
Maltose	33	Yes	
Polysaccharides			
Starch		No	
Dextrin		Slightly	
Glycogen		No	
Cellulose		No	

cies. Granules of potato starch can thus be distinguished from granules of rice, wheat, cassava, corn, or any other starch by microscopic examination of the shape and size of the granule. In addition, each of these starches has unique properties in regard to solubility, thickening power, and flavor. Nutritionally, the body does not discriminate among starches, but is able to break them all into their component glucose units for absorption and utilization by the body cells.

The animal stores a limited amount of carbohydrate as the polysaccharide *glycogen*. It is stored primarily in liver and muscle, the only two animal tissues aside from milk and blood that contain carbohydrate. The adult male stores only about three fourths of a pound of glycogen, one fourth pound as liver glycogen, and one half pound as muscle glycogen. The energy thus stored represents only enough energy to last an adult male about half a day. When excess calories are consumed in the form of carbohydrate the capacity of the liver and muscle to store glycogen may increase as much as 100%. Adipose or fat tissues may show evidence of increased carbohydrate content under such circumstances, but they will soon convert it to fat for more permanent storage in these tissues. There is virtually no glycogen in liver or muscle as they are eaten since most is converted into lactic acid at the time of slaughtering.

Dextrin, another nutritionally important polysaccharide, is the slightly soluble product resulting from the initial breakdown of a starch when the very long glucose chains may be split into shorter chains. This may be accomplished by enzymes, as occurs during digestion, or by action of dry heat on starch, such as in toasting bread or browning flour. In either case, the resulting dextrin is sweeter and more soluble than the original starch. A starch hydrolysate, dextromaltose, is often used in infant feeding since it helps prevent the formation of a heavy curd in the infant's stomach.

Cellulose, which is also composed of many glucose units linked in a slightly different manner from starch units, is an important dietary constituent. Cellulose is the structural framework of plant tissue, and the body lacks the enzyme necessary to break its monosaccharide linkages. This indigestible residue then contributes bulk to the diet and is very important in maintaining gastric motility. A minimum of 100 mg. of fiber per kilogram of body weight per day is needed to stimulate normal gastric motility and favor normal elimination. Ruminants have a bacterial enzyme system capable of fermenting cellulose linkages, which explains their ability to exist on grasses and forage crops composed largely of cellulose, whereas human beings cannot. This fermentation produces short-chain fatty acids used for energy and a useless gas, methane. Table 2-2 includes the fiber content of several foods. Newer procedures for determining fiber indicate that actual values may be several times as high as these currently accepted figures. Cellulose is the most abundant organic compound in the world. If the cellulose content of the diet is very high, it may have an adverse effect on the absorption of other nutrients by speeding the passage of food through the intestinal tract. Methyl cellulose, a synthetic product, is being used commercially in the preparation of low-calorie products. It can be used to simulate foods such as mayonnaise, cookies, or candy without providing energy.

Related carbohydrates. Mucopolysaccharides and mucoproteins are a group of compounds that are extremely important body constituents; they occur in the body but are not found in food. Mucopolysaccharides are complex combinations of two or more compounds, one of which is a carbohydrate. Many consist of loose combinations of amino sugars with protein. Some of the common mucopolysaccharides are hyaluronic acid, present in the fluid lubricating the joints and the vitreous humor of the eyeball; chondroitin sulphate in cartilage, skin, and bone; heparin, an anticoagulant; and keratosulphate, found in hard structures such as nails. Mucoproteins such as the protein in eggs and some hormones are more tightly bound polysaccharides and proteins.

DIGESTION

Before carbohydrate can fulfill its established roles in the body it must be converted into sufficiently small units to pass through the walls of the intestine into the bloodstream. The monosaccharides are the only units that normally cross the intestinal membrane. The process by which complex carbohydrates are reduced to their component monosaccharide units is digestion. Virtually all these changes are brought about by starch-splitting enzymes —*amylases.*

The amylases are present in three digestive juices—the saliva in the mouth and the pancreatic and intestinal juices in the small intestine. The salivary amylase of the saliva, which mixes with the food in the mouth, acts on the starch in a slightly alkaline medium to convert it to simpler carbohydrates, usually dextrins. If it remains in contact with the saliva sufficiently long before being acidified by the hydrochloric acid secreted in the stomach, the starch may be split as far as the disaccharide maltose. Virtually no digestion of starch occurs in the stomach, which possesses no starch-splitting enzyme. Some sucrose, in the presence of hydrochloric acid secreted in the stomach, may undergo acid hydrolysis to glucose and fructose. From the stomach the digestive mass passes to the

Table 2-2. Carbohydrate content of foods*

Food	Total carbohydrate	Fiber
	grams per 100 gm. food	
Sugar, granulated	99.5	0
Sugar, brown	96.4	0
Cornstarch	87.6	0.1
Raisins	77.4	0.9
All-purpose flour	76.1	0.3
Macaroni, dry	75.2	0.3
Chocolate fudge	75.0	0.2
Maple syrup	65.0	—
Enriched white bread	50.5	0.2
Whole wheat bread	47.7	1.6
Muffins	42.3	0.1
Rice, coated	24.2	0.1
Macaroni, cooked	23.0	0.1
Potatoes, baked	21.1	0.6
Bananas	22.2	0.5
Ice cream	20.6	0.8
Lima beans, cooked	19.8	1.8
Corn, cooked	18.8	0.7
Grapes	15.7	0.6
Apple, not pared	14.5	1.0
Ginger ale	8.0	—
Beans, green	7.1	1.0
Cabbage	5.4	0.8
Beef liver	5.3	0
Whole milk	4.9	0
Oysters, raw	3.4	0
Pears, cooked	2.0	0.6

*Based on Watts, B., and Merrill, A.: Composition of foods—raw, processed and prepared, U.S. Department of Agriculture Handbook No. 8, Washington, D.C., 1963, U.S. Department of Agriculture.

small intestine, where alkaline secretions neutralize the hydrochloric acid and create the slightly alkaline medium necessary for the action of the starch-splitting enzymes secreted into the small intestine. Pancreatic amylase attacks complex carbohydrates and converts them into the disaccharide, maltose. The final conversion of sucrose to fructose and glucose is accomplished by intestinal sucrase, of maltose to two glucose molecules by intestinal maltase, and of lactose to glucose and galactose by intestinal lactase. The long-standing belief that these enzymes act within the intestinal cavity is now being questioned. Evidence is appearing to indicate that these enzymes are not secreted into the intestinal cavity but remain in the membrane of the cells lining the intestinal cavity, where they accomplish the ultimate conversion of the disaccharides to the monosaccharides.

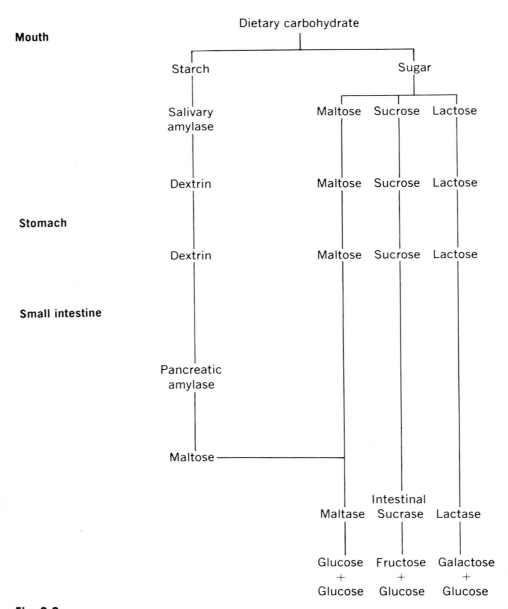

Fig. 2-2

Summary of digestion of carbohydrate.

The digestibility of carbohydrates varies with the source but ranges from 90% to 98% for most foods. The digestion of carbohydrate is summarized in Fig. 2-2.

ABSORPTION AND TRANSPORTATION

Monosaccharides pass freely across the walls of the villi, the small fingerlike projections lining the intestinal tract, but the rate varies with the sugar. Galactose is absorbed slightly faster than glucose while fructose is absorbed at less than half the rate. The rate of absorption tends to decrease with time, increase with increase in concentration of the carbohydrate solution, and increase in the presence of the hormones—insulin secreted by the pancreas and thyroxine secreted by the thyroid glands. From here the monosaccharides accumulate in the small blood vessels that eventually carry them to the portal vein. This large blood vessel carries the absorbed monosaccharides to the liver. In the liver there are two paths that may be followed by the monosaccharides glucose, fructose, and galactose. They may all be converted into glycogen up to the capacity of the liver to store glycogen, or the galactose and fructose may be converted to glucose and along with the absorbed glucose be released to the bloodstream to be carried to various cells of the body. In muscle cells some glucose may be stored as muscle glycogen. Most glucose, however, will be used as an immediate source of energy for the cells. The nerve cells of the body depend entirely on glucose as a source of energy since they are unable to utilize other energy-yielding nutrients.

METABOLISM

The liver releases carbohydrate as glucose to the bloodstream at a rate to maintain a minimum level of 100 mg. of glucose per 100 ml. of blood. Following a meal, this level of glucose may rise considerably above this but drop again as it is withdrawn by the cells. The difference between blood sugar levels in arterial and venous blood, Δ-glucose, is believed to influence the appetite-regulating mechanism, the hypothalamus of the brain. A small difference, representing depletion of blood glucose reserves, triggers the appetite. A large difference, showing an available supply of blood sugar, leads to a depressed appetite.

Glucose released from the liver is carried by the bloodstream to all tissues of the body. Here the individual cells take up the glucose through a carrier system in the cell membrane. Once within the cell the glucose is oxidized to pyruvic acid. Then, in the mitochondrion, sometimes referred to as a powerhouse of the cell, the energy stored in the carbohydrate is released to supply energy for the many needs of the body, such as heat, muscle contraction, synthesis of body compounds, and conduction of nerve impulses. Within the mitochondrion are concentrated the many enzymes necessary for the orderly and slow release of energy from glucose. Once the energy of glucose has been released, the other end products of carbohydrate metabolism, carbon dioxide and water, are released from the cell and eventually excreted from the body.

STORAGE

When carbohydrate is supplied in the diet and monosaccharides absorbed beyond the body's immediate needs for energy and its capacity to store glycogen, they cannot be excreted but must be converted into a form in which to be stored in the body. The body has an unlimited capacity to store fat. It also has the ability to convert extra carbohydrate into fat. This conversion of glucose to fatty acids occurs primarily in the microsomes of the liver. The glucose molecule is broken down into two-carbon fragments that are then synthesized into fatty acids. These are transported in the bloodstream to the adipose tissue cells, where they combine with a three-carbon

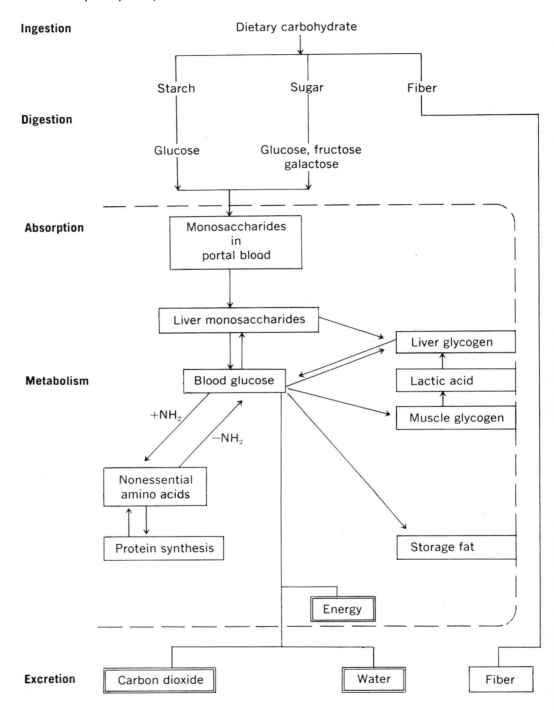

Fig. 2-3

Summary of carbohydrate digestion and metabolism. Boxed items are end products of metabolism. Changes within dotted line occur after absorption and before excretion.

compound, glycerol, also derived from glucose, to form fat.

The digestion and metabolism of carbohydrate is summarized schematically in Fig. 2-3. It is clear that carbohydrate in food can be used in one of three ways in the body:

1. Metabolized or oxidized immediately as a source of energy.
2. Converted into glycogen and stored as liver glycogen or muscle glycogen when carbohydrate intake exceeds the amount needed immediately for energy.
3. Converted into fat and stored as a reserve of energy as fat in regular cells or in special adipose cells when the carbohydrate intake exceeds the amount needed immediately for energy and when the limited glycogen reserves are saturated.

The eventual end products of carbohydrate metabolism are carbon dioxide, water, and energy. The period of time elapsing between the intake of carbohydrate and its excretion as carbon dioxide and water is relatively short; it may range from a few minutes to a few hours to several months.

FUNCTIONS

Source of energy. The major function of carbohydrate is as a source of energy. This function is not unique to carbohydrate, although it is the least expensive source of energy. Nervous tissue can use only glucose as a source of fuel, but since glucose can be produced for the body from part of the fat molecule and from some amino acids in a process called *gluconeogenesis,* even nervous tissue can get along without dietary carbohydrates. When blood glucose levels fall, the brain is deprived of glucose, its only source of energy, and reacts by firing off uncontrolled and uncoordinated impulses that produce the symptoms of convulsions.

The amount of energy provided by carbohydrate is almost constant for all forms. One gram of carbohydrate provides 4 kilocalories of energy regardless of the source—starch, sugar, monosaccharides, or disaccharides. In the typical American diet carbohydrate provides approximately 50% to 60% of the total calories. The proportion from starches has declined from 31% to 24%, and that from sugar has increased between 1930 and 1962. The percentage of carbohydrate tends to increase with a decrease in amount of money available to spend on food since it is a much less expensive source of calories than protein or fat. In some countries, such as Japan and Indonesia, where rice or cassava is the staple in the diet, as much as 80% to 85% of the calories come from carbohydrate. At the other extreme, carbohydrate provides only 8% of the energy in the high-fat diet of Eskimos. Since the calorie value of carbohydrate is the same from all sources, when a sauce can be thickened with half as much cornstarch as wheat starch it will have half the calories from starch. Similarly a sugar with high sweetening power will contribute the same degree of sweetness with less sugar and fewer calories than one of low sweetening power. Conversely, the use of a starch with a low thickening power and a sugar with a low sweetening power might help step up the caloric value of a diet without appreciably changing its character.

Dietary essential—an unexplained role. Although carbohydrate can be replaced by fat and protein as a source of energy, recent evidence indicates that a diet devoid of carbohydrate produces many undesirable symptoms. Persons on a diet of protein and fat very rapidly develop the same symptoms as persons on a starvation regime. They lose very large amounts of sodium, are unable to prevent the breakdown of body protein except at very high levels of protein intake, and develop ketosis from the accumulation in the blood and urine of abnormal products of fat metabolism by the second day of a carbohydrate-free diet. The subjects all experience loss of energy and fatigue. All these undesirable results of a lack of carbohydrate in the diet are reversed by the addition of carbohydrate, which would indicate that carbohydrate is a dietary essential. There is no evidence as to whether the need is for any carbohydrate, specifically for one group such as mono-, di-, or polysaccharides, or for a specific carbohydrate. Persons on a diet lacking in carbohydrate experience as rapid a loss of weight as do persons subjected to total starvation.

Carbohydrates or products derived from them also serve as precursors of vital body compounds such as nucleic acids and connective tissue matrix.

FOOD SOURCES

Carbohydrate is found almost exclusively in foods in plant origin. Milk, with its high lactose content, is the only important source of animal carbohydrate. Human milk contains considerably more lactose (7%) than cow's milk (4.8%). Eggs contain a very small amount, and scallops and oysters are the only other animal tissues that contain carbohydrate. The small amount in the liver is almost all converted to pyruvic and lactic acids during the slaughtering process.

Table 2-2 shows some typical sources of carbohydrate. The figures for total carbohydrate include the utilizable sugars and starches and the nondigestible cellulose or fibers. The values for fiber content represent the best currently available but may be low. When tables of food composition are used to determine the utilizable carbohydrate in the diet, the values for fiber should be subtracted from those for total carbohydrate.

It is noted that some foods, such as sugar and cornstarch, are very high in carbohydrate. Others, such as the potato and rice, commonly considered carbohydrate foods, contain a much lower percentage of carbohydrate. Most of the caloric content of the foods listed in the table is derived from carbohydrate.

The range in the amount of carbohydrate in fruits and vegetables is evident. Persons who must regulate the carbohydrate content of their diets are well aware of the classification of fruits and vegetables into exchange lists based on the carbohydrate content. The amounts of the different foods with equivalent amounts of carbohydrate are included so that a person can make substitutions.

DIETARY REQUIREMENTS

Since the body can function with considerably less carbohydrate than is present in most diets, it has been impossible to establish a dietary standard for carbohydrate. Diets low or devoid of carbohydrate are so unpalatable that there is little likelihood of their being consumed for any appreciable length of time. In addition, the fact that carbohydrate is the most economical source of calories leads to its use in sufficient quantities to insure at least a minimum intake.

ABNORMALITIES OF METABOLISM

There are several pathological conditions under which people have difficulty utilizing carbohydrate. The most common is diabetes, in which a person lacks a sufficient secretion of the hormone insulin from the pancreas to allow the cell to pick up and utilize carbohydrate from the bloodstream. Some others lack the enzyme necessary to convert galactose to glucose in the liver. Galactose appears as an abnormal constituent of the blood in a condition known as galactosemia. The lack of an enzyme needed to release stored glycogen from the liver leads to glycogen storage disease.

CARBOHYDRATE AND DENTAL HEALTH

Carbohydrate is frequently implicated in dental caries production. In the preeruptive stage when the tooth is forming and is being nourished through the bloodstream, carbohydrate has little direct effect on the tooth quality. However, if the carbohydrate in diet replaces protective foods that carry nutrients such as calcium, vitamin D, and vitamin C, which are necessary for normal tooth formation, they indirectly have an adverse effect on the health of the tooth before eruption.

In the posteruptive stage when the tooth is exposed to the oral environment and has only limited systemic connection, carbohydrate assumes importance. It has been established that before tooth decay occurs there must be present microorganisms and food for the microorganisms—carbohydrate. A carbohydrate in solution that does not adhere to the tooth surface causes relatively little harm. However, a carbohydrate-rich food, such as toffee or caramel, that tends to adhere to the tooth surface, provides the food needed by the organisms to produce the acid that ultimately facilitates the solution of tooth enamel with resultant decay of a caries-susceptible tooth. In dental health, the form of the carbohydrate is equally as important as the amount.

Carbohydrate has less detrimental effect on tooth health if it is followed by liquids or other detergent foods, such as apples, that tend to remove the carbohydrate from the tooth surface.

CARBOHYDRATE AND ATHEROSCLEROSIS

Recent research to identify a dietary factor involved in atherosclerosis, now a leading cause of death in the United States, has suggested that both the kind and amount of carbohydrate in the diet may be important factors. So far the evidence is far from conclusive but suggests that high intakes of sucrose are associated with a higher incidence of atherosclerosis, possibly through its effect in stimulating high blood triglyceride levels.

SELECTED REFERENCES

Harper, A. E.: Carbohydrates. In Food, yearbook of agriculture, Washington, D. C., 1959, U. S. Department of Agriculture.

Hodges, R.: Present knowledge of carbohydrate, Nutr. Rev. 24:65, 1966.

Krehl, W. A.: The nutritional significance of the carbohydrates, Borden Rev. Nutr. Res. (No. 6) 16:85, 1955.

Passmore, R.: Carbohydrate, the Cinderella of nutrition. In Diet and bodily constitution, Ciba Foundation Study Group No. 17, London, 1963, J. & A. Churchill, Ltd.

Review. Carbohydrate, digestion and absorption, Nutr. Rev. 21:279, 1963.

Stevens, H. A., and Ohlson, M. A.: Estimated intake of simple and complex carbohydrates, J. Am. Dietet. A. 48:294, 1966.

3

Fats or lipids

Fats, a second energy-yielding nutrient group, are a familiar item in the diet. The term *fat* is commonly used instead of the more correct term *lipid* to include fats and oils. Visible fats, such as butter, margarine, vegetable oil, and the layer of fat on meat, account for only one third of the fat in the American diet. The remainder is present as invisible fat—that marbled throughout meat fibers, in egg yolk, in homogenized milk and milk products, in nuts, and in whole-grain cereals.

The fat content of American diets has been increasing steadily. Fat was estimated to provide 32% of the calories in 1910, 35% in 1930, 38% in 1936, 42% in 1948, 44% in 1955, and 41% in 1962. About two thirds comes from animal sources, and one third comes from vegetable sources. Many racial, economic, technologic, cultural, and geographic factors influence not only the total fat intake of an individual but also the kind of fat used. For instance, intake is higher among Italians than Japanese, higher in high-income groups than in low-income groups, higher in arctic than tropical regions, and becomes lower in old age.

Not only has the amount of fat in the American diet changed, but the character of the fat has also changed. The use of butter and lard has decreased 23% from 1930 to 1962 while that of vegetable fats, such as margarine, shortening, and salad oils, is up 34%.

CHEMICAL COMPOSITION

Chemically, all food fat is composed of glycerol, a three-carbon compound that is the core of the fat molecule and to which fatty acids are attached. The physical characteristics of the fat are determined by the number and kinds of fatty acids combined with glycerol.

Glycerol is a three-carbon alcohol with the following structure:

$$
\begin{array}{c}
\text{H} \\
| \\
\text{H--C--OH} \\
| \\
\text{H--C--OH} \\
| \\
\text{H--C--OH} \\
| \\
\text{H}
\end{array}
$$

Fatty acids are straight-chain carbon compounds with an even number of carbon atoms, a methyl (CH_3) group at one end and a carboxyl (COOH) group at the other. A fatty acid can be represented by the formula $CH_3 (CH_2)_n COOH$ where n may vary from two to twenty, although most fatty acids in foods have a sixteen- to twenty-carbon chain. It is through the OH group of the carboxyl group that the fatty acid is united with hydrogen of the glycerol molecule. Water (H_2O) is split off, and the fatty acid remains attached to the glycerol core.

It is very obvious that all fats are not alike—butter fat differs from beef fat, from chicken fat, and from corn oil. Each animal has a fat that is characteristic of its own species. Chicken fat can readily be distinguished from the more solid beef fat and this in turn from the very hard white mutton fat. It is possible to modify the character of an animal's fat by modifying its diet, and animal breeders take advantage of this to market the type of fat consumers want. For instance, pigs fed peanuts produce a very soft greasy fat that is less acceptable than the harder fat resulting from a corn diet. Fats formed from carbohydrate are more likely to be saturated and hence firmer than those from protein and fat. The different characteristics are the result of the number and kinds of fatty acids included. These may vary in the length of the carbon chain from a four-carbon chain to a twenty-two–carbon chain. Only fatty acids with an even number of carbon atoms are found in foods; thus there are fatty acids with ten possible lengths of carbon chains that can be incorporated in the fat in any combination of three influence the character of the fat formed. For instance, those with short-chain fatty acids are more soluble than those with long chains. Secondly, the fatty acids may be either saturated, monounsaturated, or polyunsaturated. Saturation refers to the extent to which carbon atoms hold all the

hydrogen atoms they are capable of holding. In a saturated fatty acid each carbon has two hydrogen atoms attached to it. Saturated fatty acids provide about 42% of total fat in the diet. In a monounsaturated fatty acid one hydrogen atom is missing from each of two adjacent carbons. A double bond $-\overset{\displaystyle}{\underset{\displaystyle H}{C}}=\overset{\displaystyle}{\underset{\displaystyle H}{C}}-$ thus replaces the original $-\overset{\displaystyle H}{\underset{\displaystyle H}{C}}-\overset{\displaystyle H}{\underset{\displaystyle H}{C}}-$ structure. If two or more pairs of hydrogen atoms are removed with the formation of two or more double bonds, the fatty acid is described as polyunsaturated. There are seldom more than four double bonds in a fatty acid carbon chain. If the carbon chain folds at the double bond (cis form), it will give different characteristics to the fat in which it is incorporated than if it remains extended (trans form). Monounsaturated fatty acids contribute 41% and polyunsaturated fatty acids 17% of total dietary fat.

In addition to the type of fatty acids incorporated in a fat molecule, the number of fatty acids influences the character of the fat. Over 98% of the fat found in food and 20% of that in liver and blood is composed of triglycerides, fats in which the glycerol molecules have fatty acids attached in all three possible positions. These three fatty acids may be all the same, as in simple triglycerides, all different, or two alike, although most fats contain at least two different fatty acids and are known as mixed triglycerides. When two or more fatty acids appear in a fat molecule, the order in which they are arranged effects the fat. The remaining 2% of the fat in foods is composed of monoglycerides, glycerol to which only one fatty acid is attached; diglycerides, glycerol to which two fatty acids are attached; and phospholipids, glycerol with a phosphate and nitrogen-containing substances replacing one of the fatty acids of a triglyceride. Mono- and diglycerides are often added to baked products to improve texture and keeping qualities. In most fats, fatty acids comprise 92% to 95% of the molecule and glycerol 5% to 8%.

The general formula for glycerides may then be written as follows (FA represents a fatty acid):

$$
\begin{array}{c}
H \\
| \\
H-C-OH \\
| \\
H-C-O-FA_1 \\
| \\
H-C-O-FA_2 \\
| \\
H
\end{array}
$$

Diglyceride

$$
\begin{array}{c}
H \\
| \\
H-C-O-FA_1 \\
| \\
H-C-O-FA_2 \\
| \\
H-C-O-FA_3 \\
| \\
H
\end{array}
$$

Mixed triglyceride

$$
\begin{array}{c}
H \\
| \\
H-C-OH \\
| \\
H-C-OH \\
| \\
H-C-O-FA_1 \\
| \\
H
\end{array}
$$

Monoglyceride

The characteristics of the resulting fat depend then on the length of the fatty acid chain, the degree of saturation or unsaturation of the fatty acid, and the arrangement of fatty acids on the glycerol molecule.

The most common saturated fatty acids in foods are butyric (four carbons), pal-

mitic (sixteen carbons), and stearic (eighteen carbons); monounsaturated fatty acids are predominantly oleic with eighteen carbons and one double bond. Linoleic acid with eighteen carbons and two double bonds is the most common polyunsaturated fatty acid.

CLASSIFICATION

Fats are frequently classified as saturated or unsaturated, depending on the degree of saturation of the fatty acids present. These terms are only relative, as a triglyceride that is completely saturated or completely unsaturated is very rare. Likewise the general designation of animal fats as saturated fats and vegetable fats as unsaturated fats is not a correct classification. Most food fats have eight to ten fatty acids, some of which will be saturated and some unsaturated. Unsaturated fatty acids tend to lower the melting point of a fat and produce a fat that is liquid at room temperature. Conversely, saturated fatty acids tend to raise the melting point and saturated fats are often more solid at room temperature. Most vegetable oils are relatively high in monounsaturated and polyunsaturated fatty acids, and most animal fats are relatively high in saturated fatty acids. Exceptions are coconut oil, which is highly saturated, and poultry fat, which is highly unsaturated.

Vegetable oils, such as cottonseed, peanut, corn, safflower, and soybean, are considerably less expensive than animal fats. They can be economically and effectively changed to fats with more plastic qualities by the process of hydrogenation, in which hydrogen is introduced into the fat molecules to saturate the carbon atom with hydrogen and eliminates the double bond. Margarine and vegetable shortenings are examples of vegetable oils that have been changed by saturating at least some of the unsaturated double bonds with hydrogen to produce fats with the desired physical characteristics. The hydrogenation process can be controlled to give a fat with very specific characteristics. Competition among processors to produce the most acceptable product is evident in current advertising. As a result of hydrogenation the consumption of hydrogenated vegetable fats is rising while that of animal fats is declining. About three billion pounds of hydrogenated fat is consumed in the United States each year.

PHYSICAL PROPERTIES

Fat is insoluble in water but soluble in fat solvents such as ether, chloroform, or benzene. Fats are less dense than water so will rise to the surface of any aqueous mixture. Emulsified fats, in which fat globules are in finely divided form and kept separated from one another by an emulsifying agent, are prevented from coalescing or fusing together to form large globules. The fat dispersed through homogenized milk is an example of an emulsified fat. Egg yolk fat is a naturally emulsified fat.

Fat is not affected by temperatures normally used in food preparation; however, heating at very high temperatures, often indicated by the smoking of the fat, leads to the decomposition of fat and the production of the substance acrolein. Acrolein has a very pungent acrid fume that is extremely irritating to the nasal passages and the gastrointestinal tract. Fats are also subject to oxidation. Natural fats containing unsaturated fatty acids are very susceptible to oxidation and, like others low in antioxidants, which retard oxidation, they become rancid because of the production of peroxides of fatty acids. This is a major cause of spoilage in fats. They may become unpalatable because of their tendency to absorb odors and flavors.

DIGESTION

Before fat can enter the general circulation to be transported to the tissues of the body it must be broken down chemically into molecules sufficiently small to pass into the cells of the membranes lining the gastrointestinal tract. In most cases fat is reduced to fatty acids and glycerol, but a few monoglycerides with short-chain fatty acids can be absorbed.

Digestion of fat begins in the stomach. The enzyme gastric lipase, a component of the gastric juice secreted from the wall of the stomach, is able to break naturally occurring emulsified fat, such as that in egg yolk and homogenized milk, into fatty acids and glycerol. It is unable to attack the larger molecules of unemulsified fat found in meat, butter, and salad oils. Fatty acids liberated at this stage may be exchanged in the stomach or intestine with fatty acids of other triglycerides to modify the makeup of ingested fat. Long-chain fatty acids are more likely to be reincorporated into triglycerides than are short-chain fatty acids.

In the small intestine the bile secreted by the gallbladder acts on the larger fat molecules to break them into many smaller fat particles. This emulsification, the result of reducing surface tension on fat molecules, increases the surface area on which the digestive enzymes can act, reduces the distance through which enzymes must penetrate, and prevents the coalescing of fat molecules. Once the fat molecules are in sufficiently finely divided form, they are acted upon by both pancreatic lipase and intestinal lipase. In both cases the enzymes split the fat molecule by enzyme hydrolysis, involving the addition of water as each fatty acid is split off from the glycerol core. The breakdown of fat progresses from triglycerides to diglycerides to monoglycerides and finally the complete separation of fatty acids from glycerol. About one fifth to one half of the dietary triglycerides are completely hydrolyzed to fatty acids and glcerol. The others remain mostly as diglycerides and monoglycerides.

Most fats are between 90% and 96% digestible. The extent of digestibility depends on the length of the fatty acid chain

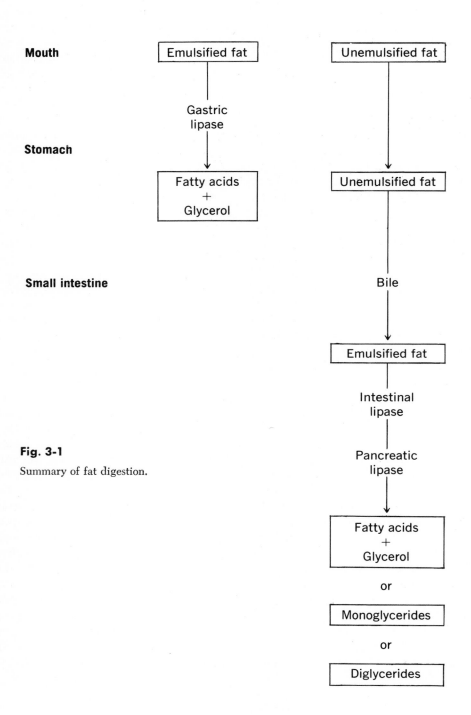

Fig. 3-1

Summary of fat digestion.

and the amount and arrangement of fatty acid in the molecule. Animal fats are more readily digested than vegetable fats. Hydrogenation will decrease digestibility only if it is carried far enough to produce significant amounts of saturated fatty acids. The changes occurring during fat digestion are shown in Fig. 3-1.

ABSORPTION AND TRANSPORTATION

The divided or digested fat molecules are taken up from the gastrointestinal tract as separate molecules of fatty acids and glycerol, as monoglycerides, as diglycerides, and as triglycerides. About 30% of the free fatty acids and glycerol are absorbed directly into the bloodstream to be carried by the portal vein directly to the liver. As soon as they pass through the epithelial cells of the lining of the intestine, many of the remaining free fatty acids unite with a different molecule of glycerol or with a monoglyceride to form fats either as monoglycerides, diglycerides, or triglycerides. About 70% of absorbed fat is resynthesized to form triglycerides. These then enter the lacteals (fat-collecting ducts for lymph) that finally carry the fat to the lymphatic system. The relationship between the lymphatic system, which is concerned primarily with collecting body fluids and returning them through the thoracic duct to the general circulatory system, is illustrated in Fig. 1-5. The fat molecules absorbed through the lacteals are transported as microscopic fat particles called chylomicrons. These are combinations of 99% fat with 1% protein that are more soluble than fat and therefore more easily transported in the blood. Some fatty acids that do not recombine with glycerol are transported bound to plasma albumin. Fat collected in the lymphatic ducts empties into the general circulation in the neck region and from there is circulated to all body cells. The presence of the chylomicrons in the blood gives a milky or turbid appearance to the blood that disappears gradually as the fat is removed by organs and tissues.

Factors affecting absorption. Absorption of fat will be decreased when there is increased motility in the gastrointestinal tract; this decreases the time in which fat is in contact with digestive juices and with the walls of the intestinal tract through which it is absorbed. Absence of bile to emulsify fat or of fat-splitting enzymes also decreases absorption, and undigested fat will appear in the feces—a condition known as steatorrhea. Longer-chain fatty acids are less well absorbed than shorter-chain ones, and saturated fatty acids less well than unsaturated ones.

METABOLISM

After the lymphatic system has deposited the chylomicrons of fat in the bloodstream, most is cleared or removed from the blood rather rapidly and stored temporarily in the liver. From the liver, fat is released into the bloodstream as lipoproteins—a soluble combination of fat with a protein. The vitamin choline or other fat-mobilizing substances facilitate the release of fat for transportation to other tissues and prevent its accumulation in the liver. The lipoproteins resemble protein more than fat and thus are more soluble in the plasma and more easily carried to the tissues. There are two types of lipoproteins involved: low-density lipoproteins with 10% protein and 90% fat and high-density lipoproteins with 45% protein and 55% fat. Fat is removed from the blood lipoproteins by various tissues and meets one of two fates. It can be oxidized (burned) through a series of complex biochemical reactions to form carbon dioxide, water, and energy or it may be stored in the fat depots of each cell or in special adipose (fat) cells for future use as a source of energy. Some fat will be used by the mammary gland during lactation in the production of milk.

When the body has need for the energy

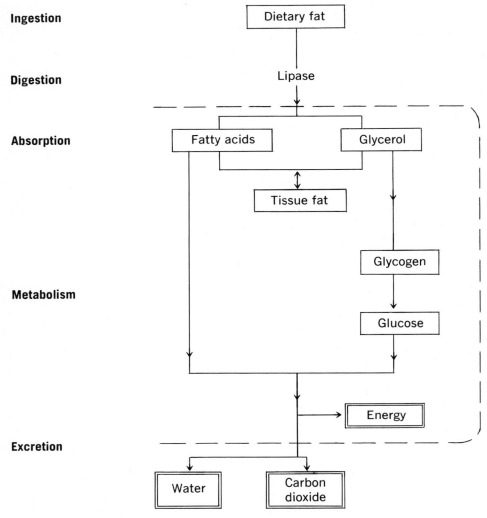

Ingestion

Digestion

Absorption

Metabolism

Excretion

Dietary fat

Lipase

Fatty acids

Glycerol

Tissue fat

Glycogen

Glucose

Energy

Water

Carbon dioxide

Fig. 3-2

Summary of fat digestion and metabolism. Boxed items are end products of metabolism. Changes within dotted line occur after absorption.

reserves, the fat stored as triglycerides is hydrolyzed by lipases within the cell to fatty acids and glycerol. The fatty acids leave the cell, become bound to the protein albumin in the bloodstream, and are carried to the tissues requiring energy. Since these fatty acids have not recombined with glycerol they are known as non-esterified fatty acids (NEFA). There is about 1% NEFA to 99% albumin. The glyc-

erol core of the stored triglycerides is oxidized as a carbohydrate.

The digestion and metabolism of fat is summarized in Fig. 3-2. This indicates that ingested fat available to the cells as fatty acids and glycerol follows one of three paths during metabolism:

1. Both fatty acids and glycerol are metabolized immediately as a source of energy.

2. Glycerol and fatty acids combine to form fat, which is stored as a reserve of energy.

3. Glycerol is converted into glucose and then metabolized in the same way as a source of energy, converted into glycogen, or converted into fat.

FUNCTIONS IN DIET

Source of energy. Fat serves as a concentrated source of energy. Each gram of fat, whether animal or vegetable, liquid or solid, provides 9 kilocalories per gram—two and a quarter times as much energy as an equal weight of either carbohydrate or protein. Fat represents the form in which the animal stores excess energy; thus the amount of fat in an animal product is determined by the energy balance of the animal. Practically all animal foods contain some fat. Even relatively lean steak is 28% fat, which contributes 70% of its calories.

Satiety value. Fat tends to leave the stomach relatively slowly, reaching maximum absorption about 3½ hours after ingestion. This delay in emptying time of the stomach helps delay the onset of hunger pangs and contributes to a feeling of satiety following a meal. The presence of fat in the duodenum stimulates the release of a hormone in the stomach, which in turn inhibits hunger contractions. Because of its high calorie value, fat intakes are frequently reduced and visible fats virtually eliminated from diets suggested for weight control. Current research shows that the inclusion of some fat—whole milk, butter on vegetables and bread, or oil on salads—increases the satiety value of low-calorie diets so that they are more easily adhered to. This more than compensates for the concentrated calorie content of the fat. Currently, moderate fat-reducing diets are considered more successful than low-fat diets.

Carrier of fat-soluble vitamins. Among the dietary essentials are four fat-soluble vitamins—vitamins A, D, E, and K. Dietary fat serves as a carrier for these nutrients or their precursors. Thus, the elimination of fat from the diet leads to a reduced intake of these nutrients. Fat also appears necessary for the absorption of vitamin A precursors from nonfat sources such as carrots. Similarly, anything that interferes with the absorption or utilization of fat, such as an obstruction of the bile duct or rancidity of fat, depresses the availability of the fat-soluble vitamins.

Source of essential fatty acids. Among the fatty acids found in some fats is a polyunsaturated fatty acid, linoleic acid, which is effective in curing the dermatitis and restoring the growth of young animals fed a diet devoid of or very low in fat. Because it cannot be produced by the body, linoleic acid is considered an essential fatty acid (EFA). Two closely related fatty acids, linolenic acid, an eighteen-carbon acid found in vegetable fats, and arachidonic acid, a twenty-carbon polyunsaturated fatty acid found only in animal tissues, can be synthesized from linoleic acid. Since the body can synthesize them they are not considered essential fatty acids even though they perform some of the same functions as linoleic acid. Linolenic acid is effective in restoring growth but has no antidermatitis effect, whereas arachidonic acid will cure dermatitis but will not promote growth. The relationship between these three is shown in Table 3-1.

Saturated fatty acids have no EFA activity and may increase the need for EFA as does an increase in dietary cholesterol. Young animals need more EFA than older animals, males more than females, and diabetics and persons with hypothyroidism more than persons under normal metabolic conditions. Needs also increase in pyridoxine deficiency. The needs for essential fatty acids are usually met when 1% of the total calories is provided by linoleic acid. Linoleic acid is present in most concentrated form in vegetable oils with some, such as corn oil, soybean oil, and safflower

Table 3-1. Relationship of related fatty acids to linoleic acid

Fatty acid	Structure	Biological role	Sources
Linoleic	18 carbons	Growth factor	Vegetable
↓	2 double bonds	Antidermatitis factor	Seed oils
Linolenic	18 carbons	Growth factor	Soybean oil
↑↓	3 double bonds		
Arachidonic acid	20 carbons	Antidermatitis factor	Animal fat
	4 double bonds		

Table 3-2. Fat and fatty acid composition of 100 gm. of selected foods*

Food	Total fat (gm.)	Saturated fatty acids (gm.)	Unsaturated fatty acids Oleic (gm.)	Linoleic (gm.)
Corn oil	100	10	28	53
Soybean oil	100	15	20	52
Olive oil	100	11	76	7
Safflower oil	100	8	15	72
Peanut oil	100	18	47	29
Mayonnaise	79.9	14	17	40
Butter	81	46	27	2
Bacon, broiled	52	17	25	5
Peanut butter	50.6	9	25	14
Cream cheese	37.7	21	12	1
Beef, rib, raw	37.4	18	16	1
Cheddar cheese	32.2	18	11	1
Ham	23	4	5	1
Chicken, raw	17.1	5	6	3
Avocado	16.4	3	7	2
Egg, cooked	11.5	4	5	1
Tuna, canned, drained	8.2	3	2	2
Milk, whole	3.7	2	1	Trace

*From Watts, B., and Merrill, A.: Composition of foods—raw, processed and prepared, U. S. Department of Agriculture Handbook No. 8, Washington, D. C., 1963, U. S. Department of Agriculture.

oil, containing over 50% linoleic acid. Lesser and variable amounts are present in hydrogenated fats or spreads made from these oils. Most diets provide many times the minimum EFA requirements. The fatty acid composition of some representative fats is given in Table 3-2. EFA deficiency occurs most frequently in bottle-fed infants fed a nonfat milk formula. The essential fatty acids requirement of infants has been set at 4% of the total calories, which is easily met by breast milk.

Palatability. The role of fat in contributing to the palatability of food is appreciated best by those forced to exist on a low-fat or fat-free diet. The use of fat for frying food, as a spread, as a base for salad dressing, and as a flavor adjunct for vegetables does much to improve the taste appeal of our meals. Many substances responsible for the flavors and aromas of food are fat-soluble. Thus, fat generally contributes to the acceptability of our meals. It has also been suggested that fat in the diet stimulates the flow of digestive juices.

ROLE IN THE BODY

Energy reserve. Body fat represents the primary form in which energy is stored in the body. Since it is an essential constituent of the cell membrane, all tissues contain some fat. Some cells, known as adipose cells, tend to store fat when excess is produced. The number of adipose cells will increase in response to a need for a storage site for fat. There appears to be no upper limit to the amount of fat the body can store as long as caloric intake continues to exceed expenditure. Once fat has been formed and deposited in the adipose tissues, the body has no way of excreting it. Thus, the only way in which body fat can be reduced is by oxidizing or burning it as a source of energy when caloric intake is less than caloric expenditure. A certain amount of body fat, about 18% to 20% of body weight for women and 15% for men, is considered normal and desirable. Reserves of fat in excess of this represent first overweight and in extreme cases obesity with all the physical, physiologic, and aesthetic disadvantages associated with it.

Body regulator. Aside from serving as a storage depot for energy, fat performs several other vital roles in the body. As an essential constituent of the membrane of each individual cell, it helps regulate the uptake and excretion of nutrients by the cell.

Insulation. Deposits of fat beneath the skin (subcutaneous fat) serve as insulating material for the body, protecting it against shock from changes in environmental temperature. Here again a certain minimum layer is desirable to prevent excessive heat loss from the body, but too thick a layer slows down the rate of heat loss during hot weather with resultant discomfort to the individual. Thick subcutaneous fat layers impede physical movement and present many aesthetic problems.

Protection of vital body organs. The fat deposits that surround certain vital organs and that are the last depots to be reduced when there is a caloric deficit serve to hold them in position and to protect them from physical shock. The kidney and heart are protected in this way.

FOOD SOURCES

The amount of fat in representative foods is shown in Table 3-2, which also indicates the amount present as saturated and unsaturated fatty acids. Some advertisers are making use of a P:S ratio to identify the nature of the fat in their product. This is an expression of the relative amounts of polyunsaturated and saturated fatty acids in their product, the assumption being that a high P:S ratio is desirable because of some evidence that polyunsaturated fatty acids are less readily converted to cholesterol than other fatty acids.

In checking the linoleic acid content of vegetable oils it is obvious that coconut oil, chocolate, and palm kernel oils contain virtually no essential fatty acid (EFA). On the other hand, wheat germ oil and walnut oil contain 57% to 73% linoleic oil respectively. Poultry and game are good sources of EFA.

The percentage of calories contributed by fat tends to be relatively high in most animal foods. In whole milk with 3.2% fat, 53% of the calories come from fat, in cheese, with 32% fat, 68%, in beef with fat, 83%, and in frankfurters containing 27% fat, 81%. Animal fats account for about two thirds of the fat eaten, much of which is invisible fat.

Vegetable foods contain less fat. Whole-grain cereals have about 2% to 9% fat, mainly in the germ. The fat in seeds ranges from 4% in corn to 17% in soybeans. Peanuts have 48% fat, and pecans have 41%. Avocado with 16% is the only fruit with any appreciable fat.

Based on its nutrient composition bacon is correctly designated as a fat food rather than a protein food. It contains 69% fat in raw form and 52% fat when cooked, although the latter figure varies with the extent of cooking.

Fig. 3-3 shows the contribution of various food groups to the total fat in the diet.

Because of the frequent suggestion in popular literature that mineral oil be substituted for vegetable oils in salad dressings it is appropriate to mention it although it has no nutritional value. It is a hydrocarbon, a by-product of the oil-refining process. The body possesses no enzymes capable of digesting it so it passes through the digestive tract unchanged. It thus acts as a lubricant and contributes no calories to the body's energy pool. However, it unfortunately acts as a solvent for the fat-soluble vitamins, which are then excreted along with the mineral oil. Since the low-calorie homemade mineral oil salad dressings are usually used on vegetable greens, one of our best sources of vitamin A, its use in the diet should be discouraged.

DIETARY REQUIREMENTS

Aside from the need for a dietary source of linoleic acid, the human does not require fat in the diet. A diet providing 1% of its calories from linoleic acid meets this requirement. However, as a concentrated source of energy it is important in allowing us to meet our energy requirements without eating large quantities of food. The current practice of obtaining as much as 40% of the calories from fat is being questioned because of the prevalence of excessive calorie intake and the possibility of an adverse effect of high fat diets in arteriovascular diseases. Nutritionists suggest that an intake of fat providing 25% to 30% of the calories is more compatible with good health.

Modification of dietary fat intake may be desirable in several conditions. In gallbladder disease, where the amount of bile necessary for the emulsification of dietary fat is limited, it may be necessary to restrict the total to as little as 10% of the calories from fat intake or to substitute emulsified fats for nonemulsified ones. Some disorders of absorption, such as sprue or ileitis (inflammation of the ileum), inhibit the absorption of fat, and the usual manifestation of this is the appearance of as much as 60 gm. of fat in the stools compared to normal levels of 2 to 5 gm. Fat in the stools is known as steatorrhea. Until the cause of the problem can be corrected the person is given as much fat as he can absorb since a restriction limits calorie intake and the absorption of fat-soluble vitamins. Hyperlipidemia, in which levels of certain fat constituents of the blood are elevated, may call for a restriction in either the kind or amount of dietary fat.

The necessity of restricting fat intake in such conditions as hepatitis, cirrhosis, and jaundice is now questioned.

RELATIONSHIP TO HEART DISEASE

The discussion of the relationship of dietary fat and atherosclerosis in an elementary text can be legitimately questioned. However, since the topic is being widely discussed in popular literature it seems appropriate to include a statement of the current interpretation of the question. This is done with the full recognition that scientific thinking on the topic may have changed direction completely in the necessary time lapse between the preparation of the manuscript and publication of the textbook.

Interest in a possible relationship be-

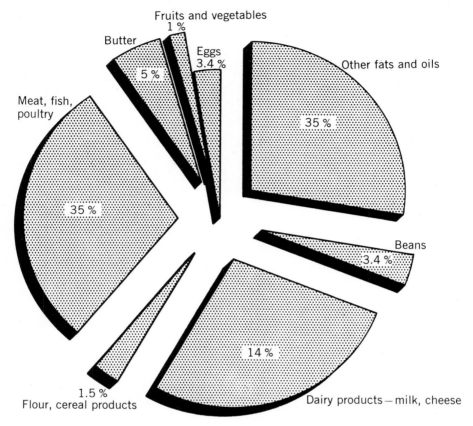

Fig. 3-3

Contribution of various food groups to total fat in American food supply. Based on Nutritive value of foods available for consumption, United States, 1909-1964. (Agricultural Research Service Publication No. 62-14, 1966.)

tween dietary factors and the incidence of heart disease was triggered by the observation that persons who suffered heart attacks almost always had above-normal levels of blood cholesterol. Cholesterol, a fat-related compound that is present in many animal foods and that the body can also synthesize, was shown to be a major constituent of the atherosclerotic plagues or precipates that form on the inside of some blood vessels, eventually narrowing the passage to the point that, if a clot forms, it closes it entirely. It was also noted that the incidence of heart disease was higher in populations that derived a higher percentage of their calories from fat than it was in populations which consumed less fat.

Efforts to lower blood cholesterol levels by dietary manipulation were made after studies on rabbits in which a restriction of dietary cholesterol resulted in lower levels of cholesterol in the blood. In human beings, however, control of dietary cholesterol by restricting the amount of cholesterol-containing foods, such as eggs, meat, and liver, led neither to lowering of blood cholesterol levels nor to a reduction in heart disease. The reason became clear when it was learned that the body can synthesize in the liver as much as 2 gm. of cholesterol from fat, carbohydrate, and protein in the diet whenever the amount of these in the diet exceeds the body's need for energy. This is considerably more than the 0.5 gm. provided from a normal diet. Since a certain amount of cholesterol is essential for the synthesis of sex hormones, for the transport of essential fatty acids, and as a constituent of the skin and covering of nerve fibers, it must be considered a normal body constituent.

Attention was next focused on the nature of fat in the diet with the observation that persons who consumed liquid fats or oils rather than solid fats had lower blood cholesterol levels than those who ate more solid animal fats. Since liquid fats differ from solid fats primarily in the proportion of polyunsaturated fatty acids (PUFA) they contain, emphasis in dietary treatment shifted towards an increased use of vegetable oils high in PUFA. This dietary modification when PUFA provided about half the dietary fat did indeed lead to a reduction in blood cholesterol levels but not to concurrent reduction in heart disease. Vast research has shown that dietary patterns and habits are reflected in blood cholesterol levels, but the need for reducing blood cholesterol has not been established.

Interest shifted to a search for another fat-related component of the blood that might reflect a tendency toward atherosclerosis. It was found that heart disease occurred only in persons who had a high blood cholesterol level coupled with a high blood triglyceride level. Triglycerides appear in the blood following a diet high in fat, but their presence also reflects the synthesis of fat from excess carbohydrate or excess protein. This situation is most likely to occur when calorie intake exceeds outgo and carbohydrate intake is high. It would appear, then, that modifying the diet to limit the carbohydrate and substituting polyunsaturated fats for saturated fats would be most likely to reduce both the triglyceride and cholesterol content of the blood, especially if accompanied by a control of caloric intake and the maintenance of optimum body weight.

Knowledge of the dietary factors involved and the balance that exists among these factors in the development of atherosclerosis is at present far from conclusive. It is felt that any drastic modification of the American diet on the basis of current information would be unwise except perhaps for middle-aged men with high blood cholesterol and triglyceride levels, with a family history of heart disease, and who are working under emotional tension—the type of person most likely to suffer from atherosclerosis. On the other hand, there would be no harm and possibly there would be benefits if the amount of fat in the diet were reduced from the present level of 40% of total calories to perhaps 25% of calorie intake.

SELECTED REFERENCES

Bronte-Stewarts, B.: Dietary fats. In Brock, J. F. (editor): Recent advances in human nutrition, Boston, 1961, Little, Brown and Company.

Council of Foods and Nutrition, American Medical Association: Regulation of dietary fat, J.A.M.A. **181:**441, 1962.

Hansen, A. E., et al.: Role of linoleic acid in infant nutrition, Pediatrics **31:**171-192, 1963.

Mead, J. F.: Present knowledge of fat, Nutr. Rev. **24:**33, 1966.

National Academy of Sciences: Dietary fat and human health, Publication No. 1147, Washington, D.C., 1966, National Research Council.

Pollock, H.: The genesis of atherosclerosis, Bull. New York Acad. Med. **40:**204, 1964.

4

Protein

The term *protein,* meaning to take first place, was introduced by Mulder, a Dutch chemist, in 1838. He attributed this to a nitrogen-containing constituent of food that he believed to be of prime importance in the functioning of the body and without which life was impossible. While it is now difficult to maintain that protein is more important than other nutrients, it is unlikely that Mulder had any conception of the extremely important roles this group of compounds play in the body nor of the number and complexity of the protein components of the body and of food. We now have evidence that protein is a constituent of every living cell and tissue. Half the dry matter of an adult is protein. One third is in muscle, one fifth in bone and cartilage, one tenth in skin, and the rest in other tissues and body fluids. All enzymes are protein in nature. Many hormones are either protein or protein derivatives. Viruses are proteins, as are the nucleoproteins in the cell nucleus responsible for the transmission of genetic information in cell reproduction. The only body compounds that normally contain no protein are urine and

bile. In the absence of protein there is a failure in body growth followed by a loss of already established body tissue. Proteins as part of every body enzyme and many hormones are vital in the regulation of body processes. When the needs for growth and repair of tissue have been met, any remaining protein is used as a source of energy, a rather expensive one, however.

Early in the twentieth century, with the availability of methods of analyzing for protein by determining the nitrogen in food and tissues, there was widespread interest in protein nutrition and especially in qualitative differences in proteins. The most significant work was done by Folin, who differentiated between *endogenous* and *exogenous* protein metabolism. He showed that endogenous metabolism (the metabolism of body proteins) was reflected in the excretion of a nitrogen-containing substance, creatinine, which remained fairly constant and appeared to reflect body mass and basal energy expenditure. On the other hand, the metabolism of the exogenous dietary protein resulted in the excretion of urea, which fluctuated with dietary intake. With the discovery of vitamins in the period between World Wars I and II, emphasis in nutrition research shifted towards a clarification of their role and structure. Again, however, in the early 1950's, interest in protein was revived. Several factors were responsible for this:

1. The recognition of a widespread protein deficiency disease, kwashiorkor, which plagues a large segment of the world's population, especially young children in developing countries.
2. Availability of radioactive isotopes, which made possible investigations of a scope not previously possible.
3. The recognition of blood and plasma transfusions as means of saving lives.

Current interest in protein nutrition is evident from the vast literature on the subject in scientific journals and books.

CHEMICAL COMPOSITION

Proteins are extremely complex substances made up of many amino acids, the structural unit of protein. These are the basic units from which protein is synthesized and into which it is converted in the course of its breakdown. The twenty different amino acids that have been identified as the building blocks for body proteins are

Table 4-1. Amino acids in food and body tissue

Classification	Amino acid or related compound
Essential for all human beings	Isoleucine
	Leucine
	Lysine
	Methionine
	Phenylalanine
	Threonine
	Tryptophan
	Valine
Nonessential	Glycine*
	Glutamic acid
	Arginine†
	Aspartic acid
	Proline
	Alanine
	Norleucine
	Serine
	Tyrosine
	Cystine
	Cysteine
Essential for infants	Histidine
Related compounds sometimes classified as amino acids	Asparagine
	Glutamine
	Hydroxyglutamic acid
	Hydroxylysine
	Hydroxyproline
	Thyroxine

*Essential for chicks.
†Essential for birds.

listed in Table 4-1. Chemically, the amino acids are composed of a carboxyl group (COOH), a hydrogen atom (H), an amino group (NH_2), and an amino acid radical (R) attached to a carbon atom as shown below.

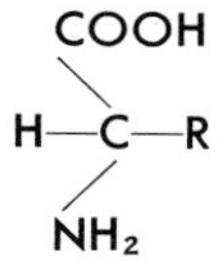

$$COOH$$
$$H-C-R$$
$$NH_2$$

The nitrogen of the amino group is unique to protein and represents an average 16% of the amino acid molecule, with a range from 15% in milk protein to 17% in cereals and 18% in nuts. Thus, most studies of protein metabolism can be based on nitrogen determinations. The carboxyl groups, the amino group, and the hydrogen atom are common to all amino acids. It is the nature of the *R group* that distinguishes one amino acid from another. *R* varies from a very simple hydrogen (H) atom as found in glycine, the simplest amino acid, to longer carbon chains of one-to seven-carbon atoms. Those in which the carbon atoms are arranged in a hexagon rather than a straight line (benzene ring) are called aromatic amino acids. Tyrosine and phenylalanine are examples. Others, such as cysteine, cystine, and methionine, also contain sulphur. Arginine, histidine, and tryptophan contain a second nitrogen atom and are thus called dibasic amino acids. Otherwise the amino acids differ from one another only in the number of carbon atoms and the arrangement of the hydrogen and oxygen atoms attached to them in the characteristic radical. It is the presence of nitrogen (N) that is unique to protein.

SYNTHESIS

Proteins are built when amino acids join together in a long chain, a peptide chain. An amino group of one amino acid joins with a carboxyl group of the next with the release of one molecule of water. Conversely, when we break the peptide linkage, as in digestion, water must be added before the amino acids can be split apart in either acid or enzyme hydrolysis. This is illustrated in Fig. 4-1. Proteins, as found in nature, consist of many amino acids linked together. The characteristics of the protein are determined not only by which amino acids are used and the number of times they are repeated but by the order in which they are joined together. Since each amino acid may be used any number of times in any relation to other amino acids, the possibility for the formation of different proteins becomes enormous. It is analogous to the number of words of fifty or more letters that could be made from an alphabet of twenty letters with no apparent limitations on the order in which they may be joined. In addition, the spatial arrangement of the amino acid chain, whether coiled, folded, or straight, influences manyfold the properties of the resulting protein and the possibilities of the

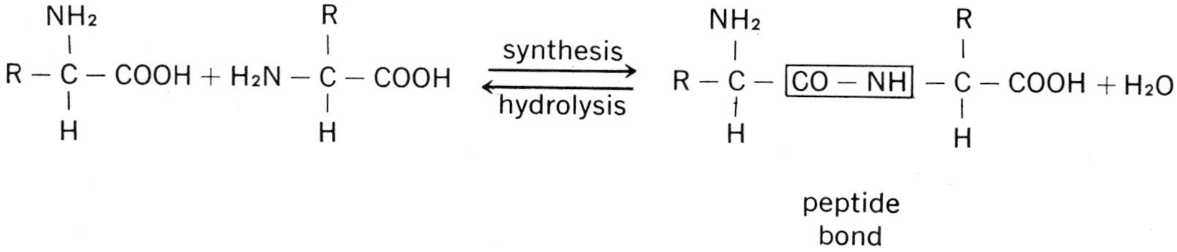

Fig. 4-1

Synthesis and hydrolysis of a dipeptide.

number of proteins. It is unlikely that anywhere near the theoretical number of proteins exists in nature, but we have evidence that a great many do. The human body contains hundreds of different proteins, some of which contain as many as two hundred amino acids. In addition, each species builds proteins characteristic of itself. Thus, while the protein hemoglobin of a horse resembles that of a duck or a dog or a human being, they differ sufficiently that they cannot be interchanged with one another. In fact, the protein of one species is frequently toxic to another if introduced into the other before being hydrolyzed into its constituent amino acids. This, of course, makes transfusion of blood from one species to another impossible. These slight differences in hemoglobin from one species to another can be used as a basis for identifying the source of a blood sample.

Only in the last decade have analytical techniques enabled us to determine the amino acid composition of a protein. It was even later before scientists could establish the order in which amino acids occurred in a peptide chain. Now the electron microscope has allowed us to determine the spatial relationship of the amino acids in a protein crystal. Myoglobin, consisting of one hundred fifty amino acid units representing nineteen different amino acids, is considered a very simple protein and is the first for which the complete composition and structure has been known. It was elucidated in 1961. There is considerable information on the structure of insulin, a hormone secreted by the pancreas composed of fifty-one amino acids, the tobacco mosaic virus with one hundred fifty-eight amino acids, hemoglobin, and ribonuclease, an enzyme with a chain of one hundred twenty-four amino acids made up of nineteen different ones. Even with the more refined techniques now available it will be a long and tedious job to elucidate the structure of even the common, relatively simple

proteins that so far have been produced in a purified form. The determination of the structure of insulin culminated ten years of work.

One of the long-term goals of biologists, nutritionists, and biochemists has been to determine how the cell knows which protein to build, that is, the kind, the order, and number of amino acids to incorporate in new protein since each cell produces specific proteins. This goal was reached in 1962 when Watson and Crick showed that the pattern for protein synthesis was present in the substance DNA (deoxyribonucleic acid), itself a special type of nucleoprotein, the gene in the nucleus of the cell. The pattern is transferred to the ribosomes, the protein-synthesizing mechanism in the cytoplasm, by the substance RNA (ribonucleic acid), also a nucleoprotein. Based on a message carried to it by a form of RNA known as messenger RNA, the ribosomes are able to produce the specific protein dictated by the code contained in DNA of the nucleus. Thus, the secret of reproducing life of a particular species has been discovered, and scientists are rapidly learning the code of bases in the RNA which identifies each amino acid.

The ultimate value of a food protein to the body lies in its amino acid composition. Actually, it is the amino acids that are the essential nutrients rather than the protein. Many foods commonly designated as proteins are more accurately called protein-rich foods, and their nutritive value lies in the amino acid composition of the various proteins that may occur in any one. Some foods, such as gelatin, contain only one protein, but many have more than one. For example, hemoglobin, myoglobin, elastin, and collagen are all found in meat; casein and lactalbumin are found in milk.

Plants are able to build protein by fixing the element nitrogen from the soil and incorporating it in the protein molecule. Bacteria are able to utilize atmospheric nitrogen, but animals have no capacity to utilize the element nitrogen. They must depend on amino acids manufactured by plants, on proteins made by herbivorous animals, or on the capacity of bacteria in their gastro-intestinal tracts to synthesize amino acids.

CLASSIFICATION

Amino acids. From a functional nutritional standpoint amino acids are classified into two groups—essential (indispensable) and nonessential (dispensable). An essential amino acid is one that cannot be synthesized by the body *at a rate* sufficient to meet the needs for growth and maintenance. In the classification in Table 4-1 it is seen that eight of the twenty amino acids must be provided by the diet. There is strong evidence that histidine is also essential for infants. Other species may require other amino acids. If sufficient nitrogen is available, the human being can synthesize the other twelve needed to build body proteins. This nitrogen, referred to as non-essential nitrogen, may come from non-essential amino acids or an excess of essential amino acids. These undergo a process called *transamination* in which the amino group is transferred to another substance, often a carbohydrate derivative, to form the required amino acid. Since the body must obtain this nitrogen from food, non-essential nitrogen is now considered a dietary essential.

Protein. Proteins in food are classified on the basis of their amino acid content. Although there is an overlap in the classification, it provides a simple basis on which to evaluate protein quality. Proteins that contain all essential amino acids in proportions capable of promoting growth when they are the sole source of protein in the diet are described as complete proteins, good-quality proteins, or proteins of high biological value. They contain about 50% essential and 50% nonessential amino acids. All animal proteins except gelatin, which lacks both tryptophan and lysine, are complete proteins. Incomplete proteins, poor-quality

proteins, or proteins of low biological value are those that lack one or more amino acids and hence are unable to provide all the amino acids for the synthesis of body proteins. When they are the sole source of protein in the diet, no new tissue can be formed, nor can worn-out tissue be replaced. An animal on such a diet loses weight rapidly. All vegetable proteins except nuts are incomplete proteins. It is possible to simulate a complete protein by choosing two vegetable proteins that supplement or complement one another or to supplement an incomplete protein with a small amount of animal protein. For instance, a combination of wheat lacking in lysine and corn lacking in tryptophan and cystine would provide a mixture containing all essential amino acids. Similarly, a small amount of milk taken with a wheat cereal would provide the missing amino acid and enhance the biological value of the wheat protein. Some proteins that contain all essential amino acids but a relatively small amount of one have sufficient amino acids to repair body tissue if they are the sole source of dietary protein, but they do not have enough to promote growth. They are designated as partially complete proteins. The amino acid present in the relatively smallest amount is called a *limiting amino acid*. Arginine is the limiting amino acid in casein, and methionine is the one in fish and eggs. A complete protein functions as a partially complete protein when it constitutes a small proportion of the diet.

Fig. 4-2 shows the results of feeding complete, partially complete, and incomplete protein to rats.

FUNCTIONS

Although we must rely on protein-rich foods as a source of amino acids, it is the eight essential amino acids that are the ultimate nutrients for the body. It is the type and amounts of amino acids provided by the dietary protein that determine how

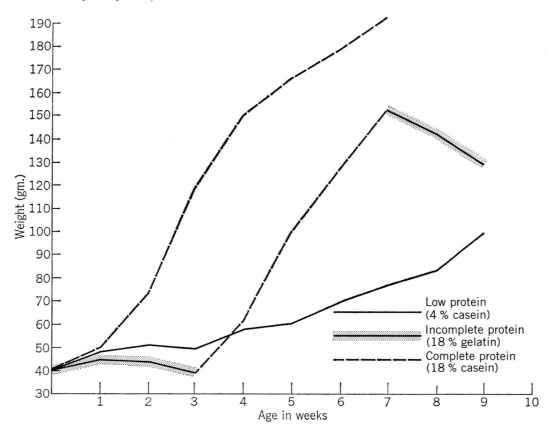

Fig. 4-2

Effect of complete, incomplete, and partially complete protein on growth of weanling rats.

effectively the body can perform the functions for which amino acids are needed. The needs for amino acids fall into six broad categories:

1. *Essential for growth.* Before cells can synthesize any new protein they must have available the eight essential amino acids plus sufficient nitrogen to incorporate with other materials to form the nonessential amino acids. Some amino acids are required to replace tissue that is constantly being broken down. If these are not available there will be a loss of total body protein that will eventually result in loss of weight and emaciation. For growth to occur amino acids must be

present in amounts over and above those needed for maintenance. The growth of some tissues calls for specific amino acids, such as the sulphur-containing amino acids characteristic of hair, skin, and nails.

Gain in body weight per se is not an adequate criterion of protein nutrition. Pups fed a diet with a wheat protein, gluten, as the source of protein gained as much weight as a group receiving egg protein. However, they were obese, inactive, and had delayed skeletal development while egg-fed pups were lean and active and had gained three times as much body protein. Rats will gain more weight on egg diet than on gluten diet, indicating that there is a correlation between weight gain in rats and tissue protein synthesis. Rather than store fat if the dietary amino acid pattern does not lead to protein synthesis, they reduce their food intake. A protein of high quality will yield maximum growth in a relatively low intake, after which weight gain per unit of protein drops and the efficiency with which protein is used also falls.

When normal body tissue fails to respond to a diet lacking in one of more amino acids, it has been found that tumor or abnormal tissue growth also subsides. This points to some hope that nutrition therapy, along with other forms of treatment, may prove useful in controlling tumor growth. If the nutrient is not available or its uptake by the cell is controlled, growth should be retarded.

2. *Formation of essential body compounds.* Hormones such as insulin, adrenalin, and thyroxine have been identified as protein substances. Each body cell contains around a thousand different enzymes, each catalyzing a specific reaction. All enzymes so far identified are protein. Coenzymes necessary for the action of enzymes have a protein structure usually associated with a specific vitamin. Hemoglobin, the substance in blood responsible for its oxygen and carbon dioxide–carrying properties so vital in respiration, is a protein complex.

The formation and replacement of these vital body compounds have high priority within the body and will suffer only in severe protein deprivation. Some tissue enzymes may be reduced 10% to 20% during protein depletion, those of brain being resistant to change and those of kidneys, skeletal muscle, and spleen showing some reduction.

3. *Regulation of water balance through the maintenance of oncotic pressure.* The distribution of fluids on either side of a cell membrane is regulated by the osmotic pressure exerted by electrolytes and the oncotic pressure exerted by protein. Since plasma protein cannot penetrate the capillary membrane, it remains in the blood when the hydrostatic pressure in the capillaries filters the plasma into the interstitial spaces to nourish the cells. At the venous end the oncotic pressure exerted by the plasma albumin exceeds the lowered hydrostatic pressure to draw the fluid back into the blood. In a protein deficiency the plasma albumin level drops, reducing the pressure to the point where the fluid accumulates in the interstitial spaces. Under these conditions the resulting soft spongy tissue is described as edematous, and the animal suffers from edema, an early sign of protein deficiency. The restoration of normal plasma protein levels with an adequate dietary intake restores normal fluid balance, the fluid being withdrawn from the intercellular spaces to restore the blood volume.

4. *Maintenance of body neutrality.* Proteins are considered amphoteric substances or buffers capable of reacting with either acids or bases. Their presence in the blood then helps prevent the accumulation of too much acid or base, either of which would interfere with normal body functioning. If an excess of base occurs, the protein acts as an acid to counteract it, and, conversely, if excess acid appears in the body fluids, the proteins of the blood act as a base to neutralize it. Thus, plasma

protein performs an important function in helping to maintain body neutrality essential to normal cellular metabolism.

5. *Stimulation of antibody formation.* The antibodies of the body responsible for its ability to combat infection are protein substances. The increased susceptibility to infection noted in low-protein diets is attributed to a lower level of antibodies capable of combatting the infective agents.

The ability to detoxify toxic material in the body is controlled by enzymes that are protein in nature. In protein depletion the ability to counteract the toxic effect of chemicals is reduced, rendering persons less resistant to certain poisons or drugs.

DIGESTION

Before protein can be absorbed through the wall of the intestine into the bloodstream, which carries it to the intercellular fluids that in turn bathe the individual cells, it must be broken down into its simplest structural blocks, the constituent amino acids. It now appears that two amino acids linked together as a dipeptide may enter the absorbing cells of the intestine but must be broken into its constituent amino acids to leave the cells in the lining of the intestine and pass into the bloodstream through the capillary wall into the intercellular spaces and through the cell membrane into the cell. This involves breaking the peptide linkages by which the amino acids are joined.

There are no protein-splitting enzymes in the saliva, so the first attack made on the peptide linkages of the complex protein is in the stomach. Here in the acid media of the gastric contents, gastric protease (pepsin), the protein-splitting enzyme of the gastric juice, attacks specific linkages in the peptide chain remote from the ends and reduces it to shorter units of amino acids known as peptones and peptides.

From the stomach the partially digested proteins pass into the small intestine where the acid is neutralized and the mixture becomes slightly alkaline. The pancreatic juice contains a protein-splitting enzyme, pancreatic protease or trypsin, which attacks very specific protein linkages—those involving carboxyl groups of lysine and arginine—but different ones from those attacked by gastric protease. The resulting shorter fragments may contain two amino acids (dipeptides) or three (tripeptides) but may also be more complex. The intestinal juice also secreted into the intestine contains enzymes capable of breaking the short protein fragments into their component amino acids. Two groups of enzymes attack the ends of the peptide chains—one known as carboxypeptidase attacks the carboxyl end, the other, an aminopeptidase, the amino end, releasing amino acids until only two remain joined as dipeptides. This final bond is broken by the action of dipeptidases—enzymes whose unique function is to separate two amino acids and which likely act in the membrane of the intestinal cells. All the protein-splitting enzymes are hydrolytic in that they require water to free the amino acids. This is a reversal of the process of synthesis in which the amino acids are joined together with the release of one molecule of water with each linkage formed. Protein digestion is summarized in Fig. 4-3.

The apparent digestibility of protein based on differences between dietary nitrogen and fecal nitrogen is 90%, but the fact that a variable amount of fecal nitrogen comes from intestinal cells and digestive enzymes makes true digestibility difficult to determine.

ABSORPTION

The amino acids formed in the process of digestion are in sufficiently simple form chemically to pass from the wall of the intestinal tract into the bloodstream either by diffusion or by the energy-requiring process of active transport. They are

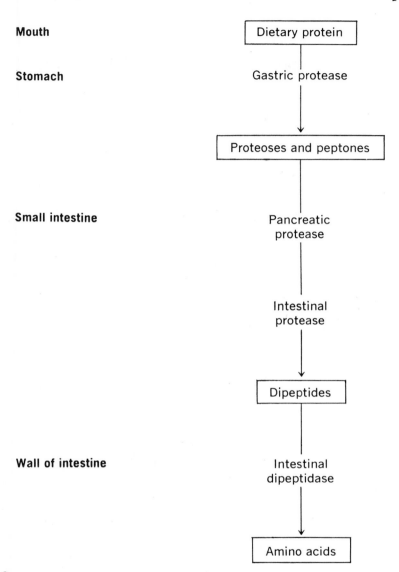

Fig. 4-3
Summary of protein digestion.

carried by the portal vein to the liver where they are released into the general circulation and carried to the various tissues and cells.

METABOLISM

The amino acids are taken up by the individual cells that use them in the synthesis of a specific protein. If the cell is to synthesize a protein, all of the essential amino acids needed for its structure must be provided simultaneously. If they are not available, the cell will release the other essential amino acids and no protein will be formed. In addition to the essential amino acids which the cell cannot manufacture, many nonessential amino acids are provided from the bloodstream. The cell will pick up at the same time any of the nonessential amino acids needed, or, if they are not available in the amino acid pool, will synthesize them, using the nitrogen of other amino acids. This process of synthesizing amino acids is accomplished by *transamination*—the transfer of an amino (NH_2) group from the amino acid to another substance frequently derived from carbohydrate to form another amino acid. It is conceivable that every cell is not capable of synthesizing all twelve indispensable amino acids but may rely on those synthesized by other cells and released into the amino acid pool of the bloodstream. For some particular cells then, there may be more than eight essential amino acids. Although very complex, the whole process of protein synthesis is very rapid, sometimes taking less than a minute. The pattern of amino acids incorporated in a synthesized protein is established by the gene present in the nucleus of the cell. The pattern is transferred from deoxyribonucleic acid (DNA) through a soluble ribonucleic acid (RNA) to the ribosomes, the site of synthesis. Thus, the particular proteins produced by any one cell are predetermined by the chromosomes of that cell.

Amino acids not needed by any of the body cells for building new protein will be released and returned to the liver where the nitrogenous group will be removed in a process called *deamination*. The nonnitrogenous residue enters the metabolic cycle for carbohydrates and fats and will either be oxidized to provide energy or will be converted into fat and stored as an energy reserve. The nitrogen portion undergoes a series of chemical changes and is finally converted into urea and excreted by the kidney in the urine. Since the kidney is called upon to excrete this urea as metabolic waste when protein is consumed in excess of needs for building body tissue and essential body compounds, it has been suggested that a high protein intake, especially when fluid intake is low, may tax the capacity of the kidney to excrete waste.

Early concepts of protein metabolism maintained that body proteins were relatively static. However, once radioactive isotopes became available, it was soon demonstrated that body proteins were in a state of dynamic equilibrium with a constant interchange of nitrogen from one tissue to another and between newly absorbed and older amino acids. Tissue proteins are continually being broken down and resynthesized—contributing to and taking away from the metabolic pools of amino acids to which dietary proteins also contribute. While there is no storage site for extra protein, the size of the liver will increase when protein is available, and some tissue proteins, such as plasma albumin, represent labile protein reserves. In a deficiency of either quantity or quality of dietary protein, it is broken down to provide amino acids for more vital uses in the body. Plasma globulin levels, however, are maintained in periods of protein depletion although they may be metabolically very active at the time albumin levels are being depleted. Liver, heart, and muscle proteins can be used as labile reserve of amino acids, but the protein of the brain is resistant to change. The labile protein reserves of the body comprise only 5% of total body protein, and the amino acid pool represents about 0.5 gm. of nitrogen per kilogram of body weight. The total amount of protein in the body does not change as long as the body is in nitrogen equilibrium, but the rate of turnover of body protein varies from tissue to tissue. Some, such as the gut, pancreas, and liver, exhibit a very rapid amino acid turnover while muscle and collagen turn over their amino acids very slowly. The rate of turnover in all tissues tends to decrease when dietary protein is limited. The half-life of total body protein is estimated at 80 days and the rate of synthesis of protein in the adult man at 0.3 gm. per kilogram of body weight per day.

Under certain conditions amino acids

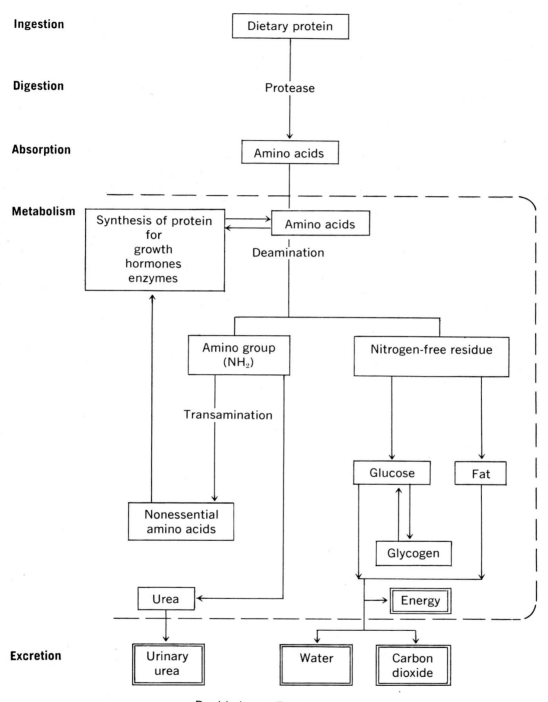

Ingestion — Dietary protein

Digestion — Protease

Absorption — Amino acids

Metabolism — Synthesis of protein for growth hormones enzymes ⇄ Amino acids — Deamination → Amino group (NH₂) / Nitrogen-free residue

Transamination → Nonessential amino acids

Amino group (NH₂) → Transamination

Nitrogen-free residue → Glucose ⇄ Glycogen / Fat

Urea

Energy

Excretion — Urinary urea / Water / Carbon dioxide

Double box = End products.

Fig. 4-4

Summary of protein digestion and metabolism. Changes within dotted lines occur after absorption and before excretion.

tend to accumulate in specific tissues. For instance, insulin stimulates uptake of amino acids in muscle cells, estradional stimulates uptake in the uterus, and epinephrine or a growth hormone increases tissue concentration.

The digestion and metabolism of protein is summarized diagramatically in Fig. 4-4. It is clear that dietary protein available to the cells as amino acids may be used in several ways.

1. If the calorie intake is adequate, amino acids are used for synthesis of protein.
2. If calorie intake is insufficient to meet energy needs *or* if more amino acids are available than are needed for synthesis of protein *or* if all the essential amino acids are not present simultaneously, amino acids are deaminated, with the amino group being excreted as urea and the nonnitrogenous fraction being used as a source of energy.
3. If glucogenic amino acids (those capable of forming glucose) are deaminated they are converted into glucose and then are metabolized as glucose, that is, used as an immediate source of energy, stored as glycogen, or stored as fat.
4. If ketogenic amino acids (those capable of forming fat directly) are deaminated they are converted into fatty acids and either used directly as a source of energy or converted into triglycerides and stored as fat.

The end products of protein metabolism are carbon dioxide, water, energy, and nitrogenous products in the urine. As with carbohydrates, the time elapsing between ingestion and excretion may vary from a few minutes to several years, depending on the intermediary steps involved.

FACTORS AFFECTING PROTEIN UTILIZATION

Amino acid balance. Equally important as the presence of all essential amino acids for protein synthesis is the balance of amino acids available to the cell. The pattern or balance of amino acids in egg protein is considered excellent for growth. Deviations from such a balance of amino acids results in less efficient growth response. It has been suggested that the limiting factor in the biological value of a protein is as frequently the pattern as the quantity of the essential amino acids. One of the hazards of supplementing a low-protein diet with a single amino acid is that an imbalance in the amino acid pattern of the total diet, which would occur if too much were added relative to the others present, may depress rather than improve the growth response. The growth depression noted in the addition of a single amino acid to low-protein diets is not noticed when a high-protein diet is supplemented. Apparently, the dietary imbalance is reflected in a proportionately high level of the amino acid in the plasma that seems to interfere with the passage of the amino acid into the cell and the ability of the cell to synthesize tissue protein.

Caloric value. The protein content of the diet cannot be adequately evaluated without a consideration of the caloric content. As the calorie value of the diet drops below a certain critical point, the retention of nitrogen drops, indicating that part of the protein was sacrificed for energy purposes. If calorie level is adequate, the level of protein utilization depends on the protein needs.

Immobility. The ability to synthesize protein appears to respond to a lack of activity. It has been observed that bedridden patients, especially older people, experience a negative nitrogen balance even when dietary protein seems adequate. Protein tissue lost in febrile illness is regained at a slower rate than that at which it is lost. In studying protein metabolism in infants, Stearns found it necessary to limit the periods of observation to a maximum of three days since further physical restraint decreased the efficiency of protein utilization.

A healthy individual in bed at rest loses nitrogen at a rate of 12 to 18 gm. per day.

Injury. Increase in nitrogen excretion after injury is well documented. It may reach as high as 20 gm. of nitrogen on a normal food intake. The use of high protein intakes immediately after injury neither prevents nor reverses the nitrogen loss. The losses are recovered once healing begins.

Emotional stability. Abnormal emotional stresses such as fear, anxiety, or anger increase the secretion of adrenaline, which in turn causes a series of changes that result in loss of nitrogen. Students lose nitrogen under the stress of examinations, as do persons experiencing severe pain, those whose work requires them to reverse normal night and day patterns, or those experiencing personal anxieties.

NITROGEN BALANCE STUDIES

Practically all proteins have a constant and equal percentage of nitrogen—16%. It does vary slightly in a few proteins, depending on their amino acid content, but it is sufficiently close that scientists have been able to use the relatively simple Kjeldahl determination of nitrogen as indicative of protein. Since nitrogen accounts for 16% of the protein molecule, values for nitrogen can be multiplied by 6.25 to give protein values. Thus, studies of nitrogen metabolism have become the basis for assessing protein metabolism. The few vitamins that contain nitrogen have so little that it does not appreciably affect the results.

Nitrogen balance studies, which involve a determination of the nitrogen content of all food taken in compared to the amount of nitrogen excreted by the body, have provided us with basic information on the overall gain or loss of body protein, although they give no information on changes among tissues. Most nitrogen is excreted either in the urine or feces. Urinary nitrogen represents both endogenous nitrogen from the breakdown of body tissue and exogenous nitrogen, which represents that from digested and absorbed amino acids in excess of the body's need to build or repair body tissue or vital body compounds. This nitrogen is that which has been removed from the absorbed amino acids so that the rest of the protein molecule can be used as a source of energy. Exogenous nitrogen will appear in the urine when protein intake exceeds the body's need for protein, when caloric intake is insufficient to meet needs of the body, or when the protein does not contain enough of the essential amino acids to allow the body to synthesize protein to replace that lost through the breakdown of body tissue. The small and fairly constant percentage of ingested nitrogen, which appears in the feces and represents undigested protein, amounts to about 8% of the total intake, although this varies with the source of protein. Table 4-2 gives the coefficients of digestibility of various proteins. Some nitrogen is also lost in perspiration and the sloughing off of

Table 4-2. Coefficients of digestibility of representative proteins

Food	Coefficient of digestibility
Eggs	97
Meat, fish	97
Milk	97
Wheat (70% to 74% extraction)	89
Fruits	85
Rice	84
Wheat cereals	79
Legumes (peas, beans, etc.)	78
Oatmeal	76
Root vegetables	74
Other vegetables	65

cells, such as the cuticle and from the surface of the body, but the difficulties involved in measuring this loss and the fact that it is likely an insignificant amount relative to the total urinary and fecal loss have not warranted its determination. Losses that range up to 0.56 gm. per square meter of body surface do assume greater importance when nitrogen balances are done in a tropical climate. Errors in nitrogen balance studies tend to overestimate intake and underestimate excretion.

When nitrogen intake equals nitrogen excretion, the individual is said to be in nitrogen equilibrium. This indicates that the protein intake is sufficient to take care of replacing and repairing body tissues but that no growth or increase in body tissue is occurring. This is a condition that should prevail in any adult who is receiving at least the minimum protein needed. It also occurs at any level above minimum where no growth is occurring. When nitrogen intake exceeds nitrogen excretion, positive nitrogen balance, tissue or vital body compounds are being built at a rate faster than that at which they are being destroyed. Under these conditions growth occurs. Positive nitrogen balance should prevail throughout the period of childhood and adolescence and during pregnancy and lactation. Nitrogen excretion in excess of intake, negative nitrogen balance, means that body tissue is wearing out or break-

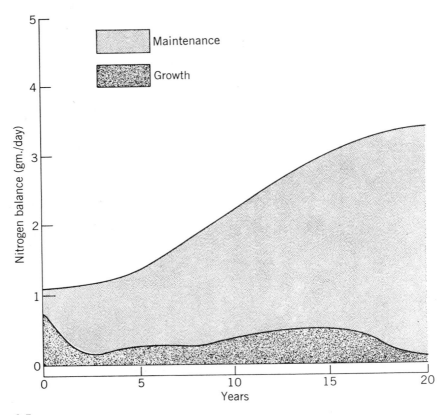

Fig. 4-5

Amounts of nitrogen needed for maintenance and growth of boys at various ages. (Adapted from Allison, J. B.: Protein malnutrition, Tr. New York Acad. Sc. **25:**293, 1963.)

ing down at a rate faster than it is being repaired. This is an undesirable situation, reflecting wasting of body tissue and loss of body protein. There is some evidence that individuals adapt to low protein intakes since low levels of intake that produce a negative balance when fed following a higher intake may eventually be sufficient to establish nitrogen equilibrium as the body adjusts toward more efficient use of the amount available. Fig. 4-5 shows the amount of nitrogen needed to maintain body tissue and the amount needed to meet needs for growth with increasing age. In infants almost equal amounts are needed for growth and maintenance, but with older persons the proportion needed for maintenance inceases and that for growth decreases until adulthood, when virtually none is used for growth. An unexplained retention of nitrogen above that needed for repair of tissue has been observed in many adults. It has been designated as nitrogen needed for adult growth although the nature of the need remains obscure.

Nitrogen balance studies yield information only on total protein mass and give no indication of a shift in body proteins from one tissue to another, which may have occurred. For instance, plasma albumin levels may drop in an individual in nitrogen equilibrium, indicating that this labile nitrogen pool has been depleted to meet needs of another tissue. Thus, it is possible for a suboptimal level of protein nutrition to prevail before it is manifest in negative nitrogen balance.

The significance of nitrogen balance data is summarized in Table 4-3.

DETERMINATION OF MINIMAL NEEDS

Nitrogen balance studies have been used to determine both minimum total protein and essential amino acid needs of the body. In this technique the subject is fed progressively lower levels of nitrogen in successive balance periods, usually of 3 to 7 days' duration. As long as the individual is in nitrogen equilibrium, we know that he is getting enough total protein, or, if one amino acid is being tested, that he is getting a sufficient amount of that amino acid. The point at which his nitrogen balance becomes negative is that at which his needs exceed his intake. His minimum protein need falls between the lowest point in which he was in equilibrium and the level at which his balance is negative. It is possible to arrive at a more precise figure by gradually increasing the protein in successive balance periods until the individual is again in equilibrium. By using this technique it has been established that the requirements for the essential amino acids are surprisingly low. It is also evident that there are wide individual differences in

Table 4-3. Summary of significance of nitrogen balance data

Condition	Measurement	Significance
Positive nitrogen balance	N intake > N excretion	Growth
Nitrogen equilibrium	N intake = N excretion	Maintenance and repair of tissue
Negative nitrogen balance	N intake < N excretion	Wasting of body, loss of weight

needs for amino acids, as for other nutrients. There is still much controversy over proposed values. In addition to the minimum amounts proposed for these amino acids, there must be sufficient nonessential nitrogen to allow for the synthesis of nonessential amino acids. With the recognition that the body needs amino acids, nitrogen, and organic acids rather than protein as such for protein synthesis, the term *protein requirement* is becoming outmoded. However, in the following discussion of requirements we will think of the amount of protein necessary to provide the amino acids and nitrogen needed by each group.

DIETARY REQUIREMENTS

Protein. The minimum nitrogen need for most adults has been set at 3.5 gm., but there is some evidence that for some people it may be as low as 2.5 gm. Since protein is 16% nitrogen, this minimum nitrogen requirement could be satisfied by an intake of 16 to 22 gm. protein or approximately 0.35 gm. per kilogram of body weight. This figure implies protein of high biological value. The National Research Council has allowed a wide margin of safety to account for variations in the biological value of the diet when they suggest one gram of protein per kilogram of body weight as a recommended level. This is justified in the United States where there is an abundant supply of high-quality protein. In areas where protein is not as available in such an ideal amino acid pattern, requirements must be modified to compensate for lower digestibility and lower biological value of the protein. Thus, the requirement for a protein that is 50% digested and has a biological value of 70 would be 1 gm. per kilogram of body weight based on the following calculations:

Protein requirement = 0.35 gm./kg. body weight

$$\times \frac{100}{50} \times \frac{100}{70} = 1 \text{ gm. per kilogram}$$

For protein diets of different biological value and different coefficients of digestibility, the requirement can be calculated.

For infants and children experiencing a rapid increase in body weight, much of which is bone and muscle growth, the recommended levels of protein intake are considerably higher per unit of body weight. Levels of 2 to 3 gm. per kilogram are proposed although one study reported positive nitrogen balance on intakes of 1 to 1.2 gm. per kilogram per day. In periods from 1½ to 3 years of age, increase in muscle accounts for half the weight gain. The amount needed to ensure normal growth is again a function of the biological value of the protein in the diet as well as the individual characteristics of the infants.

Minimum protein level needed by infants will usually be reached when protein provides 6% of the kilocalorie intake.

Up to nine years of age the skeleton grows faster than the body as a whole so that protein needs are proportionately high. As legs grow in length and center of gravity becomes farther from the floor, more muscles must be developed to maintain posture and permit activity.

For adolescents the recommendation is that 15% of the calories be provided by protein. Since protein has a physiological fuel value of 4 kilocalories per gram, a person needing 3200 calories should receive 480 calories from protein or 120 gm. of protein. One of the important considerations in establishing recommended levels for adolescents is an evaluation of the level that produces a healthy adult.

During pregnancy the NRC suggests intakes that are increased by 50% to 1.5 gm. per kilogram. This is used not only for the growth of the fetus but also for the growth of the placenta, mammary glands, and other tissue reserves for lactation. A 7-pound baby has one pound of protein acquired primarily in the last half of pregnancy. This growth calls for 4 to 6 gm. of protein per day above maintenance requirements. Restriction of protein in the mother's diet leads to the birth of shorter, lighter infants than those born to mothers on an adequate protein intake. Two thirds of the protein in the diet of pregnant women should be of high biological value. In lactation the requirement is raised to 2 gm. per kilogram of body weight. The production of 1000 ml. of mature human milk with a protein content of 1.2% involves the synthesis of 12 gm. of milk protein, mostly lactalbumin.

A comparison of protein standards recommended by various groups is given in Table 4-4.

Amino acids. In the determination of the requirements of essential amino acids based on nitrogen balance studies, amino acids must be provided in purified form and the level of all amino acids as well as that of nonessential nitrogen must be carefully controlled. The technique is costly and time-consuming. The results of experiments to assess the amino acid needs of infants,

adult men, and adult women have not been accepted uncritically. The currently accepted standards are given in Table 4-5 although it is recognized that further work will undoubtedly lead to modifications.

FOOD SOURCES

Some of the major food sources of protein and their contribution to the total protein requirement are shown graphically in Fig. 4-6. Values are expressed in terms of 100 gm. of the food and 100 kilocalories. It must be remembered that the ultimate value of a protein-rich food to the diet is determined by amino acid pattern. Generally speaking, proteins of animal origin are more adequate than those of vegetable origin, but within each group there is a wide range in biological values.

The effect of heat on the utilization of dietary protein has been the subject of much research. One attempt to show relative values of raw and overheated pork in-

Table 4-4. Comparison of protein standards for selected age groups (in grams)

	NRC recommended allowances*	Canadian dietary standards†	FAO‡	Nutrient allowances, United Kingdom§
Adult men (70 kg.)	70	50	0.59/kg.	80
Adult women (56–58 kg.)	58	39	0.59/kg.	73
Pregnancy	+20	+10	+6 gm./day	
Lactation	+40	+20	+15 gm./day	
Children 1– 3 years	32	25–30	0.88/kg.	
3– 6 years	40	30	0.81/kg.	
6– 9 years	52	40	0.77/kg.	74
9–12 years	55–60	50	0.72/kg.	
Adolescent 13–15 years (boy)	75	75	0.70/kg.	
13–15 years (girl)	62	75	0.64/kg.	

*National Academy of Sciences, National Research Council: Recommended dietary allowances, Publication No. 1146, Washington, D.C., 1964, National Research Council.
†Dietary standards for Canada, Canadian Bulletin on Nutrition, vol. 6, No. 1, March, 1964.
‡Joint FAO/WHO Expert Group: Protein requirements, FAO Nutrition Meeting Report Series No. 37, Rome, 1965, p. 22.
§Report of the Committee on Nutrition, London, 1950, British Medical Association.

Table 4-5. Minimal amino acid requirements

	Infants (milligrams per kilogram)*	Adult female (milligrams per day)†	Adult male (milligrams per day)†
Isoleucine	126	450	700
Leucine	150	620	1100
Lysine	103	500	800
Methionine	45‡	350	200‡
Phenylalanine	90§	220	300§
Threonine	87	305	500
Tryptophan	22	157	250
Valine	105	650	800
Histidine	34	—	—

(Suggested adult protein intake is 0.52 gm. per kilogram per day.)

*Holt, L. E., et al.: Protein and amino acid requirements in early life, New York, 1960, New York University Press.
†Food and Nutrition Board Committee in Amino Acids: Evaluation of protein nutrition, Publication 711, Washington, D.C., 1959, National Academy of Science, National Research Council.
‡In presence of adequate tyrosine.
§In presence of adequate cystine.

dicated that the peak level of amino acids from raw pork appeared in the blood 45 minutes after ingestion, while the peak from overheated pork was not reached for 5 hours, indicating slower digestion of the protein. Weight gain was 22% less on overheated than on raw pork. When soybeans were fed, moderate heating of the beans led to increased plasma amino acid levels, while overheating reduced them. The beneficial effects of heating were believed to be caused by greater ease in the release of the limiting amino acid methionine. On the other hand, the protein of wheat and oats is adversely affected by heat, as is that of nine out of seventeen legume seeds tested. The amount of heat used in the preparation of evaporated and dried milks seems to improve the digestibility and utilization of the protein. When heat does decrease the nutritive value of proteins the effect seems to be caused by a reduction in hydrolysis of heated proteins by digestive enzymes, indicating that heating has pro-

duced complexes resistant to the action of digestive enzymes. If heating affects the *rate* of release of amino acids from a protein, it could affect the nutritive value that is dependent on the release of all amino acids simultaneously.

Some protein-rich foods such as peanuts cannot be eaten raw as they contain either toxic substances or enzymes which must be destroyed before they are of value to the body, or are susceptible to the growth of toxic molds.

Since protein-rich foods are one of the most expensive items in the average diet, it is helpful to have information on the cost of similar amounts of protein from various sources. Such information is provided in Table 4-6, which shows the cost of one third of a day's allowance of protein for the adult male—23.3 gm. In interpreting this data it must be kept in mind that they are based on average prices in December, 1965, and may not be accurate at any specific date in the future, especially in light

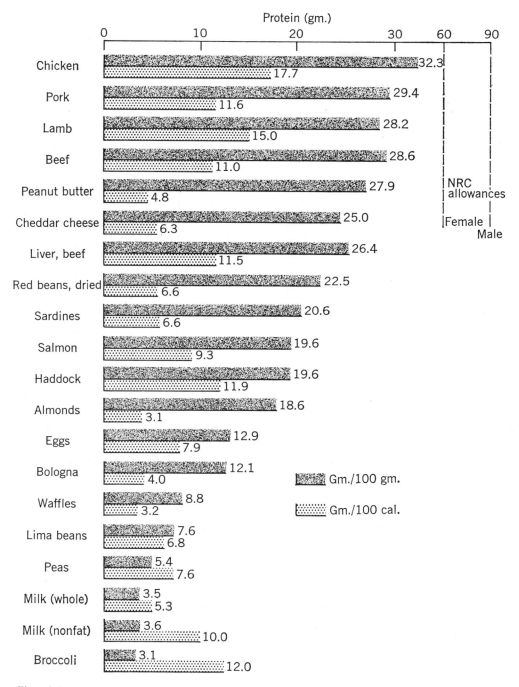

Fig. 4-6

Protein contribution of 100-gm. and 100-kilocalorie portions of some representative foods. (Based on Watts, B., and Merrill, A.: Composition of foods—raw, processed and prepared, U. S. Department of Agriculture Handbook No. 8, Washington, D. C., 1963, U. S. Department of Agriculture.)

Table 4-6. Cost of one third daily recommended allowance of protein for adult male based on average retail prices in Pennsylvania in December, 1965

Cost of portion providing 23.3 gm. protein	Food	Amount to be purchased to provide 23.3 gm. protein
<$.10	Nonfat dried milk	0.26 pound
	Dry beans	0.80 pound
	Pork liver	0.26 pound
	American cheese	0.20 pound
$.10 to $.20	Peanut butter	0.19 pound
	Cottage cheese	0.38 pound
	Turkey	0.38 pound
	Chicken	0.38 pound
	Hamburger	0.29 pound
	Beef liver	0.26 pound
	Eggs, large	0.27 dozen
	Tuna fish	0.19 pound
$.20 to $.30	Haddock fillet	0.39 pound
	Ham	0.40 pound
	Chuck roast	0.40 pound
	Frankfurters	0.42 pound
$.30 to $.40	Bologna	0.43 pound
	Round steak	0.27 pound
	Pork roast	0.46 pound
	Bacon, sliced	0.53 pound
	Sirloin steak	0.33 pound
>$.40	Pork chops	0.46 pound
	Lamb chops	0.44 pound
	Veal cutlet	0.43 pound

of the seasonal variations in costs of products such as eggs and pork. They are presented only to give some concept of relative costs. Many of the foods represented make significant contributions of other nutrients as well.

In assessing the value of a day's diet it is important to look at the distribution of dietary protein throughout the day's meals. Generally it is recommended that at least one third of the protein be from animal sources of high biological value. The typical American diet is more likely to contain 60% to 80% animal protein. But if this is not distributed so that the amino acid composition of each meal is adequate through

some complete protein or a mixture of vegetable proteins that supplement one another, the individual will be unable to use protein as a body builder and will be forced to deaminate it to use as a source of energy. Traditionally, we do use complete protein to supplement incomplete proteins in the diet. The use of milk with cereal, cheese with macaroni, meat with rice, and peanut butter with bread are examples of these complementary relationships. The increasing use of dried milk solids in commercially baked bread has a supplementary effect on the amino acid pattern of the wheat protein and improves the biological value of the bread protein.

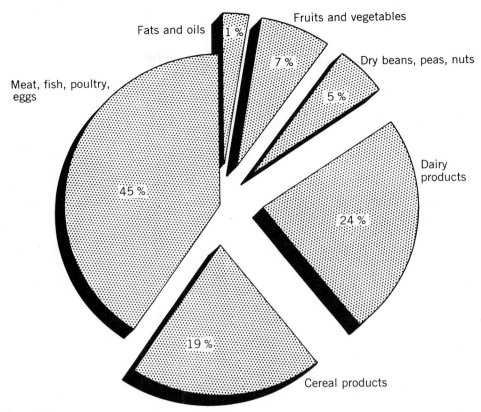

Fig. 4-7

Contribution of food groups to protein content of the American food supply. (Based on Nutritive value of foods available for consumption in United States, 1909-1964, Agricultural Research Service Publication 62-14, 1966.)

The efforts of some commercial interests to promote the addition lysine to bread and flour in the United States are likely not justified since there is no evidence of a lysine deficiency in the American diet. In addition, recent studies suggest that protein quality may be depressed rather than increased if the level of one amino acid is increased out of proportion to the others. Amino acid supplementation of a low-quality protein may be justified when it is a staple item in a total diet of low biological value, but not when protein quality is high.

The relative contribution of various food groups to the protein in the American diet is shown in Fig. 4-7.

EVALUATION OF PROTEIN QUALITY

Since the amino acid content of a protein rather than the total amount of protein in the diet determines the value of the protein the problem of measuring the relative value of various proteins as dietary constituents is very complex. Both biological and chemical methods of evaluating protein quality have been tried.

The simplest and most widely used index is the biological value (B.V.). This is a measure of the relationship of protein retention to protein absorption on the assumption that more will be retained when the essential amino acids are present in sufficient quantity to meet the needs for growth. The biological value is assessed by determining the nitrogen in the food intake and the urinary and fecal excretions. Urinary nitrogen includes that from absorbed amino acids that have been deaminated and fecal nitrogen represents that which was unabsorbed plus that from any cells that may have sloughed off the lining of the digestive tract or digestive enzymes that have not been reabsorbed. The formula for determining biological value becomes:

$$\text{B.V.} = \frac{\text{Dietary N} - (\text{Urinary N} + \text{Fecal N})}{\text{Dietary N} - \text{Fecal N}} \times 100$$

A protein with a biological value of 70 or more (that is, the body retains 70% of the intake of nitrogen) is considered capable of ensuring adequate protein nutrition, assuming that the caloric value of the diet is adequate. Dietaries with a biological value of less than 70 are not capable of supporting growth. This index may be applied to single proteins, single foods, or combinations of protein in foods. It is used extensively to determine if the protein available in a national food supply is capable of meeting the needs of the population or if some means of supplementation should be sought. The biological value of some proteins is given in Table 4-7.

Table 4-7. Biological value of representative proteins

Food	Biological value
Egg	100
Milk	93
Rice	86
Fish	75
Beef	75
Casein	75
Corn	72
Cottonseed flour	60
Peanut flour	56
Wheat gluten	44

A protein score that correlates well with biological value has been developed. In this method the amino acid pattern of a protein is compared to that of egg protein, which has a biological value of 100. The protein score represents the relative amount of the most limiting amino acid in the protein compared to that of the same amino acid in egg protein. This method has limited usefulness in that it fails to consider the total amino acid pattern.

A modified protein score, an essential amino acid (EAA) index, has been suggested. It takes into consideration the ratio of each essential amino acid in a dietary protein relative to the amount in whole egg protein. While more involved than a protein score, it gives a better picture of the overall nutritive potential of the protein.

The Food and Agricultural Organization feels that the use of egg protein as a standard for world food supplies sets an unnecessarily and unreasonably high standard. As an answer they have developed a hypothetical reference protein based on results of studies using amino acid mixtures they assumed were released simultaneously from the intestine. In this ideal aminogram, shown in Table 4-8, threonine is arbitrarily assigned a value of 1 and the amounts of other amino acids are given in reference to threonine. A comparison of this standard with the amino acid pattern of both egg protein and human milk shows that they are very similar. There is some evidence to suggest that the FAO reference protein contains too much tryptophan and methionine and too little lysine. Although needs for growth may differ from those for maintenance, an amino acid pattern that supports growth has been shown to promote repletion of depleted adult tissue. In evaluating protein quality the amino acid pattern of a specific food is compared to this arbitrary amino acid pattern based on human requirements of the amino acids.

Many other attempts have been made

Table 4-8. Aminogram proposed by Food and Agricultural Organization as a reference protein*

	Milligrams per gram of nitrogen	Grams per 100 gm. of protein
Isoleucine	270	4.2
Leucine	306	4.8
Lysine	270	4.2
Total aromatic amino acids	360	5.6
Phenylalanine	180	2.8
Sulphur-containing amino acids	270	4.2
Methionine	144	2.2
Threonine	180	2.8
Tryptophan	90	1.4
Valine	270	4.2

*FAO Committee in Protein Requirements, FAO Nutr. Stud., Series 16, 1957.

to develop a formula for evaluating protein quality. Some of the more widely used ones include the protein efficiency ratio (PER), which is based on weight gain in grams per gram of dietary nitrogen in a diet providing 10% protein; net protein utilization (NPU), which involves measurement of both digestibility and biological value of a protein; net protein utilization calories percent (NPU cal. %) in which the NPU is considered in light of the percentage of total calories coming from protein; and the plasma amino acid index (PAA) in which changes in the amino acid pattern in the blood following the feeding of a specific protein are related to fasting blood amino acid levels. The fact that so many standards have been and are being proposed is evidence that we lack any single satisfactory standard. Many standards are based on biological assays that generally are more costly and time-consuming than chemical analyses of amino acid composition. Protein metabolism is apparently so complex that a determination of chemical makeup of a

protein gives only limited information on the manner in which the animal may utilize it. Similarly, proteins that can effectively repair body tissue may have limitations as a source of growth protein.

KWASHIORKOR

The importance of protein in world nutrition has been emphasized in the last decade with the identification of the condition *kwashiorkor* as a protein-deficiency disease. This condition occurs primarily among children between the ages of 2 and 5 years who are weaned from mother's milk to a diet of starch cereal pastes practically devoid of protein. Fig. 1-2 shows kwashiorkor. This term, which was applied by the Ga tribe in Ghana to a sickness of a weanling child, means literally "first-second." It was appropriate because the first child developed it within 3 or 4 months after being abruptly weaned from the breast on the arrival of the second child, a time when milk, his only source of good-quality protein, was removed. Kwashiorkor is considered the major nutrition problem in the world today; many infants are dying as a result of it, and untold numbers are suffering from subclinical symptoms of the disease and increased susceptibility to infection. In kwashiorkor there is a deficiency in quality and quantity of dietary protein in the presence of adequate calories. *Marasmus* is the term applied to the condition resulting from both a protein and calorie deficit.

The main clinical symptoms of kwashiorkor are as follows:

1. Failure to grow in both weight and length with weak, thin, and wasting muscles.
2. Mental changes manifest as irritability and apathy.
3. Edema—the accumulation of fluid in the tissues causing them to be soft and spongy, especially in the lower half of the body.
4. Skin changes, especially in the lower part of the body. These include abnormal color in some areas, lack of color in others, and drying and peeling of the skin resulting in the formation of ulcers.
5. Changes in hair, which becomes sparse and loses its pigmentation or takes on a characteristic reddish color.
6. Loss of appetite, vomiting, and diarrhea.
7. Enlargement of the liver.
8. Anemia.

The ability of the child to combat infection is very low and death is usually attributed to an infection, such as measles or pneumonia, which would not normally be fatal.

Unfortunately, many children with kwashiorkor are never given medical help or are brought in for treatment only when the disease is well advanced. The most helpful diagnostic sign is a change in serum albumin levels, but this change does not occur in the very early stages of the condition. If diagnosed early enough prekwa-shiorkor can be treated simply by improving the amount and quality of protein in the diet. The treatment must also take into account the anorexia or loss of appetite that is common. However, in more advanced cases, extreme care must be taken to compensate for the low potassium levels that usually accompany low protein intake. Nonfat milk has been the most successful therapeutic food. It is diluted at first and increased in strength gradually until full strength can be tolerated. Once the edema has been eliminated and blood potassium levels restored, whole milk or nonfat milk with coconut and corn oil added are necessary to provide sufficient calories to stimulate growth.

The most promising attack on the problem of kwashiorkor is one of prevention, which implies the use of a diet adequate in good-quality protein and calories. Most attempts to provide sufficient animal protein are impractical where there is limited land available and where the cost of animal protein is economically out of reach of most of the population. The situation will become progressively worse as population pressures increase. The one inexpensive source of animal protein that has promise is fish, but problems of preservation in tropical climates limit the extent to which this is exploited.

Efforts are being encouraged to provide a palatable low-cost food with an adequate balance of amino acids that can be made from indigenous plant substances for use in the postweaning diet of infants to supplement the basic cereal diet. Since no one plant protein provides a desirable balance for mammalian needs, a search for such a mixture of plant proteins has been the incentive for much research. The most successful effort so far has been that of the Institute of Nutrition in Central America and Panama, commonly referred to as INCAP. They have succeeded in producing a mixture of 58% ground maize and sorghum, 36% cottonseed flour, 3% torula yeast, 1% $CaCo_3$ and vitamin A. It is sold under the name of Incaparina and has been widely accepted for use as a relatively low-bulk beverage or gruel at a cost of less than 4 cents per day. This mixture provides the critical pattern of amino acids required for child growth and at the same time corrects the nutrient deficiencies that usually accompany kwashiokor—vitamin A, riboflavin, calcium, and niacin. Other combinations of leaf protein and legumes available in other regions such as Lebanon and India have been developed and show promising results.

Some efforts have been made to enrich or fortify cereals with the limiting amino acids, such as adding lysine to wheat, lysine and threonine to rice, and lysine, threonine, and methionine to barley. This has not proved very practical, as it only improves the quality of the protein and does not solve the problem of the low protein intake. In addition, only methionine and lysine are sufficiently low in cost to begin to be economically feasible. The possibility of creating an imbalance in the amino acid pattern by the addition of too much of the limiting amino acid is another reason for caution.

A third approach has been that of supplementing basic cereal diets with small amounts of animal protein. The addition of 20% nonfat milk powder or 10% fish flour to a maize and pea mixture produced a protein equal to milk in nutritive value. The development of protein concentrates that can be incorporated into basic cereal products has been encouraging. Fish flour, with a protein content of 85% and produced from small fish that normally have no commercial value, is acceptable when it has been defatted and deodorized. Concentrates from coconut seed press cakes, other seed kernels, and cottonseed are inexpensive and promising as a partial solution to the problems of protein malnutrition. Care must be take to exclude any toxic substances that are naturally present or that develop during processing.

Other efforts have centered around the development and cultivation of more nutritive varieties of basic cereal crops in an area of low protein intake and the improvement of protein quality of the diet by processing. The possibility of using chlorella, a microscopic plankton which abounds in the sea, and a protein produced by bacteria from petroleum also have promise.

In addition to having a protein content of high biological value any food which will provide any hope for meeting the nutritional needs in developing countries must meet certain other criteria. It must be locally available or capable of being produced locally, must be within economic reach of the segment of the population needing it, must have long storage life under hot humid conditions, and must be easily transported; it must also have acceptable characteristics of taste, odor, and physical properties. On the other hand, if it is too popular it may become prestige food in the culture and be consumed by the ranking adult males rather than by children and pregnant women whose needs are greatest. The food must be free from toxic and deleterious effects in the form proposed and must not be currently used to a maximum as human food. Many foods, or combination of foods, have been suggested, but at present, in addition to fish flour, the most promising appear to be soy products with a protein value of 25%, peanut flour, sesame flour, cottonseed flour, oil seed cakes, and coconut protein. Algae and yeast, while theoretically good sources, have not proven sufficiently palatable for human use. Others have been eliminated because of their unknown nutritive value, the uneconomical aspects of their production, a limited production of the raw material, or the presence of a toxic substance.

ABNORMALITIES IN AMINO ACID METABOLISM

Some infants are born with an inability to produce the enzymes necessary for phenylalanine metabolism. These children need a small amount of this essential amino acid for protein synthesis, but have no ability to metabolize the rest with the result that phenylalanine and some of its partially oxidized derivatives accumulate in the blood and urine. They have an adverse effect on nervous tissue and the resulting condition known as phenylketonuria (PKU) is characterized by mental retardation. Early diagnosis is crucial to successful treatment in which a diet very low in phenylalanine is indicated.

A similar failure to metabolize leucine and valine is reflected as maple sugar urine disease, so named because of the characteristic odor of the urine. Failure to metabolize histidine appears related to speech defects. Other inborn errors of metabolism involving other amino acids have also been reported.

SELECTED REFERENCES

Allison, J. B., and Fitzpatrick, W. H.: Dietary proteins in health and disease, Springfield, Ill., 1960, Charles C Thomas, Publisher.

Food and Agricultural Organization: Human protein requirements and their fulfillment in practice, FAO Nutr. Stud., Series 16, 1957.

Food and Nutrition Board, National Academy of Science: Evaluation of protein nutrition, Publication No. 711, Washington, D. C., 1959, National Research Council.

Food and Nutrition Board, National Academy of Science: Evaluation of protein quality, Publication No. 1100, Washington, D. C., 1963, National Research Council.

Food and Nutrition Board, National Academy of Science: Meeting protein needs of infants and children, Publication No. 943, Washington, D. C., 1961, National Research Council.

Harper, A. E.: Some implications of amino acid supplementation, Am. J. Clin. Nutrition 9:533, 1961.

Holt, L. E., et al.: The concept of protein stores and its implication in the diet, J.A.M.A. 181:699, 1962.

5

Energy balance

ENERGY SOURCES

The energy value of food is provided entirely by the carbohydrate, fat, and protein components of the diet. These may make up from 4% of foods such as lettuce to 100% of foods such as sugar, salad oil, and dry gelatin. The remaining portion of the food consists of water, cellulose, minerals, and vitamins, none of which yield energy. In the typical American diet, carbohydrate provides 50% to 60% of the energy, protein, 10% to 15%, and fat, 35% to 45%. The source of energy in diets varies with many factors—agricultural, cultural, social, and economic. For instance, in rice-eating countries carbohydrate makes a much larger contribution, and in countries with emphasis on dairying protein assumes greater importance. Italians, with the extensive use of cooking oil, derive more energy from fats. In America, there is a trend toward greater use of protein and a concurrent decrease in carbohydrate consumption with an increase in the amount of money available for food.

Unit of measurement

The energy value of a food is expressed in terms of a unit of heat, a *kilocalorie*. This represents the amount of heat required to raise the temperature of 1 kg. (slightly over 1 quart) of water 1° C. While this unit is correctly designated as a kilocalorie to distinguish it from the smaller unit, a calorie (0.001 kilocalorie), used in most physical and chemical measurements, many nutrition sources still refer to it as the Calorie or even calorie, assuming that it is a sufficiently standardized term in nutrition that no distinction need be made. It will undoubtedly be some time before the term *calorie*, as used in popular literature, will be replaced by the more correct *kilocalorie*. Indeed, to do so might introduce undue confusion to a topic that is freely discussed but only vaguely understood by the general public.

A concept of the amount of energy or heat available from foods may be obtained by noting that 2 tablespoons of sugar provide 100 kilocalories, enough heat to raise the temperature of slightly over 4 cups of water from 0° C. (freezing) to 100° C. (boiling), assuming a high degree of efficiency in the conversion of energy. One tablespoon of fat or 4½ cups of shredded cabbage have a similar energy potential. In the body much of the energy obtained from food is converted into mechanical, osmotic, and chemical energy as well as heat. The ability of the animal to release this energy depends on the presence of minerals and vitamins that catalyze the many and complex chemical changes in the simple energy-yielding nutrients, glucose and fatty acids, until the energy is converted into a high-energy compound, ATP (adenosine triphosphate). From this form it is available in slowly regulated amounts for use within the cell. This transfer of energy to ATP takes place almost exclusively in the mitochondrion of the cell. It is used, however, in virtually all organelles of the cell for the synthesis of complex substances from simple nutrients and for all metabolic reactions that require energy.

DETERMINATION OF ENERGY VALUES
Direct calorimetry

Much of our information on the energy value of foods is determined by *direct calorimetry.* The instrument used for this measurement is the *bomb calorimeter,* a highly insulated, compact, boxlike container about 1 cubic foot in size. The essential features of a bomb calorimeter are shown in Fig. 5-1. A dried sample of food is completely burned in the oxygen-rich environment within the container, and all of the heat produced is absorbed by a weighed amount of water surrounding the combustion chamber. The change in temperature of this fluid surrounding the combustion chamber is measured. Since the amount of heat required to change the temperature of a certain volume of water is known, the amount of heat required for the observed change can be readily cal-

culated. Since the bomb is sufficiently well insulated that no heat exchange takes place with the environment, the heat necessary for the increase in water temperature must have been derived from the dried sample of food, which is completely burned and releases all its energy. A single bomb calorimeter determination takes about 20 minutes but must be preceded by very precise weighing and careful drying of the sample.

Heat of combustion

The energy value of a sample of food determined in a bomb calorimeter is known as the *heat of combustion,* the maximum amount of energy, measured as heat, the sample is capable of yielding under conditions providing for complete burning or oxidation.

As explained more fully in Chapter 15, when purified samples of carbohydrate, fat, and protein are burned in the bomb calorimeter, the amount of heat produced will vary slightly with the source and chemical composition of the nutrient, but values of 4.1 kilocalories per gram of carbohydrate, 9.45 kilocalories per gram of fat, and 5.65 kilocalories per gram of protein are generally considered representative of the carbohydrate, fat, and protein found in the American diet.

The heat of combustion represents the energy produced by the oxidation of the carbon molecule to carbon dioxide, the hydrogen to water, and the nitrogen of protein to nitrous oxide. The body is capable of releasing this energy potential of carbon through a process of *decarboxylation* or removal of carbon dioxide and that of the hydrogen through a series of reactions referred to as *coupled oxidative phosphorylation.* It cannot, however, release the energy potential of nitrogen. Thus the heat measured in the bomb calorimeter from the oxidation of nitrogen is not available when protein is utilized in the body. It is necessary then to subtract the amount of heat

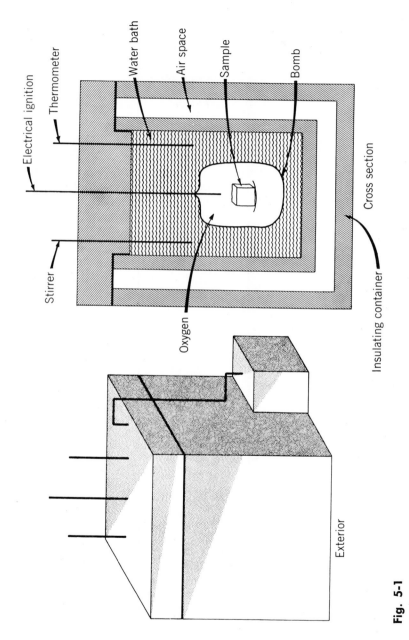

Fig. 5-1

Essential features of a bomb calorimeter. Exterior and cross section are shown.

representing the oxidation of nitrogen from the total heat of combustion of protein in estimating the amount available to the body. The oxidation of nitrogen accounted for 1.3 kilocalories of the 5.65 kilocalories per gram of protein, leaving a potential of only 4.3 kilocalories per gram of protein available to the body.

Coefficient of digestibility

Since the body is not 100% efficient in digesting (preparing food for absorption) or in absorbing food, if one wishes to determine the amount of energy available to the body from an energy-yielding nutrient one must take into account the extent to which the ingested nutrient is available to the cells. The extent of digestion varies from one nutrient to another and is also influenced by the nature of the food in which it is found. However, to calculate the potential energy from carbohydrate, fat, and protein representative *coefficients of digestibility* expressing the percentage of the nutrient ultimately available are used. For carbohydrate, which is 98% digested, fat, which is 95% digested, and protein, 92% digested, the coefficients of digestibility are 0.98, 0.95, and 0.92 respectively. While nutritionists are well aware that these factors may not be accurate for any one food, they do represent the best currently available factors to apply to the energy-yielding nutrients in the American diet to calculate the *physiologic fuel value* or the amount of potential energy available from a diet. It has been observed that other factors would be more appropriate for use in diets of other countries where the composition of the diet and its digestibility may be quite different.

Physiologic fuel value

The calculation of the physiologic fuel value of the three energy-yielding groups is summarized in Table 5-1.

The factors 4, 9, and 4, representing the amount of energy available to the body per gram of carbohydrate, fat, and protein in the diet, are widely used in nutrition and dietetics. Although they may be influenced by many factors and their use may lead to some inaccuracies, they represent a very useful tool in calculations involving energy values of diets.

Indirect calorimetry or oxycalorimetry

The energy value of a substance may also be obtained by indirect calorimetry in which the oxygen used in burning the samples and the carbon dioxide produced are measured. Results obtained in the *oxycalorimeter* correspond closely to those

Table 5-1. Calculation of physiologic fuel value of nutrients

	Kilocalories per gram		
	Carbohydrate	*Fat*	*Protein*
Heat of combustion	4.1	9.45	5.65
Energy from combustion of nitrogen unavailable to the body	—	—	1.3
Net heat of combustion	4.1	9.45	4.35
Coefficient of digestibility	0.98	0.95	0.92
Physiologic fuel value	4.0	9.0	4.0

Table 5-2. Calculation of energy value of a food from proximate analysis

Nutrient	Percent in food	Amount in 100 gm. (grams)	Energy value per gram (kilocalories)	Energy value of 100 gm. (kilocalories)
Carbohydrate	21.4	21.4	4	85.6
Fat	9.2	9.2	9	82.8
Protein	5.5	5.5	4	22.0
Total energy				190.4

from the bomb calorimeter, but this method is seldom used.

ENERGY VALUE OF FOODS
Direct calorimetry

A determination of the fuel value of a food may be obtained in two ways: by analysis or by calculation based on its carbohydrate, fat, and protein content. The bomb calorimeter is used in determining the calorie value of a food by direct calorimetry. A weighed sample of food or mixture of foods is dried to a constant weight, burned in the bomb calorimeter, and the amount of heat given off measured directly. The values obtained in this way represent the heat of combustion of the food and not its physiologic fuel value.

Proximate composition

For most foods we now have analytical data for their *proximate composition*—the percentage of carbohydrate, fat, protein, and water found in a typical sample of the food. If less precise data on the energy value of a food is needed this method is quicker and less costly than the use of the bomb calorimeter. For example, from tables of food composition we might learn that a particular food contains 9.2% fat, 21.4% utilizable carbohydrate, and 5.5% protein—the only energy-yielding nutrients in food. To calculate the energy value of 100 gm. of

the food, the procedure shown in Table 5-2 would be used.

From the information that the food sample provided 190.4 kilocalories per 100 gm. or 1.9 kilocalories per gram, one can readily calculate the energy value of a food sample of any size. Also knowing the total carbohydrate, fat, or protein content of the diet, one can readily determine the percentage of total calories contributed by any one food group. In fact, knowing the sample size and any three of the four variables, carbohydrate, fat, protein, and total energy, it is possible to calculate the unknown factor.

Variation in energy value

The energy value of a particular food is a function of its carbohydrate, fat, and protein composition. Foods with a high percentage of fat are concentrated sources of calories, as are foods with a low water content. Since small amounts of them are required to yield a certain number of calories they are often erroneously considered "fattening" foods. It is true that it is easier to eat excess calories from foods low in water or high in fat content, but the foods themselves are not to be condemned as fattening. It is only the total diet that can be described as fattening and only then when its energy value exceeds the need of the individual.

Table 5-3. Amount of food needed to provide 100 kilocalories, the size and calorie value of an average serving*

Food	Average serving	Kilocalories per serving	Amount to provide 100 kilocalories
Lettuce	¼ head	7	4½ heads
Cabbage	½ cup	12	4 cups
Asparagus	6 spears	20	30 spears
Carrots	1 medium	20	5 medium
Sugar	1 tablespoon	50	2 tablespoons
Bread	1 slice	60	1⅔ slices
Apple	1 medium	70	1½ apples
Egg	1 large	80	1¼ large
Banana	1 medium	85	1⅙ medium
Nonfat milk	1 cup	90	1 cup +
Potato	1 medium	90	1 large
Pear	1 medium	100	1
Dates	4	100	4
Whole milk	1 cup	165	⅝ cup
Butter	1 tablespoon	100	1 tablespoon
Mayonnaise	1 tablespoon	110	1 tablespoon
Salad oil	1 tablespoon	125	⅘ tablespoon

*From Home and Garden Bulletin No. 72, Washington, D.C., 1964, U. S. Department of Agriculture.

Table 5-3 presents the amounts of various foods required to provide 100 kilocalories and also the size and calorie value of an average serving. It is evident from the bulk of food required that if one wished to increase his calorie intake that foods from the bottom of the list be chosen. Conversely, if one wishes to restrict calorie intake, more satisfaction in terms of bulk in the stomach and the amount of chewing required will be obtained from using foods from the top of the list. It might be noted that items high in calories, such as sugar, flour, butter, and cheese, are often used to enhance the palatability of foods relatively low in calories. Examples of the effect of methods of food preparation on the calorie value of a food is shown in Table 5-4.

The relationship between the weight of a food and its calorie value is evident in Table 5-5. Foods low in water and high in fat have a high caloric value while those low in fat but high in water and cellulose are lower in calories.

BODY'S NEED FOR ENERGY

An individual's need for energy is a function of several factors, each of which can be estimated and which will be discussed separately—basal metabolism, sleep, nature and extent of activity, and the effect of food. All are a function either directly or indirectly of a person's size, a larger person always having higher requirements than a smaller person.

ENERGY EXPENDITURE
Basal metabolism

Basal metabolism, which represents the minimum amount of energy needed to

Table 5-4. Effect of method of preparation on energy value of an average serving of a single food

Food	Kilocalories
Apple	70
Applesauce	185
Baked apple	225
Apple Betty	350
Apple pie	330
Apple pie a la mode	440
Potato (1 medium)	
Boiled	90
Mashed with 1 teaspoon butter	120
Baked (served with 1 pat butter)	140
French fried	155
Creamed	200

Table 5-5. Calorie value of 100-gm. portions of food*

Food	Calorie value per 100 gm.
Lettuce (½ cup)	14
Asparagus (6 spears)	20
Cabbage (1 cup shredded)	24
Carrots (1½)	31
Nonfat milk or buttermilk (⅖ cup)	36
Milk (3.7% fat; ⅖ cup)	66
Peas (⅝ cup)	68
Potato (1 small)	76
Lamb (1 serving)	197
Chicken (1 serving)	208
Pork (1 serving)	236
Bread (4 slices)	250
Dates	274
Sugar (½ cup)	400
Mayonnaise (7 tablespoons)	718
Butter (7 tablespoons)	716
Salad oil (7 tablespoons)	884

*From Watts, B., and Merrill, A.: Composition of foods—raw, processed and prepared, U. S. Department of Agriculture Handbook No. 8, Washington, D.C., 1963, U. S. Department of Agriculture.

carry on the vital body processes, is an expression of the energy needs of the body during physical, emotional, and digestive rest. These vital processes, without which life is impossible, include respiration, circulation, glandular activity, cellular metabolism, and maintenance of muscle tonus and body temperature. It is well known that the rate of respiration will be increased during strenuous exercise or in the absence of sufficient oxygen as occurs at high altitudes. These changes are a response to a need for oxygen in the cells. On the other hand, a certain minimum respiratory rate is necessary to provide sufficient oxygen to maintain life at a minimum level of cellular respiration, a rate that differs from one individual to another. In measuring basal metabolic energy needs, we measure, among other things, the amount of energy needed to carry on this minimum rate of respiration. Similarly, a minimum rate of circulation must be maintained to carry oxygen and nutrients to the cells and waste products away from the cells. The energy required for this minimum rate of circulation compatible with life is included in a basal metabolism determination. As long as life continues certain glandular organs, such as the thyroid, the adrenals, the pancreas, and the liver, produce and secrete hormones that control the level and nature of cellular metabolic activity. The synthesis and secretion of these substances into the bloodstream requires energy. No matter how relaxed the person may be, there is still a state of muscular contraction or muscular elasticity. If there were not, the body would assume the form of a shapeless mass of protoplasm with no way of maintaining a normal relationship of the skeletal components of the body. The energy required to maintain this muscle tonus is also measured when basal metabolic needs are assessed. In addition, metabolic processes, such as the uptake of nutrients, the synthesis of new compounds, the excretion of waste, and the maintenance

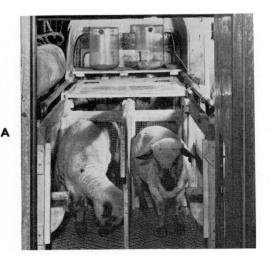

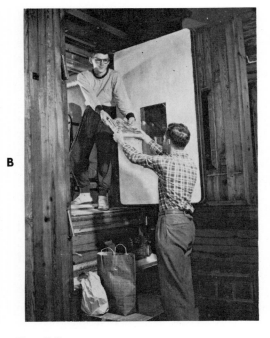

Fig. 5-2

A, Four sheep in the Armsby calorimeter participating in a metabolism experiment in animal nutrition for which the chamber was originally designed. **B,** Two men entering the same calorimeter
to participate in a 72-hour metabolism study, after
its conversion for use with human subjects in the
1950's. In both photos note the thickness of the
walls with intervening air spaces. (Photos by R.
Beese. Courtesy Dr. G. Barron, The Pennsylvania
State University.)

of internal environment of the cells, many
of which require energy, are constantly
going on within the cell as long as the cell
is living. The minimum amount of energy
to maintain this cellular activity is also
included in basal metabolism.

Measurement of basal metabolism

Basal metabolism can be measured in
two ways—by direct or indirect calorimetry.
A third test, a clinical test of the protein-
bound iodine (PBI) on a blood sample,
will give relative but not exact energy costs.

Direct calorimetry. Direct calorimetry
involves the measurement of the heat given
off by the body in a respiration chamber,
a small insulated room that operates on the
same principle as the bomb calorimeter.
By measuring the change of temperature
of a known volume of water circulating in
pipes in the top of the chamber, it is possible to determine the amount of heat
produced by a subject inside it. In addition,
a measurement is often made of the exchange of carbon dioxide and oxygen which
takes place. This allows the calculation of
a respiratory quotient, $\dfrac{CO_2 \text{ expired}}{O_2 \text{ consumed}}$, from
which one can determine whether carbo-
hydrate, fat, or protein was burned. This is
a useful piece of information in certain
clinical situations. If carbohydrate is the
sole source of fuel, the respiratory quotient
(RQ) is 1, indicating that one volume of
carbon dioxide is produced from every
volume of oxygen used in respiration. Fat
has a RQ of 0.7, protein approximately 0.8,
depending on the amino acid mixture, and
mixtures of carbohydrate, fat, and protein
have intermediate values. If the test is conducted under basal metabolic conditions,
the heat produced represents the minimum
energy need of the individual. Since the
cost of operating a respiration calorimeter
is very high and there are very few available, it is used only under carefully controlled experimental conditions. Fig. 5-2
shows subjects entering one of the few res-

piration calorimeters in the world. This one is located at the Pennsylvania State University.

A recent modification of the respiration chamber, the metabolic chamber, measures the heat given off by the subject by means of thermocouples and heat-exchange disks attached to the skin. Any changes in temperature are recorded on instruments outside the chamber. Both the chambers can be used for determinations of basal energy needs and also permit the assessment of energy costs of activities which can be performed in a limited space. Fig. 5-3 illustrates the use of one type of metabolic chamber.

Indirect calorimetry. A much simpler method involves indirect calorimetry, in which the oxygen consumption is measured to determine basal metabolism. For many years the Benedict Roth respiration apparatus was the standard machine used for this purpose. It is a closed circuit system in which the subject receives his oxygen only from a measured source of pure oxygen and exhales into a container in which the carbon dioxide and water are removed and the remaining oxygen recirculated. By measuring the difference in the oxygen level in the container before and after the standard six-minute test, one can calculate the amount of oxygen consumed. Since the use of a particular amount of oxygen represents a certain energy potential, it is possible to calculate the calorie equivalent of a known volume of oxygen. Recent studies have shown that open-circuit indirect calorimetry is equally valid. Instead of pure oxygen, it involves the use of room air and a determination of the amount of oxygen removed from it during a test period. In this, a measured amount of atmospheric air is breathed from a closed container and the exhalations are passed over soda lime, which removes the carbon dioxide. The amount of carbon dioxide removed from the exhaled air is readily measured by weighing the soda lime container before and after the test and

can be used along with oxygen figures as a basis for standardized calculations of the energy used during that period. The open-circuit method is less costly and reduces the possibility of stimulation in metabolism from the use of pure oxygen.

A determination of the energy required for basal metabolism must be made when the subject is using a minimum amount of energy for respiration, circulation, glandular activity, and maintenance of muscular tonus and virtually none for nonvital functions such as digestion, absorption, the increase in muscle tonus arising from fear or anger or other emotional states, from an uncomfortable physical environment, or from physical exertion. Some people describe the conditions under which basal metabolism is measured as those of complete physical, emotional, and digestive rest. To achieve this, the subject must be lying down, preferably immediately after a night's sleep, awake, in an environment of a comfortable temperature and humidity, in a postabsorptive state (at least twelve hours since the last meal), and at a normal body temperature. Since cellular respiration of skeletal muscle accounts for the greatest part of the oxygen consumption, it is especially important that the subject be muscularly relaxed. In some tests, drugs have been used to reduce mental and muscular tension to a minimum.

The third, a method of estimating basal metabolic needs, the protein-bound iodine (PBI) test on a blood sample, will be discussed in the chapter on iodine.

Estimation of basal energy needs

Series of basal metabolic tests have yielded sufficient data that it is now possible to estimate basal energy needs from the basic body measurements of height and weight. For persons of average body build an estimate based on body weight—1 kilocalorie per kilogram of body weight per hour—gives a value that corresponds well to those obtained on actual basal metabolic

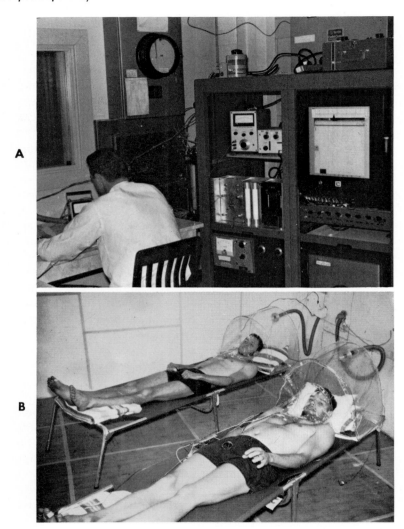

Fig. 5-3

A, Technician at control panel outside metabolic chamber at the Human Performance Laboratory at The Pennsylvania State University monitoring the oxygen consumption, carbon dioxide excretion, and the changes in surface temperature of subject in chamber behind glass. **B,** Subjects in metabolic chamber in which the effect of environmental temperature changes on oxygen consumption and skin temperature are being determined. (Photo courtesy Public Relations Department, The Pennsylvania State University.)

tests. But when this formula is applied to persons whose body build deviates from standards either in the direction of obesity or leanness it is less satisfactory, apparently because the simple measurement of body weight does not reflect body composi-

tion, which has a profound influence on basal metabolism. A better indication of basal metabolism can be obtained by calculating the metabolic or fat-free size of the body, sometimes called biological body weight. It is obtained by raising the body weight in kilograms to the 0.75 power, which gives a metabolic body size of 19 for a person weighing 50 kg., 22 for one of 60 kg., and 24 at 70 kg. Basal energy needs are then calculated as 70 (weight in kilograms$^{0.75}$). This amounts to about 1.3 kilocalories per kilogram of fat-free weight per hour. Estimates of basal metabolism obtained this way correspond very closely to those obtained on the basis of body surface area, which has long been considered the most satisfactory body measurement on which to base predictions of basal energy needs. Body surface area reflects the rate of heat transfer from the body and the rate of circulation of the blood and corresponds very closely to the level of active metabolic tissue. The use of body surface area as a standard is limited because of a lack of precise methods of estimating this measurement. It is, however, such a value based on body surface area that is the most widely used estimate of basal metabolism for people of all builds and that is still used as a standard against which to compare actual basal metabolic determinations. Metabolic body size is, however, being used with increasing frequency to predict both basal metabolism and total energy needs.

For most people, the actual basal metabolic needs fall within 10% (plus or minus) of the predicted values. When deviations occur, they are expressed as a percentage of predicted values, such as minus 12 or 12% below. Deviations may be attributed to one or more of the following factors.

Factors affecting basal energy needs

Body composition. While all body tissue is metabolically active, undergoing constant breakdown and repair, some tissues experience these changes much more rapidly than others. Muscle and glandular tissues are relatively very active, consuming relatively large amounts of oxygen per unit of weight in their normal functioning. On the other hand, bones and adipose tissue, although far from static, are relatively inactive tissues and require less oxygen to maintain normal metabolic activity. If we compare two men weighing 180 pounds, one 60 inches tall and the other 72 inches tall, we are comparing a short stocky person with less muscle and more fat to a tall thin person whose weight is composed of less fat and more muscle. The latter person would have a higher basal metabolic energy need since the muscle tissue requires more oxygen than the adipose tissue. The difference in body composition is reflected in body surface area measurements or in the measurement of metabolic body size—weight in kilograms$^{0.75}$.

Body condition. A person in good physical condition usually has developed more muscle tissue than one who has not experienced as much exercise. This time if we compare two men, both 180 pounds in weight and both 68 inches tall, one of whom is an accountant, an essentially sedentary occupation, and the other employed as a stockman, a job calling for physical activity, we would find that the weight of the sedentary individual represents less muscle and more fat than that of the physically active person. His basal metabolic needs would be lower.

Sex. Differences in body composition between a male and female of the same age, height, and weight have been documented. Women characteristically develop more adipose tissue and less musculature than men, which is reflected in a basal metabolic rate for women 5% lower than men.

Hormone secretions. The secretions of the ductless glands, the thyroid and the adrenal, have more influence of basal energy needs than any single factor. In fact, any marked deviation from predicted basal energy needs is usually attributed to an over- or undersecretion of the thyroid gland, although it is not the only possible cause. Hypothyroidism, with a below-normal secretion of thyroxine, the iodine-containing hormone of the thyroid gland, may be reflected in a basal metabolic rate depressed as much as 30%. This means that the energy required for vital body functions is 30% below that for a person with normal thyroid activity. This depressed secretion can be counteracted by the careful use of thyroid extract available only under medical supervision. Conversely, hyperthyroidism, an above-normal thyroxine secretion, may elevate basal metabolism as much as 50% to 75% or even 100%. Such a person would have an energy requirement for basal needs alone 50% to 75% above predicted levels. Hyperthyroidism is more difficult to correct. Drugs that interfere with the production of thyroxine or the uptake of iodine, an essential part of the thyroxine hormone, are sometimes used, but the results are very difficult to control. Partial thyroidectomy (removal of part of the thyroid gland) has been tried, as has a limitation in the iodine intake to reduce the amount of raw material available for thyroxine synthesis. Deviations in basal metabolism from predicted levels in excess of 20% are almost always indicative of disturbed thyroid function. A person with a very high basal metabolic rate due to excess thyroxine production is said to have *exophthalmic goiter* or *hyperthyroidism.*

The secretion of the adrenal gland, adrenalin, is produced in response to intense emotional stimuli such as anger or fear. The stimulation in metabolism resulting as more adrenalin is produced is intense but of short duration, often returning to normal levels in two or three hours.

Sleep. Measurements and estimates of basal metabolism are made, assuming the individual is awake but muscularly and emotionally relaxed. During basal metabolic tests involving the use of special breathing apparatus, it is essential that the subject be awake. During sleep, however, an individual achieves a greater degree of muscular and emotional relaxation which causes a further drop in energy needs to 10% below waking levels. This saving in

sleep amounts to 40 to 80 kilocalories per day, but is dependent upon the hours of sleep, the size of the individual, and the degree of relaxation achieved.

Some recent investigations have indicated that the energy savings due to relaxation in sleep may be counteracted by the energy expended in motion during sleep so that the values obtained from basal metabolism may well be applicable over a 24-hour period, eliminating any necessity to correct for a saving in sleep in estimating energy needs.

Age. The basal metabolic rate per unit of body surface changes with age. The rate is high at birth, increases up to two years of age, and then declines gradually except for a rise at puberty. In males it ranges from 53 kilocalories per square meter at 6 years to 41 at 20 years to 34 at 60 years of age. There is a similar gradual decline in basal energy needs for women except during pregnancy and lactation. The decline in energy needs between ages 25 and 35 amounts to only 35 kilocalories per day for a 60-kg. person, but between ages 25 and 55 it amounts to a more significant 145 kilocalories. A person who fails to adjust his calorie intake to this reduced need will experience a slow and insidious gain in weight.

The reduction in basal metabolism below values at age 25 suggested by the NRC is 2.5% in each decade between 20 and 40 years of age, 5% from 40 to 50 years of age, 7.5% from 50 to 60 years of age, 10% from 60 to 70 years of age, and 12.5% over 70 years of age. These are in close agreement with values of 3%, 5%, 7%, 7.5%, and 10% proposed by FAO.

Pregnancy. During the last few weeks of pregnancy there is an increase in basal metabolism amounting to 20% of normal values. This represents the high metabolic activity of the fetus and placenta. A decline in basal metabolic needs is observed early in pregnancy.

Previous nutritional status. Basal energy

studies in persons who have been subjected to prolonged calorie undernutrition usually yield values below predicted levels. This apparently reflects the body's efforts to conserve energy when calories are restricted. While the effect of starvation is not a significant factor among American people, it may explain the ability of persons in areas of chronic undernutrition to maintain their body weight on less than predicted caloric intakes.

Body temperature. Since heat acts as a catalyst to almost all chemical reactions, it is not surprising to find that basal metabolism increases with an increase in body temperature. An increase of 1° F. in body temperature leads to an average increase of 7% in basal metabolism although increases as high as 15% have been observed.

Environmental temperature. Lowest basal metabolism readings are obtained at an environmental temperature of 26° C. or 78° F., with higher readings being reported at both higher and lower environmental temperatures. A temporary decrease in environmental temperature, not compensated for by additional clothing, will cause shivering and a temporary increase in basal metabolic needs.

In summary, then, although many factors, such as body composition, hormone secretions, sleep, and previous nutritional status, may influence basal metabolism, for most persons an accurate estimate of needs can be made on the basis of body surface area or metabolic body size. For many people, especially those engaged in sedentary or moderately active activity, basal energy needs account for 50% to 70% of their total caloric requirements.

Activity. The energy required for physical activity above the needs for basal metabolism is usually considered to be a function of the type of activity and the size of the individual performing it. Since 75% of the energy expended in most activities is involved in moving the body it has become common practice to base estimates of energy needs for activity on body weight. As a result tables such as Table 5-6, giving the energy costs of various activities per unit of body weight, have traditionally been used in estimating energy costs. While some workers have recently published tables of energy costs of activity based on the type of activity irrespective of the size of the individual most workers continue to base requirements on body weights. These tables represent our best available estimates of energy costs, but before using them, one should be aware of the limitations in their usefulness.

First, people differ from one another in the efficiency with which they perform a particular activity either through training or innate ability so that the actual costs may vary considerably from estimates based on the tables. Calculations based on these tables should show that a 90-kg. person will use 50% more energy in performing the same task for the same length of time than a 60-kg. person, and his needs would be calculated to be the same as a 60-kg. person carrying a 30-kg. (66-pound) load on his back. In neither case would the differences be this great because of efficiencies affected by the distribution of the weight over the whole body.

Second, while many activities such as walking, swimming, or bicycling, which involve moving the body, do require an energy expenditure proportional to body size, others such as knitting, writing, and piano playing will likely not vary with body size, but rather will require about the same amount of energy for all persons.

Third, since many of the values were obtained on the basis of a very few determinations or were extrapolated from data on similar activities, they should not be considered as very precise values. For that reason the student is cautioned against attributing too much preciseness to calculations based on them. It should also be recognized that the energy expenditure attributable to the activity itself may repre-

Table 5-6. The energy cost of activities exclusive of basal metabolism and influence of food*

Activity	Calories per kilogram per hour	Activity	Calories per kilogram per hour
Bicycling (century run)	7.6	Piano playing (Liszt's	
Bicycling (moderate speed)	2.5	"Tarantella")	2.0
Bookbinding	0.8	Reading aloud	0.4
Boxing	11.4	Rowing in race	16.0
Carpentry (heavy)	2.3	Running	7.0
Cello playing	1.3	Sawing wood	5.7
Crocheting	0.4	Sewing, hand	0.4
Dancing, foxtrot	3.8	Sewing, foot-driven machine	0.6
Dancing, waltz	3.0	Sewing, motor-driven machine	0.4
Dishwashing	1.0	Shoemaking	1.0
Dressing and undressing	0.7	Singing in loud voice	0.8
Driving automobile	0.9	Sitting quietly	0.4
Eating	0.4	Skating	3.5
Fencing	7.3	Standing at attention	0.6
Horseback riding, walk	1.4	Standing relaxed	0.5
Horseback riding, trot	4.3	Stone masonry	4.7
Horseback riding, gallop	6.7	Sweeping with broom, bare floor	1.4
Ironing (5-pound iron)	1.0	Sweeping with carpet sweeper	1.6
Knitting sweater	0.7	Sweeping with vacuum sweeper	2.7
Laundry, light	1.3	Swimming (2 mph)	7.9
Lying still, awake	0.1	Tailoring	0.9
Organ playing (30% to 40% of		Typewriting rapidly	1.0
energy hand work)	1.5	Violin playing	0.6
Painting furniture	1.5	Walking (3 mph)	2.0
Paring potatoes	0.6	Walking rapidly (4 mph)	3.4
Playing Ping-Pong	4.4	Walking at high speed	
Piano playing (Mendelssohn's		(5.3 mph)	9.3
songs)	0.8	Walking downstairs	†
Piano playing (Beethoven's		Walking upstairs	‡
"Apassionata")	1.4	Washing floors	1.2
		Writing	0.4

*Courtesy Taylor, C. M., and McLeod, G.: Rose's laboratory handbook for dietetics, ed. 5, New York, 1949, The Macmillan Company, p. 18.
†Allow 0.012 calories per kilogram for an ordinary staircase with 15 steps without regard to time.
‡Allow 0.036 calories per kilogram for an ordinary staircase with 15 steps without regard to time.

sent a very small portion of the total energy used during the time since a much larger portion may be used for basal metabolism. Once the limitations are recognized, tables of energy costs are a very useful tool in nutrition studies.

Many people are disillusioned to find the relatively small amount of energy expended in performing various activities. For instance, the energy cost of walking three miles in one hour is only 2 kilocalories per kilogram of body weight above maintenance requirements. Thus, a 60-kg. (132-pound) person will expend only an additional 120 kilocalories or 96 kilocalories more than sitting in such an activity. Even one hour of skating will involve only 210 kilocalories for this same person, while bicycling requires 150 kilocalories over basal. The Canadian Dietary Standard suggests that light work such as cooking, typing, or golfing involves an average expenditure of 1.1 kilocalories per minute, while moderately heavy work such as gardening, carpentry, and swimming costs 2.6 kilocalories per minute. Heavy work such as farm chores, lumbering, or mountain climbing costs 2.8 kilocalories per minute and very strenuous work 5.1 kilocalories. These are proposed in addition to the needs for basal metabolism independent of body size.

Disillusioning as it may be, it has been established that mental effort calls for virtually no increase in energy requirements. The 3% to 4% increase sometimes recorded has been attributed to the increase in muscle tonus, the result of increased muscle tension, rather than to brain cell activity.

The decline in calorie requirements for activity that occurs with aging is proportionately greater than the decline in basal energy requirements. It decreases at 3%, 6%, 13.5%, 21%, and 31% of that at age 25 with each succeeding decade.

To estimate the caloric needs of an individual for activity, it is necessary to keep an accurate record of all activity for a specified period of not less than 24 hours. Activities are then grouped to determine the total time spent in a particular activity following the groupings given in Table 5-6. If a particular activity is not listed, a reasonable estimate can be made by classifying it with one involving a similar degree of muscular exertion. Using the energy cost factors from Table 5-6, calorie costs per kilogram for each activity can be calculated and totalled. The day's energy requirements for all activity are obtained by multiplying this total by the body weight in kilograms. The number of kilocalories needed to take care of a day's activity vary greatly from one individual to another, but for a sedentary or moderately active person usually represent from 33% to 50% of the basal energy needs. For active and very active persons, the needs for activity may equal or exceed basal energy needs.

FAO has used the formula 10.88 (weight in kilograms) + 236 to express the energy needs for activity. The Canadian Dietary Standard uses the values 23 kilocalories per unit of metabolic body size for a sedentary person, with an additional 23 kilocalories for light activity, 55 for moderate activity such as gardening or making furniture, 80 for heavy activity such as farm chores, lumbering, or active participation in competitive sports, and 107 for extremely heavy activity. These values are over and above the needs for basal metabolism.

Effect of food. It has been recognized for some time that the presence of food caused an increase in energy needs not only for the digestion, absorption, and transportation of the nutrients, but also as a result of a general stimulation in metabolism that follows the ingestion of food. This effect has been referred to as the *specific dynamic effect* of food. Experiments designed to determine the exact magnitude of this effect have produced no conclusive results. It is still generally believed that the effect of food amounts to about 10% of the total energy needed for basal metabolism and activity. In the case of a diet where protein provided almost all of the calories, this stimulation in metabolism could rise as high as 30%. Since the effect of food represents an increase in energy expenditure, it must be added to the basal needs and activity needs in calculating the total energy needs. If this factor were not considered, a diet providing only sufficient calories for basal and activity needs would lead to an inadequate calorie intake with subsequent weight loss.

Table 5-7. Factorial estimation of total energy needs

Subject: male   Weight: 60 kg.   Height: 70 inches   Age: 35

Basal metabolism: 1 kilocalorie per kilogram per hour

$$1 \text{ kilocalorie} \times 60 \times 24 = 1440 \text{ kilocalories}$$

OR

$$70 \, (\text{Wt.}_{kg.})^{0.75} = 70 \times 60^{0.75} = 70 \times 22 = 1540 \text{ kilocalories}$$

Activity needs

Activity	Time (hours)	Energy cost Kcal./kg./hr.	Energy cost Kcal./kg.
Dressing	1.5	0.7	1.05
Sitting	6.0	0.4	2.4
Skating	0.5	3.5	1.5
Walking (3 mph)	2.0	2.0	4.0
Standing relaxed	1.0	0.5	0.5
Typing	4.0	1.0	4.0
Sleeping	8.0	—	—
Playing piano	0.5	2.0	1.0
Walking upstairs	4 flights	0.036*	0.14
Walking downstairs	4 flights	0.012*	0.04
			13.88

Energy cost of activity = 13.88 kilocalories × 60   833

Total energy cost for basal metabolism and activity   2273 or 2373

Specific dynamic effect (10%)   227 or 237

Total energy requirement   2500 or 2610

*Allowance per kilogram for ordinary staircase (15 steps) regardless of time.

Estimation of total energy needs

The method used to estimate total calorie needs depends on the degree of accuracy desired. For the most precise determination, it is necessary to carry out an actual basal metabolism test and evaluate the energy cost of activity by having the subject breathe into a portable gas meter apparatus worn on his back for all activities. This expensive method is used mainly for research purposes.

Factorial method. More easily used and less expensive, but also less precise, is the *factorial method* of estimating calorie needs. It involves estimating basal metabolism from surface area measurements, or metabolic body size, activity needs from accurate activity records and an additional factor for the effect of food. The factorial method for estimating caloric needs is outlined in Table 5-7 using either body weight or metabolic body size for estimating basal needs.

Rule of thumb. For a very quick estimate of energy needs the United States Department of Agriculture suggests multiplying body weight in pounds by a factor determined by the type of physical activity in which the individual is engaged. These factors are 14 for sedentary, 18 for moderately active, and 22 for very active women. For men values of 16, 21, and 26 are used. The limitation in this method lies in the subjective judgment of the nature of a person's physical activity. The most common error is to confuse the terms *busy* and *active*. A typical college student may be very busy but very sedentary at the same time. A busy but sedentary person needs many fewer calories than a physically active individual.

Metabolic body size. The Canadian Dietary Standards propose an estimate of total energy needs based on metabolic body size. Their formula is 116 (weight in kilograms$^{0.75}$). The Food and Agricultural Organization of the United Nations (FAO) has also developed a formula from which they feel one can arrive at a figure representing the energy requirement. For men, they use 0.95 (815 + 36.6 [weight in kilograms]). The formula for women is 0.95 (580 + 31.1 [weight in kilograms]). Both these are very close to recommended levels of calorie intake in the United States.

NCR recommended allowances. The Food and Nutrition Board of the National Research Council have established the caloric allowances they believe provide sufficient energy to maintain body weight or rate of growth at levels most conducive to well-being for practically all healthy individuals. Recognizing the many factors that influence caloric requirements, they have expressed their recommendations for a reference man or woman and then indicated a basis for making adjustments.

As reference individuals they chose 25-year-old persons, representing ages 18 to 35 years, living in a temperate zone with a mean environmental temperature of 20° C. (68° F.), and who are engaged in occupations neither sedentary nor involving hard physical labor but requiring moderate physical activity. For the reference woman weighing 58 kg. (128 pounds) the allowance is set at 2100 kilocalories and for the 70-kg. (154-pound) man at 2900 kilocalories, but their values are planned primarily for assessing needs of groups rather than individuals.

Adjustment for age. Increasing age is accompanied by decreased caloric expenditures because of the progressive reduction in basal metabolic rate and usual decline in physical activity. Although there may be wide individual difference in the extent to which needs for activity are reduced with age, a decrease in total calorie needs of 5% per decade between ages 35 and 55, 8% per decade from ages 55 to 75, and 10% after age 75 is proposed as typical.

Adjustment for body size. A basic principle in physics states that the amount of work required to move a mass is proportional to the size of the mass. In assessing human energy requirements it is assumed that 75% of the energy expenditure is directly proportional to body size and 25% is independent of body weight. On this basis, formulas for caloric needs of 725 + 31 (weight in kilograms) for men and 525 + 27 (weight in kilograms) for women of 25 years of age have been developed to reflect the effect of body size on energy needs. The use of these formulas indicates a change of approximately 150 kilocalories for every 5-kg. (11-pound) deviation from the weight of the reference man or woman. The effects of body weight and age in caloric allowances are shown in Table 5-8.

Adjustment for climate. The mean environmental temperature, 20° C. (68° F.), is used in estimating calorie needs. It is applicable to persons living in most parts of the United States since modern technology in the form of air-conditioning and central heating has provided means of protecting persons against extremes of temperature. In colder temperatures an increase of 2% to 5% should be made to take care of the extra energy expended in carrying more clothing or the shivering that occurs if clothing is inadequate to protect the person. Persons who perform physical activity at temperatures over 30° C. (80° F.) have an increased caloric need of 0.5% for each degree increase in environmental temperature. For others, the tendency to re-

Table 5-8. Adjustment of caloric allowances for adult individuals of various body weights and ages (at a mean environmental temperature of 20° C. [68° F. assuming average physical activity])*

Desirable weight			Calorie allowance		
kilograms	*pounds*		*25 years*	*45 years*	*65 years*
		Men	(1)	(2)	(3)
50	110		2300	2050	1750
55	121		2450	2200	1850
60	132		2600	2350	1950
65	143		2750	2500	2100
70	154		2900	2600	2200
75	165		3050	2750	2300
80	176		3200	2900	2450
85	187		3350	3050	2550
		Women	(4)	(5)	(6)
40	88		1600	1450	1200
45	99		1750	1600	1300
50	110		1900	1700	1450
55	121		2000	1800	1550
58	128		2100	1900	1600
60	132		2150	1950	1650
65	143		2300	2050	1750
70	154		2400	2200	1850

Formulas

(1) $725 + 31W$ (2) $650 + 28W$ (3) $550 + 23.5W$
(4) $525 + 27W$ (5) $475 + 24.5W$ (6) $400 + 20.5W$
W = weight in kilograms

*From Food and Nutrition Board, National Research Council: Recommended dietary allowances, Publication No. 1146, Washington, D.C., 1963, National Research Council.

strict activity at higher temperatures counteracts the increase in needs resulting from the increase in body temperature and basal metabolic rate.

Adjustment for activity. The allowances have been established for a moderately active individual. As the degree of activity increases, the caloric cost of the activity rises proportionately but even with heavy labor caloric requirements seldom increase more than 25% above those for the reference man or woman.

Needs for pregnancy. Total energy needs during pregnancy represent normal needs plus those to meet increase in basal metabolism and the demands for the growth of the fetus, placenta, and mammary glands. During the last trimester when about two thirds of fetal growth occurs, the daily need increases by about 300 kilocalories, depending on the extent to which normal activity is decreased during pregnancy. It is estimated that 40,000 kilocalories are needed to take care of the increased energy needs for the full gestation period of 40 weeks. While the hazards of excessive weight gain during pregnancy, such as toxemia of pregnancy and complications during labor, have been known for some time, it is now recognized that the hazards of an inadequate weight increase may be equally as great, prematurity being most common. Caloric intake conducive to the optimal conditions during pregnancy should lead to a weight gain of 22 to 30 pounds. The need for other nutrients is proportionately higher, necessitating the need for great care in the selection of additional calories.

Needs for lactation. The increase in energy required for the secretion of milk amounts to 600 kilocalories for the milk and an additional 400 kilocalories to produce the milk during the first four months of lactation. The amount, of course, varies with the volume of milk secreted, approximately 120 kilocalories being needed for the secretion of 100 ml. of milk. The National Research Council recommends a caloric intake of 500 to 1000 calories above normal energy requirements.

Needs for infants and children. Growing children require a relatively high energy intake per unit of body weight to take care of the needs for maintenance, for activity, and the rapid increase that occurs in body tissue. The energy needed to meet the needs for growth fluctuates widely over even short periods of time. It must be recognized that there are wide individual differences at this age because of variations in activity patterns as well as rate of growth.

For infants the requirement at birth of 130 kilocalories per kilogram is decreased to 100 kilocalories per kilogram at the end of one year. Infants who cry a great deal have needs in excess of more tranquil infants.

CALORIC IMBALANCE

One of the major nutritional problems in the United States today is that of maintaining caloric balance. This is a problem at all stages of the life cycle but especially among adults, for whom patterns of eating and activity developed early in life are major factors in the cause and control of weight problems. As long as caloric intake is equal to caloric expenditure, there should be no change in body weight. As soon as caloric intake deviates from caloric expenditure, calories are either derived from body stores to meet a deficit or added to body stores in cases of a surplus. Persons whose intake constantly exceeds their expenditure are soon conscious of the storage of calories in the form of body fat, reflected as a gain in body weight. Persons whose intake is inadequate to meet their needs experience a weight loss as energy reserves are depleted to meet their needs. In either case, a state of malnutrition exists and the problems can be equally severe on either side of the balance. Those whose caloric intakes are inadequate are the forgotten group among our malnourished, partly because they fail to recognize their state as an undesirable deviation from a normal state and partly because social pressures on this group are not sufficient to motivate them to make an adjustment. On the other hand, those who accumulate excess poundage are confronted with a barrage of panaceas, miraculous and otherwise, to help them make the necessary weight loss painlessly. This group is in jeopardy not only because of the hazards of being overweight, but also because of the potentially dangerous weight-reducing aids to which they may unwittingly subject themselves.

To simplify an extremely complex situation, for every 3500-kilocalorie deficit in the diet, one pound of body fat will be oxidized or lost, and for approximately 3500 kilocalories in excess of needs, the weight will increase one pound, representing storage of one pound of fat or adipose tissue, which is approximately 65% fat and 35% water. It does not matter whether the imbalance is one of 700 kilocalories for each of 5 days or 10 calories for 350 days; the end result is the same.

The ease with which some people maintain caloric equilibrium is evidenced by the number of persons who maintain the same weight year after year. The fact that about 25% of the population are considered over-weight, in most cases because of an excess accumulation of fatty tissue, indicates that a large number of people fail to make the necessary adjustment.

The storage of calories will result from an excessive caloric intake or a depressed need for calories, either of which leads to a caloric imbalance. The causes, which may be many, are discussed in Chapter 20. It may be hereditary where the sensitivity of the hypothalamus, the area of the brain that regulates appetite, is reduced to the point where overeating will occur before the message to stop eating is relayed through the hypothalamus in the brain. Psychological factors may lead to overeating; the pleasure derived from eating compensates for unpleasant aspects of a personal adjustment. A reduction in physical activity which accompanies increasing age or the conveniences which are a product of the push-button age when eating practices remain the same as in an era of greater physical effort creates an imbalance. Environmental factors, such as the availability of food, the economic ability of many to buy all the food desired, the pressures of the host who sees food as an expression of hospitality, or the laden tables traditional in many cultures, create situations which tax an individual's ability to regulate intake. Physiologic factors such as a depressed basal metabolic rate resulting from decreased secretion of thyroxine may also be a contributing cause.

That individuals differ in the efficiency with which they utilize food has been suggested for some time. Recent evidence indicates that the frequency of feedings is an influencing factor. The larger the number of meals into which a day's food intake is divided, the less likely the person is to store fat. Efforts to show that the primary source of calories—carbohydrate, fat, or protein—influences the utilization of calories have indicated that there is no difference.

Regardless of the cause of a person's failure to maintain his desired body weight—physiologic, psychological, hereditary, or environmental—successful treatment involves decreasing the caloric intake to a level below caloric expenditure. Many dietary aids that may act as appetite depressants, stimulate metabolism, increase water loss through excessive perspiration or increased urinary output, and depress utilization by speeding passage of food through intestinal tract are constantly presented to the public. Some have value to some people; many are harmless but useless; and the Food and Drug Administration is constantly on guard to protect the public against harmful aids.

Equally as often, the public is given a diet designed to solve all their weight problems. The rate at which these diets appear and the diversity of ideas presented make it impossible to evaluate them individually. A few criteria may provide a basis for judging each new diet as it appears.

1. The diet must be deficient in calories. This can be determined only by comparing the caloric value of the diet with a reasonable estimate of the individual's needs. A diet that shows a deficit for one person does not necessarily do so for others. A daily deficiency of 500 kilocalories will lead to a deficit of 3500 in one week, which should result in the loss of one pound of body weight. The tendency of the body to replace this fat with water temporarily often masks the loss of fat and is a source of discouragement to the reducer. If the regime is continued sufficiently long the total predicted loss eventually occurs.

2. The diet should be adequate in all other nutrients except calories. While this criterion is difficult to check precisely, a fairly good indication may be gained by checking the diet to see that it includes servings from each of the four major food groups, each of which must be present if a diet to

approach adequacy in most nutrients. There should be at least two servings each from milk and dairy products; fruits and vegetables; cereal products; and meat, fish, poultry, or eggs. At a level of 1400 kilocalories, it is possible with a careful choice of foods to achieve a diet that meets the National Research Council recommended allowances for all nutrients. As the calories drop, it is increasingly difficult to choose an adequate diet and if energy intake is restricted to less than 1000 kilocalories, the diet should be supplemented with a protective level of the minerals and vitamins likely to be lacking in the diet.

3. The diet should have satiety value. Diets containing moderate amounts of fat and high levels of protein delay the onset of hunger pangs for a longer time than isocaloric diets composed primarily of carbohydrate. It is easier to adhere to a diet of high satiety value than one that leaves the stomach rapidly.

4. A diet should be one that can be adopted readily from family meals and which can be obtained in public eating places. Any diet that sets the dieter apart from others with whom he eats or imposes extra preparation on the person preparing meals is less likely to be followed than one which allows a person to eat inconspicuously with the family or friends in all social situations.

5. The diet should be reasonable in cost. If it makes use of seasonal foods and staple dietary items, it will be more acceptable than one that calls for expensive, out-of-season, unfamiliar foods.

6. It should be one that can be adhered to for a sufficient period of time to achieve the desired weight loss. It is recommended that except in extreme obesity that the rate of weight loss not exceed one to one and a half pounds per week. Thus, a person wishing to lose 20 pounds should try to accomplish this over a period of at least fifteen weeks. Crash diets, which limit the dieter to a restricted list of foods, such as cottage cheese and peaches or steak, eggs, and tomatoes, are not only nutritionally inadequate, but are so monotonous that the psychological appeal that they have lasts only a short time and it is almost impossible for a person to remain on such a limited selection of foods to achieve the desired weight loss.

7. Most important of all if the dieter is to achieve long-term success, the diet should represent a sufficient departure from his former pattern of eating that he will be retrained in a new set of eating habits to which he can expect to adhere, with slight modifications, as a maintenance diet for a lifetime. The failure of the once-popular liquid formula diets to achieve any permanent weight loss can be attributed partly to their failure to substitute a new socially acceptable pattern of eating for the old one that led to the weight gain.

SELECTED REFERENCES

Buskirk, E. R.: Problems related to the caloric cost of living, Bull. New York Acad. Med. **36**:63, 1960.

Food and Agricultural Organization: Calorie requirements, FAO Nutr. Stud. **15**, 1957.

Kleiber, M.: The fire of life, an introduction to animal energetics, New York, 1961, John Wiley and Sons, Inc.

National Academy of Science: Recommended dietary allowances, Publication No. 1146, Washington, D. C., 1964, National Research Council.

Symposium on energy balance, Am. J. Clin. Nutrition **8**:527-774, 1960.

6

Mineral elements

It had been demonstrated in the middle of the nineteenth century that a mixture of the known constituents of food—the proximate principles, carbohydrate, fat, protein, and water—was not capable of supporting growth. Scientists then looked to the noncombustible fraction of food or the mineral ash for a clue to the growth-promoting properties of natural food absent in the synthetic mixtures they had fed to animals unsuccessfully. Although mineral residue when added to a synthetic diet did not stimulate growth or prevent death in animals and hence did not stimulate much interest in the 1880's, it has since been shown to be composed of many mineral elements that play many vital roles in human nutrition.

Distribution in the body

The elements carbon, hydrogen, and oxygen, the components of carbohydrate, fat, and protein (all of which can be oxidized to carbon dioxide and water), the nitrogen of protein, and water comprise 96% of the body weight. The remaining 4%, about six pounds in the adult male, is made up of many mineral elements. Approximately fifteen of these different mineral elements have been proved essential in human nutrition but an analysis of mineral ash may reveal an additional twenty or thirty present because of contamination from the environment—the soil, air, or water.

Essential elements

It is very possible that some elements now believed to be contaminants will be established as dietary essentials as techniques for studying their metabolism are further developed. For instance, there is now some evidence to suggest that chromium may be closely bound to the DNA molecule responsible for the genetic code in the nucleus of the cell. Minerals occur in the body in combination with organic compounds as does the iron in hemoglobin, with other inorganic ions as does the calcium phosphate of bone, or as free ionized ions such as the calcium in the intercellular fluids.

Progressive refinement in the techniques used to study mineral metabolism—spectroscopy, colorimetry, the use of radioactive isotopes, and flame photometry—has made possible studies of progressively smaller concentrations of minerals in biological tissue and has helped elucidate roles for mineral elements that have established their essential nature. A mineral is considered essential if there is a demonstrable improvement in the health and growth of the animal upon addition of the mineral to a purified diet, if the removal of the element from a diet containing adequate but not toxic amounts of all other dietary essentials results in clear-cut evidence of defi-

ciency symptoms, and if a low intake can be correlated with subnormal levels of the element in blood or other tissues. Even when it is determined that an element is a part of an essential enzyme system it must still be established that the reaction cannot be catalyzed by some other means.

Classification

The essential mineral elements are often grouped as macronutrient elements, those present in relatively high amounts in animal tissue, and micronutrient elements or trace elements present as less than 0.005%

Table 6-1. Classification of mineral elements

Classification	*Elements*	*Percent of body weight*
Macronutrient elements essential for human nutrition (> 0.005% body weight or 50 ppm)	Calcium	1.5 to 2.2
	Phosphorus	0.8 to 1.2
	Potassium	0.35
	Sulphur	0.25
	Sodium	0.15
	Chlorine	0.15
	Magnesium	0.05
Micronutrient elements essential for human nutrition (< 0.005% body weight)	Iron	0.004
	Zinc	0.002
	Selenium	0.0003
	Manganese	0.0002
	Copper	0.00015
	Iodine	0.00004
	Molybdenum	
	Cobalt	
Elements for which essentiality has not yet been established although there is evidence of their participation in certain biological reactions	Vanadium	
	Barium	
	Fluorine	
	Bromine	
	Strontium	
Elements found in the body but for which no metabolic role has been elucidated	Gold	
	Silver	
	Aluminum	
	Tin	
	Bismuth	
	Gallium	

(50 parts per million) of the body weight. Although there is not complete agreement about this categorization, it is presented in Table 6-1 as a basis for our discussion. It is entirely possible that with the increasingly sensitive analytical techniques available that biological roles will be discovered for at least some of the elements in the last group.

While most of these are also essential for plant growth some, such as cobalt, sodium, and iodine, are not essential but do occur in foods of plant origin, which then become a major source of these elements in the human diet. The amount of a mineral element in an animal tissue reflects the amount present in the plants it eats, and this in turn is a function of the amount of the element present in the soil and the ability of the plant to concentrate it. The presence of some of these elements in animal tissue may represent contamination from the environment.

The complex interrelationships that exist among the mineral elements as they function in the body suggest a discussion of the general functions of minerals. Some elements have been studied extensively and will be discussed individually. The ones on which the most information has been acquired are those most likely to be lacking in the diet and for which specific deficiency conditions have been recognized. This does not minimize the role of the other mineral elements, which are equally as important in maintaining normal body function.

General functions of mineral elements

Maintenance of acid-base balance. The cells of the body, in which a tremendous number of biological reactions take place, can function only in a very specific external and internal environment. Just as the enzymes of the digestive juices require a specific acidity or alkalinity, the enzymes that work within the body cells can perform their task only when the fluid in the cells is essentially neutral in reaction. Anything that changes the reaction of pH of the cell environment will influence the reaction of the cell contents and may inactivate or change the level of activity of the cellular enzymes once the capacity of the cell membrane to regulate the uptake of nutrients has been overtaxed. Inactivation of the enzymes results in cellular starvation and death of the cell. Among the many factors that influence the reaction of the cell is the nature of the minerals in the extracellular fluids.

Some minerals are considered acid-forming since they have the potential of creating an acid medium. These elements are chlorine, sulphur, and phosphorus. The acid-forming properties are determined by the components of the noncombustible mineral ash of the food and not by the presence of organic acids in food, which may give them an acid taste but which are generally oxidized in the body to carbon dioxide, water, and energy and hence do not influence acid-base balance. The acid-forming elements predominate in foods containing protein, such as meat, fish, poultry, eggs, and cereal products, which in turn are designated as acid-forming foods.

Mineral elements that are basic or alkaline in reaction are calcium, sodium, potassium, iron, and magnesium. These elements tend to predominate in fruits and vegetables. Thus even citrus fruits such as grapefruit, lemons, and oranges that have an acid taste because of the presence of organic acids, are base-forming since their organic acids are metabolized in the body and the mineral residue predominates in potentially basic or alkaline elements. A few foods, such as cranberries, rhubarb, cocoa, and tea, are acid-forming because they contain acids the body cannot metabolize—benzoic, oxalic, and tannic acid. The acid potential of these overbalances the base-forming mineral elements and makes them acid-forming foods.

Milk, which contains an internal balance

of base-forming calcium and acid-forming phosphorus, and pure carbohydrates and fats that contain virtually no minerals do not influence the acid-base balance of the body.

Most mixed diets contain a slight surplus of acid-forming mineral elements, but the body has mechanisms by which it can counteract this potential acidity. The excretion of carbon dioxide through the lungs and of a slightly acid urine through the kidneys helps rid the body of excess acid and help maintain the neutrality of the internal environment of the body. However, strict vegetarians who consume a diet with a predominantly basic residue, persons on a very high-protein diet with a predominantly acid residue in the mineral ash, and those who make frequent use of sodium-containing antacids, especially when combined with a high milk intake to create an alkaline balance, may tax the body's ability to maintain neutrality. The maintenance of body neutrality is so important to the survival of body cells that there are several ways in which an excess acid or excess base can be neutralized. The blood contains buffers, such as carbonates, phosphates, and proteins, that can react with either excess acid or excess base to prevent them from influencing the reaction of the blood and hence that of the fluids bathing the tissues. Bone can also release phosphates to act as buffers and remove hydrogen ions from surrounding fluids. If the buffers cannot take care of the excess acid or base, the body can form a reserve acid (carbonic acid) from the carbon dioxide and water of metabolism, which are normally excreted, to neutralize excess alkali-forming elements and prevent alkalosis. Excess acid may be neutralized by a reserve base formed from the NH_2 from the deamination of protein and water to prevent acidosis.

Catalysts for biological reactions. Mineral elements are catalysts for many biological reactions. As such they are not part of the initial compounds or the end products but are essential for the reaction to take place. Minerals that catalyze the action of many of the body's enzymes are sometimes thought of as the vital link between an enzyme and its substrate. They catalyze many of the separate steps involved in the catabolism of carbohydrates, fat, and protein to carbon dioxide, water, and energy and in the anabolism or synthesis of fat and protein in the body. The synthesis of essential body compounds such as hemoglobin depends on the presence of several mineral elements other than those that may become a part of the substance. The clotting of blood depends on the catalytic effect of calcium.

Fig. 6-1, which is by no means a complete tabulation, indicates the role of minerals in the metabolism of carbohydrate, fat, and protein in the body. It is obvious that many reactions are mineral-dependent and that some of the elements listed are involved at several different stages.

The transport of substances across biological membranes, as in absorption of nutrients from the gastrointestinal tract or uptake of nutrients by the cell, is often a mineral-dependent reaction. For instance, calcium facilitates the absorption of cobalamin or vitamin B_{12}, and magnesium and sodium facilitate the absorption of carbohydrate. Several digestive enzymes are activated by minerals, such as the activation of pancreatic lipase by calcium and magnesium.

Components of essential body compounds. Many of the hormones, enzymes, and other vital body compounds that are synthesized in the body and regulate body functioning contain minerals as integral parts of their structure. In the absence of the required mineral, the body will be unable to produce adequate amounts of the essential substance.

The production of thyroxine, which regulates energy metabolism, depends on an adequate supply of iodine to the thyroid

CATABOLISM

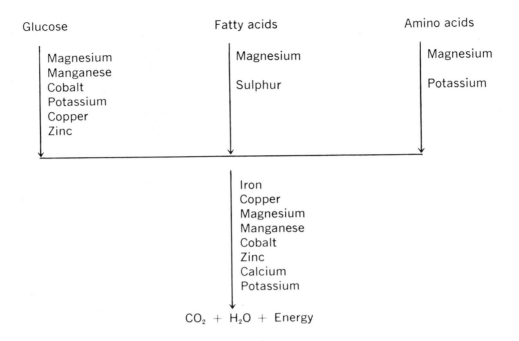

ANABOLISM

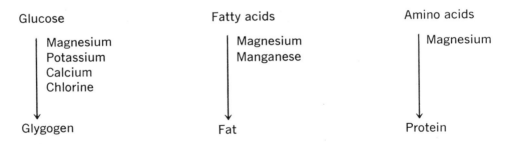

Fig. 6-1

Role of minerals as catalysts to biological reactions.

gland. The production and storage of insulin, which regulates carbohydrate metabolism, usually involves zinc. Hemoglobin, essential for the transport of oxygen to and carbon dioxide from the cells, is an iron-containing compound. Chlorine must be available for the production of hydrochloric acid for secretion into the stomach to create the acid environment necessary for the action of digestive enzymes in the stomach.

Minerals are an integral part of many enzymes in the body. These mineral-containing enzymes are sometimes designated

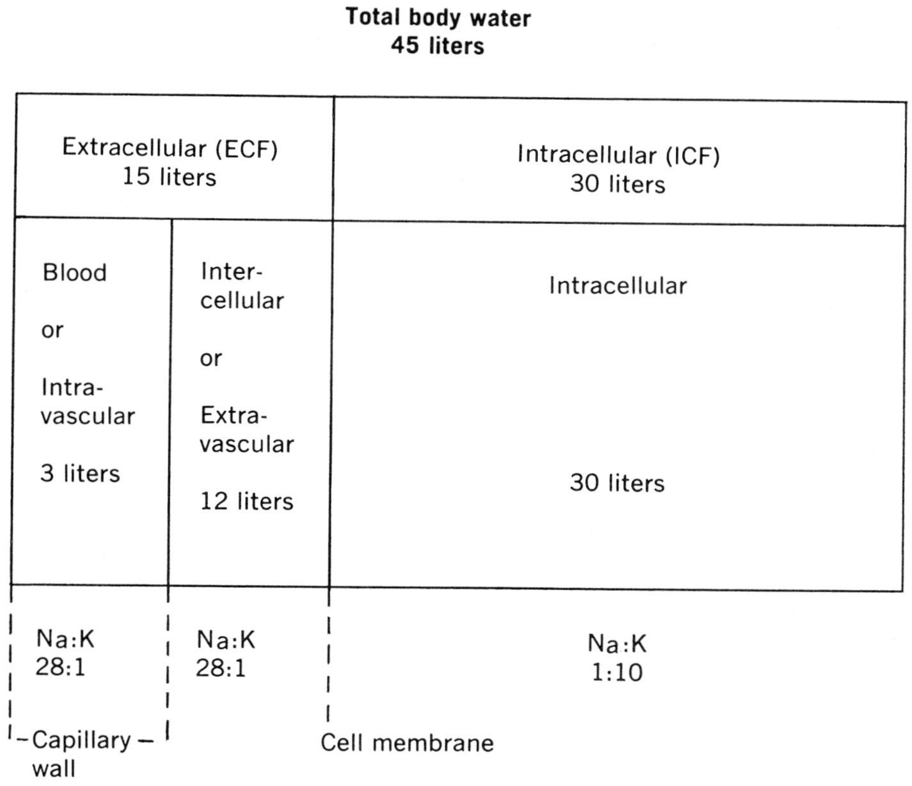

**Total body water
45 liters**

Extracellular (ECF) 15 liters		Intracellular (ICF) 30 liters
Blood or Intra- vascular 3 liters	Inter- cellular or Extra- vascular 12 liters	Intracellular 30 liters
Na:K 28:1	Na:K 28:1	Na:K 1:10

– Capillary –
wall
                Cell membrane

Fig. 6-2

Diagrammatic representation of three major fluid compartments of the body. A fourth division, the transcellular fluid compartment, is a subdivision of the extracellular fluid and includes water in collagen, connective tissue, bone, synovial fluid, and digestive secretions.

as "metaloenzymes" since if the metal is removed the enzyme loses its effectiveness. To cite but a few examples: both copper and iron are part of the enzyme cytochrome oxidase involved in release of energy; molybdenum is part of xanthine oxidase needed to release liver stores of iron for use by other tissues; and zinc is part of a protein-splitting enzyme, carboxypeptidase, secreted in the intestinal juice.

In addition to the carbon, hydrogen, oxygen, and nitrogen that are part of the vitamins most essential for body functioning, some, such as thiamine with sulphur and cobalamin with cobalt, have minerals as integral parts of their structure.

Maintenance of water balance. Water,

which comprises approximately 72% of the fat-free weight of the body and 60% of the total body weight, may be considered to be present in three "compartments" in the body, each of which is separated from the other by a semipermeable membrane. The compartmentalization is shown diagramatically in Fig. 6-2. The intravascular compartment includes the fluid in all parts of the vascular system—arteries, veins, and capillaries. The walls of the vascular system separate the intravascular fluid from the intercellular or extravascular fluid that bathes the individual cells and tissues and which provides the external environment from which the cells are nourished. The fluid or nutrients in the intercellular compartment must cross the cell membrane to enter the cell and become a source of nourishment for the cell in the intracellular fluid. The intercellular compartment acts as a buffer area; its volume will change to prevent changes in the volume of intravascular and intracellular fluid. The term transcellular fluid has been applied to a fourth compartment—fluids such as the synovial fluid lubricating joints and the vitreous humor of the eyeball—but these represent a very small portion of total body water and are not usually responsive to shifts in electrolyte or mineral balances.

The movement of fluid from one compartment to another is governed to a large extent by the concentration of minerals on either side of the membrane separating the compartments. When the same number of molecules and ions per exact volume of fluid is present on either side of the membrane, the osmotic pressures are the same and the total amount of fluid on either side remains relatively constant. Much of the osmotic pressure in the fluid compartments of the body is determined by the concentration of minerals in the fluid. If for any reason the mineral concentration in any one compartment becomes greater than that on the other side, fluid will cross the semipermeable membrane in such a direction as to establish osmotic equilibrium since many of the other ions cross the membrane only with difficulty.

Under most circumstances the body is able to cope with shifts in electrolyte concentrations so that there is no marked change in water balance. However, in some cases the homeostatic mechanisms of the body are taxed, resulting in a noticeable shift of fluids. For instance, when the sodium intake exceeds the ability of the kidney to excrete it, the level of sodium in the blood and in the interstitial fluid increases. Since the cells cannot function in such a hypertonic environment a series of changes occur to restore normal electrolyte levels. The thirst center is stimulated to increase the water intake, and fluid is withdrawn from the cells to dilute the intercellular fluid. This causes an increase in the volume of blood and interstitial fluid. The former results in an elevated blood pressure and the latter in the accumulation of fluid in the intercellular spaces to produce a soft, spongy, edematous tissue. Conversely, if sodium levels fall there is a contraction of blood volume, a drop in blood pressure, a decrease in intercellular fluid, and fluid is restored to the cells.

When sodium is lost from the extracellular compartment, as it may following excessive perspiration, potassium is pumped out of the cells to replace the lost sodium, and at the same time some water leaves the cell. Loss of water and potassium from the cell produces symptoms of weakness in the subject so common in heat prostration.

The mineral elements within each compartment vary, sodium being present in higher concentrations outside the cell, and potassium within the cell. Chlorine, which crosses the cell membrane easily, quickly establishes an equilibrium between the cell contents and the extracellular fluid and so plays a minor role in the exchange of body fluids.

Transmission of nerve impulses. Minerals play a vital role in the mechanism by which nerve impulses are conducted through nerve fibers. A nerve impulse is essentially an electrical stimulus that passes through a nerve fiber. During excitation or stimulation of nerve fibers the permeability of the membrane of nerve cells changes, allowing sodium to enter the cell more freely and potassium to leave. This creates a temporary change in the electrical charge on the membrane. This in turn changes the permeability of the next segment of the membrane, which changes the electrical charge again, and the message is passed down the membrane. It is, then, the exchange of sodium and potassium ions across the cell membrane that is responsible for the transmission of a nerve impulse.

Anything that changes the mineral concentration of the fluids bathing nerve cells may interfere with their ability to transmit nerve impulses. The effect a disruption in nerve stimulation can have on muscular contraction is evident from the uncontrolled contraction and relaxation of muscles that occurs in tetany where the calcium content of the extracellular fluids drops relative to magnesium, sodium, and potassium levels.

The transmission of a nerve impulse from one nerve cell to another is dependent on the presence of acetylcholine at the junction of the two fibers. The release of this compound is regulated by calcium.

Regulation of contractility of muscles. The muscles of the body are constantly bathed in a fluid—the interstitial fluid. For normal functioning of these muscles in contraction and relaxation, the composition of the interstitial fluid must represent a certain balance between elements that tend to stimulate muscular contraction, such as calcium, and those that exert a relaxing effect, such as sodium, potassium, and magnesium. This balance is steadfastly maintained under normal conditions. An upset in this balance is usually caused by the effect of the parathyroid hormone on the calcium levels. A drop in calcium levels without a concurrent decrease in the levels of the relaxing elements leads to a state of spasmodic contractions known as tetany. Conversely, an increase in calcium levels relative to the relaxing elements produces a state of tonic contractions known as calcium rigor. This effect of high calcium in fluids surrounding heart muscle in prolonging contraction and inhibiting relaxation of heart muscle is the basis of one test for ionized calcium.

During muscular contraction there is a release of potassium from the muscle cell, which is subsequently restored during the resting period. This seems to indicate an essential role for potassium in muscular contraction.

Growth of body tissue. Some mineral elements, such as calcium and phosphorous, occur in large concentration in bones and teeth and can rightly be considered as building constituents of body tissue. An absence of these raw materials will be reflected as stunted growth or in the development of tissue of inferior quality. Indirectly, many minerals are involved in the growth process through their catalytic action on many reactions involved in the synthesis of body compounds or in the release of energy.

In the following chapters the macronutrients will be discussed first, followed by a general discussion of all micronutrients and then a more detailed presentation of the information available on the most extensively studied microelements.

SELECTED REFERENCES

Council on Foods and Nutrition: Some inorganic elements in human nutrition, Symposium, Chicago, 1955, American Medical Association.

Hoekstra, W. G.: Recent observations on mineral interrelationships, part I, Fed. Proc. **23:**1068, 1964.

7

Macronutrient elements

CALCIUM

Calcium is the inorganic mineral element usually associated with bone and tooth formation. The use of the term calcification to describe the process by which these structures assume strength and rigidity has tended to reinforce ideas of the importance of calcium in bone formation. Whereas calcium does play an important role in this process, it is only one of many nutrients necessary for effective bone and tooth formation. In addition, the role of calcium in bone and tooth formation is only one of several very vital biological functions it performs. Although many writers have chosen to discuss calcium and phosphorus together because of their intimate relationship in bone and tooth development, we will emphasize their unique and independent roles by discussing each separately.

Distribution in body

The adult body contains between 1.5% and 2% of its weight as calcium. Of this 850 to 1400 gm. in the adult body 99% is present in hard tissues, bones, and teeth. The remaining 10 gm., about one third of which is closely bound to protein, is broadly distributed in the extracellular fluids bathing the cells and in the intracellular material of soft tissue, where it is vital to normal cell functioning. Much of the calcium in soft tissue is concentrated in muscle, although the membrane and cytoplasm of every cell contain calcium. The roles of calcium in these fluids are so important that calcium will be mobilized from bones to maintain a functional level. For this reason, calcium deficiency symptoms are virtually unknown, although it has been established that extensive decalcification of bones can occur on low calcium intake.

In spite of the fact that specific deficiency symptoms can rarely be attributed to a lack of dietary calcium, we do have concrete evidence of several specific roles of the mineral in body metabolism. The great reserve of calcium in the skeleton, which can be released to meet the needs of extracellular and soft tissues, and the mechanisms by which the body adapts to low dietary intakes by absorbing more and excreting less calcium have minimized the effects of intakes below the recommended allowances. So far, attempts to find a method of evaluating the extent of calcification of bone sensitive enough to reflect dietary intake have been unsuccessful. Only when the mobile reserves of calcium in the bone have been depleted will changes resulting from a lack of calcium be apparent in other tissues. Because of calcium's limited distribution in foods, intakes below recommended levels are frequently recorded but cannot be assessed on the basis of tissue changes.

Functions

Bone formation. Early in fetal development a strong but flexible protein (collagen) matrix or pattern for bone is formed. It bears the same general shape as the mature bone and is capable of growth but lacks strength and rigidity. The matrix remains rather flexible until after birth, possibly to facilitate the birth process and reduce damage to both the fetus and mother. Shortly after birth this matrix becomes strong and rigid, primarily as the result of the deposition and growth of calcium phosphate and calcium carbonate crystals in the protein matrix in a process known as *ossification.* Since calcium and phosphorus are the predominate mineral elements in these crystals of the physiologically stable compound, hydroxyapatite, an adequate supply of both minerals must be present before they can precipitate from the fluids surrounding the bone matrix to grow in the bone tissue.

Calcification apparently occurs when the product of the level of calcium and phosphorus in the blood and extracellular fluids exceeds 36, i.e., milligrams of phosphorus × milligrams of calcium per 100 ml. of blood > 36. The availability of phosphorus is increased by the action of the enzyme phosphatase, which can split off phosphorus from some of the many organic compounds in which it occurs and free it to participate in calcification of bones. As bone matures water is lost, and the bone becomes more dense. An increase in blood phosphatase levels corresponds with the period of bone growth. This process of bone growth is also catalyzed in an unexplained way by vitamin D.

The shaft of the bone becomes quite rigid and strong, capable of supporting the weight of the body before the infant begins to walk, sometimes as early as eight months of age. Throughout the entire growth process there is a constant lengthening of this bone shaft as the formation of new collagen matrix is followed by its calcification. The ends of the long bones retain a porous lacelike structure known as the *trabeculae.* The trabeculae contain a high proportion of red marrow and a liberal supply of calcium, which can be readily mobilized to maintain the critical blood calcium levels when dietary levels drop. Only when calcium reserves of the trabeculae have been depleted will decalcification of other parts of the bones occur. Under these conditions the pelvis and the spine are the first to release calcium.

During growth and throughout adult life there is a constant remodeling and reshaping of the bone in response to changing stresses from the weight of the developing body. It is estimated that about 20% of bone calcium is resorbed and replaced each year; thus every five years the calcium in the bone has been completely replaced. The knowledge of this dynamic or changing state of bone metabolism was possible only with the use of radioactive isotopes of calcium that could be traced in their path through the body. From these studies we have learned that even in adults approximately 600 to 700 mg. of calcium are deposited each day in newly formed bone, replacing that which has been resorbed. About one third of the calcium in the adult bone appears to be in equilibrium with that in the extracellular fluids; the rest is in a more stable complex.

The amount of calcium needed to meet

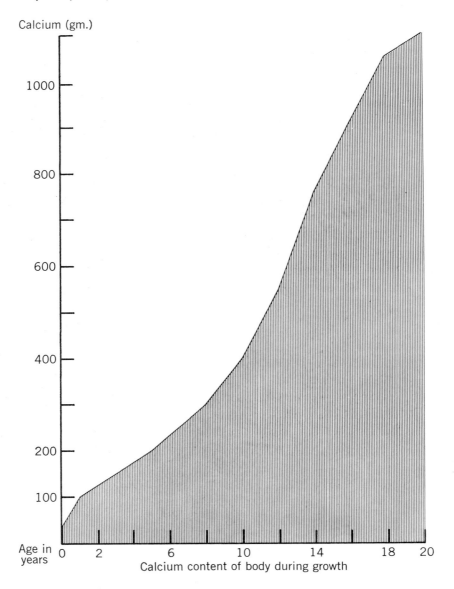

Fig. 7-1

Rate of accumulation of calcium in the body during growth.

demands for bone growth varies with the rate of skeletal development. The increase in calcium content of the body from 0.8% of body weight at birth (about 28 gm.) to 1.7% at maturity (about 1200 gm.) represents an average daily increment of 165 mg. with a reported range of 70 to 400 mg., depending on the stage of bone growth. Maximum needs occur between 13 and 14 years of age when the body requires about 90 gm. of calcium per year, representing an increase of about 300 to 400 mg. per day in body calcium. The rate at which body calcium accumulates with age is shown in Fig. 7-1. The need for calcium reflects growth in body height rather than body weight.

In addition to calcium and phosphorus, vitamin A, magnesium, manganese, choline, vitamin C, vitamin D, and protein have been shown to affect bone growth.

Tooth formation. The mineral of dentine and enamel is the same hydroxyapatite found in bones, but the crystals are more dense and the water content lower. The protein in enamel is keratin whereas that in dentine is collagen. In contrast to bones, which are relatively active metabolically, teeth undergo an almost imperceptible change once they have erupted into the oral cavity. The very slow rate of exchange between the tooth calcium and that of the body is confined almost entirely to the dentine layer, although evidence is accumulating to suggest that there may be some microchemical reaction involving calcium exchange between the tooth enamel and saliva that is accentuated once tooth decay has been initiated.

Calcification of deciduous teeth begins by the twentieth week of fetal life, although it is completed only shortly before eruption into the oral cavity. Permanent teeth begin to calcify when the child is between three months and three years of age while wisdom teeth, the last to erupt, may not begin to calcify until the eighth to tenth year of life. A full complement of adult teeth contains only 11 gm. of calcium or about 1% of total body calcium.

Since teeth do not have the ability to repair themselves once they have erupted, there is no further need for a dietary source of calcium to maintain or repair teeth. A deficiency of calcium during the formative period for teeth may be reflected as a weakness in structure with increased susceptibility to tooth decay even though the teeth appear normal histologically. As in the case of bone, the integrity of tooth structure involves many nutrients in addition to calcium.

Growth. While failure in growth is not a specific response to a dietary calcium deficiency, the observation that the stature of some persons, such as Orientals raised on a diet traditionally low in calcium, is frequently shorter than that of persons of the same race raised in a part of the world where the diet is adequate in calcium has led to the suggestion that calcium is necessary for normal growth. Certainly height will increase only when sufficient calcium is available for bone growth. Since diets low in calcium also are frequently low in protein and since protein is a specific growth factor it is difficult to argue that a lack of calcium is a primary cause of growth failure, although it may be a contributing factor.

Blood-clotting. The role of calcium in the blood-clotting mechanism is one of the more clearly understood of its functions. Once cells have been injured ionized calcium, representing about half the total blood calcium, stimulates the release of thromboplastin from the blood platelets. Thromboplastin in turn catalyzes the conversion of prothrombin, a normal blood constituent, to thrombin. Thrombin then aids in the polymerization of fibrinogen to fibrin, the clot. The process is illustrated in Fig. 7-2. A schematic representation of the blood-clotting mechanisms shows that calcium must be present to initiate a series of changes needed for the formation of the clot. Under normal conditions blood calcium levels are maintained at a sufficiently high level to facilitate the blood-clotting process so that an increase in dietary calcium will have little direct effect on blood-clotting time.

Catalyst for biological reactions. Calcium is vital to normal body functioning through its role as a catalyst in many biological reactions. The absorption of cobalamin (vitamin B_{12}) through the intestinal wall is dependent on calcium. The fat-splitting enzyme of pancreatic lipase is activated by calcium, as are many of the

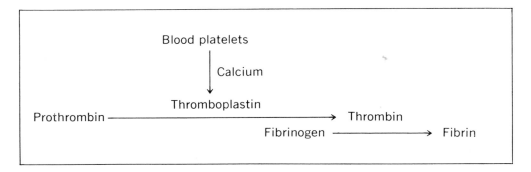

Fig. 7-2
Schematic representation of the blood-clotting mechanism.

enzymes involved in the release of energy from carbohydrates, fat, and protein. In addition the formation of acetylcholine, the substance necessary for the transmission of an impulse from one nerve fiber to the next, is dependent on calcium. The level of calcium needed to facilitate these reactions will be maintained at the expense of skeletal calcium so that as in blood-clotting the level of dietary intake will not have a direct effect on these reactions.

Regulation of permeability of cell membrane. Calcium occurs in the cell membrane closely bound to the fat-related substance lecithin. Here in an antagonistic relationship with other ions it governs the permeability of the cell membrane to various nutrients and thus controls the uptake of nutrients by the cell. In much the same way, it plays a role in regulating the contraction and relaxation of muscle fibers and the transmission of nerve impulses.

Regulation of strontium uptake. With the increased amounts of strontium 90 available to humans and animals as a result of radioactive fallout, the possible protective value of a high-calcium diet in preventing the uptake of strontium has received much attention. Although similar chemically, calcium and strontium behave differently physiologically. The uptake of strontium by the body is often undesirable since it can replace calcium in bone formation

where it may continue to cause irradiation. Present evidence indicates that if sufficient calcium is available the body will preferentially absorb calcium by a factor of 9:1, but if less calcium is available strontium will be taken up and become an undesirable substitute for calcium in many compounds. The body also excretes strontium in preference to calcium in the urine, and preferentially transfers calcium to milk and across the placental barrier to the fetus. Thus, when dietary calcium is high the body absorbs less strontium and excretes more, reducing the amount retained by the body compared to conditions of limited calcium intake. The relative value of calcium from various sources in protecting against strontium uptake is being investigated.

Absorption

In comparison to the rat, which can absorb 100% of dietary calcium, the human is very inefficient, absorbing a maximum of 40% to 60% under optimal conditions and greatest need. Normally an absorption of 20% to 30% of ingested calcium is considered good, and frequently it is as low as 10%. Most of this occurs in the upper end of the small intestine where the digestive mass is more likely to be acid. Here calcium is absorbed either by active transport, an energy-requiring process, or by passive diffusion, in which absorption occurs when calcium goes from an area of high concentration (intestine) to one of lower concentration (the blood). Before being absorbed calcium must be separated from any complex in which it may occur in food and be ionized. Whatever food calcium is unabsorbed passes on through the digestive tract and is excreted as exogenous fecal calcium.

The efficiency with which calcium is absorbed is a function of many factors, some of which favor and some of which depress calcium utilization. Under any set of conditions, there are wide individual differences in the efficiency of calcium absorption.

Factors favoring calcium absorption

Vitamin D. The effectiveness of vitamin D in facilitating the uptake of calcium from the intestine has been recognized since the early 1920's, but only recently has there been any evidence as to how it operates. First, it appears to increase the permeability of the intestinal membrane to calcium. Since not all minerals are more readily absorbed in the presence of vitamin D it seems that the effect is specific for calcium. In addition, when vitamin D is present calcium is absorbed throughout a greater length of the intestine than when it is absent; thus more calcium will be absorbed before the food moves on to the colon, where no absorption occurs. There is evidence also that vitamin D activates the active transport system by which some calcium is also absorbed.

Acidity of digestive mass. Calcium is more soluble in acid and hence is more readily absorbed from an acid than from an alkaline medium. Since calcium is absorbed primarily from the small intestine in which the contents must be rendered slightly alkaline before the intestinal enzymes can function, anything that increases the acidity of the digestive mass entering from the stomach and prolongs the time before the acid is neutralized should in-

crease the possibility of calcium absorption. Hydrochloric acid normally secreted in the stomach is responsible for the acidity of the contents of the digestive tract as it enters the small intestine. When hydrochloric acid secretion is reduced, as it often is in old age, calcium absorption may be depressed. This can be partially compensated for by an increased intake of foods rich in ascorbic acid, which can contribute to the acidity of the stomach and intestinal contents. The suggestion that the fermentation of lactose to lactic acid in the lower intestinal tract accounts for the improved utilization of calcium on diets high in lactose have not been substantiated experimentally. The increase in calcium absorption noted on diets high in protein has been attributed by some to the action of the amino acids, the products of protein digestion, in forming a soluble complex with calcium to facilitate its absorption, or by preventing its precipitation as an insoluble complex. Although we have no explanation of why it is effective there is experimental evidence to show that a high intake of lysine will increase calcium absorption as much as 50%.

Lactose. There is ample evidence that the absorption of calcium is improved in the presence of the disaccharide lactose, with reports of increases ranging from 15% to 50%. Attempts to explain this effect on the basis of changes in the growth of micro-organisms in the lower gastrointestinal tract, its slower rate of absorption, or changes in the acidity of intestinal contents occurring in the presence of lactose have failed. Recently it has been suggested that the beneficial effects are caused by the formation of a soluble sugar-calcium complex in the intestine that keeps the calcium in a form in which it can be transported to and possibly across the intestinal wall. This complex also prevents the precipitation of calcium as an insoluble and hence unabsorbable complex as the contents of the gastrointestinal tract change from acid to alkali in the intestine. A relatively high ratio of lactose to calcium is necessary to form the soluble complex. Other sugars such as the five-carbon monosaccharide, ribose, and the six-carbon monosaccharide, fructose, also enhance calcium absorption, but lactose is the most effective. The benefits of obtaining calcium from milk, a food also high in lactose, are obvious.

Calcium-phosphorus ratio. The relationship between calcium and phosphorus levels in the diet plays an important role in the absorption of both. A dietary ratio of 2 parts of phosphorus to 1 part calcium promotes the highest level of absorption, while a 1:1 ratio is considerably better than a 1:2 proportion. An upset Ca:P ratio is unlikely to occur on a normal diet, so its effect is of theoretical rather than practical interest, although it has been used in experimental diets to study calcium metabolism.

Fat. The evidence of the effect of fat on calcium absorption is somewhat contradictory. Some research indicates an improved absorption resulting from the slower passage of food through the digestive tract. On the other hand, the formation of insoluble soaps of calcium with fatty acids is reported to reduce the amount of calcium available.

Emotional stability. The efficiency with which the food calcium is absorbed can be influenced by the emotional stability of the individual. In one study, a group of emotionally distressed young women were found to require a higher intake of calcium to maintain calcium balance than a comparable group of happy relaxed women. Another study of calcium metabolism of college men indicated a lowered absorption and increased excretion under conditions of stress such as examinations.

Need for calcium. The extent to which calcium is absorbed may be influenced by the body's need for calcium. During pregnancy and lactation and during adolescence, when needs are greater, absorp-

tion rates as high as 60% of ingested calcium have been observed. Similarly, on consistently low calcium intake the body is able to compensate by absorbing a high percentage. When the demands for calcium are lower, a smaller portion of the ingested calcium will be absorbed.

Factors depressing absorption

Oxalic acid. Oxalic acid is an organic acid that is found in several fruits and vegetables, such as rhubarb, spinach, chard, and beet greens. It combines in the digestive tract with calcium to form an insoluble complex, calcium oxalate, from which the body cannot release the calcium for absorption. In most foods containing oxalic acid there is also present sufficient calcium to tie up all the oxalic acid, leaving no surplus to bind calcium from other foods eaten at the same time. There is no evidence, for instance, to suggest that the oxalic acid of spinach will interfere with the absorption of the calcium in milk taken at the same time. The presence of 5% to 6% unbound oxalic acid in lower grades of cocoa led to reservations about the use of chocolate milk for children. Early misgivings were based on results of studies on rats where the addition of a low grade cocoa to the diet caused a depression of calcium utilization by as much as 27%. More recent work on college women at the University of Illinois showed that women could tolerate a maximum of one ounce of cocoa without nausea—an amount that could not be shown to cause any significant depression in calcium utilization on either a low or high calcium intake. Comparable studies have not been done on children but one would expect results comparable to those on women, indicating no reason for condemning chocolate milk on the basis of decreased calcium utilization.

Phytic acid. Another organic acid, phytic acid, found predominantly in the outer husks of cereals, has been shown to lower utilization of calcium by binding it in an insoluble complex. Studies comparing the utilization of calcium on diets containing comparable amounts of farina, low in phytic acid, and oatmeal, high in phytic acid, show up to 33% poorer utilization on the oatmeal diet. The human being lacks the enzyme phytase, which some species have, to hydrolyze the phytate group and release the calcium. Only in cases where the consumption of calcium-rich foods is in conjunction with foods high in phytic acid would this inhibitory effect become a practical problem. There is evidence, too, of a rapid adaptation to diets of high phytic acid so that the depressing effect of phytic acid on calcium absorption is minimized.

Increased gastrointestinal motility. Anything that increases the rate of passage of food through the intestinal tract decreases the absorption of calcium by reducing the time in which the contents of the intestinal tract are in contact with the intestinal wall. Laxatives and foods high in bulk may have this effect.

Lack of exercise. Persons who receive little exercise and bed-ridden persons who are essentially immobilized experience a loss of body calcium and a reduced ability to absorb calcium to replace it. This may be a cause, or at least a complicating factor, in the decalcification of bone so often experienced by older people. Evidence now indicates that it is the lack of weight on the legs rather than immobility per se that causes negative calcium balance during bed rest.

Table 7-1 summarizes the factors affecting calcium absorption.

Metabolism

Once calcium has been absorbed through the wall of the intestine, it is transported by the bloodstream and released to the fluids bathing the tissues of the body. From there the cells pick up whatever calcium is needed for their normal functioning and growth. Some calcium becomes a part of the digestive secretions into the stomach and intestine, but much of this calcium appears to be reabsorbed. As the calcium in the blood passes through the kidney most of it is resorbed and retained in the body although some leaves the body in the urine. Any calcium from the breakdown of bone in excess of vital body needs is excreted also by the kidney.

As indicated earlier, most of the absorbed calcium is used in the calcification

Table 7-1. Summary of factors influencing calcium absorption

Classification	Factor
Factors favoring absorption	Adequate vitamin D
	Acidity of digestive mass
	Calcium : phosphorus ratios of 2 : 1
	Presence of dietary fat
	Need for calcium
Factors depressing absorption	Oxalic acid
	Phytic acid
	Increased gastrointestinal motility
	Lack of exercise or weight bearing
	Emotional instability

of bones. When the amount of calcium and phosphorus in the fluids bathing the bone cartilage cells exceeds a critical concentration, calcium phosphate precipates and becomes attached to this bone matrix through the phosphate portion of the molecule. It then grows as a crystalline structure that gives strength and rigidity to the bones. The deposition of calcium in the bones is facilitated by vitamin D and the enzyme phosphatase, which releases phosphorus from other compounds to combine with calcium and precipitate out of the blood.

The calcium in the blood is in equilibrium with bone calcium, about one third of which is available to provide calcium to maintain blood calcium levels of at least 7 mg. per 100 ml. If blood calcium falls below this level the parathyroid gland secretes a hormone, parathormone, which stimulates the release of some of the exchangeable calcium from the bone. This usually occurs as the result of the release and metabolism of some of the carbohydrate in the bone to citric acid in which the bone calcium is very soluble. This in turn increases the level of calcium in the blood and intercellular fluids to the point where it again is adequate for normal blood coagulation, the transmission of nerve impulses, and the contraction of muscles. At the same time the parathyroid stimulates the release of stored calcium, it causes the kidney to resorb more of the calcium, which might normally be excreted in the urine, and it stimulates a greater absorption of calcium from the gastrointestinal tract. When blood levels return to normal, the secretion of the parathyroid returns to normal and calcium is mobilized from the bone to maintain blood levels at a normal rate. Opposing the action of parathormone in a second hormone, *calcitonin*, believed to be secreted by the thyroid gland under stimulation from the parathyroid in hypercalcemia, which acts to lower blood calcium levels. Thus the parathyroid gland,

through its effect directly or indirectly on the secretion of these two hormones, is responsible for maintaining the level of calcium in the blood within the very narrow limits demanded by the body.

The regulatory effect of the parathyroid hormone is integrated with the action of vitamin D, which also stimulates the absorption of calcium from the intestinal tract, increases the retention of calcium by the kidney, and allows the release of bone calcium to maintain blood levels. An excess of vitamin D in some individuals will stimulate the decalcification of bone and produce high blood calcium levels.

The paths of the absorption and metabolism of calcium are shown schematically in Fig. 7-3.

Calcium requirements

Controversy. In attempting to establish a recommended level for calcium intake, nutritionists have become involved in an intense controversy. Proponents of a lower allowance maintain that we have no evidence of adverse effects from low intakes, that there is no evidence that low calcium is a deterrent to growth, and that no clinical condition can be classified as a calcium deficiency. They maintain that conditions that have been classified as calcium deficiency diseases are in reality the result of inadequate vitamin D. Those who feel that the present standard should be maintained are convinced that persons who have been on a restricted intake in their early years are more susceptible to osteoporosis as they grow older, that there is no evidence of harm from moderate intakes, that not all people are able to adapt to low intakes, and that the larger amounts are readily available in the food supply to provide these levels for the American population. Where less calcium is available in the food supply and the population has adapted to lower intakes, a lower dietary standard is justified.

Calcium balance studies. Estimates of

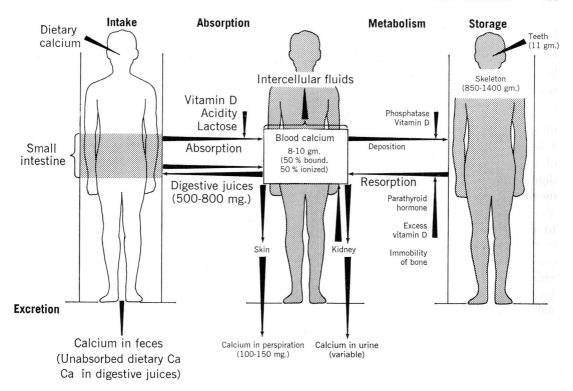

Fig. 7-3

Absorption and metabolism of calcium.

calcium needs have been based on the results of calcium balance studies in which the calcium content of the diet is compared to the amount of calcium excreted in the urine and feces. Urinary calcium represents calcium obtained from the resorption of bone, which, in the adult, approximates 175 mg. per day plus any absorbed dietary calcium that is not resorbed as the blood flows through the kidney. Fecal calcium includes some of the endogenous calcium secreted into the small intestine in the digestive juices (at least 125 mg. per day) plus any unabsorbed dietary calcium, which is referred to as exogenous calcium. This may represent from 40% to 90% of ingested calcium. It has been assumed that when calcium intake exceeds calcium excretion the body is in positive calcium balance and storing calcium. When

intake equals excretion the body is in calcium equilibrium and is neither accumulating calcium nor losing it. In negative calcium balance the excretion exceeds the intake, indicating that the body is releasing more body calcium than it is replacing, resulting in a net loss from the body that reflects decalcification of bone tissue in most cases.

Limitations. There are several limitations to the use of calcium balance data as currently obtained as a basis for requirements. Measurement of intake seldom involves a determination of the calcium in water, which in tropical areas with a hard water supply is an appreciable amount. Nor does it take into account the nonfood sources of calcium such as lime ingested by betel chewers and by persons eating Mexican tortillas made from lime-treated corn. An appreciable amount of calcium may be lost in perspiration and tears which are seldom analyzed because we have not developed techniques to do so. In a tropical climate this may amount to 140. mg. per day, sufficient to make a difference between positive and negative balance in many studies. Since some people adapt to a low calcium intake by conserving calcium either through a higher rate of absorption, a lower rate of excretion, or lessened secretions in the digestive juices, calcium balance data are meaningful only if there is information about dietary history. A person accustomed to an intake of 500 mg. could maintain calcium balance on 400 mg. more easily than could a person whose customary diet provided 1000 mg. The length of time required for adaptation varies. Some persons adapt within two months to a lower intake, others

much more slowly, and some, never. In addition Ohlson observed that a positive or negative balance that had prevailed for weeks could be reversed without any dietary change in adult women. Calcium balances have been reported to reflect the emotional state of the individual becoming negative under stressful circumstances and positive again as stress passes. Some evidence suggests that calcium balance data are useful only if considered in light of phosphorus balance data and a recent study has shown that the level of sodium in the diet also has a marked influence on calcium utilization.

In spite of the reservations that many scientists have expressed about the validity of calcium balance studies, they remain a widely used criterion for establishing a standard for calcium intake. The recom-

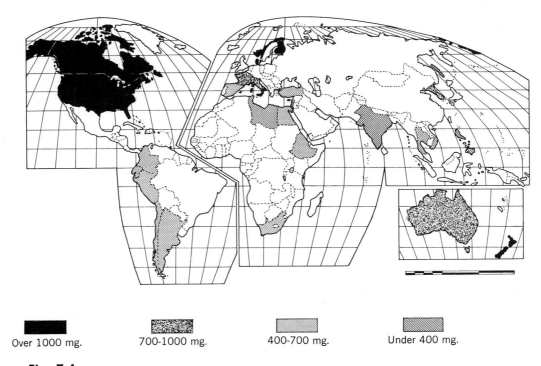

Over 1000 mg.   700-1000 mg.   400-700 mg.   Under 400 mg.

Fig. 7-4

Amounts of calcium per capita available in food supply in different parts of the world. (Based on data from Calcium requirements, WHO Publication No. 230, Geneva, 1962, World Health Organization.)

mended allowances proposed by the Food and Nutrition Board of the National Research Council in 1964 have been set at a level the Council believes will meet the needs of essentially all healthy individuals and one that can be readily achieved from the national food supply.

The Food and Agricultural Organization have released suggested practical calcium allowances. They feel these lower values represent a level that can more readily be achieved by a larger segment of the world's population, many of whom consume low amounts of calcium because of its limited availability in their national food supplies. The wide variation in the calcium available in the diets of various countries is evident from Fig. 7-4. The determination of these figures is complicated by the

fact that there is little relationship between values obtained by calculations from tables of food composition and those obtained by actual analysis. A comparison of American, Canadian, British, and FAO recommendations listed in Table 7-2 shows that there is no general agreement as to the optimal level of calcium intake. The FAO group, after evaluating all available data, suggests that there is no evidence that when vitamin D is adequate there are any harmful effects from diets containing below 300 mg. or more than 1000 mg. of calcium per day.

Calcification of soft tissues does not occur in normal, healthy individuals solely as a result of high intakes of calcium. If, however, blood calcium levels become high because of increased bone resorption, it may

Table 7-2. Comparison of standards for calcium intake for selected age and sex groups

	Age	Canadian dietary standard (1962)* (milligrams per day)	British† (milligrams per day)	NRC recommended dietary allowances (1964)‡ (milligrams per day)	FAO/WHO suggested practical allowances§ (milligrams per day)
Children	7–12 months	500	1000	700	500– 600
	10–12 years	1200	1300	1100	600– 700
Males	16–19 years	900	1400	1300	500– 600
	Adult	500	800	800	400– 500
Females	16–19 years	900	1300	1300	500– 600
	Adult	500	800	800	400– 500
	Pregnancy	1200	1500	1300	1000–1200
	Lactation	1200	2000	1300	1000–1200

*Dietary standards for Canada, Canadian Bulletin on Nutrition, vol. 6, No. 1, March, 1964.
†British Medical Association: Report of the committee on nutrition, London, 1950, British Medical Association.
‡FAO/WHO calcium requirements, Technical Report Series No. 230, Geneva, 1962, World Health Organization.
§Recommended dietary allowances, Publication No. 1146, Washington, D.C., 1964, National Research Council.

be helpful to reduce dietary calcium in an effort to reduce the amount available for calcification of soft tissue such as the kidney. The abnormal deposition of calcium in soft tissues is more likely a result of low magnesium than of high calcium.

Infants. There is relatively little data available on calcium needs of infants. It is assumed that the breast-fed infant who receives about 30 mg. of calcium per 100 ml. of milk and who absorbs two thirds of it receives adequate calcium. For the artificially fed infant who absorbs about 35% of the 160 mg. per 100 ml. in cow's milk formula, an intake of 700 mg. is suggested.

Children. The daily retention of 75 to 150 mg. of calcium per day requires a daily intake of 800 mg. of calcium for children one to nine years of age. The rapidly growing skeleton of adolescents requires as much as 400 mg. of calcium per day, calling for an intake of 1400 mg. for boys and 1300 mg. for girls.

Adults. Balance studies show that the average person achieves calcium equilibrium on an intake of 10 mg. per kilogram of body weight; however, the wide individual variations indicate that 18 mg. per kilogram would be needed to meet the needs of 95% of the population and 22 mg. if one were to be assured of meeting the needs of 99% of the population.

Pregnancy and lactation. Although the child is born with very poorly calcified bones, the full-term fetus contains approximately 28 gm. of calcium, which must be provided from the mother's reserves. There is need for an increased maternal intake, not only for the calcification of the fetal teeth and bones that occurs during pregnancy, but also to build the storage reserves of the mother to meet the high demands during lactation. Calcium is deposited in the fetal tissue at the rate of 25, 50, 84, 125, 175, 235, and 300 mg. per day during the last 7 months of pregnancy. Over half of the calcium deposited in the fetus is transferred from the mother between the thirty-fourth and fortieth week of pregnancy. Studies using radioactive isotopes of calcium in mothers' diets show that 85% to 90% of the calcium in the fetal skeleton and in human milk came from the mother's diet while 10% to 15% was withdrawn from maternal reserves. Indications are that the ability to absorb calcium increases with need and that the pregnant woman may absorb up to 40% of dietary calcium. Even so the National Research Council has recommended an additional 500 mg. a day over normal requirements to meet both fetal and maternal demands. A retention by the mother of two to five times fetal needs has been reported in sixth and seventh months, indicating that maternal reserves are being built up at this time. Research also suggests a sharp reduction in the muscular cramps frequently encountered in pregnancy upon administration of both vitamin D and calcium.

The transfer of calcium from mother to infant is greater during lactation than during pregnancy, about 50 gm. being secreted in milk during a six-month lactation period. Human milk contains about 30 mg. calcium per 100 ml. To meet this demand for 200 to 300 mg. per day for the production of 850 ml. of milk without causing a severe depletion of mother's reserves or a decrease in milk production, a maternal intake of 1300 mg. has been advised. At a 40% utilization rate, 750 mg. would be needed for milk production alone. This requires the use of large amounts of dairy products (a minimum of one and a half quarts of milk or its equivalent) plus generous use of other calcium-rich foods. Very few women maintain calcium equilibrium during lactation but draw on the calcium reserves built up during pregnancy to help provide the 50 gm. of calcium transferred to milk in a six-month lactation period. The ability of some women to maintain a successful level of lactation on very low calcium intakes is unexplained.

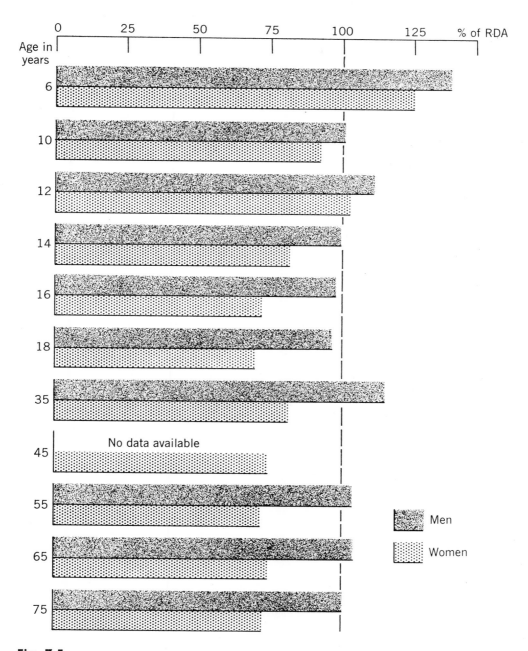

Fig. 7-5

Adequacy of calcium in the American diet expressed as percentage of recommended dietary allowances at various ages.

Old age. There is no basis on which to suggest an increase in calcium need with age, but all evidence points to the need for maintaining the adult intake of 800 mg. per day throughout the later years to reduce the likelihood of demineralization of the skeleton frequently observed, especially in women over 65 years of age.

Adequacy of calcium in American diet. If the NRC recommended allowances are used as a criterion for adequacy, it is apparent from many studies of dietary intake that many persons in the United States fail to meet this standard. The extent to which the diets of Americans meet the National Research Council Standards is shown in Fig. 7-5. This shows that men and boys are much more likely to consume adequate amounts than are women and girls. Milk was a major source of calcium in all diets, providing about three fourths of the calcium in most of the diets evaluated. Persons who do not drink milk, especially those who also restrict their use of other dairy products, find it virtually impossible to consume a diet reaching NRC standards. The decreased intake in calcium in the diets of older women is of special concern be-

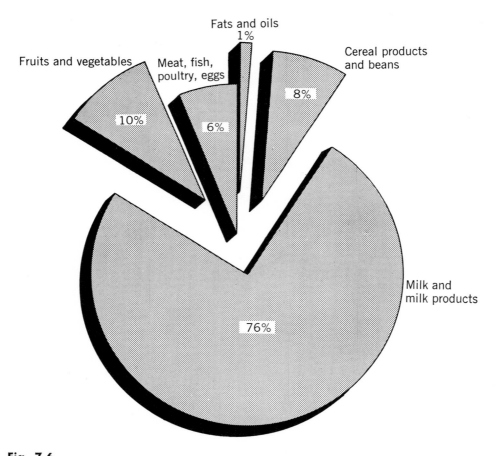

Fig. 7-6

Contribution of various food groups to the calcium content of the American diet. (Based on Nutritive value of foods available for consumption, United States, 1909-1964, Agricultural Research Service Publication 62-14, 1966.)

cause of the increased likelihood of osteoporosis in this group.

Food sources

Calcium is present in significant amounts in a very limited number of foods. Fig. 7-6 shows the contribution of various food groups to the total calcium in the American diet, which has increased steadily from 0.86 gm. in 1906 to 1.16 gm. per capita per day in 1962. Milk and dairy products are the most dependable sources because of the many ways in which they can be consumed, their availability, and their relatively low cost. In addition, the calcium in milk is in complexes from which it is readily released. It becomes obvious from Fig. 7-7, showing the relative amounts of calcium from various food sources on the basis of 100 gm. and 100 kilocalories of food, that should dairy products be excluded from the diet, the bulk of other foods needed to supply comparable amounts of calcium would make their use as a major source of calcium very difficult. As sources of calcium they are also very expensive.

Fish flour made from whole fish, including bones, has an extremely high calcium value both per 100-gm. portion and per 100 kilocalories. While it may assume major importance as a source of both calcium and protein in countries where milk is not available, the possibility of its widespread use in the American diet is remote. Only a limited amount could reasonably be incorporated into a day's diet, and technically there are still many problems relative to flavor and keeping qualities to be solved.

Foods of low water content, such as sardines and almonds, have an appreciable amount of calcium in terms of 100-gm. portions, but their value to the diet is limited when one considers their contribution relative to calories—an especially important consideration for people on diets restricted in calories.

The most useful sources of calcium then become milk and milk products. The ultra-high temperature sterilization of milk does not affect the availability of milk calcium; nor do the more common practices of pasteurization or homogenization. The adding of chocolate to milk does not reduce significantly the availability of calcium. It is seen that nonfat milk and buttermilk are slightly better than whole milk as sources of calcium. This may be explained by the fact that when the fat portion, which is almost devoid of calcium, is removed it is replaced by the calcium-containing portion of milk. Where cost is a prime consideration, nonfat products will provide calcium at one fourth to one third the price of whole milk. One ounce of cheddar cheese provides as much calcium as a cup of milk and often finds greater acceptance than milk as a source of calcium for adults. Cottage cheese is a variable source of calcium, depending on the method of processing used. Rennin coagulation retains more calcium in the curd than either a combination of acid and rennin coagulation or acid coagulation alone. All methods are used commercially. Cream cheese is a poor source, being made from the fat portion of milk that is low in calcium. Ice cream, a popular form of milk product, can be substituted at a level of one cup of ice cream for one half cup of milk as a source of available calcium.

The amount of calcium in milk from a particular species varies with the rate of growth of the offspring. It ranges from 0.02% in the milk of human beings, whose babies double birth weight in 180 days, to 0.12% in the milk of cows, whose calves double their birth weight in 47 days, and 0.32% in the milk of dogs, who achieve the same proportionate increase in weight in seven days.

The calcium of goat's milk contains slightly more calcium than cow's milk and often is substituted when an infant is allergic to cow's milk. Where cow's and goat's milk are not available or not tolerated by young infants, soybean milk prep-

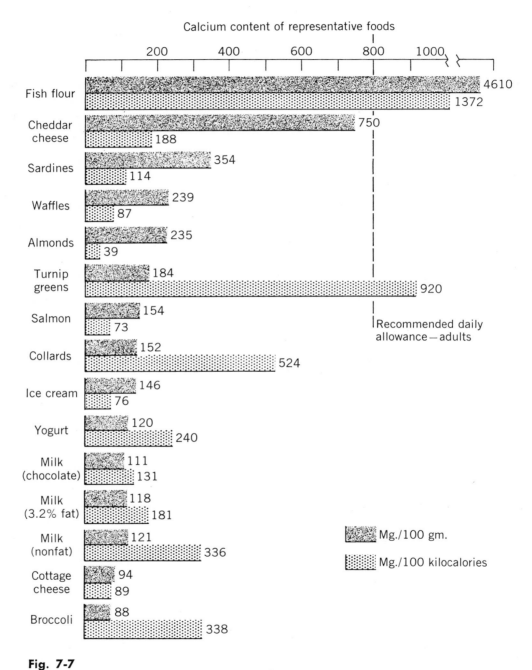

Fig. 7-7

Calcium content of some representative foods. (Based on Watts, B., and Merrill, A.: Composition of foods—raw, processed and prepared, U. S. Department of Agriculture Handbook No. 8, Washington, D. C., 1963, U. S. Department of Agriculture.)

arations in either powdered or liquid form may be substituted as a satisfactory source of calcium.

Next to milk products, green leafy vegetables such as broccoli, turnip greens, and kale, which do not contain oxalic acid, have the most appreciable amounts of available calcium. The utilization of vegetable calcium is not as high because the increased gastric motility caused by the bulk of the vegetable increases rate of passage through the intestinal tract. In the case of the green leafy vegetables the fact that calcium is contained within the cell whose cellulose wall is digested with difficulty often limits the availability of this calcium. Considerable calcium may be lost in preparation of vegetables if thick skins are removed or the dark green leaves discarded.

Soybeans become a significant calcium source when consumed in large amounts. In Indonesia, for instance, a fermented soybean product, tempeh, and a dried soybean milk powder, saridele, are being advocated as potential sources of calcium and protein. In Oriental countries soy sauce may represent a significant source of calcium.

While bread has not been traditionally considered a source of calcium, the current trend toward use of dried milk solids and calcium-containing mold inhibitors raises its available calcium to the point where many adults receive as much as one seventh of their day's requirement from bread. Similarly the calcium value of baked products such as muffins, waffles, and cakes should not be overlooked. There is also the potential for increasing their calcium value by adding additional milk solids up to the point where the product remains palatable.

In tropical areas where milk products are produced and consumed by only a small segment of the population, other less traditional sources of calcium may assume much greater importance, although we have virtually no information as to the extent to which they are utilized by the body.

Where water consumption is high, as is common in the tropics, and its mineral content high (50 mg. or more per liter), water may provide up to 200 mg. or more per day. Small whole fish or fermented fish pastes are high in calcium. The mill powder used in grinding rice may adhere to the kernel in sufficient quantities to contribute to the overall calcium intake. Lime used in making tortillas adds a significant amount of calcium to diets of Mexicans. Similarly lime used by betel chewers adds to the calcium intake of these individuals, as does the ground rock, cal, used in porridges by the Peruvians. Even sweet potatoes, when they are a staple item in the diet as in the Papuan highlands, provide sufficient calcium to meet minimum dietary needs. In China eggs may contribute a substantial proportion of the limited total calcium consumed, and in Malaya pregnant women eat a small shellfish, which is ground up and eaten whole. These represent but a few of the possible ways in which various populations possibly acquire sufficient calcium although they consume practically no dairy products.

Many diet supplements contain calcium salts, such as calcium carbonate, calcium gluconate, calcium lactate, and calcium citrate. These seem to be well utilized and may be of value during times of very high need such as pregnancy and lactation. They should be considered a supplement to a calcium-rich diet but not a replacement for dietary calcium. Purveyors of special food-blending devices are constantly promoting the consumption of pulverized eggshell as a feasible method of obtaining an adequate calcium intake. An eggshell does contain 2 gm. of calcium, but since we have no data on the utilization of calcium from this source, one can question the reliance on such a source, especially where adequate calcium is available from more conventional sources.

For people who have a restricted food budget, knowledge of the cost of a nutrient

Table 7-3. Relative costs of one third the adult daily calcium allowance from various food sources

Food	Amount required in ounces	Cost*
Dried nonfat milk	0.67	$ .02
Cheddar cheese	1	$ .04
Fresh whole milk	8	$ .06
Chocolate milk	8	$ .07
Ice cream	6	$ .09
Sardines	2.5	$ .13
Cottage cheese	9	$ .19
Broccoli	10	$ .25
Almonds	3.5	$ .36

*Based on prices prevailing in Northeastern United States, Spring, 1965.

from various sources may be helpful in planning an adequate intake at minimum cost. Table 7-3 gives such information for some representative sources of calcium.

High calcium intake

Although we have no evidence of deleterious effects from excessive intakes of calcium per se, popular literature is suggesting with increasing frequency that a high intake of calcium is undesirable. In the several studies that have been undertaken to assess the effect of high oral calcium intakes, it was found that diets high in calcium (2 gm.) had no effect on the level of calcium in the urine of normal subjects although they would result in high urinary calcium levels (hypercalcuria) in numerous disease states. In addition there is no evidence that high dietary calcium levels have any effect on kidney stone formation nor do they lead to deposition of calcium in other soft tissues in the absence of metabolic abnormalities. Work on animals has suggested that excessively high intakes of calcium have a depressing effect on the utilization of other nutrients, such as phosphorus, fat, iodine, zinc, magnesium, and iron, when the latter are present at minimal levels. However, the ratios at which this can occur are far beyond those calcium intakes which might be encountered in a normal diet. In adults, high intakes of calcium lead to increased total absorption of calcium although the efficiency of absorption is decreased. In children, however, an intake of 2300 mg. of calcium and 2400 mg. of phosphorus resulted in a depressed retention of calcium. This was accompanied by a marked increase in fat excretion in feces and may be caused by an inhibition of the fat-splitting enzyme pancreatic lipase in the presence of high calcium concentration in the intestine.

Once high urinary calcium levels occur as the result of some metabolic abnormality, such as hypothyroidism, which stimulates calcium absorption, the restriction of dietary calcium to the levels considered adequate but not in excess of those required to meet body needs is likely a rational therapeutic approach.

Thus while we have no evidence of additional benefits to be derived from calcium intakes in excess of recommended levels, neither can we point to any evidence of detrimental effects except for individuals in whom there is a tendency to deposit calcium in soft tissues.

Assessment of body calcium reserves

The major problem in assessing body nutriture in respect to calcium is the lack of feasible method which is sensitive to changes in body calcium. Blood calcium levels are readily determined but the action of the parathyroid gland in mobilizing bone calcium to maintain blood calcium at a level of at least 7 mg. per 100 ml. means that a drop in blood calcium is a more sensitive measure of the efficiency of the parathyroid than of calcium status. The hazards and cost involved in the use of radioactive isotopes of calcium limit its usefulness to controlled studies on limited numbers of subjects. Considerable work has been done to develop an x-ray measurement of bone density that will reflect the degree of mineralization of bone. Bones of the heel and finger, which have been investigated, do not show sufficient variation in mineralization within the normal range of human calcium intake to be of any use in assessing calcium nutriture. From 10% to 40% demineralization of bone may have occurred before the change will be reflected in x-ray measurements. The problem is further complicated by the fact that so far no deficiency symptoms can be attributed to a lack of dietary calcium.

Abnormalities of calcium metabolism

Osteoporosis. Osteoporosis is a condition found primarily among middle-aged women in which the absolute amount of bone in the skeleton has been diminished but in which the remaining bone mass is of normal composition. This is reflected in a shortening of stature and symptoms of low backache. It affects a minimum of 10% of the population over 50 years of age, and several studies have reported

as high as 50% incidence. It is estimated that in 1963 there were over four million cases of severe osteoporosis in the United States, 80% of which were in women. Until recently osteoporosis was considered inevitable in older people, in the belief that it was either an endocrine disorder or a protein deficiency state that resulted in a diminished formation of the bone matrix. It is now believed that the rate of bone formation is normal but that bone resorption occurs at an accelerated rate. The increased rate of bone resorption may occur to maintain normal blood levels of calcium where dietary intake is low or where dietary needs are abnormally high because of poor absorption. It also appears that a reduction in bone mass can occur only after prolonged periods in which calcium losses exceed calcium uptake and may not be diagnosed until bone mass has been reduced as much as 30%. People with osteoporosis have usually been found to have had a lower than normal intake of calcium over a long period of time. Older people have been shown to absorb less calcium than younger people and people with osteoporosis less than those free of the disease; in some cases they also excrete more but in all cases the gain in body calcium has failed to compensate for the losses which has led to a resorption of bone tissue to maintain normal blood levels. People with osteoporosis do not have the ability of normal people to reduce urinary calcium excretion when dietary intake is low. Thus it appears that the people who develop osteoporosis are those who cannot adapt to a low level of dietary intake, those who have impaired absorptive mechanisms, or those who persistently lose body calcium. Treatment of osteoporosis with a diet high in calcium (15.5 mg. per kilogram of body weight) and with adequate vitamin D has been shown to arrest the resorption of the bone and has led to the observation that the prevention of osteoporosis with lifelong adequate calcium intakes is the best treatment. The high incidence of bone fracture among osteoporotic patients may be due to spontaneous fractures in which the break precedes the fall rather than being caused by falls. Osteoporotic bone breaks at loads 40% less than normal, and the healing period for fractures is considerably longer than normal.

The use of cortisone in the treatment of patients with arthritis, which has increased the tendency to osteoporosis, is thought to increase the urinary excretion of calcium. The tendency has been compensated for by a diet high in calcium and adequate in vitamin D.

Osteomalacia. Osteomalacia, on the other hand, is a condition in which there is a reduction in the mineral content of the bone but not in the total amount of bone. Sometimes referred to as adult rickets, it is most likely to occur among women living in areas of low sunshine, those whose clothing prevents exposure to sunlight, those whose diets are low in calcium, and in those for whom the demands of successive pregnancies and prolonged lactation have depleted their mineral resources.

Hypercalcemia. Hypercalcemia in infants, which is being reported with increasing frequency, is attributed to a sensitivity to high levels of vitamin D. The hypercalcemia can be corrected best by reducing the vitamin D rather than by limiting the calcium in the diet.

Tetany and calcium rigor. When the level of calcium in the blood and hence in the extracellular fluids drop below a critical level, there is a change in the stimulation of nerve cells, resulting in increased excitability of the nerve and spasmodic and uncontrolled contractions of muscle tissue, a condition described as tetany. When calcium levels rise above normal, the muscle fibers enter a state of tonic contraction known as *calcium rigor*. Neither of these conditions is the result of abnormal dietary levels of calcium but rather reflects an abnormality in parathyroid functioning.

PHOSPHORUS
Distribution

Since phosphorus constitutes 22% of the mineral ash in an adult body or 1% of body weight, it is classified as a *macronutrient* element. Its role as a major constituent of bones and teeth is recognized by even the casual student of nutrition. The fact that it is often discussed in connection with calcium has further emphasized its role in the formation of hard tissues with the result that its other very vital roles are often overlooked or underestimated.

It is estimated that the adult body contains 12 gm. of phosphorus per kilogram of fat-free tissue. This amounts to about 670 gm. of phosphorus in the male and 630 gm. in the female. Of this phosphorus 85% to 90% is in the form of the insoluble calcium phosphate (apatite) crystals that give rigidity and strength to bones and teeth. The remaining 10% to 15% is distributed throughout all living cells of the body with about half present in striated muscle. Specifically, it is a part of the nucleus and the cytoplasm of every living cell, where it plays an essential role in many body processes and as a structural component. In fact practically all biological reactions involve phosphorus to some extent since it is vital to any reaction that involves the uptake or release of energy.

Functions

Regulates the release of energy. It is a phosphorus-containing substance, phosphate, that is responsible for the controlled release of energy resulting from the combustion or oxidation of carbohydrate, fat, and protein. A third phosphate molecule is attached to the compound ADP or adenosine diphosphate to form ATP, adenosine triphosphate, in a bond or linkage that stores energy. This linkage is referred to as a high-energy phosphate bond. As energy is needed, the ATP is changed to ADP, and a phosphate molecule and the energy that held it to ADP is released to supply energy slowly for many body re-actions. If the cells were unable to convert energy into these high-energy bonds for storage, they would be incapable of regulating the rate at which it is avail-able. Phosphate, and hence phosphorus, appears many times in the chemical re-actions that occur in metabolism within the cell.

Facilitates absorption and transportation of nutrients. Phosphate is attached to many substances such as monosaccharides in a process known as phosphorylation to facili-tate their passage through cell membranes. This occurs in absorption from the intestine, release from the bloodstream to the inter-cellular fluids, uptake into the cell, and uptake by the organelles of the cell. Fats that are insoluble in water are transported in the bloodstream as phospholipids, a com-bination of phosphate with the fat mole-cule that renders the fat more soluble. When glycogen is released from the liver or muscle storage sites to be used as a source of energy it appears as a phos-phorylated glucose compound, another manifestation of the essential nature of phosphorus.

Part of essential body compounds. The active form of some vitamins is one con-taining phosphorus—thiamine pyrophos-phate, B_1, is an example. Since all enzymes are proteins and many proteins contain phosphorus, the essentiality of this mineral is obvious. Even more crucial is the role of phosphate as an integral part of the nucleic acids, DNA and RNA, both of which are essential for cell reproduction through their vital roles in protein syn-thesis.

Calcification of bones and teeth. The use of the term *calcification* to describe the process in which calcium and phosphorus precipitate from the fluids bathing the bone cell matrix and crystallize as apatite in the organic framework of the bone to give it strength and rigidity has led to the errone-ous belief that a lack of calcium is a major

cause of failure of the process. Although bones contain half as much phosphorus as calcium failure of bone calcification is as often the result of unavailability of phos-phorus as of calcium. In cases of poor cal-cification of bone, there is an increase in the enzyme phosphatase that facilitates the release of phosphorus from organic tissue compounds into the blood to create the proper calcium phosphorus rates for bone growth. The initiation of the calcification process involves the fixation of phosphate to the matrix, indicating a primary role of phosphorus bone formation. The low phos-phorus levels in the body are more likely a reflection of excessive excretion of phos-phorus in the urine than of inadequate dietary phosphorus. It is well beyond the scope of this presentation to attempt to enumerate all the biological reactions in which phosphorus plays a key role. Those mentioned merely illustrate the diversity of reactions in which phosphorus partici-pates.

Metabolism

In addition to being associated in bone and tooth structure, both calcium and phosphorus metabolism are influenced by the same factors. The parathyroid, which regulates the level of calcium in the blood, affects the levels of phosphorus in the blood and its rate of resorption from the kidney. Vitamin D, which facilitates the absorption of calcium from the gastro-intestinal tract, also increases the rate of resorption of phosphorus from the kidney. In this way the levels of both calcium and phosphorus needed for calcification of bone are raised simultaneously. Blood levels of phosphorus range from 35 to 45 mg. per 100 ml., of which 3 to 5 mg. is in the form of inorganic phosphorus. Like calcium, phosphorus is constantly being released and rebuilt into bone tissue in the re-modeling processes typical of bone. Evi-dence now indicates that the phosphorus of tooth enamel is exchanged with phos-

Table 7-4. Phosphorus content of representative foods*

Food	Phosphorus (milligrams per 100 gm.)
Cheddar cheese	478
Peanuts	401
Cod, broiled	274
Beef, lean round	250
Pork, lean	249
Halibut, broiled	248
Bread, whole-wheat	228
Eggs	205
Cottage cheese	152
Peas, fresh	116
Milk, whole	93
Bread, white enriched	90
Lima beans	67
Oatmeal	57
Rice, cooked	28

*Based on Watts, B., and Merrill, A.: Composition of foods—raw, processed and prepared, U.S. Department of Agriculture Handbook No. 8, Washington, D.C., 1963, U.S. Department of Agriculture.

phorus in the saliva and that in the dentine with that of the blood supply.

Food sources

Foods rich in protein are also rich in phosphorus content. Thus we find meat, fish, poultry, eggs, and cereal products are the primary sources of phosphorus in the average diet.

Whole-grain cereals contain phytic acid, a phosphorus-containing organic acid that is not available to the body. This phytic acid may combine with calcium in an insoluble complex from which neither nutrient can be absorbed. The amount of phosphorus in some representative foods is given in Table 7-4.

Requirements

The NRC recommended allowances suggest a phosphorus intake of at least 800 mg., equal to the calcium allowance indicated for the growth period. Diets adequate in protein invariably provide an adequate amount of phosphorus—about one and one half times the calcium intake considered more than satisfactory for older adults. Experimental diets with a very low P:Ca ratio have been used to produce rickets, but an upset phosphorus to calcium ratio in human diets rarely occurs. About 10% of dietary phosphorus is absorbed.

POTASSIUM
Distribution

Potassium is a monovalent cation with chemical properties similar to sodium but physiologically unlike sodium in that it is concentrated inside the cell rather than in the extracellular fluid. A sodium:potassium ratio of 1:10 is maintained within the cell, compared to 28:1 in the extracellular fluids. Thus most of the 250 gm. normally present in the body is within the cells, where it is a major factor in maintaining the osmotic pressure of the cell. Its presence within the cell is an important factor in the maintenance of acid-base balance, although it is not as readily mobilized as sodium to offset excess of acid-forming elements. It also plays a role in the transmission of nerve impulses and exerts an influence on water balance.

The amount of potassium in the blood plasma seems to reflect the nature of cellular metabolism rather than body reserves. Plasma potassium rises when there is a breakdown of body tissue (catabolism) and also in acidosis as an indication that potassium is leaving the cell. It decreases when the rate of protein synthesis or glycogen deposition within the cell increases or in alkalosis, indicating that potassium is entering the cell. If the level of potassium in the blood and hence in the extracellular fluids increases to too high a level, muscular coordination is disturbed, and in severe cases cardiac arrest occurs. This is usually the result of failure of the kidney to excrete potassium. Potassium acts along with magnesium as a muscular relaxant in opposition to calcium, which stimulates muscular contraction.

Functions

Within the cell potassium acts as a catalyst in many biological reactions, especially those involved in the release of energy and in glycogen and protein synthesis. If the sodium level increases in the intracellular material it may counteract the catalytic effect of potassium and interfere with cellular metabolism, especially protein synthesis, leading to the death of the cell.

Potassium levels in the body have been found to reflect body composition, the levels increasing with an increase in lean body mass. This relationship has become the basis of a fairly simple and promising method of determining lean body mass, *the whole body counter.* In this method an estimate of the amount of radioactive potassium 40 in the body is made by a special Geiger-counting device. Since potassium 40 represents a constant percentage of the total dietary potassium, it is assumed that the same ratio holds in the body. By determining the amount of radioactive potassium in the body and from this the total amount of potassium, it is possible to estimate the amount of lean body mass. A comparison of this value with total body weight provides information on total body fat. A drop in body weight without a concurrent drop in total body potassium indicates a loss of adipose tissue rather than lean body mass.

Deficiency

Potassium-deficiency symptoms are fairly well documented but seldom occur as a result of suboptimal dietary intakes. A deficiency state may occur in infants suffering from diarrhea where the passage of the intestinal contents is so rapid that there is a decreased absorption of dietary potassium and an increased loss of the potassium that is not resorbed from digestive secretions. The body is less efficient in conserving or resorbing potassium than many other constituents when blood passes through the kidney so that there is normally a loss of about 7% of blood potassium in the urine. Overall muscle weakness, poor intestinal tonus, heart abnormalities, and weakness of respiratory muscles are characteristic. Infants suffering from the protein-deficiency disease, kwashiorkor, respond to treatment only when potassium therapy is given along with an increased protein intake.

Because of the antagonistic relationship between sodium and potassium an excessive intake of sodium may have the same effect as a suboptimal level of potassium.

Table 7-5. Potassium content of some representative foods

Food	Milligrams per 100 gm.
Halibut	525
Baked potato	503
Lima beans	422
Pork, cooked	390
Beef, cooked	370
Lamb, cooked	290
Cabbage, raw	233
Asparagus, cooked	183
Waffles	145
Milk, whole	144
Egg, cooked	140
Grapefruit	135
Apples	110
White bread	85
Cheddar cheese	82

Requirements

The amount of potassium in the American diet has been variously estimated as 1 to 4, 2 to 4, and 6.5 grams per day or 0.8 to 1.5 gm. per 1000 calories. Since potassium is distributed in a great many foods, its presence in the diet tends to parallel the caloric value of the diet. While it has been established that potassium is a dietary essential, there is little information on minimal needs, but there is no evidence that the amount generally found in the diet is suboptimal. The potassium content of some representative foods is shown in Table 7-5. Potassium in food occurs in very soluble form, increasing the possibility that a considerable amount may leach into the cooking water.

Plants are rich in potassium and it is sometimes necessary to provide salt licks for herbivorous animals, such as cattle and sheep, to provide sodium in the diet to prevent a sodium-potassium imbalance.

SULPHUR

Sulphur, which represents 0.25% of body weight, is present in every cell of the body. It is concentrated in the cytoplasm. The highest concentration of sulphur is found in the hair, skin, and nails, as evidenced by the characteristic odor of sulphur dioxide given off when these keratin-containing tissues are burned. The sulphur-containing amino acids, cystine and methionine, are in high concentration in these tissues and are characteristic of keratin.

Sulphur in combination with hydrogen (SH) plays a very important role in metabolism since it is readily oxidized, a reaction essential for the formation of a blood clot. It is also able to form high energy compounds that make it important in the transfer of energy. It is part of at least four vitamins—thiamine, pantothenic acid, biotin, and lipoic acid—which act as coenzymes necessary to activate the action of several enzymes. Compounds containing sulphur act as detoxifying substances by combining with toxic substances to convert them into harmless compounds that are excreted.

Sulphur is available to the body through the organic sulphur in the amino acids, methionine and cystine, since inorganic sulphur or the sulphur as sulphate cannot be used. Any excess of the element is excreted in the urine.

SODIUM

The necessity of salt, a major source of sodium, has been recognized for centuries, and many of the major conquests of the world revolved around a search for a salt supply. Trading in salt has had many social, political, and economic consequences. In spite of a long history, not until 1937 was the role of sodium as a dietary essential established. Salt is practically the only food not prepared in the home, although in many countries the only source of salt is the evaporation of sea water, frequently carried out on a very small scale.

Distribution

Sodium is a monovalent cation present in the body primarily in the extracellular fluids—the vascular fluids within the blood vessels, arteries, veins, capillaries, and the intercellular fluids surrounding the cells. About two ounces or 50% of the total body sodium is found in these fluids, where it represents an important part of the cell's environment. Under normal conditions as little as 10% of body sodium is present within the cell, although the body has to work constantly to pump sodium out of the cell. The remaining 40% of body sodium is found in the skeleton, where about half of it acts as a reserve of exchangeable sodium available to the extracellular fluids when less dietary sodium is available or when losses from the body are high. In infants the bone cartilage can act as a reservoir of sodium. Except where low intakes occur in conjunction with increased demand, it takes a long period of sodium restriction to use up all the body reserves.

Absorption and metabolism

Normally from 3 to 7 gm. of sodium are ingested daily, although the amount varies greatly with the extent to which table salt (sodium chloride) is added during cooking and at the table. The body has an ability to handle considerably larger amounts, although sodium can be toxic if consumed in excessive amounts. However, levels sufficiently high to become toxic are extremely unpalatable and unlikely to be consumed voluntarily.

A very small portion of sodium is absorbed in the stomach, but most of it is absorbed very rapidly from the small intestine. The absorption of sodium is an active (energy-requiring) process. Absorbed sodium is carried through the bloodstream to the kidney where sodium is filtered out and returned to the bloodstream in the amounts to maintain the blood levels within the narrow range required by the body. Any excess, which usually amounts to 90% of ingested sodium, is excreted in the urine. This regulation of sodium metabolism is controlled by aldosterone, a hormone secreted by the adrenal gland. The level of sodium in the urine reflects dietary intake—being high when intake is high and low when intake is low. Some sodium is also deposited in the bone to become a reservoir available in time of need.

Since there is a limit to the amount of sodium that can be excreted in a certain volume of urine, blood levels and extracellular fluid levels will rise if dietary intake exceeds the kidney's ability to excrete it. When blood sodium levels rise, it is believed that the thirst receptors in the hypothalamus of the brain react by stimulating the thirst sensation. This leads to greater fluid consumption, which in turn allows the kidney to excrete more urine and more sodium. Sodium blood levels drop, followed by a diminution of thirst.

Sodium is also lost from the body through perspiration. Normally these losses are minimal, but under environmental conditions that lead to excessive perspiration the loss of sodium by this route may be appreciable, one investigator reporting losses of 5 to 6 gm. of sodium chloride per day in the summer in the tropics. If losses through the skin become great, the hormone aldosterone stimulates the kidney to retain more sodium and help minimize the effects from this sodium loss.

The loss of body sodium leads to low levels in the extracellular fluids. In an attempt to equalize the osmotic pressure from electrolytes on either side of the cell membrane, potassium leaves the cell. It is this loss of potassium from the cell that causes the feeling of fatigue that accompanies sodium depletion.

Sodium is an integral part of digestive secretions such as gastric juice, bile, and pancreatic and intestinal juices. A large amount (20 gm. per day) is secreted into the gastrointestinal tract by this route, but most of this is reabsorbed. Only under abnormal conditions, such as diarrhea, where the digestive mass passes through the digestive tract very rapidly, is there a major loss of sodium through fecal excretions.

A loss of body sodium will occur in the fluid exuded by burned areas, but this is not an appreciable source of loss except in a very few instances.

Functions

Sodium plays a very vital role in performing the general functions of minerals discussed in Chapter 6.

As a cation in the extracellular fluids it helps maintain osmotic pressure on the outside of the cell membrane to counteract the similar effect of potassium within the cell and maintain normal water balance within the cell. If the sodium concentration within the cell rises, water will be taken in to dilute the sodium to normal concentrations; the resulting waterlogged cells are described as edematous.

As a base-forming element sodium helps to maintain body neutrality by counteracting the acid-forming elements. When an excess of acid-forming elements appears in the body fluids, sodium can be released from the sodium reserves in the bone to offset the acid. One of the major causes of alkalosis is the ingestion of excess sodium-containing antacid preparations.

In the transmission of nerve impulses, a change in the permeability of the nerve cell membrane allows sodium to enter and for a very temporary period this changes the electrical charge on the membrane. This electrical charge travels down the nerve fiber as a nerve impulse or message. If the balance between sodium outside and inside the cell were not normal, this transmission of nerve impulses could not occur.

Sodium is also essential for the absorption of glucose and may be involved in the transport of other nutrients across membranes.

Food sources

Dietary sources of sodium fall into two main categories: that present in food naturally and that added primarily as salt (sodium chloride) during processing and preparation.

Sodium is present in food in widely varying amounts, more generally being found in foods of animal origin than in those of plant origin. The sodium content of some representative foods is shown in Table 7-6. The amount found in a diet is as much a function of the amount of salt added in processing as of the amount present in the food. For instance, raw potatoes have only 0.001 mg. per 100 gm. while the same weight of potato chips has 0.340 mg. Cured ham has twenty times as much sodium as raw pork. The amount of sodium in the average diet is variously reported as 3 to 7 gm. per day. Five grams will meet the needs of most people.

In some areas the sodium content of the water supply may be sufficiently high to make water a major source of sodium, perhaps exceeding that supplied by food. Many of the ion exchange units used as water softeners also produce water with

Table 7-6. Sodium content of representative foods*

Low sodium	Milligrams per 100 gm.	Moderate sodium	Milligrams per 100 gm.	High sodium	Milligrams per 100 gm.
Apples	1	Milk	50	Graham crackers	670
Asparagus, cooked	1	Chicken		Cheddar cheese	700
		Light meat	64		
		Dark meat	86		
Grapefruit	1	Celery	100	Sauerkraut	750
Pineapple	1	Egg	122	Cornflakes	1000
Egg noodles	5	Tomato juice, canned	200	Processed cheese	1100
Sweet potato	10	Cottage cheese	290	Cured ham	1100
Broccoli, frozen	15	Sardines, canned	510	Olives, green	2400
Raisins	25				
Carrots	50				

*Based on Watts, B., and Merrill, A.: Composition of foods—raw, processed, and prepared, U.S. Department of Agriculture Handbook No. 8, Washington, D.C., 1963, U.S. Department of Agriculture.

a high sodium content. There is some evidence associating high sodium levels in the water with the incidence of atherosclerosis.

Sodium restriction

Under certain conditions, such as hypertension and kidney disorders, it has been considered important to restrict dietary sodium intake. The degree of restriction varies with the severity of the condition. Mild restriction, with intake limited to 500 to 700 mg., can often be accomplished by limiting the use of salt at the table. For very strict restriction to 200 mg., it may be necessary to choose foods naturally low in sodium, to eliminate all foods in which sodium is used in processing, and to use sodium-free salt substitutes and low-salt milks from which much of the sodium has been removed by a process in which there is an exchange of ions. Spices, except celery salt, parsley flakes, and vegetable salts, may be used since they contain virtually no sodium.

The long-standing use of low-sodium diets to treat toxemia of pregnancy is now being challenged. Clinical studies on humans indicate that high-sodium rather than low-sodium diets are effective in preventing or relieving the symptoms of toxemia—high blood pressure, edema, dizziness, and blurred vision. Extensive studies in rats have indicated an increased need for sodium during pregnancy, as evidenced by a decreased excretion of the element. The animals were better able to maintain normal bone and muscle sodium levels and gave birth to more and healthier young on elevated rather than reduced sodium intakes. Those on restricted intakes showed signs of sodium deficiency—general lethargy, debility, and a reduced amount of sodium in the blood and tissues.

CHLORINE

Chlorine, present as 0.15% of body weight, is widely distributed throughout the body, but is found in highest concentration as chloride in the cerebrospinal fluid and in the secretions into the gastrointestinal tract. Muscle and nerve tissue are relatively low in chlorine.

As a part of hydrochloric acid, chlorine is necessary to maintain the normal acidity of the stomach contents necessary for the action of gastric enzymes. It is an acid-forming element, and along with the other acid-forming elements, phosphorus and sulphur, helps maintain acid-base balance in the body fluids. Chloride ions are able to pass out of the red blood cell into the blood plasma very easily. They contribute to the ability of the blood to carry large amounts of carbon dioxide to the lungs and release it without changing its own reaction by moving in and out to balance the levels of carbon dioxide as carbonate in either the plasma or erythrocytes. This ready transfer of chloride in and out of the red blood cell is called a chloride shift.

Chlorine in the diet is provided almost exclusively by sodium chloride, so that when salt intake is restricted the chlorine level, first in urine and then in the tissue, drops. Whenever there are excessive losses of sodium, as in diarrhea, sweating, or vomiting, there are concurrent losses of chloride ions.

MAGNESIUM

The presence of magnesium in living organisms has been known since 1859, but practically all of the information on its biological functions has been gathered since 1950. By 1926 it had been identified as a dietary essential for mice and by 1932 as an essential for rats, but its role in human nutrition was much more difficult to establish. The sizeable reserve of magnesium in bone, some of which can be liberated to help meet the demands of the soft tissues, and the capacity of the kidney to reabsorb magnesium when needed have increased the difficulty of depleting magnesium levels in human beings sufficiently to study the effects of a deficiency. In plant life it is an essential part of the green pigment chlorophyll, which differs from the hemoglobin of the blood only in that magnesium replaces iron as the mineral in its structure.

The 0.5 to 0.6 gm. of magnesium in the infant at birth increase in the adult to 21 to 28 gm. (1 ounce), 60% of which is concentrated in the bone, primarily on the bone surface. In the soft tissues it is concentrated within the cell with a very small amount in the extracellular fluids. Bone ash is 0.5% to 0.7% magnesium, while the total body magnesium represents 0.43% of the fat-free tissue. Very little magnesium is excreted in the feces, but urinary losses range from 60 to 200 mg. per day.

Functions

Within the cell magnesium plays a very important role as catalyst to several hundred biological reactions, a major portion of which take place in the mitochondrion of the cell. It activates the production of ATP by oxidative phosphorylation and all changes of ATP to ADP. This change is necessary in all reactions involving the expenditure or release of energy, such as synthesis of body compounds, the absorption and transportation of nutrients, and any physical activity. The importance of magnesium in cellular metabolism is evidenced by the fact that the level of magnesium in metabolically active muscle tissue and liver is seven times that in the blood. Magnesium is crucial in cellular respiration, although in some reactions it may be replaced by other divalent elements such as manganese or cobalt. There is some evidence that magnesium also influences protein synthesis through an influence on the arrangement of the protein-synthesizing organelles of the cell, the ribosomes.

Magnesium is one of the minerals involved in providing the proper environment in the extracellular fluid of nerve cells to promote the conduction of nerve impulses and to allow normal muscular contraction. In this situation magnesium and calcium play antagonistic roles, calcium acting as a stimulator and magnesium as a relaxor substance. The competitive nature of the calcium-magnesium interrelationship is further evident during absorption and excretion. When a large amount of one is being absorbed or excreted there is usually a reduction in the amount of the other.

Adequate magnesium may increase the stability of calcium in tooth enamel. It also influences the secretion of thyroxine and the maintenance of normal basal metabolic rate and facilitates adaption to cold.

Deficiency symptoms

A recently recognized form of magnesium deficiency is a low magnesium tetany very similar to that produced when blood calcium level drops. The body's control over the contractions and relaxations of body muscles is lost. The individual suffers from uncontrolled neuromuscular activity diagnosed early as tremors but becoming increasingly involved until convulsive seizures occur in the more severe deprivation. These symptoms most often arise when a low dietary intake is superimposed on conditions that reduce the absorption and increase the excretion of magnesium. Alcohol increases the rate of magnesium excretion and may partially explain the loss of neuromuscular control diagnosed as magnesium tetany in alcoholics. Others who experience magnesium deficiency symptoms are infants suffering from kwashiorkor, persons maintained for long periods on magnesium-free fluids, as may occur postoperatively, or persons suffering prolonged losses because of nausea or diarrhea. High intakes of calcium aggravate the symptoms of low magnesium levels by favoring its excretion.

In the absence of adequate magnesium the cardiovascular system and the renal system are also affected, with symptoms such as vasodilation and skin changes frequent. Intramuscular injections of magnesium sulphate relieve these symptoms as well as the neuromuscular symptoms.

Assessment of reserves

Blood levels of magnesium do not provide a sensitive indication of the level of magnesium in cells since about 35% of the blood magnesium is bound to a protein and not measured with current analytical techniques. Tissues may be depleted of magnesium while serum levels remain normal.

Bone formed when there is adequate magnesium available contains about 16% of its magnesium as a reserve that can be released to maintain blood levels when dietary magnesium drops. However, bone formed when little magnesium was available will have little or no magnesium and will tend to take up magnesium when it becomes available from the diet, thus keeping blood levels low for a longer time.

The high levels of magnesium found in the red blood cells of mentally retarded children suggest that their ability to regulate magnesium metabolism is impaired.

Dietary needs

Although it has been contended for some time that a typical western diet provides sufficient magnesium, recent evidence from balance studies indicates that an intake of 6 mg. per kilogram of body weight (420 mg. for a 70-kg. man) is necessary to maintain positive magnesium balance. When the diet is high in calcium and protein and is supplemented with vitamin D, the magnesium requirements may increase to 7 to 10 mg. per kilogram. These values are well in excess of the 230 to 300 mg. found in typical American diets. When intakes were increased to 10 mg. per kilogram in an experimental situation there was a period of large retentions of magnesium, which later dropped, apparently after body stores were replenished.

The absence of magnesium deficiency symptoms in the American population, which apparently consumes too little to

Table 7-7. Suggested magnesium needs

Age	Milligrams of magnesium
Birth to 10 years	150
10 to 12 years	200
13 to 19 years	250 to 300
Adult men	300 to 400
Adult women	300
Pregnancy	350 to 400
Lactation	400

meet its needs, may be explained by the fact that it experiences a very slight deficit that becomes significant only when a condition of stress is superimposed. Such situations may be the increased excretion that occurs with alcohol consumption, the impaired absorption accompanying the increased use of diuretics, or the decreased intake of magnesium of patients on fluid feedings.

No recommended dietary allowances have been established for magnesium, but there is sufficient evidence accumulating to justify some suggestions. Suggested magnesium requirements are presented in Table 7-7.

Food sources

Only recently have analytical methods provided satisfactory analyses of the magnesium content of foods. Table 7-8 classifies some common foods on the basis of their magnesium content. Precise figures are not given, since in several instances only single determinations have been made. The high chlorophyll content of green leafy vegetables accounts for their value as a source of magnesium. The rate of absorption of ingested magnesium is not well established, with reports ranging from 24% to 85%, less being absorbed from a larger dose. Absorption is reduced in

Table 7-8. Classification of some representative foods as sources of magnesium

Rich sources (> 100 mg. %)	Good sources (50 to 100 mg. %)	Fair sources (25 to 50 mg. %)	Poor sources (<25 mg. %)
Cocoa	Clams	Oysters	Lobster
Nuts	Cornmeal	Crab	Pork
Soybeans	Spinach	Fresh peas	Lamb
Whole grains		Liver	Milk
		Veal	Eggs
			Veal
			Cod
			Most fruits and vegetables
			Fowl

diets high in phytic acid normally found in the outer husks of cereal grains such as rice or oats. The magnesium in foods high in oxalic acid may be found in an insoluble complex.

Although milk is a relatively poor source of magnesium it appears adequate to meet the needs of either breast- or bottle-fed infants.

Oriental diets that include appreciable amounts of magnesium, which is high in rice, soybeans, and fish, provide sufficient amounts to maintain magnesium balance. This observation is more interesting in light of recent findings that show that those persons with high magnesium intakes are less susceptible to cardiovascular diseases than those on low intakes. Men have lower magnesium stores than women or Orientals, both of whom are less susceptible to cardiovascular disease and the adverse effects of cholesterogenic diets.

The increase in the undesirable calcification of soft tissues in magnesium deficiency may reflect the incease in calcium absorption that occurs when less magnesium competes with calcium for the common carrier that transports them across the intestinal wall. This is often accompanied by an increase in the amount of calcium mobilized from the bone, which also increases the calcium available for deposition for soft tissues. High-calcium and low-magnesium diets also lead to an increase in magnesium excretion, further aggravating the antagonistic effects of these two elements.

SELECTED REFERENCES

Calcium

American Institute of Nutrition: Symposium on effects of high calcium intakes, Fed. Proc. **18:** 1075, 1959.

Council on Foods and Nutrition: Symposium on human calcium requirements, J.A.M.A. **185:**588, 1963.

Johnston, F. A.: The controversy regarding the calcium requirement, New York J. Med. **59:**3635, 1959.

Leitch, I., and Aitken, F. C.: An estimation of calcium requirement; a re-examination, Nutrition Abstr. & Rev. **29:**394, 1959.

Lutwak, L., and Whedon, G. D.: Osteoporosis—a disorder of mineral metabolism, Borden Rev. Nutr. Res. (23) 4:45, 1962.

Lutwak, L., and Whedon, G. D.: Osteoporosis—a mineral deficiency disease?, J. Am. Dietet. A. **44:**173, 1964.

Neuman, W. F., and Neuman, M. W.: Recent advances in bone growth and nutrition, Borden Rev. Nutr. Res. (21) 4:37, 1962.

Ohlson, M. A.: The calcium controversy, J. Am. Dietet. A. 31:333, 1955.

Thorangkul, D., Johnston, F. A., Kine, N. S., and Clark, S. J.: Adaptation to a low-calcium intake, J. Am. Dietet. A. 35:23, 1959.

WHO Technical Report Series No. 230: Calcium requirements, Geneva, 1962, World Health Organization.

Sodium

Block, M. R.: Social influence of salt, Scient. Am. 208:88-99, 1963.

Pike, R. L.: Sodium intake during pregnancy, J. Am. Dietet. A. 44:176, 1964.

Potassium

Darrow, D. C.: Physiological basis of potassium therapy, J.A.M.A. 162:1310-1315, 1956.

Magnesium

Council on Foods and Nutrition: Some inorganic elements in human nutrition, Symposium 1, Chicago, 1955, American Medical Association.

Hathaway, M. L.: Magnesium in human nutrition, Home Economics Research Report No. 19, Agricultural Research Service, Washington, D. C., 1962, U. S. Department of Agriculture.

Seelig, M. S.: The requirement of magnesium by the normal adult, Am. J. Clin. Nutrition 14:342, 1964.

Shils, M.: Experimental human magnesium depletion. I. Clinical observations and blood chemistry alterations, Am. J. Clin. Nutrition 15:133, 1964.

Wacker, E. C., and Vallee, B. L.: The magnesium deficiency tetany syndrome in man, Borden Rev. Nutr. Res. 22:51, 1961.

Wacker, E. C.: Magnesium metabolism, J. Am. Dietet. A. 44:362, 1964.

8

Micronutrient elements

IRON

The mineral element iron is present in relatively small amounts in the body but plays vital roles in human metabolism. The adult body contains 0.004% iron, representing a total amount of approximately 3 to 5 gm., the actual amount varying with age, sex, nutrition, general health, and size of iron stores. This amount is concentrated primarily in the blood, but some iron is present in every living cell of the body. The ability of iron to act as an oxygen carrier establishes its role in cellular respiration, during which oxygen must be made available for oxidative reactions necessary for life.

Distribution in the body

The distribution of iron throughout the body is shown in Table 8-1. Of the 3 to 5 gm. of iron in the human body 60% to 75% or 2 to 3 gm. is present in the iron-containing pigment of the blood, hemoglobin. Hemoglobin is a complex substance made up of the protein globin and the iron-containing substance, heme, in which iron

represents 3.4% of the molecule. Myoglobin, a similar iron-containing substance in muscle that differs from hemoglobin only in the nature of the protein portion, contains 3% of total body iron. The primary sites for iron storage—the liver, spleen, and bone marrow—contain 20% (0.5 to 2.5 gm.) of body iron. In the liver iron is present either as ferritin, a soluble iron-protein complex with 20% iron, or as hemosiderin, an insoluble iron-protein complex which contains up to 35% iron. The remaining 5% to 15% of body iron is found distributed as a respiratory substance throughout all living cells of the body where it is part of many enzymes—notably cytochrome and cytochrome oxidase involved in the release of energy from glucose and fatty acids in the cell mitochondrion. In addition to the iron in hemoglobin, the blood also contains about 4 mg. of iron which is present in the plasma as iron in transport, practically all of which is bound to the blood protein transferrin. Although the plasma contains a small amount of transport iron, the turnover is so rapid that about 35 to 40 mg. is

Table 8-1. Distribution of iron throughout body

	Percent	*Approximate amount in grams*
Hemoglobin	60% to 75%	2.0 to 3.0
Myoglobin	3%	0.1
Storage iron (liver, spleen, and bone marrow)	20%	0.5 to 1.5
Tissue iron	5% to 15%	0.300
Transport iron		0.004

exchanged each day. Women usually have a lower total iron content per unit of body weight than men.

Studies of iron metabolism have shown that the body is very efficient in its use of the mineral. Since there is no pathway for excreting iron, it is salvaged and reused when iron-containing substances wear out and are broken down. The residue is then either oxidized or excreted.

Function

Carrier of oxygen and carbon dioxide. The major function of iron in the body is as a carrier of oxygen. As part of the hemoglobin molecule it carries oxygen to the cells and as part of respiratory enzymes such as cytochrome oxidase, peroxidase, and catalase it makes the oxygen available in regulated amounts for the oxidation of glucose and fatty acids in the mitochondrion of the cell. Myoglobin within the muscle cells acts as a readily available source of oxygen for muscle contraction.

After releasing oxygen to the cells, iron-containing substances are capable of picking up carbon dioxide, a waste product of metabolism, and carrying it to the lungs to be excreted.

Red blood cell formation and metabolism. Over 60% of the body iron is contained in the hemoglobin molecule, which is the pigment in the red blood cells. The measurement of levels of hemoglobin in the blood is an easy and relatively sensitive indication of the state of iron nutrition. The red blood cells or erythrocytes are formed in the bone marrow where they begin as nucleated immature cells known as erythroblasts. The production of erythroblasts is stimulated when the oxygen-carrying capacity of the blood drops, creating a demand for more red blood cells signalled by the formation of *erythropoietin* by the kidney. As the erythroblasts mature in the bone marrow, heme, an iron-containing compound made from the amino acid glycine and iron, is synthesized in the presence of vitamin B_6. Heme unites with globin, a protein, made simultaneously from other amino acids, to form hemoglobin. These hemoglobin-containing immature red blood cells, known as reticulocytes, undergo loss of nucleus and are released into the bloodstream as mature unnucleated red blood cells capable of carrying oxygen to the tissues from the lungs and carbon dioxide from the tissues to the lungs. The iron in the hemoglobin is responsible for its ability to carry oxygen since it can be reversibly oxidized. Without a nucleus the red blood cells cannot synthesize new enzymes and so live only as long as the enzymes available at maturity last.

Normal adult male blood contains 15 gm. of hemoglobin per 100 ml. of blood, while women have 13.6 gm. as a standard. Thus the male body with a total blood volume of approximately 5 l. or 5000 ml. contains 750 gm. of hemoglobin into which has been incorporated about 2500 mg. of iron, since hemoglobin contains 3.4% iron. The red blood cells have a life expectancy of only 4 months or 120 days since they cannot live longer without a nucleus and must be replaced at that time. This involves the incorporation of 1/120 of the 2500 mg. or 20 mg. of iron into new red blood cells every day since approximately 1/120 of the red blood cells are destroyed every day. As the red blood cells die they are removed by the liver and bone marrow and by the spleen, which removes the iron and amino acids. The iron is returned to the iron pool in the bone marrow or to storage sites and the amino acids to the general circulation where they may be used again in the synthesis of protein or be deaminated in the liver and used as a source of energy. The dead erythrocytes are excreted in the bile. In this way the iron is not lost but is available to be reused in the synthesis of more hemoglobin in the bone marrow. The destruction of hemoglobin occurs at a slightly greater rate during sleep than during periods of activity.

The rate of destruction of red blood cells is faster when certain dietary deficiencies prevail, such as a lack of vitamin C, vitamin B_{12}, which leads to pernicious anemia, or vitamin E, which reduces with the stability of the cell membrane. All cause an accelerated rate of destruction of red blood cells, which in turn stimulates the bone marrow to produce mature red blood cells faster, at a rate that may reach six times normal.

Need for iron

Replacement of losses of body iron. Although the body avidly conserves the iron from the breakdown of hemoglobin there is still some loss of iron from the body. Since iron is present in all living cells of the body, when surface or epithelial cells die and desquamate or slough off from the surface of the body or into the gastrointestinal tract from its lining or when the hair or nails are cut, iron is lost. A small number of red blood cells find their way into the urine and into the gastrointestinal tract, from which they are lost in the feces. Other iron losses occur through perspiration. The fecal losses are estimated at 0.5 mg. per day, and the loss in urine, sweat, and desquamated cells amount to 0.2 to 0.5 mg. per day. These small losses of 0.7 to 1 mg. per day represent the only losses experienced by adult men. For women, however, there is need to replace the iron loss in menstruation where the amount varies widely from one individual to another with reported losses ranging from 2 to 32 mg. per month. The losses recorded for any one woman appear fairly consistent from one menstrual period to the next. If the average menstrual losses amount to 16 to 32 mg. of iron, representing an excretion of 0.5 to 1 mg. per day calculated over a 28-day menstrual cycle, women then need a dietary source of iron to replace 1.2 to 2 mg. of iron per day, a need almost twice that of men.

Growth. During growth there is an additional need for iron that has been difficult to assess quantitatively. The total increase in body iron from 0.5 gm. at birth to 5 gm. in the mature adult represents an accumulation of 4.5 gm. during the 20-year growth period. Assuming a uniform accretion of iron during this period, growth needs account for 225 mg. per year or 0.6 mg. of iron a day.

Iron needs are summarized in Table 8-2.

Absorption

Mechanism. Iron is obtained from food, where it occurs primarily in the oxidized form, ferric iron (Fe^{+++}), although some ferrous iron (Fe^{++}) has been found. Both

Table 8-2. Summary of iron requirements

Age group	Losses in feces	Losses in urine, perspiration, and desquamation	Needs for menstrua- tion	Needs for growth	Needs for pregnancy	Total needs
		Milligrams per day				
Adult men	0.5	0.2–0.5				0.7–1.0
Adult women	0.5	0.2–0.5	0.5–1.0			1.2–2.0
Pregnant women	0.5	0.2–0.5			1.0–2.0	1.7–3.0
Children	0.5	0.2–0.5		0.6		1.3–1.6
Adolescent girls	0.5	0.2–0.5	0.5–1.0	0.6		1.8–2.6

are attached to organic compounds from which they must be released before being absorbed. The body can utilize either form but evidence indicates that naturally occurring ferrous iron is used more efficiently than ferric iron and that most iron is reduced to ferrous iron before being absorbed. The absorption of iron occurs in regulated amounts in the upper part of the gastrointestinal tract, usually in the duodenum. Some is taken up in the stomach. The rapid rate of absorption has been indicated by studies with radioactive iron, which showed that significant amounts were absorbed within four hours after ingestion and appeared in the erythroblasts within 24 hours. Under most circumstances about 10% of the iron content of food is absorbed. The many factors which influence this will be discussed later.

Since the body has no mechanism for excreting iron, the iron content of the body is regulated through a controlled absorption. The exact nature of the mechanism is not too clear, but it now appears that dietary iron from the gastrointestinal tract passes into the epithelial or mucosal cells lining this area attached to a carrier substance such as the carbohydrates, fructose and sorbitol, or some amino acids. These substances are usually called chelating agents, and the combination with iron, iron chel-

ates. Within the epithelial cell the iron may remain attached to the carrier substance or be transferred to a larger molecule, apoferritin, as long as there is free apoferritin present within the epithelial cells. The combination of iron and apoferritin is known as ferritin, the form in which much iron is temporarily stored in the epithelial cells. The rate at which iron is released from the epithelial cell to the general circulation depends on the amount of a protein carrier substance transferrin or B-globulin in the blood. This substance, capable of binding two atoms of iron per molecule, is able to carry iron to the tissues, bone marrow, and storage sites. When transferrin is saturated up to about one third of its total iron-binding capacity, TIBC, no more is absorbed from the mucosal cells except under conditions of excessive intakes. However, whenever there is more of this unbound transferrin, the iron in the epithelial cell recombines with a carbohydrate or amino acid carrier to again form an iron chelate. This iron-containing complex passes from the epithelial cell into the blood plasma, where it releases its iron to transferrin. The uptake of iron from the intestinal tract apparently depends on the presence of a suitable carrier, and its release into the bloodstream is believed to be regulated by the amount of transferrin present. The total transferrin in the blood is usually capable of transporting 2 to 3 mg. at once. If the iron is needed it passes quickly into the bloodstream. If not needed it remains in the epithelial cells and will be lost from the body through fecal excretion when these cells die and slough off from the wall of the intestinal tract as they do at a rate of 50 to 80 gm. per day, as complete renewal of the lining of the gastrointestinal tract occurs in less than two days.

Factors affecting absorption

The body's need for iron. The need for iron is reflected in the unbound transferrin level of the blood. When this rises, indicating that iron has been removed from the blood to the tissues or storage sites, more iron is absorbed to maintain a constant level in the blood. When the transferrin is saturated with iron, representing a decreased demand for iron on the part of the body cells, less is absorbed. Thus the iron absorption mechanism responds to the body's need for iron. A person with normal hemoglobin levels absorbs from 2% to 20% of dietary iron. A person with low hemoglobin levels and probably high demands for iron may absorb as much as 60% of dietary iron. One study using the whole body counter for radioactive iron showed that iron-deficient subjects absorbed 29% of ingested iron while normal subjects absorbed 10%. Increased iron absorption is noted in the later half of pregnancy when the demands of the fetus on maternal iron are great for the estimated daily transfer of 3 to 4 mg. to the fetus. Children may also absorb iron at a rate up to twice that of adults.

Form of iron. Although the body can absorb both the reduced ferrous (Fe^{++}) and the oxidized ferric (Fe^{+++}) iron, absorption is greater when iron is available in the reduced ferrous form. The ferric iron that predominates in food is usually reduced to the ferrous form prior to absorption although during absorption it may be oxidized and reduced several times. The presence of any reducing substance such as acid is believed to enhance iron absorption. The hydrochloric acid secreted in the stomach keeps iron in the more readily available reduced form. Decreased iron utilization is sometimes noted in persons with a decreased secretion of hydrochloric acid in the stomach known as achlorhydria, often associated with increasing age or with the consumption of alkaline powders in large amounts, as by ulcer patients. The addition of hydrochloric acid to the diets of people suffering from achlorhydria had no beneficial effect on iron absorption, suggesting that the decreased hydrochloric acid secretion may well be a result of and not a cause of poor iron absorption. Organic acids in food such as ascorbic acid (vitamin C), found in citrus fruits, enhance iron absorption by helping reduce ferric to ferrous iron. It may play an important role in diets of older people where it may compensate for the reduced hydrochloric acid level. Since studies have shown that an increase in dietary vitamin C without an increase in iron is beneficial in iron-deficiency conditions, vitamin C is often included with iron supplements.

Bulk in diet. High bulk in the diet depresses the utilization of iron, which may account for the reports of poor absorption often noted from green leafy vegetables such as spinach. On the basis of this it has been suggested that iron supplements be taken before meals to minimize the interference the bulk of the diet may exert on iron absorption.

Size of dose. The percentage of absorption of iron varies inversely with the size of the dose. An intake of iron at a level of 0.25 mg. per kilogram of body weight resulted in 32% utilization whereas at an increased level of 4 mg. per kilogram only 4.1% was utilized. The administration of supplemental iron in smaller divided doses three or four times a day at a level commensurate with the body's ability to absorb it results in much better utilization than a single large dose.

Other factors. Phytic acid is an organic acid found in some whole-grain cereal products, such as oatmeal, which combines with iron to form an insoluble iron complex that the body cannot utilize. The presence of phytic acid is not a cause for concern in a normal mixed diet, but should oatmeal become a staple item in the diet, then the adverse effects of phytic acid on iron absorption might become significant. Excess phosphorus may also have an inhibitory effect on iron absorption.

Steatorrhea, an abnormal condition in which higher than normal amounts of fat appear in the feces, is associated with a decreased rate of iron absorption.

The altitude at which a person lives also influences extent of iron absorption. An increase occurs at high altitudes, while less is absorbed at lower altitudes.

Transportation and metabolism

Once iron has been absorbed from the epithelial cells into the blood it is carried throughout the body bound to the protein carrier transferrin. From the blood it may be removed by several pathways. In response to the demands of all body cells it will be released for use in the synthesis of respiratory enzymes and other vital cellular constituents that require iron. Much of the iron in transit in the blood plasma, which may come either from dietary sources, from the breakdown of body cells, and/or from the storage depots, will be removed by the bone marrow to be used in the manufacture of the hemoglobin for red blood cells. About 20 mg. of iron is used in the 7 to 8 gm. of hemoglobin liberated daily from the bone marrow in the newly formed red blood cells. Iron in excess of immediate needs of cells and bone marrow will be deposited in the iron storage depots of the body. Of approximately 1000 mg. (1 gm.) of iron stored in the body

at any one time 30% is in the liver, 30% in bone marrow, and the rest in the spleen and muscles.

On the other hand, if the dietary iron absorbed from the intestinal tract coupled with that obtained from the breakdown of red blood cells is not adequate to meet the needs of the bone marrow for hemoglobin synthesis and of other body cells for respiratory enzymes or cell growth, iron will be mobilized from the reserves in the liver, bound to transferrin in the blood, and recirculated throughout the body. Only when the body's reserves of iron have been depleted will there be any evidence of iron deficiency symptoms. In infants the liver stores are adequate to last three to six months. A reserve of 1000 mg. in the adult lasts a male 1000 days and a woman over 500 days. The absorption and metabolism of iron are summarized diagrammatically in Fig. 8-1.

Recommended dietary allowances

Adults. The National Research Council recommended allowances for iron for adults are based on the assumption that an adult male must obtain approximately 0.7 to 1 mg. of iron a day to replace body losses and the adult female 1.2 to 2 mg. per day. Since the average rate of iron absorption is 10% of ingested iron it has been recommended that men obtain 10 mg. and women 15 mg. from dietary sources. For women whose needs range from 1.2 to 2 mg. per day this represents a very narrow margin of safety and may actually fail to meet the needs of some women.

Pregnancy. During pregnancy the recommended intake remains unchanged because the elimination of menstrual losses counterbalances the demands of the fetus, which amount to approximately 400 mg. for a full-term infant. Iron is stored rapidly in fetal tissue during the latter half of pregnancy, when the fetus is parasitic on the mother for iron. Iron will be transferred to fetal blood in an irreversible

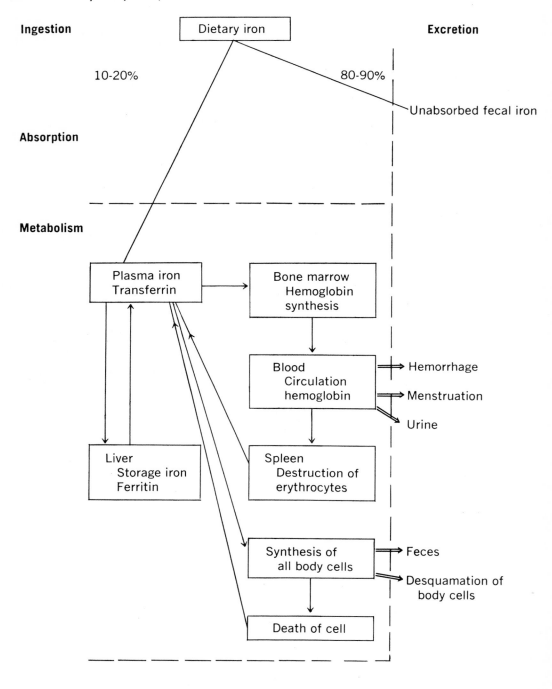

Fig. 8-1

Schematic representation of the absorption and metabolism of iron.

fashion even if the mother's hemoglobin levels drop. The apparent drop in hemoglobin levels of the mother during pregnancy often reflects an increase in blood volume rather than an absolute drop in the amount of hemoglobin. Twins who must share a maternal iron supply and premature infants who have been deprived of part of the period in utero of maximum transfer of iron to the fetus are usually born with hemoglobin levels below the normally high infant levels of 17 to 20 gm. per 100 ml. of blood. Since their reserve of iron is usually lower also, it may be necessary to supplement their diets with iron at an earlier age than for a full-term infant.

Lactation. Milk contains relatively little iron; thus the demands for iron during lactation are not increased above needs for pregnancy. Although human milk contains about 50% more iron than cow's milk, the addition of iron to the maternal diet has been ineffective in raising the amount transferred during lactation.

Infants and children. The reserve of iron in the liver of a full-term infant is sufficient to last from three to six months, during which time the infant doubles its birth weight. Thus the National Research Council sees no need to recommend a dietary source of iron other than milk until at least three months of age. The very high hemoglobin values of 17 to 20 gm. per 100 ml. of blood found in newborn infants drops rapidly to 12 gm. at four to six months of age, and is maintained close to this level throughout childhood and then rises in late adolescence to adult levels.

There is apparently no advantage in maintaining the high birth levels. In fact, attempts to supplement the infant diet to prevent this drop have been unsuccessful, since little iron is absorbed in early infancy unless there is a physiologic need for it. The current trend of adding iron to prepared infant formula is of limited usefulness until the infant has a need for a dietary source at about three months of age.

For infants over three months of age, dietary iron should be provided in adequate amounts to take care of the synthesis of hemoglobin required by the increasing blood volume and the demands of newly formed cells for iron. Needs of infants for dietary iron are greater per unit of body weight than are adult needs and remain relatively high during childhood. Recommended iron intakes then increase in proportion to the increase in body size up to physical maturity, after which iron is needed only for replacement of iron lost from the body.

Food sources

The iron content of some representative foods in the American diet is given in Fig. 8-2. Liver is the only very rich source of iron, and it is noted from Table 8-3 that there is quite a difference depending on the type of liver used. In any species the amount found in the liver will reflect the recent dietary intake of iron by the animal.

Since nutritionists have been only partially successful in increasing the popularity of liver in the American diet, most peo-

Table 8-3. Iron content of different types of cooked liver*

Liver	Milligrams of iron per 100 gm.
Chicken	8.5
Beef	8.8
Calf	14.2
Lamb	17.9
Pork	29.1

*From Watt, B., and Merrill, A.: Composition of foods—raw, processed and prepared, U. S. Department of Agriculture Handbook No. 8, Washington, D. C., 1963, U. S. Department of Agriculture.

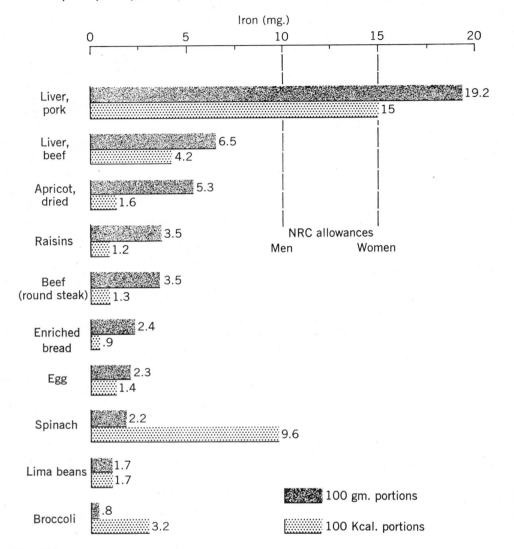

Fig. 8-2

Iron content of 100-gm. and 100-kilocalorie portions of representative foods. (Based on Watts, B., and Merrill, A.: Composition of foods—raw, processed and prepared, U. S. Department of Agriculture Handbook No. 8, Washington, D. C., 1963, U. S. Department of Agriculture.)

ple depend on other sources. As there are virtually no other very rich sources, a variety of moderately good sources must be combined to meet needs.

From Fig. 8-3, showing the contribution of various food groups to the day's iron intake, it is clear that no one group is responsible for a large share of the iron in the diet, but that the meat, cereal, and fruit and vegetable groups make comparable contributions.

Because of wide differences in the degree to which iron from various sources is absorbed, knowledge of the iron content of foods does not always give a true picture of its availability. There are difficulties in-

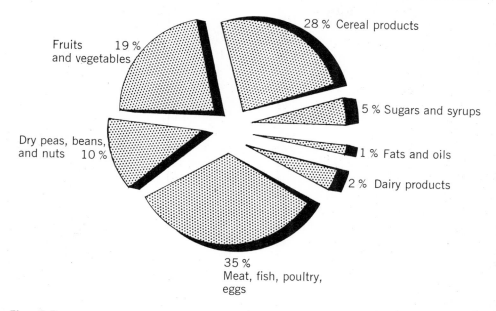

28 % Cereal products

Fruits 19 %
and vegetables

5 % Sugars and syrups

Dry peas, beans,
and nuts 10 %

1 % Fats and oils

2 % Dairy products

35 %
Meat, fish, poultry,
eggs

Fig. 8-3

Relative contribution of various food groups to total iron intake in the American food supply. (From Nutritive value of food available for consumption, United States, 1909-1964, Agricultural Research Service Publication 62-14, 1966.)

herent in the determination of the utilization of iron that make it very difficult to get agreement in data on iron absorption even with the use of radioactive isotopes of iron and even when balance studies are done with meticulous care. In all cases absorption by iron-deficient subjects averaged 20% while that from subjects with normal hemoglobin levels averaged 10%, but there is a wide range of values reported for each food tested.

The iron found in meat reflects the iron in both blood and muscle hemoglobin and is well absorbed. In eggs the iron is concentrated almost entirely in the yolk, but only about 4% is absorbed. The iron in chicken is very well absorbed, with values up to 30% reported.

Fruits and vegetables are fairly good sources of iron, but many times the bulk of the cellulose they also contain results in relatively poor utilization. The iron content of vegetables is influenced by soil and cli-

matic conditions so that there is a wide range of values reported for the same product. Vegetables provide about three times as much iron in the American diet as do fruits. Fruits and juices are rated as poor iron sources, potatoes and green stalks and leaves as good sources, and leguminous plants as excellent sources. Studies to determine the utilization of iron from various vegetable sources have not given consistent results. The pulp of fruits such as tomatoes and oranges contains twice as much iron as the juice. Occasionally canned fruits and vegetables or acid foods cooked in an iron container will pick up additional iron, which is equally as available as naturally occurring iron. Legumes such as peas and beans are relatively good sources especially when the dry mature seed, which has had a prolonged growing period during which to accumulate iron, is used.

Raisins and other dried fruits are often

recommended for their iron content. They will have no more iron than the original fruit from which they were derived. It should be remembered that the amount of dried fruit needed to make a significant contribution of iron also makes a significant contribution of calories. For instance, one fourth cup of raisins, which provides 1.4 mg. of iron, also provides 115 calories.

Cereals, either enriched or whole-grain, provide small amounts of iron per unit of weight, but because of the extent to which they may be consumed by certain groups, such as adolescent boys and families on restricted food budgets, they often make a significant contribution to the day's iron intake. For enriched bread, macaroni, and corn grits, for which enrichment standards have been set to provide a maximum as well as a minimum amount that can be added, the products contain slightly less iron than the whole-grain cereal from which they were derived. It is estimated that the use of enriched bread and cereals in place of refined cereals has increased the iron content of the diet by 14%. It makes little difference what form of iron salts are added. For other cereal products, however, iron can be added at any level within safe limits as long as the amount is declared on the label. Processors of such products as infant cereals and some prepared dried cereals have chosen to enrich their products at an extremely high level. This likely represents excessive enrichment for trade advantages with little benefit accruing to the consumer.

The only food group characterized as a poor source of iron is milk and milk products. The small amount of iron in milk is very well utilized but still makes an insignificant contribution to the total dietary intake.

Some food sources which are relatively rich in iron but which do not make a major contribution to the diet because of the infrequency with which they are consumed are oysters (6.3 mg. per serving), clams (6.1 mg.), and cocoa (1 mg. per tablespoon).

In some areas iron in the drinking water may be a significant source to the body, especially when iron values of water exceed 5 mg. per liter.

Blackstrap molasses, a by-product of the sugar-refining process, and so widely extolled by food faddists, contains about 2.5 mg. per tablespoon. Because of the bitter flavor of the product it is questionable if it can be considered a significant dietary item.

In 1959 the average per capita consumption of iron was placed at 16.3 mg. per day. Of all families 90% reported an intake of over 12 mg. per person per day and 42% reported over 20 mg. per day, indicating intakes capable of meeting the needs for most adults.

Effect of cooking. Loss of iron in cooking arises from loss by solution into cooking water, which is discarded, and the removal of peelings, with the loss of the iron concentrated near the skin. Any cooking method that minimizes the possibility of iron dissolving in the cooking water, such as the use of relatively large pieces of food, cooking with skins on, and the use of simmering rather than boiling water, will increase the amount of iron available in the diet. Steamed vegetables have more iron than boiled vegetables; those cooked for a short time in a small amount of water have more than those cooked in a large amount of water and for a longer period; and those cooked in their skins have more iron than peeled ones. The use of vegetable stock in soups or gravies also helps minimize iron losses.

Deficiencies

Since the body is so efficient in conserving iron supplies, simple iron deficiencies occur only during the growth period or when intake fails to meet needs following loss of blood from the body or in women who have experienced frequent pregnancies in rapid succession. *Anemia,* a condition in which there is a deficiency in the quantity and/or quality of the red blood cells, is the most common manifestation of iron deficiency.

Diagnosis. Anemia can be diagnosed by comparing blood hemoglobin levels measured as grams of hemoglobin per 100 ml. of blood and red blood cells counts measured as the number of red blood cells per cubic millimeter of blood to established standards. Standards for hemoglobin are 15 gm. of hemoglobin per 100 ml. of blood for men and 13.6 gm. for women. Clinical laboratories frequently report hemoglobin levels as a percentage of the standard. Thus a hemoglobin level of 90 means that the blood contained 90% of the standard, or, in the case of men, 90% of 15 gm. or 13.5 gm. Red blood cell standards are 5 million red blood cells per cubic milliliter of blood for men and 4.5 million for women. The total number of red blood cells in the body is so large that it defies comprehension—over 25 trillion. The number replaced every second is 2.5 million.

A third measurement, the color index, is useful in diagnosing the type of anemia. It involves the ratio of hemoglobin value expressed as a percentage of the standard to the red blood cell count expressed as a percentage of that standard. Thus:

$$\text{Color index} = \frac{\text{percent normal hemoglobin}}{\text{percent normal red cell count}}.$$

Under normal conditions the color index is approximately 1. A value of more than 1 indicates a deficiency in the number of red blood cells with normal amounts of hemoglobin; a value of less than 1 indicates a lack of hemoglobin in presence of an adequate number of cells.

Recent advances in techniques for measuring enzyme levels in living tissue have cast doubt on earlier beliefs that tissue respiratory enzymes had first call on iron reserves and that enzyme levels would drop only after a decrease in hemoglobin levels. There is now considerable evidence that the determination of tissue enzyme levels may be a valuable diagnostic tool in identifying iron deficiency in the absence of a drop in hemoglobin levels.

Anemia can be classified into two categories based on the underlying cause—nutritional and hemorrhagic.

Nutritional anemia. Nutritional anemia is caused by the absence of any dietary essential involved in hemoglobin formation or by poor absorption of these dietary components. The most likely causes are lack of dietary iron or high-quality protein. But anemias have been reported associated with a lack of pyridoxine (vitamin B_6), which catalyzes the synthesis of the heme portion of the hemoglobin molecule, of ascorbic acid, which influences the rate of iron absorption and the release of iron from transferrin to the tissues, and of vitamin E, which effects the stability of the red blood cell membrane. Experimentally the omission of copper from the diet causes low hemoglobin values. Copper is not part of the hemoglobin molecule but apparently facilitates its formation by influencing either the absorption of iron or its incorporation into a hemoglobin molecule.

Nutritional anemia is usually characterized as hypochromic and microcytic. This broad classification suggests a lack of the pigment hemoglobin and the presence of small cells. Failure of the cell to grow in the absence of hemoglobin synthesis produces the small cells. As a result nutritional anemia can be identified by a low color index and occurs primarily during the growth period where demands of growing cells and increased blood volume are not met by dietary intake of nutrients needed for hemoglobin synthesis. It is most pronounced in adolescent girls where the growth demands superimposed on the menstrual losses are difficult to meet by dietary means. This condition is sometimes described as *chlorosis* because of the greenish cast it gives the skin. A cursory diagnosis of hemoglobin status can often be made by a visual examination of the mucous membranes, especially on the underside of the eyelid or in the mouth, where the blood vessels are close to the epithelial surface. Pale membranes usually signify low hemoglobin values.

In adult men nutritional anemia is not very likely to develop once normal levels have been reached because of the minimal need for iron and the relatively large liver reserves. Even on a diet devoid of iron it would take over six years to deplete the liver reserves and cause a sufficiently large drop in hemoglobin values to lead to a diagnosis of anemia. In adult women a comparable situation could arise in four years.

Nutritional anemia does occur frequently in young infants who are maintained on a diet consisting solely of milk for a period of time exceeding the three- to six-month period during which fetal liver reserves are adequate. Infants utilize little dietary iron during the first four months of life, but after that the addition of enriched cereal, egg yolk, and meat to the infant's diet all provide good sources of iron. One study reported an incidence of anemia in 42% of breast-fed infants and 70% of bottle-fed infants at one year of age. Another study of nutritional intake of infants showed that unless the diet contained enriched cereals, it would fail to meet the recommended allowances for iron. Meat, fruits, and vegetables in the amounts consumed by these infants was not sufficient to meet the iron need without the use of cereal products.

Pernicious anemia. Pernicious anemia, a form of nutritional anemia in which the number of red blood cells and not the hemoglobin level is low, as shown by a high color index, is caused primarily by failure in the absorption of vitamin B_{12} or cobalamin rather than lack of a nutrient. It will be discussed in Chapter 12.

Hemorrhagic anemia. Hemorrhagic anemia is caused by an excessive loss of blood. This may occur following surgery, bleeding of wounds, internal hemorrhaging, excessive menstrual losses, blood donations, or in the presence of intestinal parasites. Following a blood loss the blood volume is restored almost immediately, followed by an increase in the number of red blood cells and finally by the restoration of hemoglobin levels. A low color index also prevails in hemorrhagic anemia.

With the loss of one pint of blood there is a loss of 250 mg. of iron. Even with the increased rate of iron absorption that occurs after blood loss, it takes at least 50 days to restore normal hemoglobin levels. This period may be reduced to 35 days if iron supplements and ascorbic acid are given. The wisdom of limiting blood donations to 4 to 6 pints per year, especially for women, is obvious.

Treatment. Where iron-deficiency anemia with its symptoms of pallor, easy fatigue, decreased resistance to infection, soreness in mouth, achlorhydria, and palpitation after exercise is diagnosed, the use of a diet high in iron-rich foods with a concurrent intake of appreciable amounts of ascorbic acid is indicated. The use of iron salts in therapeutic doses is likely justified to speed the restoration of hemoglobin levels to normal, and in many cases is the only way in which hemoglobin synthesis is adequately stimulated. Many iron salts, both organic and inorganic, such as ferrous gluconate, ferrous sulphate, ferrous citrate, ferric ammonium citrate, and ferrous fumarate, have been promoted by pharmaceutical firms. So far no preparation has been shown to be superior to ferrous sulphate, which contains 36% iron and is the least expensive of all these forms, costing from 1 to 15 cents per daily dosage. Therapeutic doses may contain as much as 250 mg. of iron, which may be absorbed at the rate of 150 mg. per day to bring about a maximum rate of increase in hemoglobin levels of 0.3 gm. per day. To provide this level of iron, it takes 0.8 gm. of ferrous sulphate or 1.2 gm. of ferrous gluconate. It is wise to build up therapeutic dosages slowly to develop a gradual tolerance to the iron and prevent gastrointestinal upsets. Once normal hemoglobin levels are reached the continued use of iron salts is not justified from either a nutritional or an economic point of view.

Excess

The theory that the absorption of iron was regulated in the intestinal mucosa suggested that the uptake of excess iron was impossible. This theory was questioned when it was reported that an African tribe, the Bantu, suffered from siderosis or hemochromatosis, a disease in which the iron reserves were found to be up to thirty times the normal 1-gm. reserve. The source of their iron, which amounted to 200 mg. per day, is thought to be the kettles in which the large amounts of beer they consume are fermented. An excess absorption as small as 3 mg. per day will result in 1 mg. of storage iron per day, which can accumulate to a sizeable amount over a period of years. A similar iron toxicity has been reported among persons who are overzealous in their use of therapeutic iron so readily available on the open shelves in drugstores. There are many reports of ferrous sulphate toxicity in infants who have had 3 to 10 gm. of ferrous sulphate.

In siderosis, iron increased in the mitochondria of cells, reflecting increased tissue iron; serum iron increased, and the bone marrow became hyperplastic. The failure of the absorption mechanism to regulate iron absorption occurs at very high levels of iron intake. Under these circumstances the transferrin of blood is saturated at three times its normal level and is incapable of binding all the absorbed iron in a harmless complex.

Some evidence of iron overload has been noted in persons who have had successive blood transfusions. Even although the transfused blood is providing iron, they continue to absorb iron in a manner characteristic of an iron-deficient individual.

IODINE

Distribution. The essential trace mineral element, iodine, is present in the body in very minute amounts, about 0.00004% of body weight, which amounts to 15 to 23 mg. in a healthy human adult. Like iron, iodine is present in every living cell of the body with 70% to 80% or about 10 mg. concentrated in a single tissue, the thyroid gland. The level of iodine in the thyroid gland is twenty times that of the blood that supplies it. The thyroid gland is a tissue consisting of two lobes or parts located in the neck on either side of the trachea just below the larynx and weighing about 25 gm. or 0.2% of body weight. The two sides of the thyroid gland are joined by a thin strip of tissue sometimes called the thyroid isthmus. Bile, hair, ovaries, and skeletal muscle rank next on the basis of the concentration of iodine they contain.

Our knowledge of iodine metabolism has been advanced recently with the use of radioactive isotopes of iodine, especially I^{131}, and the development of analytical methods sufficiently sensitive to determine the minute amounts of this element found in biological material.

Absorption

Iodine occurs in food primarily in the reduced iodide form but also as inorganic iodine or as an organically bound iodine complex. The latter is freed from its organic component, and the free iodine reduced to iodide before absorption. Inorganic iodide is absorbed in all parts of the gastrointestinal tract but primarily in the small intestine. Some organically bound iodine is not absorbed and may be excreted in the feces, but it represents a maximum of 2% of ingested iodine. Iodine may also be absorbed through epithelial cells of skin.

Once absorbed the iodine appears immediately in the bloodstream where it constitutes the major part of the "iodide pool"—all extracellular iodide. About 30% of the iodide in the blood plasma is absorbed by the thyroid gland, where the concentration is about twenty times that in the plasma, and the rest taken up by the kidney and excreted in the urine. The excretion of iodine not used by the thyroid gland provides a protection against toxic levels in other tissues.

Metabolism

The iodine picked up or "trapped" by the thyroid gland is immediately oxidized to iodine within the thyroid gland. In this form one or two molecules unite with the amino acid tyrosine, which is attached to thyroglobulin, a mucoprotein rich in this amino acid, and leucine, which is present in the center cells of the thyroid gland. The iodated tyrosine molecules unite to form either thyroxine with four atoms of iodine or thyronine with three atoms of iodine. These active hormones are released from thyroglobulin by a protein-splitting enzyme and enter the circulation. Thyronine is a much more active form of the hormone than thyroxine but is present in relatively small amounts in the blood. There is some evidence that once thyroxine enters the individual cell it becomes deiodated by the removal of one atom of iodine to form the more active thyronine with three atoms of iodine.

Function

Part of thyroxine. As part of the thyroid hormone, thyroxine, secreted into the circulating plasma iodine, plays a major role in regulating the growth and development of the organism and its rate of metabolism. The stimulating effect of thyroxine on metabolism can be appreciable, with the effects of a single dose persisting for six days

or more. When the rate of metabolism increases, more oxygen is used up by the cells, indicating that more energy is being released from glucose and fatty acids to take care of the needs of the more active cells.

Although most attention has been focused on the role of thyroxine in energy metabolism an increasing number of direct and indirect effects of thyroxine in metabolic functions are becoming apparent. The conversion of carotene, the precursor of vitamin A, to the active form of the vitamin, the synthesis of protein by ribosomes, and the absorption of carbohydrate from the intestine are more efficient when thyroxine production is normal. The synthesis of cholesterol is influenced by thyroxine levels with above-normal cholesterol levels occurring in hypothyroidism and below-normal levels in hyperthyroidism.

Secondary to the effect of thyroxine in stimulating metabolism is its effect on nitrogen excretion. When energy needs increase, more of the calories from protein must be used as a source of energy rather than for growth or maintenance of tissue, leading to increased loss of nitrogen from the body. The rapid breakdown of body tissue that occurs with protein catabolism leads to extreme body weakness that can be attributed to the loss of potassium and hence sodium that accompanies protein loss. If food intake is not increased to take care of increased energy expenditure body reserves of protein and fat will be depleted to meet the need with a resultant loss of weight. Before the Food and Drug Administration ruled that thyroxine preparations would be available through prescriptions only, unscrupulous peddlers of weight-reducing aids were incorporating thyroid extract on the theory that they facilitated weight loss. They do indeed, but the undesirable side effects that accompany their uncontrolled use make such a practice potentially hazardous.

Since the only known function of iodine

is in thyroxine formation much of the discussion of iodine metabolism and needs centers around the activity of thyroxine and the thyroid gland.

Requirements

The Food and Nutrition Board of the National Research Council has suggested that an intake of 1 μg. of iodine per kilogram of body weight is adequate for most adults. To assure a margin of safety to take care of individual variations they recommend a daily intake of 100 to 150 μg. per day. For pregnant and lactating women the need is higher. If, as is often recommended, the salt intake is restricted during pregnancy, eliminating a major source of iodine in the diet, precautions should be taken to see that sufficient iodine is available from other sources.

The need for growing children, especially girls, may exceed the suggested level of 1 μg. per kilogram of body weight.

Food sources

Both food and water provide iodine in the human diet. The amount present in the water varies from one area to another and tends to parallel the iodine content of the soil. Iodine contents of less than 2 μg. per liter are associated with iodine-deficiency conditions and those of 2 to 15 μg. with the absence of iodine deficiency. In the United States the iodine content of the water varies from 0.01 to 73 ppm.

Seafoods such as lobster, shrimp, and oysters are among the richest dietary sources, but because of the relatively minor role they play in the diet, except among people living in coastal regions, they do not make a major contribution to the iodine content of many diets. Salt-water fish contain 300 to 3,000 μg. of iodine per kilogram of flesh compared to 20 to 40 μg. in fresh-water fish. Fresh river water contains 0.5 to 2 μg. per liter; sea water contains 17 to 50 μg. Salt-water fish have an amazing capacity to concentrate this rela-

tively small amount of iodine within their tissue.

The amount of iodine in dairy products and eggs is extremely variable and reflects the iodine content of the soil on which the rations of the animals have been grown and the season of the year. The iodine content of milk rapidly reflects addition of iodine to the cow's diet. Most cereal grains, legumes, fruits, and vegetables are low in iodine content, but they fluctuate with the iodine content of the soil in which they were grown. In general the leaves of plants have higher iodine concentrations than the roots. Spinach leaves are especially concentrated and have the highest iodine content of all plants. Corn is extremely low in iodine, which may make corn-eating people more susceptible to iodine deficiency conditions.

The variation in iodine content of vegetables from various sources can be illustrated by values of 240, 407, and 1283 μg. per kilogram of dry weight of carrots grown in Florida, Oklahoma, and Louisiana respectively. Modern marketing practices in which the food supply of any one community comes from widely separated geographical areas have done much to assure a more uniform and more nearly adequate level of iodine for the average American.

The use of iodized salt in cooking has proven the most effective method of assuring sufficient iodine in the diet. It is added to salt as potassium iodide at a level of 100 mg. per kilogram or 1 part per 10,000 parts of salt, a level established to be completely safe and yet valuable in combatting goiter. This provides the person who consumes 6 gm. of table salt with 500 μg. per day. Some countries, such as Canada, Guatemala, and Colombia, have passed legislation to require the iodization of salt at 1 part iodine to 10,000 parts salt. In Europe 1 part iodine to 100,000 parts salt is used. Mandatory iodization has been recommended by the Food and Nutrition Board in the United States, but currently it is a voluntary measure on the part of the salt producers, who must comply only with the labelling requirements of the Food and Drug Administration. Currently only half of the salt sold in the United States is iodized, although 75% of all families report using it and only 4% say they never use it. A more stable iodate may replace potassium iodide as the enrichment agent, especially in countries where salt is moist, making iodide unstable.

Other methods of increasing the iodine intake of population groups in low-iodine areas have met with varying degrees of success. The addition of iodine to water supplies has been abandoned because of its failure to benefit people in rural areas and others with private water supplies. Iodized tablets or candies are rarely satisfactory even though they provide measured amounts of iodine because they depend on complete cooperation of a number of people. Where little baking of bread at home is done and where bread is a staple in the diet, the use of iodized salt in bread has been fairly effective.

In countries such as Japan where seaweed, which has a capacity to concentrate iodine from sea water, is consumed as a regular dietary item, it is a major source of iodine, containing 0.4% to 0.6% iodine on a dry weight basis. The value of recommending seaweed for use in a culture unaccustomed to its use is doubtful.

One of the few studies based on the chemical analysis of iodine content of American diets showed intakes varying from 65 to 529 μg. per day, the principal contribution being from vegetables and dairy products.

EVALUATION OF NUTRITIONAL STATUS

Since the dietary intake of iodine includes that in water as well as in food, the difficulties in conducting iodine balance studies to assess iodine nutriture are greater than for other nutrients that are provided only by food. In order to obtain some assessment of the adequacy of iodine nutrition, use has been made of the determination of the iodine excretion in a single sample of urine in relation to the amount of creatinine excreted. In areas where available iodine is low there is an excretion of from 25 μg. of iodine per gram of creatinine whereas in areas of high available iodine the excretion was at least 50 μg., indicating a daily intake of at least 50 μg. Some excretion rates were as high as 1000 μg. per gram of creatinine.

Thyroxine

Since most of the iodine in the body is used in thyroxine synthesis, a convenient way to study iodine metabolism is to study thyroxine metabolism.

Measurement. The rate of thyroxine production can be measured in several ways. The basal metabolic rate as determined by indirect calorimetry (described in Chapter 5) is closely related to the level of thyroxine production. A basal metabolic rate elevated at least 15% above the level predicted in the basis of body surface area or metabolic body size indicates a state of hyperthyroidism, an excess production of thyroxine. On the other hand, a depressed basal metabolic rate reflects a state of hypothyroidism, a decreased rate of thyroxine production.

More recently a simpler, less costly method of assessing thyroxine level, the protein-bound iodine (PBI) test on less than 1 ml. of blood, has been developed. This method has an advantage over basal metabolism in that it is not influenced by previous meals or activity and is less costly. There is a positive relationship between the amount of iodine bound to protein circulating in the blood and the level of thyroxine produced, since 90% of the protein-bound iodine is in thyroxine, which is 65% iodine by weight. Normally PBI levels are 4 to 8 μg. per 100 ml. of blood. PBI blood levels above 11 μg. per 100 ml. are indicative of hyperthyroidism and levels below 3 μg. of hypothyroidism. It is not possible to calculate the exact extent to which energy needs are increased using this method, but the relative level of metabolism can be determined.

Radioactive isotopes have proven useful in assessing the state of thyroxine production. Radioactive iodine is administered orally. The amount taken up by the thyroid gland is determined by measuring the radioactivity in the neck region and that taken up by other tissues by a radioactivity reading in the thigh area. In hyperthyroidism there is a very rapid uptake of iodine by the thyroid followed by a gradual drop after 24 hours. Under conditions of normal thyroid function the uptake of radioactive iodine is gradual. In hypothyroidism the rate of uptake is rapid, and the iodine remains in the thyroid gland for much longer periods.

Regulation. The functioning of the thyroid gland is controlled by a thyroid-stimulating hormone (TSH) secreted by the pituitary gland when the level of thyroxine in the blood drops. This in turn is a response to the availability of iodine for thyroxine synthesis. There are many factors that may influence the amount of TSH produced and hence the activity of the thyroid gland. When dietary iodine falls below 20 μg., which is inadequate for sufficient thyroxine synthesis, more TSH is produced. This leads to hypertrophy or increase in size of the thyroid gland, known as simple goiter, in which both the size and number of thyroid cells increase.

Several antithyroid drugs have much the same effect in stimulating TSH production by inhibiting thyroxine formation. They may either interfere with the ability of the thyroid gland to trap iodine, block the oxidation of iodide to iodine, or block the organic binding of iodine. In any case, drugs such as thiourea or thiouracil stimulate the pituitary gland to secrete more thyroid-stimulating hormone. Thiocyanates used in the treatment of hypertension inhibit the ability of the thyroid gland to concentrate iodine and so increase the work involved in producing thyroxine.

Certain foods contain substances called goitrogens because their presence predisposes a person to the iodine-deficiency disease goiter. They act in much the same way as the antithyroid drugs blocking the absorption or utilization of iodine. Foods of the cabbage family, such as rutabagas, turnips, and cabbage, contain a heat-stable substance, *pregoitren,* and a heat-labile activator that converts pregoitren to goitren. In raw foods the goitren that interferes with iodine utilization is formed; in cooked foods the conversion cannot take place unless an activator is formed by bacterial synthesis. There is increasing evidence of the presence of such an enzyme in the gastrointestinal tract, which means that the pregoitren in cooked foods may also be converted to a goitren.

Ground nuts contain a substance, *arachidoside,* that also interferes with iodine utilization. The presence of this substance is one of the drawbacks to the use of nuts to improve the protein quality of the diet in areas where the diet consists of low-quality protein.

Sulphonamides, widely used antibiotics that reduce the conversion of iodide to iodine, are potentially goitrogenic but at the levels used in treating infection have little effect on thyroid activity. The extensive use of the vitamin-like substance para-amino benzoic acid (PABA) has a similar effect. There is some evidence also to support the theory that a high-calcium diet may be goitrogenic. A diet very high in iodine may also be goitrogenic by limiting iodine absorption.

The salivary gland may play a role in regulating the level of thyroxine in the blood. It has the capacity to remove iodine (deiodate) from thyroxine thus inactivating it. The iodine is secreted in the saliva and can be reabsorbed in the gastrointestinal tract.

Goiter

In 1920 iodine was recognized as an effective agent in the treatment of simple goiter, a condition in which the thyroid gland enlarges and causes a swelling in the throat, an effect evident from a profile view. A deficiency of iodine is the primary but not the only cause of simple goiter. Goiter may also be caused by factors that interfere with the availability of dietary iodine, impose abnormal demands on the thyroid gland, or interfere with the utilization of iodine by the thyroid. These interfering substances include chemicals naturally present in some foods or purposely introduced for therapeutic reasons or defects in an enzyme system necessary for the synthesis and release of thyroxine. In these cases the thyroid gland enlarges to compensate for the lack of iodine needed for its normal functioning. Of the estimated 200 million cases of simple goiter in the world today, the majority are caused by a

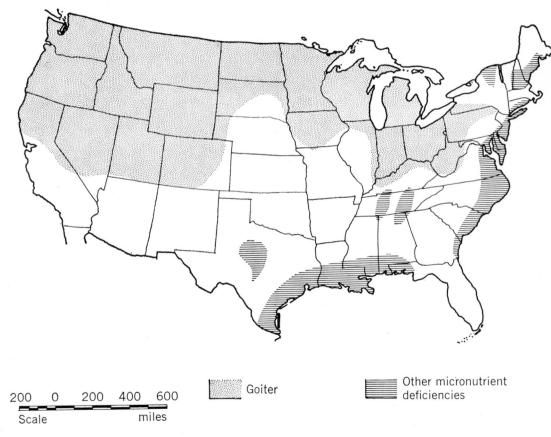

200 0 200 400 600
Scale   miles

Goiter

Other micronutrient deficiencies

Fig. 8-4

Distribution of micronutrient element deficiencies in the soil in the United States. Some other micronutrient deficiencies also occur in scattered parts of goitrous areas. (Adapted from Beesom, K. C.: The relation of soils to the micronutrient element content of plants and to animal nutrition. In Lamb, C. A., Bentley, O. G., and Blathic, J. M.: Trace elements, New York, 1958, Academic Press Inc.)

dietary lack of iodine and tend to occur in definite geographic regions.

Incidence. It has been established that the incidence of goiter is regional, occurring primarily in areas where the soil is of glacial origin or where flooding or tropical rains have leached the iodine from the soil. It is nonexistent in areas when iodine-laden vapors from the sea condense and deposit iodine on the soil. As shown in Fig. 8-4, in the United States areas of highest incidence are the areas bordering the Great Lakes—Michigan, Wisconsin, and Ohio—and the Rocky Mountain states. Coastal areas are relatively free of the condition, as are the southern states. Studies of the iodine content of the soils and water supplies of goitrous areas showed a very low concentration. Since simple goiter is not an incapacitating disease and in its early stages is a problem merely from an aesthetic point of view, people suffering from the condition were not motivated to seek medical help. Consequently little at-

tention was paid to the disease. The increasing incidence reported by 1915 led to the first large-scale study on the control of goiter in human beings in Ohio from 1916 to 1920. There the addition of iodine tablets to the water supply twice a year effectively reduced the incidence of goiter in adolescent girls, the group most susceptible to the disease. Other methods have been tried, such as feeding iodized salt to cows to increase the iodine content of their diet in an effort to increase the amount appearing in the milk, and the iodization of the water supply and the iodization of salt. Of these, only the iodization of salt proved an effective method for reaching the majority of the population. The cost of adding iodine to the salt supply is so small that in most cases the manufacturers absorbed the cost.

In Michigan, where goiter among 47% of school children in 1921 constituted a major public health problem, an intensive educational campaign to promote the use of iodized salt was launched. The results were

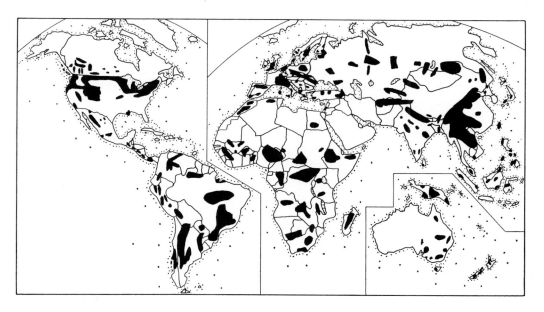

Fig. 8-5
Goiter areas of the world.

very encouraging. By 1925, the incidence had dropped to 32% and by 1951 only 1% of the population had simple goiter. Michigan's experience, however, has shown that it is necessary to maintain the educational program to keep the condition under control since a letup in their educational efforts in 1951 resulted in a temporary increase.

The incidence of goiter is about six times as high in females as males, and the most susceptible groups are adolescent girls and pregnant women.

The distribution of goiter areas in the world is shown in Fig. 8-5.

Treatment. Most goiters respond to iodine therapy, and it is now obvious that the effective agent in the successful use of sponges in treating goiter, reported as early as 1280, was iodine. The use of iodine salts in the treatment of goiter was recognized as early as 1820, although it was ten years later before it was suggested that a lack of iodine in the diet might be a cause of simple goiter. Thirty years later the lack of iodine was associated with low iodine levels in the soil and water but the suggestion of the French botanist Chatin that iodine be added to water in areas where there was an occurrence of goiter was not then accepted. However, toward the turn of the century when it was shown that iodine was a normal constituent of the thyroid gland and that the normal levels of 10 to 15 mg. drop as low as 1 mg. in endemic goiter, there was a renewed interest in the use of iodine therapy in the treatment of goiter. Several investigations confirmed that endemic goiter was primarily the result of an iodine deficiency and could be controlled by raising dietary iodine intakes.

The most effective method is one of prevention, and the use of iodized salt has proven most useful in controlling the incidence of goiter. Simple goiter is a painless condition that has some undesirable effects on physical appearance, since once a simple goiter is formed in an adult it cannot be reduced in size with iodine therapy. If the simple goiter continues to grow, the hazards increase until there is danger of blocking off the trachea due to pressure from the growth of thyroid tissue on either side. Under these circumstances treatment involves thyroidectomy, the surgical removal of part of the thyroid gland, an operation complicated by the fact that the parathyroid gland so vital in the control of calcium metabolism is embedded in the surface of the thyroid gland. Ligating (or tying off of an artery leading to the thyroid) has occasionally been effective in controlling the growth of the gland.

Other abnormalities of iodine metabolism

Among children born to mothers who have had a limited iodine intake during adolescence and pregnancy and who live in areas when iodine deficiency has prevailed for years and where goiter is endemic, the condition cretinism is frequently encountered. Cretins who suffer from hypothyroidism are physically dwarfed, mentally retarded, and have enlarged protruding abdomens. If treatment is started soon after birth many of the symptoms of cretinism are reversible, but if the conditions persist beyond early childhood permanent mental and physical retardation cannot be prevented.

Adults who have had symptoms of hypothyroidism throughout their developmental period suffer from myxedema. These people have coarse sparse hair, dry yellowish skin, a poor tolerance for cold, and a low husky voice.

Both cretinism and myxedema are still found but the use of iodized salt has greatly reduced the incidence in countries such as Switzerland where the soil and water is extremely low in iodine. A similar program in the Andes would undoubtedly lower the incidence in this mountainous low-iodine area.

Hyperthyroidism in which the basal metabolic rate may be elevated as much as 100% above normal is also known as Grave's disease and exophthalmic goiter. Persons suffering from the overactivity of the thyroid gland experience nervousness, weight loss, increased appetite, intolerance to heat, tremors when the hand is outstretched, and protruding eyeballs. The increased rate of metabolism that accompanies increased thyroxine production puts an increased load on the cardiovascular system.

OTHER MICRONUTRIENT ELEMENTS
Essentiality

In addition to the seven macronutrient elements discussed in the previous chapter and the micronutrient elements iron and iodine discussed in this chapter there are six other mineral elements present in the body in small and variable amounts which have been shown to play an essential role in metabolism in human beings.

A trace element is considered essential when there is a repeated demonstration of a significant growth response to dietary supplements of this element alone, the development of a deficiency state on diets otherwise adequate and a correlation of the deficiency state with the occurence of suboptimal levels of the element in the blood or tissues of animals.

Seven others whose essential nature has not yet been established on the basis of these criteria may perform some functions similar to those deemed essential. Because some aspects of metabolism are common to many of them they will be discussed as a group, followed by a brief discussion of unique aspects of several of them.

The use of the term *trace elements* to describe this group is unfortunate since it may imply a lack of nutritional importance. Its use stems from the era when analytical techniques were sufficiently sensitive to detect their presence but not able to measure the minute amounts needed. The extremely small concentrations at which these elements are functional is illustrated by the fact that one atom in 10 million is active. The occurrence of micronutrient element deficiencies in the United States is shown in Fig. 8-4.

Role in body

The small amounts needed bear no relationship to importance; a lack of one of these micronutrients can be equally as serious as the lack of one needed at a level many hundreds of times higher. Some are catalysts to biological reactions acting as a link between the enzyme and its substrate, others are part of essential body compounds such as hormones and enzymes, and others are incorporated in the growth of tissue.

Because of the varied geographical sources of food in the average diet and the fact that the amount of these micronutrient elements present in food is a function of the soil on which they are grown there is virtually no evidence of dietary deficiencies of these nutrients. In fact it has been impossible to purify experimental diets to the point where an inadequate level of one nutrient and an adequate amount of all others is present. As a result most of our evidence of the biological role of trace elements has been the result of animal studies in which the source of food has been from a geographically restricted area where a deficiency of the element in the soil is reflected in a very limited amount in the crops grown on these soils. Once the role of the nutrient has been elucidated in animals it has often been possible to demonstrate a similar function in human nutrition. Frequently it is necessary to interfere with the absorption of an element as well as eliminate it from the diet for long periods to demonstrate a deficiency.

Interrelationships

One of the major difficulties in acquiring precise information on the function of many mineral elements has been the extent to which the presence or absence of one element may influence the role of a second and modify the requirement of another.

The interactions between minerals may occur in the diet, in the intestine, at the sites of excretion in the kidney, intestine, or lungs and at specific sites within the body cells.

As an example of interrelationships it may be noted that an increase in the molybdenum content of the diet without a simultaneous increase in the copper or sulphate content results in depressed growth and restricted hemoglobin production. The copper-molybdenum antagonism is apparently reciprocal. As further examples, increased copper interferes with iron and zinc metabolism, high manganese affects iron metabolism, and excess cobalt interferes with the synthesis of the iodine-containing hormone thyroxine. Zinc-deficiency symptoms can be precipitated by diets high in calcium and low in zinc and relieved by correcting the imbalance. The fact that abnormally high levels of some elements can displace other elements that are essential parts of enzymes can lead to the replacement of a biologically active enzyme with one that is not only inactive itself but one that may block the use of the effective one. The utilization of one mineral element can be evaluated only in light of the availability and utilization of other nutrients with which it may have a close metabolic interrelationship.

The ability of one element to replace another in key compounds is one of the hazards of some of the multimineral supplements on the commercial market. Too often the basis of the formula is maximum profit to the promoter rather than any consideration of the nutritional needs of the individual. Unbalanced mineral supplements are potentially harmful. The Food and Drug Administration suggests that calcium, iron, and iodine are the only mineral elements that can be justified in dietary supplements.

Because of the complexities of the interrelationships among trace mineral elements it is necessary to assess the whole nutritional environment in studies of deficiency, toxicity, or requirements. Simple and uncomplicated deficiencies of single micronutrient elements seldom occur under normal conditions.

Toxicity

Some trace mineral elements essential in small amounts may be toxic when present at high levels. Most of the cases of toxicity from trace minerals have been the result of exposure to an environment saturated with the element since minerals can enter the body through the respiratory tract and the skin as well as through the gastrointestinal tract. The manganese and selenium toxicity found among miners is believed to be caused by aspiration of air containing above normal concentrations of the element. Fluoride toxicity, which takes the form of a dental fluorosis or mottled enamel, is the result of ingesting large quantities of water containing over 2.5 ppm of naturally occurring fluoride.

Selenium poisoning in animals is common in areas where the selenium content of the soil is high. High urinary levels are found in humans in the same area although there is no definite evidence of selenium poisoning in man.

Deficiencies

Deficiencies of most trace mineral elements become evident only after prolonged dietary inadequacies and then usually only when associated with some defect in absorption and a change in other dietary components that leads to increased need. Usually the first evidence of an inadequacy appears in a reduction of enzymes of which the mineral is an essential part or a reduction in the activity of enzymes that are catalyzed by the element. Changes in blood levels of trace elements usually reflect the level of body stores rather than dietary intake as body stores will be mobilized to maintain blood and tissue levels in the event of a dietary deficiency. Only when these are depleted will blood levels drop.

Human requirements

The human requirements for most of the trace mineral elements has not been established. Their widespread presence in foods, the minute amounts involved, the absence of any deficiency states that can be attributed directly to the lack of the nutrient, and the interrelationships among trace elements has made the assessment of dietary needs impossible with the techniques currently available. In addition modification of the level of other elements of the diet such as protein may influence the amount of the element needed.

Food sources

The amount present in vegetable foods is primarily a function of the amount present in the soils in which the crops were grown. In the case of animal foods, the amount of some elements reflects the diet of the animal while for others the animal may regulate the amount present in its tissue. In any case the ultimate source of the mineral content of food is the soil. The possibility of a trace mineral element deficiency is greatly reduced with modern marketing techniques that lead to the consumption of a diet from widely scattered areas rather than from a restricted geographical region. Some mineral elements are also introduced into foods through contamination during processing.

Milk is a relatively poor source of most micronutrient elements. This may be one reason to suggest the introduction of a wider variety of foods into the infant's diet after three or four months.

ZINC

Zinc has been recognized as an essential for fungi growth for almost 100 years and for rat growth since 1934, but only in the last five years have we had evidence that a suboptimal intake of zinc by humans may

well be a cause of growth retardation. A recent review suggests that either a low dietary intake of zinc or a defect in its absorption and utilization may be a cause of retarded physical development in the United States. In animals retardation of growth may precede a drop in the activity of enzymes of which it is a part. Related to its effect in growth may be its role in the absorption and utilization of thiamine, which is impaired in a zinc deficiency.

Biological roles

Zinc is important as the metal constituent of many enzymes involved in digestion and metabolism. Among these is carbonic anhydrase, which contains 0.33% zinc and which is necessary in many body reactions requiring the addition or transfer of carbon dioxide. This enzyme is vital in respiration. In addition it acts as an activator of many other enzymes especially those involved in protein metabolism.

Zinc is normally associated with the hormone insulin secreted by the pancreas and necessary for carbohydrate metabolism. Since it is possible to produce an active zinc-free insulin it is suggested that it is not an essential part of the insulin molecule but may help to hold or bind it in the pancreas until needed.

There is some evidence that zinc, like many other mineral elements, plays a role in the contraction and relaxation of muscles.

Distribution in the body

Zinc is widely distributed in the body, which contains about 2 gm. The high concentrations found in the hair, skin, nails, and testes suggests a special function for zinc in these tissues. The highest concentrations occur in the retina of the eye, but so far we have no explanation for this.

In the blood 85% of the zinc appears in the red blood cells with the remaining 15% occurring in the serum. The serum levels decrease in infection, pernicious anemia, hyperthyroidism, and liver cirrhosis from normal levels of 120 mg. per 100 ml. to 70, the loss being reflected by increased urinary excretion.

Requirement

The body's need for zinc appears to be met by intakes of 0.3 to 0.6 mg. per kilogram of body weight, but the requirements increase with an increase in dietary protein. High calcium levels depress the absorption of zinc necessitating higher dietary levels.

Food sources

The zinc content of the diet varies but most provide 10 to 15 mg. per day. Diets high in protein and whole-grain products are usually higher. The zinc content of some representative foods is shown in Table 8-4. The zinc content of plant protein such as soybean or sesame oil meal is less available than that in the animal protein casein. Phytic acid depresses the absorption of zinc, as shown by an increase in the excretion in the feces.

The zinc concentration of human milk is 20 mg. per liter, but drops to 0.65 mg. per liter at six months. This is less than the level in cow's milk.

Toxicity

Toxicity from excessive intakes of zinc that may occur when galvanized utensils are used in processing of acid foods or when carbonated beverages are sold in metal containers has been reported. Among the metabolic changes are a loss of iron from the liver which may amount to 50% in three days, followed by a loss of copper much later. Both of these changes are reflected in anemia.

SELENIUM
Biological role

Recent interest in selenium stems from the recognition in 1957 of its ability to replace vitamin E in some metabolic reactions, such as those dependent on its antioxidant properties. In addition to replacing vitamin E in these reactions, selenium acts with vitamin E in preventing certain conditions and under some circumstances, such as promoting normal growth and fertility, has very specific functions of its own. Within the body the liver and kidney contain four to five times as much selenium as muscles and other tissues.

In a study of dental caries in children it was observed that the DMF index increased with an increase in the urinary excretion of selenium although as yet we have no theory to explain this observation.

Food sources

The selenium content of foods reflects the level of the mineral in the soil in

---

Table 8-4. Dietary sources of zinc

Rich sources (> 3 mg. per 100 gm.)	Moderate sources (1 to 3 mg. per 100 gm.)	Poor sources (< 1 mg. per 100 gm.)
Maple syrup	Beef	Lettuce
Oysters	Clams	Butter
Peas	Corn	Oranges
Whole-wheat cereals	Peanut butter	
Liver	Milk	
Oatmeal	Egg yolk	

which plants are grown. Since cereals have a greater ability to concentrate selenium than do vegetables they generally have a higher concentration and within the cereal, the bran and germ have the highest amounts.

Toxicity

At high levels of intake (5 to 10 ppm) selenium is toxic, apparently because of its capacity to replace sulphur in biological compounds and to inhibit the action of some enzymes. Likelihood of selenium poisoning in human beings is confined to persons exposed to industrial dusts containing the element. Toxicity is reduced by diets high in protein and prevented completely in animals by arsenic. However, because of the fact that it too is toxic, arsenic can be used only in limited amounts.

Selenium found in cereal products is more toxic than selenium salts, which are only slightly soluble and poorly absorbed. Once absorbed, selenium is excreted in the urine. Expired selenium, along with fecal selenium, reflects unabsorbed minerals.

MANGANESE
Biological role

Manganese has been identified as an essential nutrient on the basis of its role as a catalyst to a large number of enzymes, although no known human deficiency symptoms can be attributed to a lack of manganese. There is some evidence that a lack of manganese leads to a underdevelopment of bones, especially the long bones. It is part of the enzyme arginase necessary for urea formation. Adequate manganese increases the storage of thiamine.

Food sources

Whole-grain cereals and green vegetables are among the better sources of manganese but the amount present depends on the part of the plant and the geographic source. Tea (150 to 900 ppm) is an extremely rich source and in English diets is estimated to proviae 3.3 mg. of manganese. Relative manganese values of common foodstuffs are given in Table 8-5. There is no evidence of dietary deficiencies of manganese in spite of the fact that it is very poorly absorbed especially in the presence of large amounts of calcium and phosphorus, but for children an intake of 0.2 to 0.3 mg. per kilogram or 3 to 5 mg. per day is considered adequate to provide the store of 12 to 20 mg. present widely distributed in the adult man. Liver and pancreas have the highest level.

Toxicity

Diets containing 1000 to 2000 ppm of manganese have had a very depressing effect on hemoglobin regeneration and have led to reduced concentrations of iron in liver, kidney, and spleen apparently because of its interference with iron absorption.

Table 8-5. Dietary sources of manganese

Rich sources (> 20 ppm)	Moderate sources (1 to 5 ppm)	Poor sources (< 1 ppm)
Nuts	Green leafy vegetables	Animal tissues
Whole-grain cereals	Dried fruits	Poultry
Dried legumes	Fresh fruits	Dairy products
Tea	Nonleafy vegetables	Seafood

COPPER
Functions

A lack of copper, recognized in animal tissues over a century ago, has been associated since 1924 with a lack of hemoglobin in the red blood cells even though copper is not a part of the hemoglobin molecule. Instead of catalyzing hemoglobin formation as previously believed it now appears that copper is more likely involved in promoting the maturation of red blood cells and increasing their survival time in the bloodstream. Thus it may be an essential associated with red blood cells rather than hemoglobin alone. There is some evidence from animal studies that copper may have a favorable influence on iron absorption. In fact, liver iron levels are more indicative of copper status than are determinations of blood or liver copper. In addition to its role in the prevention of anemia, whether through its effect on iron absorption, hemoglobin formation, or on red blood cell metabolism, copper helps maintain the integrity of the myelin sheath surrounding nerve fibers, is part of certain enzymes such as cytochrome oxidase and catalase involved in cellular respiration, plays an unexplained role in bone formation, helps maintain normal fertility, and may be involved in the formation of the melanin pigment of hair and skin through its role in tyrosine metabolism.

Absorption and metabolism

Slightly over 30% of dietary copper, or 0.6 to 1.6 mg. of the 2 to 2.5 mg. consumed, is absorbed in the intestine, where uptake is facilitated by acid. From there it enters the bloodstream where it exists in two forms. Copper in transport is loosely bound to the blood protein albumin in a complex containing 2 mg. of copper, representing 7% of the plasma copper. This copper is quickly distributed to the liver, bone marrow, kidney, cerebral spinal fluid, and other tissues, which contain about 66 mg. altogether. In the liver, copper is used in the

synthesis of a copper protein complex, cereluplasmin, which is 0.32% copper and which is secreted into the bloodstream where it represents 93% of the 110 μg. per 100 ml. found in the blood serum. The blood levels of copper increase during pregnancy, iron deficiency, and infection; they decrease in Wilson's disease, a hereditary disease involving the central nervous system. Within the red blood cells copper occurs in two forms—60% as a protein complex, erthyrocuprein, synthesized in the bone marrow cell, and the remaining 40% in some unidentified nonerythrocuprein form. The level of copper within the red blood cells does not seem to be influenced by serum levels of copper nor does it reflect dietary intake or loss of blood from the body. Copper in cerebral spinal fluid is in equilibrium with blood plasma. Total body copper has been estimated at 80 to 150 mg., with highest concentrations found in the brain, liver, heart, kidney, and blood. Bones, with 23 mg., and muscles, with 65 mg., contain 50% to 75% of total body copper.

Excretion

Copper is excreted from the body in small amounts, about 80% of which leaves in the feces as a result of the bile secretion, while 16% appears in the feces as a result of direct loss through the intestinal wall, and a mere 4% is lost in the urine. Unabsorbed copper, of course, appears in the feces also.

There is evidence of trace mineral interrelationships that influence copper excretion. Zinc increases its excretion, and a relatively high molybdenum in conjunction with high sulphate intake decreases copper absorption or increases its excretion.

Requirements

The dietary requirement of copper has not been established, although it is suggested that 0.05 mg. per kilogram of body weight is adequate. Actually no one has demonstrated an uncomplicated copper deficiency in adults, but an anemic condition in young children has responded to copper therapy in a manner to suggest an essential role for copper.

High reserves of copper, about five times adult levels, found in the liver at birth are sufficient to meet the infant's needs until the diet becomes varied enough to provide adequate amounts. The transfer of copper to the fetus in prenatal life is the result of very high plasma copper levels found in pregnant women.

Food sources

Content of copper in food varies widely; it is to a certain extent a function of the copper content of the soil in which it is raised and ranges up to 400 ppm. A general categorization of the copper content of foods is given in Table 8-6.

Deficiency

Low blood levels of copper (hypocupremia) have been found in infants. These are usually the result of an abnormally high loss of copper, disturbances in protein metabolism, and a secondary effect of an iron deficiency rather than of a low intake, even though milk is very low in copper.

Toxicity

Copper is likely toxic to man but only at levels at least ten times that found in a normal diet. Only where copper in the environment is as high as it might be in industrial circumstances is copper toxicity a hazard.

Abnormalities of metabolism

Copper metabolism is abnormal in two diseases of man—nephrosis and Wilson's disease. In Wilson's disease, a hereditary condition, the body continues to absorb copper; it accumulates in the tissues after a failure in the production of ceruloplasmin, which regulates the level of plasma copper.

MOLYBDENUM
Biological role

It has been clearly established that molybdenum is an essential part of two enzymes—xanthine oxidase, which is involved in the formation of uric acid from xanthine, a purine, and which also aids in mobilizing iron from liver reserves and aldehyde oxidase. It has not been confirmed, however, that the body cannot perform these changes by other means. On this basis there has been a reluctance to classify molybdenum unequivocally as an essential nutrient. Evi-

Table 8-6. Dietary sources of copper

Rich sources (> 8 ppm)	*Intermediate sources* (2 to 8 ppm)	*Poor sources* (< 2 ppm)
Organ meats	Leafy vegetables	Milk
Shellfish (especially oysters)	Eggs	Butter
	Muscle meat	Cheese
Nuts	Fish	Sugar
Dried legumes	Poultry	Fresh furits
Cocoa	Peas	and vegetables
Cherries	Beans	
Mushrooms	Fresh fruit	
Whole-grain cereals	Refined cereals	

dence of molybdenum toxicity at high levels includes diarrhea, anemia, and a depressed growth rate.

Interrelationships

Most of the interest in molybdenum nutrition has centered around its metabolic interrelationships with copper and sulphate. The observed toxicity manifest in animal diets as depressed growth and hemoglobin production from high levels of molybdenum obtained from ingestion of crops grown in soils high in molybdenum can be overcome by the addition of copper to the ration. Similarly a high molybdenum intake can induce a copper deficiency. High intakes of molybdenum alter the activity of alkaline phosphatase and produce certain bone abnormalities.

Absorption

Molybdenum is readily absorbed from the gastrointestinal tract and is excreted mainly in the urine, but the amount absorbed and excreted is influenced to a large extent by the amount of sulphate in the diet. High-sulphate diets increase urinary but not fecal excretion levels.

Food sources

Peas and beans with contents of 3 to 9 ppm are relatively rich; whole-grain cereals and dark green leafy vegetables, good (0.2 to 0.6 ppm); and fruits and vegetables with less than 0.1 ppm, poor sources.

COBALT
Biological role

In human nutrition the major role of cobalt is as an essential part of vitamin B_{12} or cobalamin, which is necessary to prevent pernicious anemia. The human being does not have the ability to synthesize the vitamin and must thus depend on animal sources of the nutrient. These have been synthesized by microorganisms in the intestine of animals that can incorporate the cobalt obtained from the plants they eat.

Thus cobalt is a direct dietary essential for animals and indirectly for humans. The cobalt content of plants reflects the cobalt content of the soil in which it is grown.

Food sources

The 5 to 8 μg. of cobalt in the adult diet appears to be about ten times the cobalt present in the cobalamin required by the body, and since human tissues cannot synthesize vitamin B_{12}, very little is retained from other than animal sources. Cobalt content of some representative foods is given in Table 8-7, but it must be remembered that the amount present is dependent on the cobalt in the soil in which plants are grown.

Toxicity

There is some evidence that high intakes of cobalt may have toxic effects. One that has been observed is the goitrogenic effect following the prolonged ingestion of cobalous chloride. The enlarged thyroid gland returns to normal following the cessation of cobalt administration. High intakes in animals have been observed to cause polycythemia, an increase in the number of red blood cells, and hyperplasia (increase in quantity) of bone marrow, which is believed to be related to the production of

Table 8-7. Dietary sources of cobalt listed according to micrograms per grams dry weight

Excellent (> 5)	Good (1.5 to 5)	Poor (< 0.05)
Liver	Lean beef	Cereal grains
Kidney	Lamb	Leguminous seeds
Oysters	Veal	Green leafy vege-
Clams	Poultry	tables
	Salt-water fish	Yeast
	Milk	

erythropoietin that stimulates red blood cell formation in the bone marrow.

VANADIUM

The role of vanadium in human nutrition has been studied only recently, and as yet there is insufficient evidence to consider it a dietary essential.

Some workers maintain that vanadium is necessary in prenatal life for calcification of bones and teeth, but they have been unable to identify a relationship between dietary vanadium and dental caries rate. It is possible that vanadium replaces phosphorus in apatite crystals and increases the hardness of the tooth enamel.

Some evidence was advanced in 1954 to suggest that vanadium in the diet of humans at a level of 100 to 125 mg. per day inhibits the synthesis of cholesterol, although the effect does not exist at lower levels of intake. Vanadium may counteract the stimulating effect that manganese exerts on cholesterol synthesis.

So far we have no reason to attribute any toxic effects to vanadium, although there have been extensive investigations of its role in bone marrow, liver, kidney, or adrenal tissue.

FLUORINE

On the basis of our criteria for establishing the essentiality of nutrient there is little justification for including a discussion of fluorine as an essential micronutrient element. However, because of the widespread interest and frequent controversy regarding the nutrient in the popular press, it is felt that it should not be ignored and that its role in the human nutrition should be clarified. In fact some workers do consider it a dietary essential.

Historical background

Interest in the possible nutritional role of fluorine dates back to 1931 when it was established that the water in communities where people had a remarkable freedom from tooth decay but suffered from an undesirable brownish appearance on the tooth surface contained considerably more of the mineral element fluorine than did most communal water supplies. The efforts to identify the factor had started in 1902 when a dentist in Colorado Springs became curious about the brown stain known as *Colorado brown stain* on the teeth of many of his patients.

Once fluorine had been identified as the substance in the water supply responsible for the brown staining and the absence of dental caries, other studies soon showed that somewhat lower levels of fluorine in the water were responsible for a markedly lower incidence of tooth decay without the undesirable mottling of tooth enamel (dental fluorosis) illustrated in Fig. 8-6. The relationship between the fluoride content of the water and the rate of tooth decay was established in 1942. A water supply containing one part per million (1 ppm) of fluorine produced a 50% to 60% reduction in tooth decay without any opacity or chalkiness in the tooth enamel. Only when the fluorine content of the water rose above 2.5 ppm was there evidence of dental fluorosis.

Recognizing dental caries as a major public health problem and seeking some effective means of controlling it, the United States Public Health Service in 1945 initiated a study to determine if the addition of sufficient fluorine to the water supply to raise the natural fluoride content to 1 ppm would afford the same degree of protection against tooth decay as would a natural fluoride level of 1 ppm. Newburgh, a city on the Hudson River in New York, was chosen as the experimental city with Kingston, a city across the river with a population of similar economic, racial, and cultural background and a fluoride-free water supply, serving as a control. Careful records were kept of the incidence of tooth decay in both cities, and at the end of a ten-year period a report was made available. It showed that children under ten years of age had received the greatest protection, having a DMF index (total number of decayed, missing, and filled teeth) 60% to 65% below those of their counterparts in Kingston. Children 12 to 14 years old who had consumed fluoridated water from early childhood but not since birth had a 48% reduction in tooth decay, while 16-year-olds who had been on it for an even shorter time had only a 40% reduction. A 15-year report on the same communities showed a similar degree of protection with no detectable adverse effects. A comparison of six-year-olds in the two communities in 1962 showed that 33.9% of those in Newburgh were caries-free compared to 16.4% in Kingston. In addition comparable DMF rates were 0.09 and 0.65 per child respectively. These findings, showing that the earlier a child has an available source of fluorine the greater the protection it will provide, have since been confirmed and reconfirmed in fluoridation studies in many other communities. The child whose mother is drinking fluoridated water during pregnancy appears to receive maximum protection, although evidence shows that fluorine passes the placental barrier with difficulty.

The effect of the fluoridation of the water supply on the dental health of children in various communities is shown in Table 8-8. The observed reduction of 50% to 60% approaches that observed in communities whose natural fluorine content is similar.

Recently several reports have been re-

Table 8-8. Reductions in decayed, missing, and filled permanent teeth reported among children in communities after ten years of fluoridation*

Community	Age studied	Percentage reduction
Grand Junction, Colo.	6	94.0
New Britain, Conn.	6 through 16	44.6
District of Columbia	6	59.1
Evanston, Ill.	6-7-8	91.3-64.6-62.6
Fort Wayne, Ind.	6 through 10	>50.0
Hopkinsville, Ky.	? (Children)	56.0
Louisville, Ky.	First 3 grades	62.1
Hagerstown, Md.	7, 9, 11 & 13	57.0
Grand Rapids, Mich.	6-7-8	75.0-63.0-57.0
Grand Rapids, Mich.	9-10	50.0-52.0
Newburgh, N. Y.	6-9	58.0
Newburgh, N. Y.	10-12	57.0
Newburgh, N. Y.	13-14	48.0
Newburgh, N. Y.	16	41.0
Charlotte, N. C.	6-11	60.0
Chattanooga, Tenn.	6-14	70.8
Marshall, Texas	7-15	54.0
Brantford, Ont.	6-7-8	60.0-67.0-54.0
Brantford, Ont.	9-10	46.0-41.0
Brantford, Ont.	11-13	44.0
Brantford, Ont.	14-16	35.0

*From Dunning, J. M.: Current status of fluoridation, New England J. Med. **272**:30, 1965.

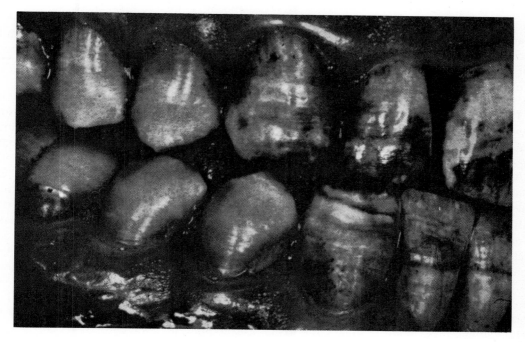

Fig. 8-6
Appearance of teeth in dental fluorosis. (Courtesy Duckworth, R.: Fluoridation, Proc. Nutrition Soc. **22:**79, 1963.)

leased showing an increase in tooth decay when a community dropped a fluoridation program that had been in effect for several years. Such reports that indicate beneficial effects from the addition of fluorine and a reversal of these in its withdrawal help establish the fact that the benefits are caused by fluorine rather than other unidentified factors.

Aside from the benefits a pregnant woman may pass on to her child by drinking fluoridated water, there is little advantage as far as dental health is concerned from the consumption of fluoridated water by adults. However there may be other benefits that accrue to the adult from the ingestion of fluoride-containing water. For instance, fluoride, by increasing the stability of the skeleton, may protect it against losses of calcium that often occur at menopause, under conditions of immobility, and, as recently observed, in space flight. The incidence of osteoporosis, an abnormality of bone metabolism that affects older people, is less among persons with fluoridated than low-fluorine water supplies.

Metabolism

Soluble fluoride is absorbed very readily from the intestine although some may be taken up by the stomach. About 90% of that ingested appears in the bloodstream. Of this, about 50% is excreted in the urine, and the other half is taken up readily by bones and teeth, where it apparently becomes an integral and important part of the tooth and bone structure. Regardless of the amount ingested, blood levels remain amazingly constant. Failure of blood plasma levels of fluoride to increase with an increase in dietary fluorides reflects the ability of the kidney to control the levels in body tissues by excreting amounts in excess of the body's needs. None appears in the soft tissues. The amount of fluorine appearing in other tissues, such as saliva, milk, and fetal blood, parallels that in the blood but at a slightly lower level.

Insoluble calcium and aluminum salts of fluorine retard the absorption of fluorine.

The affinity bone has for fluorine has given rise to concern over possible skeletal toxicity from the deposition of excess fluorine in the skeleton following ingestion of water with a high fluorine content. The homeostatic mechanism that maintains blood levels at a constant value undoubtedly prevents such a situation. Efforts to identify such an effect have shown that a lifelong ingestion of water containing 4 ppm of fluorine has no detrimental effects on bone formation. With continued exposure to high fluorine intakes, the bone ceases to take up more fluorine. There is some evidence that fluorine delays the excretion of calcium, a factor that is of advantage in maintaining calcium balances. In fact, a dose of 50 mg. of fluorine per day has proven effective in improving calcium balance and preventing osteoporosis without any toxic effects.

Mode of action

The mechanisms by which fluorine imparts greater resistance to tooth decay have been studied extensively. It appears that where fluorine is available some crystals of fluoroapatite replace the calcium phosphate crystals of hydroxyapatite that are normally deposited during tooth formation. Fluoride at high concentrations may also replace some of the carbonate usually found in bone. These substances are apparently less soluble in acid and more resistant to the cariogenic action of acids in the oral environment. Fluorine is known to stimulate the action of some enzymes and inhibit that of others. Consequently it may act in this way to reduce the formation of acid by the action of bacteria on carbohydrate in the mouth, thus reducing the likelihood of the solution of tooth enamel. It is known that

both the dentine and the enamel of teeth that have formed when fluorine is available do contain more fluorine than otherwise, indicating that fluorine does become an integral part of the tooth structure.

The enamel surface is still capable of taking up fluorine shortly after eruption during the final stages of tooth calcification. Fluorine available in the saliva is presumably preferentially absorbed on the tooth surface, adding strength and rigidity. In addition there is some evidence that fluorine promotes the precipitation of calcium phosphate from saliva, which may facilitate the remineralization of teeth following decalcification in oral environment during the initial stages of tooth decay. Larger, more nearly perfect crystals in bone have been observed as fluoride concentration of human bone increases. As much as 5000 to 6000 ppm in bone does not constitute a physiologic hazard.

Sources

In addition to water, from which an adult usually ingests 1.5 mg. fluorine per day, another 1.3 to 1.8 mg. comes from tea and solid food high in fluorine content. The determination of the fluorine content

Table 8-9. Fluorine content of some representative foods[*]

Food	Milligrams per 100 gm.
Tea	0.475
Coffee	0.250
Rice	0.07
Buckwheat	0.17
Soybeans	0.40 to 0.67
Spinach	0.02
Onions	0.05
Lettuce	0.01

[*]From Gordenoff, T., and Mender, W.: Fluorine, World Rev. Nutr. Diet. **2:**213–42, 1962.

of food is very tedious. Results of some efforts are shown in Table 8-9.

Fluoridation of public water supplies

As soon as communities began to consider the fluoridation of their water supplies, groups of people began to oppose it for a wide variety of reasons, most of which revolved around its hazards, its ineffectiveness, and ethical considerations of so-called compulsory medication. Social issues assumed more importance than health issues. The opponents claimed that fluorine was toxic, that fluoridation of water supplies was a violation of the rights of the individual, and through a variety of highly emotional attacks on the program created doubt as to the motives of the proponents of the measure. Any possibility of fluorine toxicity has been thoroughly investigated by the United States Public Health Service, which has been unable to find any evidence of detrimental effects from the addition of 1 ppm of fluorine to the drinking water no matter how large the water consumption. Based on the health records of 2 million people in artificially fluoridated areas, there is no evidence of increased deposition of fluorine in soft tissues such as the kidney or heart, no increase in mortality and morbidity rates, no growth depression or abnormalities, no increase in cancer or nephritis, and no increase in the mongolism birth rate, all of which have been claimed by the antifluoridation forces. Claims that fluorides interfered with cell growth and protein synthesis have been discredited by studies showing that cellular reproduction continues in the presence of an amount of fluoride far in excess of the amount that can be brought into the circulating fluids by oral intakes of fluoride. On the contrary, in addition to a reduction in tooth decay, a reduction in the amount of peridontal disease, a 30% reduction in the incidence of malocclusion and among older people a decreased incidence of the bone abnormality osteoporosis was found.

Fluorine is toxic but only at levels well beyond that at which it is added to communal water supplies. Mottled enamel or dental fluorosis, which presents only aesthetic problems, may occur at concentrations 2 to 8 ppm, osteosclerosis at 8 to 20 ppm, growth depression at 50 ppm or more and fatal poisoning at 2500 times recommended levels. Extreme precautions and constant surveillance of the level of fluoride in the water assure the public that the level in their water could not approach toxic levels. As an added precaution, it is suggested that in tropical areas where water consumption may be higher that the level of fluoridation be reduced to 0.7 ppm.

In spite of the evidence that the addition of fluorine to the water supply to provide a total fluorine content of 1 ppm, the endorsement of fluoridation by every medical and dental group in the United States, the United States Public Health Service, and many Asian and European countries, and the lack of any evidence of adverse effects at this level, fluoridation remains a very controversial issue. These antifluoridation groups have become so vocal that in many cases where fluoridation has come up for a public referendum it has been defeated. Of 56 communities voting on fluoridation in 1960, 43 rejected it. In a few cases fluoridation has been terminated after a period of successful use. In spite of the efforts of the antifluoridation forces in 1965, 55 million people in over 2800 communities were consuming water to which fluorine had been added and another 7 million drank water in which the natural fluoride content was at a protective level. With the decision to fluoridate the water supply of New York City in 1965 another 8.5 million persons will receive the benefits of a fluoridation program. In all cases where it has been introduced there has been a significant reduction in tooth decay among children, a protection that carries over into adulthood.

Different forms of fluoride, sodium fluoride, sodium silicofluoride, and fluorosilisic acid—have all been used effectively to provide the fluoride ions as active agents in the water supply. None of these appear to influence the odor, taste, color, or hardness of the water, and all can be readily introduced into the community water system without causing a depreciation in plumbing equipment. The cost of fluoridation varies, depending on the chemical chosen and the engineering complexity of the water system, but most cities report a cost of 5 to 15 cents per person per year. In light of the fact that 99% of the population experience tooth decay and will stand to benefit financially as well as through a reduction in physical discomfort accompanying tooth decay, the cost seems small. In Philadelphia it was estimated that fluoridation had saved 360,000 teeth valued at over 2 million dollars in dental bills during a 13-year period. In Newburgh the cost of the initial dental care of five-, six-, and seven-year old children who had been on fluoridated water all their lives was less than half and annual dental costs slightly more than half that of their counterparts in Kingston. Defluoridation or the removal of natural fluoride from the water has been undertaken in some communities where fluorine is naturally present at a level that causes mottling of tooth enamel. It has cost one dollar per person per year.

Other methods of acquiring fluorine. Fluoridation of the water supply has proven the most feasible means of providing protection against tooth decay, but for persons who either do not have access to a community water supply or who live in communities that have not introduced it, other methods of obtaining the benefits of fluorine have been tried. The most frequent method is the use of sodium fluoride tablets. A year's supply of 2-mg. tablets to be taken daily that will release 1 mg. of fluorine cost only 15 cents a person, but distribution costs add another $3.50 per year. A major deterrent to the success of tablets is the failure of parents to continue

to provide them throughout the whole growth period or at least for the first ten years. In Hawaii, where tablets were distributed free, 90% of the parents provided them for their children at the beginning of the program but four years later only 12% were still using them. In Switzerland the use of tablets proved more successful with a 20% to 35% reduction reported. For infants, they must be dissolved in the formula or fruit juice, and care must be taken to see that they do not inadvertently get an overdose. Many of the commonly used infant supplements have fluorine added, but in areas where the water supply is fluoridated their sale is restricted to prescription distribution.

Topical applications of 8% stannous fluoride solution to the dry surface of teeth shortly after they erupt has been a relatively successful means, providing about 40% protection against caries, but the professional time involved makes the yearly treatment relatively expensive and hence unavailable to many who would benefit most. Most recently the application of a phosphate fluoride every two years has resulted in a 70% reduction in caries. While successful, these methods have limited value because of a shortage of dentists needed to carry out the process. In Switzerland an attempt to add fluorine to salt was unsuccessful, especially since infants who need fluorine are seldom given salt. Attempts to add fluorine to the milk supply were also of limited usefulness.

The value of fluoridated dentifrices that contain about 0.1% fluoride is still being evaluated, and at the present time the evidence seems controversial. One problem revolves around the observation that fluoride content decreases with storage. It is possible that fluorine inhibits the action of enzymes or bacteria involved in the formation of acid in the mouth. It has been shown that the plaques that form on teeth on which it is believed that bacteria act to produce the acid which initiates the solution of enamel and tooth decay contain almost twice as much fluoride where there is a 2 ppm in the water supply compared to a fluoride-free area. Apparently the enamel surface is capable of taking in some fluoride ions from the fluids to which it is exposed in the mouth.

A proposal that a fluoride can be injected into the gum area just prior to the time that the teeth erupt, when they are most receptive to the uptake of fluoride ions, has received some scientific backing.

SELECTED REFERENCES

Micronutrient elements

Davis, G. K.: Trace mineral dietary interrelationships, Borden Rev. Nutr. Res. **18**:83, 1957.

Mills, C. F.: Metabolic interrelationships in the utilization of trace elements, Proc. Nutrition Soc. **23**:38, 1964.

Underwood, E. J.: Trace elements in human and animal nutrition, ed. 2, New York, 1962, Academic Press Inc.

Iron

Brown, E. B.: The absorption of iron, Am. J. Clin. Nutr. **12**:205-213, 1963.

Brown, E. B.: The utilization of iron in erythropoiesis, Am. J. Clin. Nutr. **12**:77-87, 1963.

Charley, P. J., Still, C., Shore, E., and Soltman, P.: Studies in the regulation of intestinal iron absorption, J. Lab. & Clin. Med. **61**:397, 1963.

Editorial. Iron overload, J.A.M.A. **191**:668, 1965.

Finch, C. A.: The role of iron in hemoglobin synthesis, Conference on hemoglobin, Publication No. 557, Washington, D. C., 1957, National Academy of Sciences.

Hallberg, L., and Solvell, L.: Absorption of hemoglobin iron in man, Am. J. Digest. Dis. **9**:787, 1964.

Kasper, C. K., Whissell, V. E., and Wallerstein, R. O.: Clinical aspects of iron deficiency, J.A.M.A. **191**:359, 1965.

Scheffer, L. M., Price, D. C., and Cronkite, E. P.: Iron absorption and anemia, J. Lab. & Clin. Med. **65**:316, 1965.

Vitter, R. W.: Vitamins, minerals and anemia, J.A.M.A. **175**:152, 1961.

Wadsworth, G. R.: Nutritional factors in anemia, World Rev. Nutr. Diet. **1**:149, 1959.

Woodruff, C. W.: Iron, Borden Rev. Nutr. Res. **20**:61, 1959.

Iodine

Matovinovic, J.: Endemic goiter, J. Am. M. Women's A. **17**:427, 495, 571, 646, 1962.

Review. Endemic goiter, Nutr. Rev. **21**:73, 1963.

Vought, R. L., and London, W. T.: Iodine intake and excretion in healthy nonhospitalized subjects, Am. J. Clin. Nutr. **15**:124, 1964.

Vought, R. L., and London, W. T.: Dietary sources of iodine, Am. J. Clin. Nutr. **14**:186, 1964.

Zinc

Mayer, J.: Zinc deficiency, a cause of growth retardation, Postgrad. Med. **35**:206, 1964.

Sullivan, J. F., and Lankford, H. G.: Zinc metabolism and chronic alcoholism, Am. J. Clin. Nutr. **17**:57, 1965.

Vallee, B. L.: The metabolic role of zinc, J.A.M.A. **162**:1053, 1956.

Luecke, R. V.: Significance of zinc in nutrition, Borden Rev. Nutr. Res. **26**:45, 1965.

Selenium

Hadjimarkos, D. M., and Bonhorst, C. W.: The selenium content of eggs, milk and water in relation to dental caries in children, J. Pediat. **59**:256-264, 1961.

Copper

Cartwright, G. E., and Wintrobe, M. M.: Copper metabolism in normal subjects, Am. J. Clin. Nutrition **14**:224, 1964.

Gubler, C. J.: Copper metabolism in man, J.A.M.A. **161**:530, 1956.

Review. Copper deficiency in malnourished infants, Nutr. Rev. **23**:164, 1960.

Sturgeon, P., and Brubaker, C.: Copper deficiency in infants, Am. J. Dis. Child. **92**:254, 1956.

Vanadium

Dimond, E. G., Caravaca, J., and Benchumol, A.: Vanadium excretion, toxicity and lipid effect in man, Am. J. Clin. Nutrition **12**:49, 1963.

Fluorine

Ash, D. B., and Fitzgerald, B.: Effectiveness of water fluoridation, J. Am. Dent. A. **65**:581, 1962.

Ash, D. B., Cows, N. C., Carlos, J. P., and Maiwald, A. A.: Time and cost factors to provide regular periodic dental care for children in fluoridated and nonfluoridated areas, Am. J. Pub. Health **55**:811, 1965.

Blomquist, C. H., Singer, L., Pollock, M. E., McLaren, L. C., and Armstrong, W. D.: Sodium fluoride and cell growth, Brit. M. J. **1**:486, 1965.

Bransby, E. R., and Forrest, J. R.: Dental effects of fluoridation of water with particular reference to a study in the United Kingdom, Proc. Nutrition Soc. **22**:84, 1963.

Duckworth, R.: Fluoridation, Proc. Nutrition Soc. **22**:79, 1963.

Dunning, J. M.: Current status of fluoridation, New England J. Med. **272**:30, 84, 1965.

Foster, R. D.: Self-application of topically applied stannous fluoride, J. Am. Dent. A. **70**:329, 1965.

Hodge, H. C.: Safety factors in water fluoridation based on toxicology of fluoride, Proc. Nutrition Soc. **22**:111, 1963.

Review. Attitudes toward fluoridation, Nutr. Rev. **22**:291, 1964.

Schlesinger, E. R.: Dietary fluorides and caries prevention, Am. J. Pub. Health **55**:1123, 1965.

Sognnaes, R. F.: Fluoride protection of bones and teeth, Science **150**:989, 1965.

Weech, A. A.: Fluoridation, Am. J. Dis. Child. **108**:571, 1964.

9

Water

If it is possible to say that one essential nutrient is more essential than another, one would have to concede that it is water. And yet it is the nutrient most often taken for granted—so much so that some writers even fail to include it in a list of essential nutrients. The human being can live for weeks and even years before death will result from a failure to consume some essential vitamins and minerals but will survive only a few days in the absence of water, even though the body possesses rather involved mechanisms for conserving water when the supply is short. The longest time man has survived without water is seventeen days, but two or three days is the usual limit.

Distribution in body

Water constitutes 60% of the total body weight and 70% of the lean body mass. Water as a constituent of every cell of the body contributes volume and form to the soft tissues. It is present in widely varying concentrations in various tissues, constituting 72% of muscle, 20% to 35% of adipose tissue, and 10% of bone and cartilage.

The distribution of fluids in the body is described in terms of an intracellular compartment representing the water within the cells, which accounts for 65% of total body water and 33% of total body weight, and an extracellular compartment, comprising the other 35% of body water. This extracellular component can be further subdivided into four compartments: the intravascular, the intercellular, the transcellular, and the dense connective tissue, bone, and cartilage compartment. Exchange of fluids between the intracellular and intercellular compartments and between the intercellular and intravascular compartments, all of which are separated by a semipermeable membrane, occurs quite freely and is regulated by many factors, including the relative concentrations of protein and of electrolytes such as sodium and potassium. The direction and the rate of exchange are determined by osmotic and hydrostatic pressures on either side of the membrane. The other fluid compartments do not participate as extensively in the dynamic exchange of fluid.

The intravascular fluid includes the water

169

in the blood vessels, arteries, veins, and capillaries and accounts for 4.5% of body weight and 7.5% of total body water. The intercellular (or extravascular) fluid includes that which has left the blood vessels and is present in the spaces surrounding each cell. The intracellular fluid, representing the largest amount of water, is enclosed inside the cell membrane of each individual cell. Transcellular water is that which is present in such fluids as the spinal fluid, the ocular fluid in the eyeballs, the synovial fluid that lubricates joints, and the fluids in the mucous secretions of the linings of the respiratory tract, the gastrointestinal tract, and the genitourinary tract. It comprises 2.5% of total body water. The water in dense connective tissue, cartilage, and bone is part of its structural material and accounts for 15% of total body water.

Functions

Three to five liters of fluid are present in the bloodstream—arteries, veins, and capillaries—where the fluid acts as a solvent for the nutrients, monosaccharides, amino acids, fats (as phospholipids), vitamins, and minerals and for the hormones secreted by the glands, all of which must be transported to all parts of the body if the individual cells are to be adequately nourished. This intravascular fluid also acts as a solvent and transporter of the waste products of metabolism such as carbon dioxide, ammonia, and electrolytes, which must be carried from the cells to the lungs, skin, or kidney to be excreted.

Twelve liters of fluid are in the extravascular or interstitial compartment of the body. This is the fluid, carrying nutrients, that has left the blood vessels and surrounds each cell to bring in close proximity to its membrane the nutrients that must gain entrance to the cell if it is to live. It also collects waste products excreted from the cell and hormones or other substances that may be secreted by the cell. Much of this fluid reenters the circulatory

system, being pulled back by the osmotic pressures built up by the blood proteins that do not leave the bloodstream. Any remaining intercellular fluid in excess of normal amounts is accumulated by the lymphatic system and eventually returned to the bloodstream. The amount of water in the extravascular or intercellular compartment fluctuates more than that in other compartments since it can tolerate greater variations than other compartments. The blood volume is usually maintained at a fairly constant level at the expense of the intercellular fluid. Similarly the intracellular fluid, which must also be maintained at a constant level to prevent the swelling or shrinking of cells, draws on the intercellular fluid. The intercellular fluid may thus be thought of as a buffer zone.

Within the cell, intracellular water is used as body builder, being incorporated into a new material as it is synthesized. Glycogen, the form in which carbohydrate is stored, accumulates only in the presence of water. The deposition of fat involves the accumulation of an additional 20% water. Water also acts as a catalyst in many biological reactions within the cell and as a solvent for nutrients that must be transported from one organelle to another within the cell and for the waste products that must be eliminated.

In the transcellular fluids, such as saliva, water acts as a lubricant, facilitating the passage of food down the esophagus. In the stomach and small intestine, where digestion of food occurs, the water is necessary for the hydrolytic reactions required to break the complex nutrients into their simpler component parts since most of these reactions are hydrolytic or water-requiring. Some of this water is derived from food and beverages, but a great deal of it comes from the digestive juices secreted into the gastrointestinal tract. In the synovial fluid of joints, the prime function of water is to act as a lubricant.

In addition to the well-established roles

of water in the body that we have already discussed, it is becoming increasingly evident that the amount of water in the diet exerts a very definite influence on the metabolism of other nutrients. When 20% water was added to diets containing 6%, 9%, or 12% protein, there was a significant gain in the protein efficiency ration (PER). PER is the weight gain per gram of protein. Some work has indicated that the appetite control center in the hypothalamus of the brain is in reality a thirst-control center and that the intake of food is a response to the intake of fluid. Under circumstances where thirst is depressed food intake may also be reduced.

Studies to determine limiting factors in the work output of an individual suggest that a lack of water has a much more profound effect on work production than does a lack of food.

Another important role of water, beyond acting as a solvent and transporter for nutrients and metabolic waste products and as a lubricant, is in the regulation of body temperature. The evaporation of water from the surface of the body is the most effective method of ridding the body of extra heat produced in the metabolism of carbohydrate, fat, and protein. Some of this heat is required to maintain body temperature at 98.6°, the temperature at which all enzymes crucial to metabolic processes operate most effectively. But the metabolism of energy-yielding nutrients to provide energy for muscular, chemical, and osmotic work in the body yields as a by-product more heat than is necessary to maintain normal body temperature. If this is not released from the body promptly, the body temperature increases beyond a point compatible with life and the individual dies, since all cellular enzymes will be inactivated. The evaporation of fluid from the skin requires energy in the form of heat, which is a by-product when energy-yielding nutrients are metabolized, and the body is constantly cooling itself by causing

water to be lost through evaporation. The loss of heat through the skin represents about 25% of the total caloric expenditure of the body. This water loss, which amounts to 350 to 700 ml. per day under normal conditions of temperature and humidity, is referred to as "insensible perspiration loss." The greater the body surface area, the greater the amount of heat that can be lost through the skin. A layer of subcutaneous fat that acts as an insulating material, reducing the speed with which heat is lost from the body, is an advantage in the winter and a disadvantage in the summer.

Water balance

Sources of body water. Water is essential for normal body functioning. In contrast to all other nutrients, which must be provided in food, water is available to the body from various sources.

The major source is the fluids consumed as beverages. The amount in fluids will vary from one individual to another. Infants consume more per unit of body weight than do adults. Persons living in the tropics where there is greater evaporation from the skin consume more than persons in temperate climates, and persons engaged in strenuous physical activity consume more than sedentary individuals. The amount consumed by adults as fluids varies from 900 to 1500 ml., with an average of 1100 ml. under normal circumstances.

So-called solid foods vary in their water content from none to 96% water. The water content of some representative foods is given in Table 9-1, from which it is evident that many foods conceived as solid foods contain over 70% water. A 2000-kilocalorie diet chosen according to a typical food plan provides from 500 to 800 ml. of water.

The end products of combustion of carbohydrate, fat, and protein include water in addition to carbon dioxide and energy. A constant amount of water is released during the oxidation or burning of each of

Table 9-1. Water content of representative foods*

Food	Percent of water
Lettuce	95
Asparagus	92
Milk	87
Oranges	86
Potatoes	80
Cottage cheese	79
Veal	66
Chicken	63
Beef	47
Cheddar cheese	37
Bread	36
Butter	15
Gelatin	13
White sugar	0.5

*From Watts, B. K., and Merrill, A. L.: Composition of foods—raw, processed and prepared, U. S. Department of Agriculture Handbook No. 8, Washington, D. C., 1963, U. S. Department of Agriculture.

these—1 gm. of carbohydrate yielding 0.6 gm. of water, 1 gm. of protein, 0.42 gm. of water, and 1 gm. of fat yielding 1 gm. of water. This amounts to 15, 10.5, and 11.1 gm. respectively from the ingestion of 100 calories from carbohydrate, protein, and fat. Thus, for an individual utilizing 2000 kilocalories a day, 50% of which came from carbohydrate, 35% from fat, and 15% from protein, the water of metabolism would amount to 260 ml. per day, as shown in the following calculation in Table 9-2.

Thus on this 2000-kilocalorie diet a person will normally have available 262 ml. of water from metabolism. This amounts to 13.1 gm. per 100 kilocalories.

Loss of body water. Counterbalancing the intake of water there are several pathways by which water is lost—urinary losses, respiratory losses through the lungs, and evaporation losses through the skin.

Most of the ingested water is absorbed very rapidly through the walls of the intestinal tract—so rapidly that we find little relationship between the amount of water ingested and the amount found in the stomach.

Once absorbed, water is taken up by the bloodstream and carried to the kidney, where it becomes a solvent for waste products from the body and is excreted as urine. The fluid is filtered through the kidney tubule at the rate of 125 ml. per minute, which amounts to 120 to 190 l. per day. Here sufficient water is reabsorbed to retain normal blood volumes and the rest is excreted in the urine. If the fluid intake is high, urine volume is increased above the normal level of 1 to 2 l. and the concentration of excretory products in the urine will be low. Such a urine has a low specific gravity. When fluid intake is low, much of it must be resorbed to maintain blood volume, and a much smaller amount will be used in the urine as a solvent for the excretory products. Since there is a limit to the extent to which the kidney can concentrate urine, there is a minimum urine volume necessary to rid the body of waste products. This minimum has been estimated at somewhere between 300 and 500 ml. If less than this amount of fluid is available for urine formation, waste products of metabolism will be retained in the tissue, where they may concentrate up to toxic levels. Under circumstances such as disasters and manned space flights where the fluid available is very limited and must be conserved, the mandatory excretion through the kidney can be reduced by limiting the intake of foods that normally give rise to metabolites, which must be excreted in the urine. Restricting protein and salt intake are the easiest, most effective methods of reducing the necessary urine volume. Very young infants with poorly developed kidney function can excrete very small amounts of electrolytes.

Loss of water through the skin, which is

Table 9-2. Calculation of water of metabolism produced on a 2000-kilocalorie diet

Source of calories	Percent of calories provided	Distribution of calories in 2000-calorie diet	Weight of nutrient (gm.)	Water of metabolism per gram	Total water of metabolism
Carbohydrate	50	1000	250	0.6	150
Fat	35	700	77	1.07	78
Protein	15	300	75	0.42	32
					260

the way in which the body regulates its internal temperature, amounts to 350 to 700 ml. per day. It has been reported as high as 2500 ml. per hour, and 500 ml. per hour is not uncommon. Infants experience a high rate of evaporation from the skin, which compensates for small urinary losses.

Water is constantly being lost along with carbon dioxide through the lungs. The amount released this way amounts to 300 ml. but will increase at high altitudes, which lead to increased respiration rates. Where the atmosphere is unusually dry the total lost through the lungs and skin usually equals urinary losses.

During a 24-hour period as much as 8 to 10 l. of water (with 3700 ml. considered a minimum) may be secreted into the digestive tract as digestive juices. Practically all of this is reabsorbed as it passes down the gastrointestinal tract so that as little as 200 ml. will be excreted in the feces. These secretions include saliva, gastric juices, intestinal and pancreatic juice, bile, and secretion of lymph glands. The volume of digestive juices secreted is determined to a certain extent by the moisture content of the food. When food is dry, the secretion of saliva is increased to exert a maximum lubricating effect on the food to facilitate swallowing and the action of di-

gestive enzymes. Secretion of bile is stimulated by ingestion of large amounts of fat, and the volume of the gastric, pancreatic, and intestinal juices may fluctuate in response to the variation in moisture content of the food.

The sources of water in the gastrointestinal tract in a 24-hour period for a normal adult are shown in Table 9-3.

Summing up, it becomes obvious that to compensate for water losses in the urine

Table 9-3. Water exchange in gastrointestinal tract

Source	Milliliters
Saliva	1500
Gastric juice	2500
Bile	500
Pancreatic juices	700
Intestinal juices	3000
Water intake	2000
Absorbed	10,000
Fecal	200
Total	10,200

Table 9-4. Typical water balance in adult

Sources and loss	Milliliters
Sources of water	
Liquid food	1100
Solid food	500–1000
Water of oxidation	300– 400
Total	1900–2500
Loss of water	
Urine	1000–1300
Perspiration and evaporation from skin	800–1000
Feces	100
Total	1900–2500

and feces and through the skin and lungs, there must be a fluid intake of at least 2 l. from food and beverages. About 40% of the liquid comes from tap water; the rest comes from milk and other beverages. Table 9-4 summarizes the factors involved in water balance within the body.

Requirements

The need for fluid in relation to body weight varies with the age; the younger the person, the greater the fluid requirement per unit of body weight. Fluid requirements under various conditions of age and environmental temperatures are shown in Table 9-5.

As a guide it is suggested that 1000 ml. of water must be consumed for every 1000 kilocalories in the diet of adults and 1500 in infants to meet this demand. Usually about two thirds of this comes from beverages and the remainder from solid food. This is considerably less than the 4700 to 17,000 ml. of water that may be turned over in the body each day, indicating that the

body has extensive mechanisms for conserving water.

Regulation of body fluid. The regulation of body fluid content is a function of the kidney, which reabsorbs a sufficient amount to maintain blood volume at a normal level. When the sodium concentration of the blood rises by as little as 1%, as it will when the volume diminishes, the thirst-regulating center of the brain is stimulated and the individual consumes more water.

Disturbances in water metabolism. Water is an essential part of cell cytoplasm, and the functioning of the cell is dependent on a certain concentration of nutrients in the internal environment of the cell. Any loss or accumulation of fluid in cells can lead to acute metabolic difficulties. This may result from abnormal loss such as in diarrhea, nausea, or fever, abnormal retention, a defect in intestinal absorption, or an altered distribution of fluids within the body. When body fluids are reduced as much as 10% symptoms of severe dehydration appear; an increase to levels 10% above normal represents edema.

Under conditions of high environmental temperature the body loses very large amounts of water (up to 2500 ml. per hour) through perspiration. Along with the water loss there is an appreciable loss of sodium. The loss of water will stimulate the thirst center in the hypothalamus of the

Table 9-5. Fluid requirement per kilogram of body weight

Classifications	Milliliters
Infants	110
10-year-old children	40
Adults	
72° F.	22
100° F.	38

brain, leading to an increased consumption of water to replace that lost in perspiration. If this water intake is not accompanied by a source of sodium to replace that lost in perspiration along with the water, the individual suffers from a condition known as *water intoxication,* in which the sodium concentration in the fluids becomes very diluted. Industries in which men work at high temperatures frequently require that their employees take salt tablets when they drink water. Travellers in tropical areas who are unaccustomed to high heat may find it necessary to use salt tablets to avoid the weakness that accompanies a loss of sodium from the body.

Another form of water intoxication, in which the intake of water exceeds the maximum rate of urine flow of 16 ml. per minute, is caused by an uptake of the extra water by the cells, again causing a dilution of the cellular constituents in addition to the swelling of cells. When this occurs in brain cells, convulsions, coma, and death can result.

SELECTED REFERENCES

Brooke, C. E.: Oral fluid and electrolytes, J.A.M.A. 179:792, 1962.

Walker, J. S., Margolis, F. J., Teate, H. L., Weil, M. L., and Wilson, H. L.: Water intake of normal children, Science 140:890, 1963.

10

Vitamins

DISCOVERY

Vitamins were the last group of dietary essentials to be recognized. This is easy to understand since they are needed in such very small amounts. Their presence in food is correspondingly low and hence was easily overlooked in the early analysis of foods. The minimum need for vitamins varies from a low of a few micrograms to a high of 30 mg., those needed in the smallest amounts being equally as important as those needed at one hundred or one thousand times that level.

Vitamins are now defined as organic substances needed in very small amounts for normal functioning of the body that must be provided in the diet of the animal. Those substances considered vitamins for one species that cannot synthesize them may not be vitamins for another species that has the ability to synthesize its own. For instance vitamin C must be provided in the diet of man, monkeys, and guinea pigs, but is synthesized by rats, rabbits, dogs, and other animals; thus they do not need to have them provided in the diet.

The term *vitamine* was coined by Casimir Funk in 1912. He was searching for the elusive substance in rice bran that had great power to cure the condition beriberi. He confirmed Eijkman's hypothesis that disease could be caused by a lack of a dietary constituent. These substances he correctly believed to be necessary for life (vita) and, in the case of the antiberiberi factor, nitrogen-containing (amine). Hence the term *vitamine*. He suggested that it was likely that there were vitamins to protect against pellagra, scurvy, and rickets. Subsequent work showed that there were many "vitamines" and that only a few were "amine" in nature, so the final *e* was dropped to give us the familiar term *vitamin*.

Shortly after Funk postulated his vitamin hypothesis McCollum and Davis and Osborne and Mendel, working independently, reported an elusive, unidentified substance in fat that was necessary for growth and reproduction in animals. This they designated fat-soluble A to differentiate it from the water-soluble B believed to be respon-

Table 10-1. Discovery, isolation, synthesis, and nomenclature of vitamins

	Discovery	Isolation	Synthesis	Other names
Water-soluble vitamins				
Ascorbic acid (C)		1932	1933	Antiscorbutic factor Cevitamic acid
Thiamine (B$_1$)*	1921	1926	1936	Aneurine Antineuritic factor Antiberiberi factor
Riboflavin (B$_2$)	1932	1933	1935	Yellow enzyme Vitamin G Lactoflavin Hepatoflavin Ovoflavin
Niacin*	1936	1936		Nicotinic acid Nicotinamide or niacinamide Pellagra-preventative factor
Pyridoxine (B$_6$)*	1934	1938	1939	Pyridoxic acid Pyridoxal Pyridoxol Pyridoxamine
Folacin	1945	1945	1945	Adermin Folic acid Citrovorum factor Pteroylglutamic acid *Lactobacillus casei* factor Vitamin M Vitamin B$_c$ Factor U
Cobalamin (B$_{12}$)	1948	1948	1955	Antipernicious anemia factor Cyanocobalamin Hydroxycobalamin Erythrocyte maturation factor
Panthothenic acid	1933	1938	1940	Animal protein factor (A.P.F.) Pantotheine Antichromomotriclia factor
Biotin		1935	1942	Antiegg white injury factor Bios II Vitamin H
Choline	1930	1962		
Inositol	1928	1928		Muscle sugar

*Since the preparation of this manuscript the IUB Commission on Nomenclature has ruled that the correct designation of these vitamins be changed to thiamin, nicotinic acid, and pyridoxol (J. Biol. Chem. **241**:287, 1966). The names used above are used throughout the text, however.

Continued.

Table 10-1. Discovery, isolation, synthesis, and nomenclature of vitamins—cont'd

	Discovery	Isolation	Synthesis	Other names
Fat-soluble vitamins				
Vitamin A	1915	1937	1946	Axerophthol Retinoic acid Retinal Retinol Dehydroretinol
Vitamin D	1918	1930	1936	Antirachitic factor Cholecalciferol Ergocalciferol
Vitamin E	1922	1936	1937	Tocopherol Antisterility factor
Vitamin K	1934	1939	1939	Phylloquinine Farnoquinone Antihemorrhagic factor Menadione (synthetic) Synkovite (synthetic) Hykanone (synthetic)

sible for preventing and curing beriberi.

From this very simple classification of vitamins has grown a list of four completely different fat-soluble vitamins and eleven water-soluble substances that have been grouped together as the vitamin B complex and vitamin C. As our knowledge of the chemical and physical properties and the physiologic roles of the vitamins has grown and the unique features of each member of the B complex has been clarified, there has been an effort to drop such designations as vitamin B_1, B_2, B_6, which imply a common functional or structural relationship. Since virtually no direct relationship exists except that they are all water-soluble and most operate as coenzymes in metabolic reactions, terms that more adequately designate their composition or structure, such as thiamine, riboflavin, pyridoxine, and cobala-min, are being used now. To a certain extent the B complex vitamins have much the same natural distribution in foods. It will undoubtedly be some time before the old terminology disappears from the literature, but by pointing out the various systems of nomenclature we hope to minimize the confusion.

Table 10-1 presents in historical sequence the discovery of vitamins. Gaps in the alphabetical and numerical designations can be explained by the fact that scientists, thinking they had discovered a new nutritional principle, would label it as a vitamin only to discover later that it did not have vitamin activity or was identical with another factor. It is clear that no new vitamins have been elucidated in the last fifteen years, and biochemists, physiologists, and nutritionists feel that they can establish normal growth, reproductive capacity, and a high level of health by feeding a synthetic diet of the now known nutritional principles in which the balance of nutrients approximates that in natural foods. However, one can never dismiss the possibility that other factors will be discovered. This is especially true as biochemical technique and instruments become more refined and sensitive.

In spite of the fact that individual members of the fat-soluble group (vitamins A, D, E, and K) and the water-soluble group (all others) have unique functions, there are a few characteristics that generally differentiate the two groups. These are summarized in Table 10-2.

Related substances

Two groups of compounds chemically related to vitamins are of nutritional importance—vitamin precursors or provitamins and antivitamins.

Provitamins or precursors are substances chemically related to the biologically active form of the vitamin but which have no vitamin activity until the body converts it into the active form. The conversion of the precursor to the active form takes place in different parts of the body with different degrees of efficiency, depending on the form of the precursor and the complexity

of the reactions required to convert it to the active form. For instance, carotenes are converted to vitamin A in the intestinal wall, 7-dehydrocholesterol to vitamin D in the skin catalyzed by the ultraviolet rays from the sun, and tryptophan to niacin in the liver. Folic acid or folacin, as it occurs in food, is actually the precursor of the biologically active citrovorum factor. In this case the conversion which likely occurs in the cell requires two other vitamins—ascorbic acid and niacin.

Antivitamins, vitamin antagonists, or pseudovitamins are chemically related to the biologically active vitamin. In this case the body does not discriminate between the useful form of the vitamin and the antagonist and so incorporates either into essential body compounds. The active vitamin as part of enzymes or coenzymes allows biochemical reactions to occur normally. The antagonist not only does not function in the enzyme system but stubbornly refuses to be replaced by the proper substance, which would allow the reaction to proceed. The situation is analogous to putting the key in a lock only to find that it does not work and cannot be removed so that the proper key can be used. Vitamin antagonists have been used to produce experimental vitamin deficiencies, especially of nutrients so widespread in nature that it is difficult to

Table 10-2. General properties of fat-soluble and water-soluble vitamins

Fat-soluble vitamins	*Water-soluble vitamins*
Soluble in fat and fat solvents (water-miscible derivatives are available)	Soluble in water
Intake in excess of daily need stored in the body	Minimal storage of dietary excesses
Not excreted	Excreted in urine
Deficiencies slow to develop	Deficiency symptoms often develop rapidly
Not absolutely necessary in diet every day	Must be supplied every day in diet
Have precursors	Generally do not have precursors

produce a diet sufficiently low in them to establish deficiency symptoms or to determine their metabolic role. Medically, these are also proving useful in retarding the undesirable growth of tissues. A folacin antagonist, for instance, has shown some promise in retarding the growth of the rapidly growing leucocytes in leukemia but must be used with caution since it also inhibits the growth of desirable cells.

Functions

In spite of our knowledge of the chemical structure of the vitamins and observations on the effects of their absence on body biochemistry, scientists still have been unable to determine the exact biochemical role of many of the vitamins. Those whose functions have been determined serve primarily as coenzymes needed to facilitate action of enzymes. The chemical changes that occur in the products of digestion of food after it has been absorbed, which lead either to its incorporation into body structure or to the release of its energy, take place in individual cells. Each cell contains at least 500 enzymes that catalyze these changes. Some enzymes work alone to bring about the required changes; others require the help of coenzymes, most of which are vitamins or vitamin complexes. If the vitamins are not available to form the coenzymes, the sequence of chemical changes cannot proceed and the product whose change is blocked accumulates in the tissues or blood or metabolism is diverted in another direction. In many cases the accumulated intermediary product of the biochemical changes that occur in a normal pattern is responsible for many of the symptoms associated with lack of a specific vitamin.

Deficiencies

Vitamin deficiencies may arise from one or several causes. Most common is the lack of the nutrient in the diet. Individuals show wide variation in normal needs; an amount adequate for one person may be insufficient for another. For instance, some adults can function with 0.2 mg. of thiamine while others require as much as 0.8 mg. It is to take care of the needs of the latter that has led the National Research Council to allow such a wide margin of safety over average needs in establishing its recommended dietary allowances.

Failure of the body to absorb the nutrient provided in food makes it unavailable to perform its function in the cell. For instance, persons whose secretion of bile is limited or absent usually absorb lower amounts of the fat-soluble vitamins than persons who have an adequate amount of bile to facilitate fat absorption. A defect of gastric acid secretion precludes the absorption of cobalamin. Rapid passage of food through the gastrointestinal tract also inhibits absorption.

Increased need for a vitamin may precipitate symptoms on an intake that would normally be adequate. For instance, alcoholics experience an increased need for thiamine, persons with tuberculosis need more vitamin C, and now evidence is suggesting that an infant can be conditioned to need an abnormally high amount of pyridoxine or vitamin C if maternal tissues were saturated during fetal development.

Unusually high losses from poor methods of harvesting, storage, or preparation of the food reduce the actual content of the diet below expected levels.

Supplements

Knowledge of the beneficial effects that occur when vitamin intake is adequate and the detrimental effects associated with inadequate intake have resulted in an undue concern over the vitamin content of the diet. Many purveyors of vitamin supplements have capitalized on this concern and have created doubts on the part of the American public as to the possibility of obtaining sufficient amounts of vitamins from food. Beyond this they market supplements that contains vitamins at levels well beyond any conceivable need. As a result many persons are buying and consuming vitamins in excess of their daily needs. Aside from the economic waste involved there is little harm from excess amounts of the water-soluble vitamins. However, as will be discussed later, excessive intakes of fat-soluble vitamins may have definite harmful effects, and indiscriminate use of such supplements should be discouraged. It is interesting and perhaps appalling to find that the United States produced 1200 pounds of ascorbic acid in 1962, enough to provide 20 mg. per person per day for a year for everyone in the world. Some was used in food preservation to preserve and maintain food quality eventually to end up in the diet, but an undue amount went into vitamin pills to be consumed by an overzealous public.

11

Fat-soluble vitamins

VITAMIN A

Shortly after Casimir Funk designated the then-unknown accessory substances in food as "vitamines," two groups of scientists working independently recognized a fat-soluble substance in food as necessary for growth in animals. This "vitamine," the first to be identified, was designated as fat-soluble A. It is still known as vitamin A, but it has since been established that there is a complex of chemically related substances that have varying degrees of vitamin A activity rather than one single active compound. The term *axerophthol*, reflecting the use of one form of the vitamin in treating a condition known as xerophthalmia, has been applied occasionally to this same substance.

In 1912 Osborne and Mendel, working at Yale, reported that animals grew normally on diets containing milk fat but failed to grow when the milk fat was withdrawn. Growth failure was followed by an eye disease. Simultaneously, at the University of Wisconsin, McCollum and Davis were studying the growth of rats on a purified ration of carbohydrate, casein, minerals,

and lard. They observed that after periods ranging from 70 to 120 days growth ceased. They were able to restore growth and relieve the eye symptoms with an ether extract of either butter, cod-liver oil, or egg yolk. Both groups concluded that a fat-soluble substance was necessary for normal growth in animals. In 1915 they named it fat-soluble A to distinguish it from the water-soluble B that had been detected about the same time.

It was not until 1919 that Steenbock, also working in Wisconsin, recognized a similar growth-promoting property in diets containing a yellow vegetable pigment. He was stimulated in his work by Wisconsin dairy farmers' reports of better growth and improvement in fertility when cows were fed yellow corn rather than white corn. As a result of his observations, he was able to attach nutritional significance to the yellow coloring matter in plants such as corn, carrots, and sweet potatoes. Carotene, one of the yellow pigments of plants, was identified as a potent precursor of vitamin A in 1928.

The vitamin A activity of plant and animal foods is measured in terms of International Units (I.U.) or United States Pharmacopeia Units (U.S.P.), which are equal in potency and represent the amount of vitamin A or its precursor that will cause a specific growth response in rats whose reserves of vitamin A have been depleted. These bioassays have been standardized to that amount.

Chemical properties

In spite of its early discovery, it was not until 1930 to 1932 that Swiss and British scientists chemically identified vitamin A. In 1937 it was crystallized from halibut-liver oil, which has a potency ranging from 2,000,000 to 36,000,000 I.U. per gram. By 1946 a method of synthesizing vitamin A had been developed, but only recently has it been economically feasible to produce synthetic vitamin A rather than crystallizing it from natural sources. Synthetic vitamin A has a potency of 4,500,000 I.U. per gram at a cost of slightly over one dollar and is now used in many enriched products.

Beta-carotene, a vitamin A percursor with a pronounced yellow color in its purified form, has been produced synthetically and is currently one of the few yellow pigments approved by the Food and Drug Administration for the artificial coloring of food. It is used extensively in gelatin, margarine, soft drinks, cake mixes, and cereal products.

Vitamin A is active in a variety of chemical forms, some of which are specific for certain physiologic reactions. It is transported to the liver as an ester, usually in combination with palmitic acid, stored in the liver as an ester, primarily vitamin A acetate, and transported from the liver as vitamin A alcohol. In its role in visual pigments it is active in the aldehyde form. More recently the metabolic roles of vitamin A acid and possibly other derivatives have been discovered. In an effort to simplify and standardize nomenclature, vitamin A alcohol has been designated as *retinol*, vitamin A aldehyde as *retinal,* and vitamin A acid as *retinoic acid.* Retinol or retinal can be reversibly oxidized and reduced, but, as shown in Fig. 11-1, retinoic acid cannot be converted back to the other two. Vitamin A acid, which prevents some signs of vitamin A deficiency, cannot be stored and disappears very rapidly, possibly by being converted into derivatives of vitamin A acid such as anhydroretinoic acid. Since vitamin A acid is

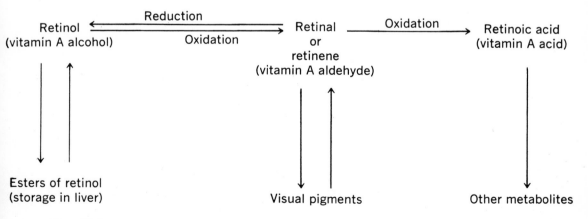

Fig. 11-1

Relationship of biological forms of vitamin A.

capable of performing some but not all of the functions of vitamin A_1 it has been referred to as a partial vitamin.

The biologically active form of vitamin A_1 is found only in foods of animal origin with the exception of a small amount found in spinach. A related form designated vitamin A_2 is found only in livers of fresh-water fish and is of little practical significance. Many plants, however, are rich in a group of compounds chemically related to vitamin A that are known as precursors or provitamins. These substances belong primarily to a group of compounds known as carotenoids, ten of which have been identified in food. Of these, alpha-, beta-, and gamma-carotene and crytoxanthine are the most important in human and animal nutrition. It is from these carotenoid compounds that animals are able to synthesize vitamin A. The presence of the biologically active provitamins parallels the presence of green and yellow pigments in fruits and vegetables—a direct relationship existing between degree of pigmentation and potential vitamin A value. Yellow pigments such as lycopene in tomatoes and xanthophyll in corn do not have vitamin A potential although both these foods do contain other vitamin A precursors.

Vitamin A is an almost colorless substance soluble in fat or fat solvents and very stable under normal conditions of storage and food preparation.

Both carotene and vitamin A are relatively insoluble in water so that practically none is lost in cooking water. They are stable to heat, acid, and alkali but unstable to oxidation. Thus vitamin A is seldom lost in food preparation except when fat becomes rancid and is followed by the oxidation of vitamin A.

Functions

The metabolic roles of vitamin A appear to be numerous but are not well understood, in spite of the fact that it was the first vitamin to be discovered and has been chemically identified for over thirty years. The fact that we are only now gaining some information on it reflects the complexity of its biological role. It has been positively identified as participating in at least five distinct metabolic reactions and it is felt that there must be a common metabolic factor in its effect on cartilage, bone, and epithelium, but so far no one has been able to identify the biochemical nature of its role. The clinical effects of vitamin A are many and seem to involve all human cells in one way or another.

Maintenance of visual purple for vision in dim light. The biochemistry of the action of vitamin A in dark adaptation is the only one of its functions that has been clearly defined. Vitamin A in the form of the aldehyde, retinol, or retinene is essential to combine with the protein scotopsin for the formation of visual purple, the photoreceptor pigment in the special cells known as rods, in the retina of the eyes, which are responsible for vision in dim light. As light strikes the retina the visual purple is bleached to visual yellow and retinene or retinal is separated from scotopsin. With this action a stimulus is transferred from the retina through the optic nerve fibers to the brain. During the process some vitamin A, which is split off from the protein, is reduced to retinol, most of which is reconverted to retinal to recombine with scotopsin to regenerate visual purple or rhodopsin. A small amount of retinol is lost, and vitamin A to replace it must come from the blood. The amount available in the blood determines the rate at which the rhodopsin is regenerated and is available to act again as a receptor substance in the retina. Until the cycle has been completed vision in dim light is not possible. The mechanism involved is shown in Fig. 11-2.

Two good examples of this phenomenon are the visual reaction of persons on entering a dimly lit theater from a brightly lit street and the temporary blindness experienced by a driver at night after meeting a

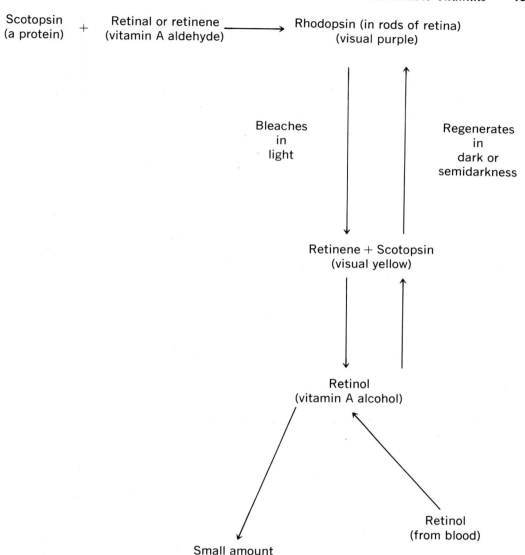

Fig. 11-2

Role of vitamin A in dark adaptation.

car with bright headlights. In both cases the bright light has caused excessive bleaching of rhodopsin, and vision in dim light such as in the relatively dark theater or unlit road will be possible only when a sufficient amount of visual purple has re-formed to facilitate vision. This is illus-trated in Fig. 11-3. The speed with which the eye adapts after exposure to bright light is believed to be directly related to the amount of vitamin A available to regen-erate rhodopsin. The "dark adaptation" test, the speed of recovery of visual acuity in dim light as measured by an especially

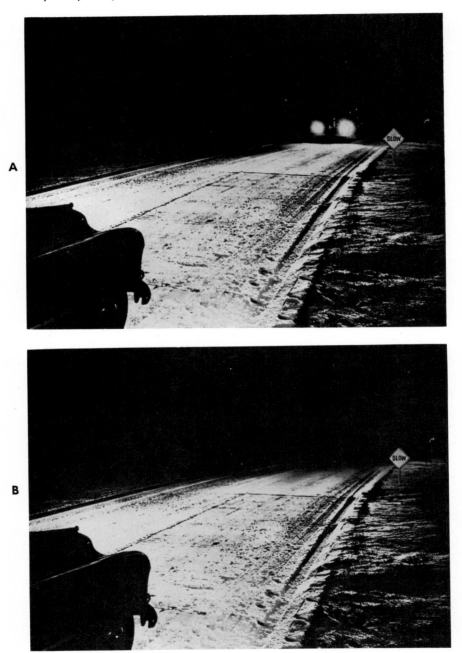

Fig. 11-3

Night blindness. Night blindness is a useful and early diagnostic sign of vitamin A deficiency. This loss of visual acuity in dim light following exposure to bright light is illustrated here. **A,** Both the normal individual and the vitamin A–deficient subject see the headlights of an approaching car. **B,** After the car has passed, the normal individual sees a wide stretch of road. **C,** The vitamin A–deficient subject can barely see a few feet ahead and cannot see the road sign at all. (Courtesy Upjohn Company, Kalamazoo, Mich.)

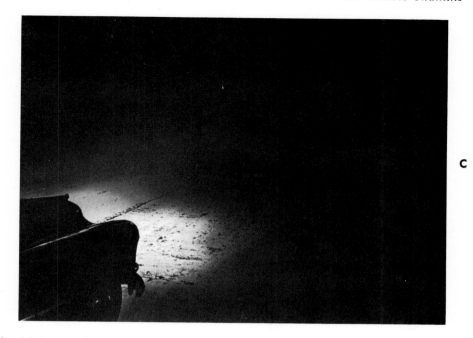

C

Fig. 11-3, cont'd.

For legend see opposite page.

designed apparatus, was long considered the most sensitive measure of vitamin A status. It is now believed to be of limited usefulness.

Vitamin A is also part of another photoreceptor substance, iodopsin, in the cells in the retina known as cones, which are responsible for vision in bright light. The cones, however, are not as sensitive to changes in the amount of vitamin A available as are the rods.

Growth. The effect of vitamin A on growth is best illustrated by the fact that an animal deprived of vitamin A will cease to grow once vitamin A reserves have been depleted (Fig. 11-4). Growth failure shows up before any other symptoms. Bones fail to grow in length, and the remodelling process, an essential phase of bone growth, slows down. Since there is not a concurrent decrease in growth of nervous tissue there may be undue pressure on brain and other parts of nervous tissue whose growth is not depressed in vitamin A deficiency and which are protected by a bony framework that fails to grow fast enough to accommodate it. Bone growth is stimulated when vitamin A is made available again.

Evidence is accumulating to suggest that there may be a degeneration or defective formation of nervous tissue independent of the effect of a deficiency of vitamin A on bone growth. One theory is that in the absence of vitamin A the protective layer of tissue surrounding nerve fibers does not form satisfactorily.

Reproduction. The role of vitamin A in promoting fertility in animals was one of the first discovered. Either vitamin A alcohol (retinol) or its aldehyde derivative (retinal) is necessary for normal reproduction in rats. In its absence there is an absence of spermatogenesis in the male, and fetal resorption occurs in females. The exact biochemical mechanism is unknown, but it has been shown that while the alcohol

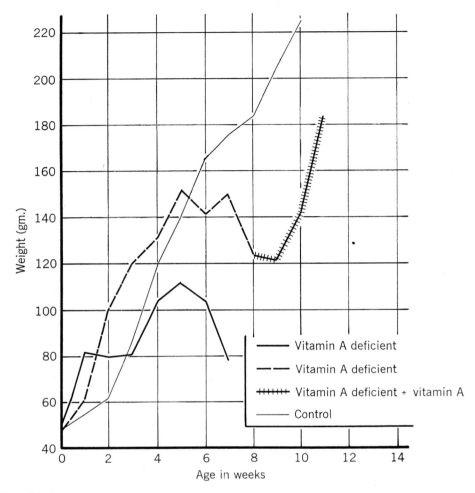

Fig. 11-4

Growth response of weanling albino rats to a diet deficient in vitamin A.

form of vitamin A is effective in stimulating normal reproduction, vitamin A acid will permit conception but will not prevent fetal resorption.

Health of epithelial cells. Epithelial cells constitute not only the outer protective layer of skin but also the linings of all openings from the body, such as the respiratory tract, the gastrointestinal tract, and the genitourinary tract. In many cases these epithelial cells normally secrete mucus. The fact that certain sequences of degenerative changes occur when vitamin

A is lacking supports the belief that vitamin A is essential to biochemical reactions necessary to preserve health of epithelial cells.

During a deficiency there is a drying or keratinization of the layer of cells, followed by a loss of cilia and the ability of the cells to secrete mucus. This depressed secretion of mucus is believed to be due to the fact that vitamin A is necessary for the synthesis of the carbohydrate, mucopolysaccharide, a normal constituent of mucus, as well as the fact that ducts may become

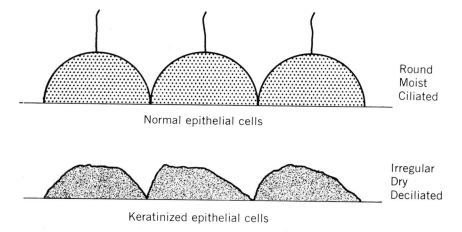

Normal epithelial cells — Round / Moist / Ciliated

Keratinized epithelial cells — Irregular / Dry / Deciliated

Fig. 11-5

Schematic representation of changes in epithelial cells in vitamin A deficiency.

clogged by keratinized plugs. Finally the outer layers pile up, leaving a layer of horny keratinized cells in place of the moist, rounded, ciliated cells of normal epithelium. The changes in epithelial cells are shown diagrammatically in Fig. 11-5. A large number of body processes are affected when there is inadequate vitamin A to promote the normal health of epithelial cells. These will be discussed as results of deficiency of vitamin A.

Other functions. Studies have indicated that vitamin A (either as acid or alcohol) is necessary for the release of proteolytic or protein-splitting enzymes from particles in the cell known as lysosomes or perinuclear dense bodies. These enzymes must be released to act on the cartilage of bone tissue during bone remodelling to cause a breakdown of the protein structure and the dissolution of the matrix itself. An excess of vitamin A may cause complete disintegration of the matrix by releasing too many enzymes too fast. An imbalance between the rate of breakdown of bone and bone formation is reflected in abnormal bone structure.

Both vitamin A and vitamin A acid have been shown to be effective in the synthesis

of the hormone corticosterone from cholesterol in the adrenal cortex. In the absence of vitamin A and with reduced corticosterone synthesis there is a loss of the ability of the body to synthesize glycogen, the storage form of carbohydrate.

Absorption and metabolism

The absorption of vitamin A and its precursors takes place through the wall of the intestine into the lymphatic system. Since both are soluble in fat, factors that facilitate absorption of fat facilitate the absorption of vitamin A, and conversely factors depressing fat absorption also depress the utilization of fat-soluble vitamins.

Before vitamin A can be absorbed it must be separated from the ester in which it usually occurs in food. This separation is usually accomplished by an enzyme secreted by the pancreas but if this is not present enzymes in the intestinal wall will cause the separation. Once it is in the walls of the intestine, vitamin A combines with a fatty acid, most often the long-chain saturated palmitic acid, to form vitamin A palmitate. This then attaches to a protein to render it more soluble, is released into the lymphatic system, and carried to the blood and then to the liver. The absorption of vitamin A, which is facilitated by the presence of bile salts and which increases as protein increases, usually takes place three to five hours after ingestion.

Vitamin A is withdrawn by the liver as vitamin A palmitate or stearate and stored until it is released into the blood as retinol attached to a protein to meet the metabolic demands of other tissues. Protein appears necessary for the mobilization of vitamin A reserves from the liver. This may explain low blood levels of vitamin A found in kwashiorkor or prekwashiorkor, a protein-deficiency disease, which respond when protein and no additional vitamin A are given. Normal blood levels for vitamin A are approximately 130 I.U. per 100 ml. Any drop in plasma vitamin A levels reflects a depletion of liver reserves and a prolonged dietary deficiency rather than immediate dietary intake.

The four major vegetable precursors of vitamin A—alpha-, beta-, and gamma-carotene and cryptoxanthine—are absorbed in the presence of bile salts from the intestine after being released from the plant cell during digestion. They are converted in the intestinal wall to vitamin A. The conversion of carotene to vitamin A is not complete, with some carotene absorbed unchanged, entering the circulation where normal carotene levels approximate 150 I.U. per 100 ml. of blood. Carotene levels reflect dietary carotene and do not reflect storage of vitamin A so that in decreased intakes there is a rather rapid drop in carotene values. Unconverted carotene is stored in the fat depots rather than in the liver of human beings.

The amount of vitamin A formed from the precursor depends on the form of the precursor. Beta-carotene is a symmetrical molecule made up of two vitamin A molecules. Although it could theoretically be changed into two molecules by breaking it in the center evidence now shows that it is more likely to be broken down in a step-wise fashion from one end to give only one molecule of vitamin A. The other precursors can yield only one molecule of vitamin A, but usually yield less than beta-carotene. Approximately one third of the carotene in food is converted to vitamin A; carotenes in carrots and root vegetables undergo less than one fourth conversion and those in leafy vegetables about one half. The conversion of carotene to vitamin A occurs primarily in the intestinal wall, although some may take place in liver and lungs. In any case the conversion is stimulated by thyroxine. Once converted into vitamin A, it is handled in the same way as the preformed vitamin.

The absorption of vitamin A from foods is decreased in liver injury, which decreases bile formation, or in any condition in which there is an obstruction of the bile duct. Mineral oil has an affinity for vitamin A, and since it is unaffected by digestive enzymes and passes through the digestive tract it will carry with it much of the potential vitamin A in the diet. For this reason the practice of using mineral oil as a source of fat for low-calorie salad dressings on salad greens, one of the potentially good sources of vitamin A activity, is to be condemned. The intake of polyunsaturated fatty acids with carotene results in rapid destruction of carotene unless antioxidants are also present.

The concentration of vitamin A in human liver reflects long-term dietary intakes. The small number of studies reported have given values from 100 I.U. per gram in Great Britain, through 766 I.U. per gram for Americans, to a high of 1000 I.U. per gram among New Zealanders who live on a diet high in butter. It is estimated that a healthy person stores 500,000 I.U. in his liver, an amount that may last him several years.

Food sources

The vitamin A value of some representative foods is shown in Fig. 11-6.

Preformed vitamin A is available only in

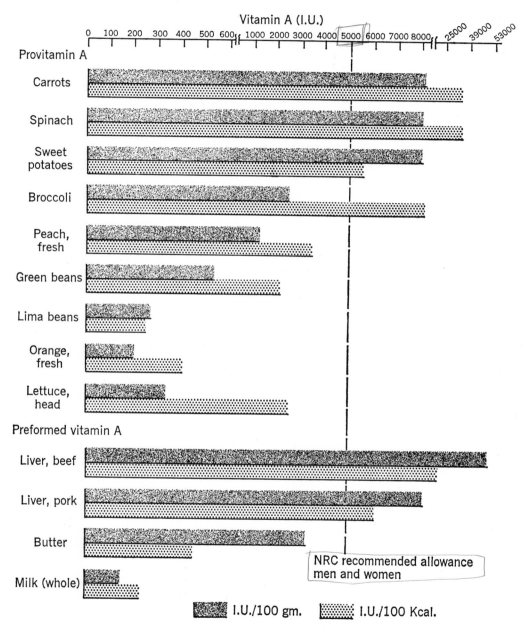

Fig. 11-6

Vitamin A value of 100-gm. and 100-kilocalorie portions of some representative foods. (Based on Watts, B., and Merrill, A.: Composition of foods—raw, processed and prepared, U. S. Department of Agriculture Handbook No. 8, Washington, D. C., 1963, U. S. Department of Agriculture.)

animal products in which the animal has metabolized the carotene of its food into vitamin A and concentrated it in certain tissues. Liver, representing the storage site for vitamin A, reflects the dietary intake of the animal. It ranges from 2,000,-000 I.U. per 100 gm. in polar bear liver to 45,000 I.U. in beef liver to 19,000 I.U. per 100 gm. in pork liver. Fish-liver oils are extremely rich, and until very recently concentrates of these were the most widely used therapeutic sources of vitamin A.

Egg yolk with 2000 to 4000 I.U. per 100 gm. is a good source of vitamin A in the form of retinol and is the one usually introduced first into the diet to replenish the fetal reserves of a young infant. Since preformed vitamin A is colorless, the color of the yolk is no indication of its potency in the yolk. A deep yellow color may reflect unconverted carotene, but more often it is xanthophyll with no vitamin A activity and which varies with the breed of the animal. It is possible to increase the amount of vitamin A in an egg yolk by increasing the amount fed to the hen.

The vitamin A value of butter varies with the breed of animal and its diet and shows a definite seasonal variation. In winter butter averages 9000 I.U. per pound while in summer values may exceed 15,000 I.U., the amount with which margarine is usually fortified. In neither case is color an indication of vitamin A value.

In milk the vitamin A is present in the fat portion; this is absent in nonfat milk. Average values for milk are 390 I.U. per cup, which is relatively low, and the loss of vitamin A when nonfat milk replaces whole milk becomes important only when milk is the sole item in the diet, as it is in very young infants. Any yellow color in milk is due to presence of carotene, reflecting inefficient conversion on the part of the cow. Fresh fluid nonfat milk and homogenized whole milk is often enriched with vitamin A. The amount of vitamin A in cheese is the same as that in the milk from which it is made.

Aside from milk products, eggs, and liver, animal products contain virtually no vitamin A. Muscle meats are devoid of vitamin A value.

Fruits and vegetables contain no pre-

Table 11-1. Vitamin A values of representative foods

Food	I.U. of vitamin A activity
Fruits and vegetables	
Spinach (½ cup)	10,600
Carrots, diced (½ cup)	9065
Broccoli (½ cup)	2550
Kale (½ cup)	4610
Asparagus (½ cup)	910
Peas (½ cup)	575
Brussels sprouts (½ cup)	260
Lima beans (½ cup)	230
Cabbage, cooked (½ cup)	75
Apricots, dried (½ cup)	8195
Apricots, canned (½ cup)	2260
Papaya (½ cup)	1595
Watermelon (2-pound wedge)	1265
Peaches, raw (½ cup)	1115
Orange (1 medium)	290
Banana (1 medium)	95
Pineapple, raw (½ cup)	90
Dairy products	
Milk, fresh whole (1 cup)	390
Milk, fresh nonfat (1 cup)	10
Cheese, cheddar (1 ounce)	378
Cheese, processed cheddar (1 ounce)	300
Butter (1 tablespoon)	230
Margarine (1 tablespoon)	230
Meat, fish, poultry, and eggs	
Egg, whole	590
Egg yolk	580
Liver (3 ounces)	
Beef	45,450
Lamb	43,000
Chicken	27,000
Calves	19,000
Pork	12,000

formed vitamin A but only precursors. Because of this, tables of food composition report vitamin A activity or vitamin A value of foods, reflecting the potential vitamin A available from the food based on ability of the body to make the conversion.

Generally, as seen from Table 11-1, the vitamin A value of fruits and vegetables is directly proportional to the amount of carotene or chlorophyll present in the food. In addition, if one examines the vitamin A values of a food such as a head of lettuce one finds a tenfold increase as one progresses from the inner bleached leaves to the outer leaves higher in chlorophyll and carotenoids. Unfortunately a high concentration of chlorophyll is often accompanied by an astringent bitter taste, as in very dark green endive leaves, so that a potentially rich source of vitamin A is unpalatable. Some fruits such as mangoes increase their carotene content with storage.

The yellow pigments, lycopene, found in watermelon and tomatoes, and xanthophyll, found in corn and egg yolk, do not have vitamin A value. Another yellow pigment, cryptoxanthine in corn, does have vitamin A potential of about 3.5 I.U. per gram. In countries where red palm oil is used in cooking its carotene content represents a major source of vitamin A activity.

The ability of the body to utilize carotene varies with the food and the form in which the food is ingested. For instance, grated carrots have greater value than carrot slices. Utilization varies from 30% to 70% of available vitamin A.

Vitamin A is very stable to heat, light, acid, and alkali, and very little is lost under normal conditions of food preparation. Excessive temperatures in frying oils high in carotene such as palm oil, used extensively in tropical countries, may cause its destruction, as will the oxidation that occurs in rancid fats. The very small amount of green and yellow pigment that may appear in cooking water from fruits and vegetables represents an insignificant portion of that present in the food. Sun-drying of fruits may lead to some loss of vitamin A.

The contributions of various food groups to the vitamin A content of the American diet are shown in Fig. 11-7.

In the United States there is an average daily intake of over 10,000 I.U., 50% of which comes from vegetable sources, compared to about 4300 I.U. in Britain, two thirds of which is from animal sources. In Central and South America, 93% of the vitamin A comes from the precursor and one third of this from yellow maize. India has an intake of less than 1000 I.U. per day, and the simultaneous low protein intake keeps the level of utilization low.

Recommended allowances

The National Research Council recommended allowances for vitamin A have been established in relation to body weight and to the source of vitamin A—whether the active form or the precursor. When the sole source is the preformed form the minimum requirement is 20 I.U. per kilogram of body weight, whereas 40 I.U. per kilogram is suggested when carotene is the sole source. Assuming that one third of the vitamin A value of a mixed diet comes from animal sources and two thirds from vegetable sources, the recommendation allowances have been set at 5000 I.U. for an adult per day. If preformed vitamin A from animals is the sole source, 3000 I.U. is considered sufficient. During pregnancy the recommendation is increased to 6000 I.U., and in lactation 8000 I.U. is deemed adequate. The recommended amounts for other age groups are shown in Appendix C.

The discrepancies in recommended levels of vitamin A intake in various standards result from assumptions of different proportions of vitamin A and carotene in diets and different interpretations of the efficiency with which carotene is converted into vitamin A.

The need for vitamin A varies from individual to individual under varying con-

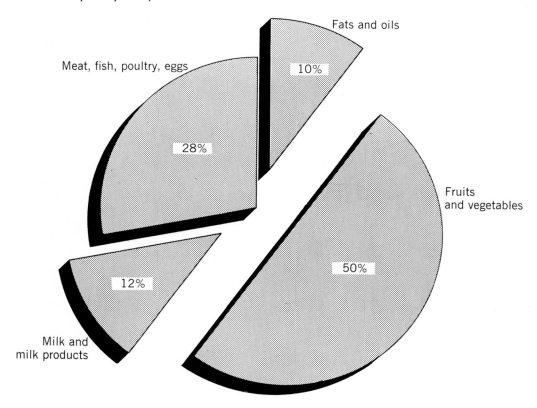

Fig. 11-7

Contribution of various food groups to the vitamin A content of the American food supply. (Based on Nutritive value of food available for consumption, United States, 1909-1964, Agricultural Research Service Publication 62-14, 1966.)

ditions. Tiring work, especially in hot weather, tends to raise needs. This may be a manifestation of the decreased ability to convert carotene into vitamin A at higher temperatures. Also, more vitamin A is needed after removal of gallbladder, in hypothyroidism, and in conditions of impaired intestinal absorption.

Results of deficiency

Vitamin A deficiency symptoms will show up only after liver reserves have been depleted, the period of time depending on the extent of the reserves determined by previous dietary intake. In animals, growth ceases when the reserves of vitamin A have been used up. Most symptoms of a vitamin

A deficiency as seen in human beings are a reflection of its role in maintaining the health of epithelial cells. They may result from low dietary intakes, interference with absorption and storage, interference with conversion of carotene to vitamin A, or rapid loss of vitamin A from the body.

Night blindness. One of the earliest symptoms of vitamin A deficiency is night blindness. In low intakes the liver reserves drop, followed by a drop in blood levels and a subsequent drop in the level available in the retina of the eye, which eventually shows up in a slow dark adaptation time and finally night blindness.

Changes in eye. The cornea of the eye is affected early. The lachrymal gland fails to secrete, possibly as a result of decreased ability to synthesize mucopolysaccharide or of a blocking of the lachrymal duct. This is followed by a keratinization and opacity and sloughing of epithelial cells of the cornea with eventual rupturing of the corneal tissue. Infection apparently sets in, pus is exudated, and the eye will hemorrhage. This condition is known as Bitot's spots in its mildest form, as xerosis conjunctivae in moderately severe form, and as xerophthalmia in advanced stages. These conditions were prevalent in children in Denmark during World War I when occupation troops deprived them of dairy products, their most dependable source of vitamin A. It is now reported frequently in Indonesia and other tropical countries where a low protein intake may also be a contributing factor. Typical eye symptoms of severe vitamin A deficiency are shown in Fig. 11-8. Total blindness is a frequent result and most frequently affects children. It is suggested that many children succumb to other forms of vitamin A deficiency before xerophthalmia develops.

Respiratory infections. Vitamin A has often been designated as the anti-infective vitamin because of high incidence of respiratory ailments associated with a vitamin A deficiency. Since vitamin A does not directly attack the infective organism the use of this term has been questioned by some. However, there is evidence that when the epithelium of the trachea and bronchi become keratinized, deciliated, and deprived of their mucous secretions and a break occurs in the integrity of the mucous membranes, they become a good harbor for microorganisms that would not normally penetrate a healthy epithelial layer. In animals the changes in epithelium during vitamin A deficiency usually lead to terminal bronchial pneumonia. Recovery among tuberculosis patients has been more rapid when diet is high in vitamin A. Efforts to relate susceptibility to the common cold to vitamin A intake have shown no

relationship, but those on diets high in vitamin A have had colds of shorter duration.

Changes in skin. A dry rough skin, especially in the area of the shoulders, may be an early sign of a vitamin A deficiency. This condition, known as folliculosis, in which there are simply eruptions near the base of the hair follicle that subsequently undergo a keratinization, is used as an indication of possible vitamin A deficiency in many nutritional status studies.

Changes in genitourinary tract. Keratinization of epithelial cells seems to favor calcium deposition and may well predispose to kidney stones.

Changes in gastrointestinal tract. Many disturbances in the gastrointestinal tract, such as diarrhea, have been linked by various investigations to the changes in epithelial tissue that takes place in the absence of vitamin A.

Failure of tooth enamel. The integrity of the enamel layer of teeth may reflect the adequacy of vitamin A at the time the ameloblast cells of epithelial origin are forming, in most cases no later than the fifth year of life. In vitamin A deprivation in animals the enamel layer of teeth is absent where growth during avitaminosis A was depressed.

Changes in nervous tissue. The paralysis that affects the extremities and that has been identified with vitamin A deficiency may conceivably be caused by a degeneration of nervous tissue, but more likely is the result of pressure on nervous tissue resulting from failure of bone growth in the spine and brain.

Toxicity

The possibility that excessive amounts of vitamin A may produce detrimental rather than desirable results has been recognized only recently. Symptoms have appeared as a result of the use of polar bear liver, which has a very high vitamin A potency, the treatment of a skin disorder in adolescents with daily doses of vitamin

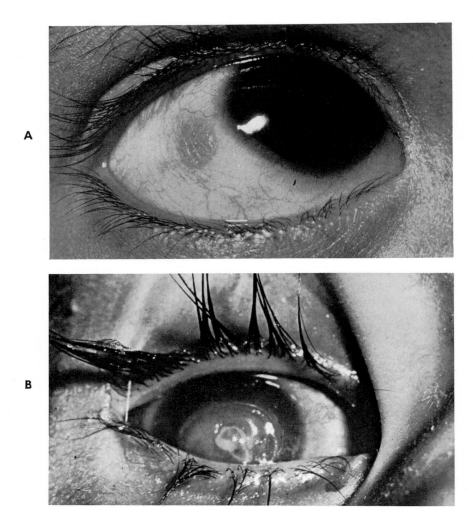

Fig. 11-8

Changes in the eyes characteristic of severe vitamin A deficiency. **A,** Early corneal xerosis with infiltration in lower central cornea. **B,** Keratomalacia—softening and protrusion of whole central area of cornea. **C,** Generalized xerosis with clearly demarcated Bitot's spots. (From McLaren, D. S., Shirajan, E., Tschalian, M., and Khuory, G.: Xerophthalmia in Jordan, Am. J. Clin. Nutrition **17:**117, 1965.)

A of 50,000 to 100,000 I.U. and the use of large doses of vitamin A supplements for infants by overzealous mothers. The symptoms of vitamin A toxicity are many, ranging from headache, drowsiness, nausea, loss of hair, and diarrhea in adults, to a scaly dermatitis, weight loss, anorexia, and skeletal pain in infants, to loss of hemo-globin and potassium from red blood cells, cessation of menstruation in young girls and women, and rapid resorption of bone in adults. The period between the initiation of high intakes and the onset of symptoms varies from six to fifteen months. There seem to be wide individual differences in sensitivity to high levels, some

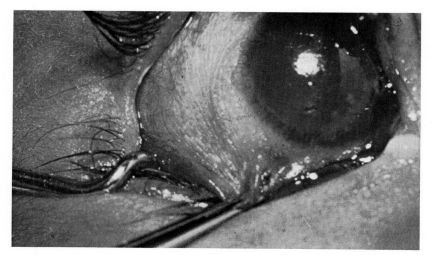

C

Fig. 11-8, cont'd.

For legend see opposite page.

persons showing symptoms after long-term dosages of 50,000 I.U. per day while others have exhibited a reaction only at levels of 150,000 to 200,000 I.U. daily. There is a rapid and complete recovery on withdrawal of excess intake, with symptoms subsiding in 72 hours in many cases. Toxic reactions can occur only from overconsumption of the preformed vitamin but not with the precursor. Permanent effects of vitamin A toxicity are rare. Some workers are concerned that long-standing high intakes on the part of the mother, resulting in storage levels in the liver of 1000 I.U. or more per gram, may have harmful effects in the fetus even if the mother has not exhibited a toxic reaction herself. In animals, single injections of vitamin A in the pregnant female have produced congenital skeletal abnormalities in her young. Even though vitamin A acid cannot be stored it can contribute to toxic reactions and thus there are suggestions that toxicity is caused by oxidation of the acid.

The Food and Drug Administration has become sufficiently concerned to ask that a ceiling be placed on the amount of vitamin A that can be included in a multivitamin preparation available without a prescription. The availability of vitamin A supplements of high potency at a low price often leads people to oversupplement the diet. This, coupled with the widespread practice of enriching food products for trade advantages, increases the possibility of a person receiving a toxic dose. The possibility of this occurring in a normal mixed diet is quite remote.

VITAMIN D

Vitamin D is now officially designated as cholecalciferol (vitamin D_3) or ergocalciferol (vitamin D_2), depending on whether it is derived from animal or vegetable sources. It had been known previously as the *sunshine vitamin* because sunshine is one of its sources to the body and the *antirachitic factor, or rickets-preventative factor* because of its effectiveness in curing rickets.

Since vitamin D_3 can be produced in the body it is technically a hormone, but if insufficient amounts are produced in the body, either vitamin D_2 or vitamin D_3 must be supplied by the diet, in which case they are technically vitamins. Vitamin D is necessary for all animals with a bony skeleton since it facilitates the absorption and utilization of calcium and phosphorus for normal bone formation. Like vitamin A, vitamin D is measured in terms of international units defined in terms of a biological response to the administration of the vitamin to a depleted animal. One I.U. of vitamin D weighs 0.025 μg. and 1 mg. contains 40,000 I.U.

Rickets

Rickets is a condition that has plagued infants in the temperate zone for many years. It was so common in England that some writers referred to it as the *English disease*. Before a dietary factor was implicated as causative agent, many environmental factors had been investigated. The fact that it occurred more frequently among people living in the crowded, smoky, industrial areas of cities where standards of sanitation were often poor suggested that rickets was a disease of bacterial origin. Dark-skinned people moving from the tropics to the temperate zone were very susceptible to rickets. Since they frequently lived in crowded industrial areas, there seemed to be more support for the environmental theory. From time to time there were suggestions that sunshine had a curative effect on rickets but the relationship between sunshine and rickets was not established until the late 1920's, after the nature of vitamin D had been clarified.

Rickets is essentially a disease of defective bone formation that manifests itself in many ways. The bones, which are normally poorly calcified at the time of birth, remain soft and pliable. Deformities develop when these poorly calcified bones are called upon to perform functions for which they are not sufficiently strong. Bowing of legs occurs when a child starts to walk before the bones have become sufficiently rigid to support the weight of the body. The ends of the long bones become enlarged, causing difficulties in movement.

Knock-knee is a manifestation of this enlargement, which results from the flattening that occurs when the poorly calcified ends of the bones are subjected to the weight of the body. Deformities of the ribs result in a concave breast (pigeon breast) that causes crowding in the chest cavity. Ribs also develop irregularly spaced areas of swelling that take on the appearance of beading, which has led to the use of the term *rachitic rosary* to describe this syndrome. The failure of the fontanel of the skull to close allows rapid enlargement of the head, sometimes interpreted as a sign of a health in a child as witnessed by the number of rachitic infants who have been judged "best baby in the show."

Teeth erupt later, are less well formed than is normal, and decay earlier. Growth is generally retarded, but the severity of the disease as measured by other symptoms is frequently greater in children who have undergone rapid growth.

Rickets is a condition that primarily affects children. The symptoms are very slowly reversible, so that some symptoms produced during early childhood may remain throughout adulthood. There are very few reports of anyone over two years of age developing rickets, but this does not mean that there is any decrease in the need for vitamin D. The term *adult rickets* is sometimes applied to the disease osteoporosis, which reflects a defect in bone formation but not a vitamin D deficiency.

Discovery

The discovery of vitamin D followed by six years the identification of fat-soluble A. In 1918 a British nutritionist, Mellanby, presented the first evidence of a fat-soluble substance with antirachitic properties. By 1919 scientists had produced rickets experimentally by feeding animals diets in which vegetable or animal fats replaced cod-liver oil. By 1922 the recognition that the antirachitic properties of cod-liver oil were not destroyed by oxidation that destroyed its vitamin A value led to the suggestion that there was a second fat-soluble vitamin, soon identified as vitamin D.

The existence of provitamin D, which could be activated by the short ultraviolet rays of the sun, was discovered in 1922. This antirachitic factor was isolated in a crystalline form in 1930, twelve years after the first report of the substance.

Functions

The chemistry of vitamin D has been known since 1930 and its role in promoting normal calcification of bones has been evident for some time. However, the mechanism by which vitamin D operates is still not clear and the search continues to elucidate a theory which will satisfactorily explain the physiologic changes which occur in a vitamin D deficiency and which are reversed or prevented by the use of vitamin D. These include:

1. Reduced intestinal absorption of calcium and phosphate.
2. Reduced resorption of phosphate and amino acids by the kidney.
3. Hypocalcemia (low blood calcium levels) and a failure to mobilize bone calcium.
4. Reduced concentrations of citrate (an organic compound intermediary in cellular respiration) in body fluids and bones.
5. Increase in level of the enzyme alkaline phosphatase in the blood.

The role of vitamin D in intestinal absorption is possibly one of activating a system of transporting calcium across the cell membrane. Since the absorption involves overcoming a concentration difference and an electrochemical potential in the cell membrane, energy must be involved in the transport. This effect of vitamin D in facilitating absorption by active transport seems to be greatest in the lower end of gastrointestinal tract. There is also evidence that vitamin D increases the permeability of the cell membrane to calcium ions and possibly to other divalent ions such as magnesium and cobalt. It does not, however, increase the permeability to monovalent ions such as sodium and potassium. The effect of vitamin D on cell permeability extends throughout the whole gastrointestinal tract.

The fact that there is a delay after the administration of vitamin D before improvement in absorption of calcium is noted led to research that suggested that vitamin D was necessary for the synthesis of a protein that acted as a carrier for calcium during absorption.

Failure of calcification of bone is more often caused by an inadequate supply of phosphate than of calcium, although the term calcification to describe the deposition of calcium phosphate crystals in the bone matrix implies that calcium is primarily involved. The addition of vitamin D to the diet increases the rate of absorption of phosphate as well as calcium, but likely of greater importance is that it increases the resorption of phosphate from the tubules of the kidneys. In the absence of vitamin D much phosphate is lost in urinary excretions and the blood levels of phosphate and hence the rate of calcification drops. Vitamin D also influences the rate of resorption of amino acids in the kidney tubules. Recent evidence indicates that the level of amino acids in the urine (aminoaciduria) is a fairly sensitive indication of vitamin D status, increasing in a deficiency and decreasing when vitamin D restores normal rate of resorption.

The importance of maintaining blood calcium levels at a level of at least 7 mg. per 100 ml. is so great that the body mobilizes calcium from the bone matrix to hold this level even in a dietary calcium deficiency. In a vitamin D deficiency the mechanisms for mobilizing calcium fail to function with a resultant drop in blood calcium levels (hypocalcemia).

The adequacy of dietary vitamin D and

the calcification of bone is reflected in the level of citrate in body fluids. In vitamin D deficiency citrate levels drop and are restored in the administration of vitamin D.

A discussion of the role of vitamin D would be incomplete without mention of the antagonistic relationship between vitamin D and hydrocortisone, a hormone secreted by the adrenal gland and used therapeutically in the treatment of many conditions. Hydrocortisone can depress the high blood levels of calcium associated with excessive intakes of vitamin D. It can also decrease the permeability of the intestinal membrane and hence calcium absorption when administered along with normal levels of vitamin D.

As noted in the discussion on calcium, the parathyroid hormone also influences the mobilization of calcium from reserves of exchangeable calcium in bones. Vitamin D appears to permit or regulate the action of the parathyroid hormone. It is evident that three factors—vitamin D, hydrocortisone, and the parathyroid hormone—all operate to regulate calcium balances and bone metabolism. The nature of the interrelationship is not clear. In the case of the effect on kidney resorption of phosphates, the action of vitamin D, which favors the resorption of phosphate, is antagonistic to the action of the parathyroid hormone, which inhibits the resorption of phosphate.

The absence of vitamin D is known to have undesirable effects on the calcification of bone. It is believed that the presence of vitamin D operates to facilitate the absorption of calcium and phosphorus from the intestinal tract and also their deposition as an insoluble complex in the organic bone matrix. The details of the mechanism, however, have not been clearly established, but it has been postulated that this calcification is facilitated by two enzymes—phosphorylase, which accumulates in the ends of bones close to calcification centers, and alkaline phosphatase, which is produced in large amounts on the growing surface of bones to release phosphate from organic compounds. Measure of the alkaline phosphatase level of the blood is frequently used as an indication of the extent of calcification occurring. High values, showing active calcification, and low values, showing poor calcification, reflect vitamin D levels.

The rate of absorption of calcium is greatly increased in the presence of adequate dietary vitamin D; a rate of 10% absorption without vitamin D may be increased to 33% in the presence of the vitamin.

Absorption

Vitamin D is absorbed in the intestinal tract in the presence of bile. Absorption is complete, regardless of the form of the vitamin—cholecalciferol or ergocalciferol—or of the medium in which it is presented—oil or aqueous. Conditions in which fat absorption is reduced, such as steatorrhea or obstructive jaundice, result in a decreased rate of absorption of vitamin D. In contrast to vitamin A, vitamin D is stored in only limited amounts in mammals, with most of it being stored in the liver, kidney, adrenal glands, and bone. Rachitic bone has a greater affinity for it than nonrachitic bone. Vitamin D is excreted through the bile and the intestinal wall.

Dietary requirements

Because of the two sources of vitamin D, the evaluation of minimum requirements is difficult. Indications are that between 100 and 400 I.U. of vitamin D will protect against rickets and promote growth. Increased intake appears to provide no greater protection against rickets and at too high levels may have detrimental effects, reversing the beneficial effects of lower levels. Both breast- and bottle-fed infants should receive a dietary supplement of vitamin D by two weeks of age to provide the NRC recommended intake of 400 I.U. per day.

During pregnancy and lactation an intake of 400 I.U. is deemed desirable. Otherwise adults appear to obtain sufficient amounts if they are exposed to some degree of sunshine and have a varied diet. If occupational or clothing habits are such that exposure to sunlight is limited, a dietary source for adults is recommended.

In older children and adults who seldom develop rickets, it is much more difficult to evaluate minimal needs since no other criterion of adequacy of vitamin D has been established.

Premature infants whose calcium reserves are much lower than those of full-term infants, in whom half the calcium is deposited in the last six weeks of fetal life, have a need for vitamin D to facilitate the absorption of the high level of calcium needed to meet the demands of their rapid growth. Apparent ineffectiveness of dosages of 400 I.U. of vitamin D in breast-fed premature infants may be a function of the low calcium content of breast milk rather than an increased need for vitamin D.

It is only when exposure to sunlight is inadequate, dietary intake of vitamin D is restricted, and needs relatively high that deficiency symptoms develop.

Sources

Irradiation of precursor in skin. Vitamin D is available to the body by two quite separate pathways. The skin normally contains a fat-related substance, dehydrocholesterol, which constitutes 0.15% to 0.42% of the sterols in the skin and which performs no biological function. However, when exposed to the short ultraviolet rays, from 275 to 300 mμ in length from the sun or from sunlamps, it is converted into the biological active substance vitamin D_3 or cholecalciferol. This is then absorbed from the skin into the general circulation, in which it is carried to all body tissues. It is still not clear whether the conversion takes place in the epithelial cells of the skin or on the surface of the skin, but evidence seems to favor the latter. The amount of vitamin D available through the irradiation of the precursor in the skin is influenced more by the amount of ultraviolet light to which the individual is exposed than by a limit in the amount of the precursor present. In the summer in the temperate zone ultraviolet rays may penetrate sufficiently far north for a maximum of four hours in the middle of the day. In winter this time may be reduced to less than an hour. Ultraviolet rays are incapable of penetrating fog, smog, clouds, smoke, ordinary window glass, window screening, clothing, or skin pigment. The presence of any or all of these reduce the potential vitamin D available through irradiation. The pigment in the skin, which acts as a protection against overproduction of vitamin D in the skin of dark-skinned people living in the tropics, reduces the benefits from the much smaller amount of irradiation available in the temperate zone to the point that the incidence of rickets among dark-skinned infants in the temperate zone is much higher than among light-skinned infants and among dark-skinned infants in the tropics. Some protection against overirradiation is necessary since it can lead to the production of potentially toxic substances such as tachysterol, toxisterol, and suprasterol.

A special window glass, mercury quartz, permits the transmission of ultraviolet rays. The benefits from its use in windows in hospital nurseries where patients are unable to be taken out-of-doors may justify the additional cost, which is over ten times that of regular glass.

Although milk is the only product that has been endorsed for fortification, vitamin D is being added to many other products, such as infant cereals, prepared breakfast cereals, milk flavorings, margarine, bread, and even some beverages. If one consumed even one serving of each of these along with one quart of fortified milk a day, the intake could readily reach 1000 I.U. per day.

In the temperate zone, where neither sunshine nor a diet of nonfortified products can be relied upon to provide enough vitamin D for protection from rickets, it has become standard pediatric practice to introduce a supplementary source of vitamin D in infants diets. The use of cod-liver oil, which was traditional since the early 1920's, has been almost completely replaced by water-miscible preparations of vitamin D. This overcomes the increasing problem of lipoid pneumonia in infants from aspirating the oily cod-liver oil. The odor of the cod-liver oil was much more objectionable to mothers than to infants, as was the problem of oil-stained clothing. Water-miscible preparations traditionally contain vitamin A and also ascorbic acid. Most drug companies had voluntarily reduced the recommended dosage to provide only 400 I.U. of vitamin D per dose rather than the 800 I.U. previously suggested before the Food and Drug Administration made it mandatory in 1965.

Cod-liver oil preparations, which are still used, are standardized to provide 85 I.U. per gram or 340 I.U. per teaspoon.

A solution of irradiated ergosterol (ergocalciferol) in a neutral oil is marketed as viosterol, a very concentrated source of vitamin D that makes the likelihood of an overdose greater.

The presence of calcium salts with vitamin D in therapeutic preparations may adversely effect the stability of vitamin D. Distributors of mineral-vitamin preparations are being discouraged from combining vitamin D with mineral supplements even though it might seem a logical combination.

In Europe, where the habit of using daily supplements of vitamin D or foods enriched with vitamin D has not been established, physicians have found that massive injections of 300,000 I.U. of vitamin D at intervals of six weeks to three months is an effective way to control rickets. There are apparently no adverse effects from such large doses, but in the United States smaller daily doses are preferred.

Dietary intake. The other source, and in the temperate zone the major source of vitamin D, is ingested vitamin D. Some foods of animal origin, such as eggs, milk, butter, and fish-liver oils, constitute the major sources of the preformed vitamin, but they are characteristically poor and unreliable sources, the amount present varying with the diet and breed of the animal. Even when all potential dietary sources are included it is possible to obtain only about 125 I.U. per day. This would include egg yolk with 2 to 5 I.U. per gram, butter with 0.1 to 1.0 I.U. per gram, and milk with 0.02 I.U. per gram. As a result, it is now customary to rely on foods enriched with vitamin D or nutritional supplements during periods of maximum need for vitamin D.

Milk, a carrier of both calcium and phosphorus, needed for calcification of bones, is the food most commonly fortified with vitamin D. Evaporated milk, irradiated to provide 400 I.U. per quart of reconstituted milk, was the first food to be sold as an irradiated product. Now practically all homogenized milk and nonfat milk has vitamin D added. Regular milk, in which a cream layer rises to the top, is not enriched because the fat-soluble vitamin D would concentrate in the cream layer. About 85% of all milk sold in the United States is fortified with vitamin D at a level that will permit maximum utilization of the calcium and phosphorus of milk.

Many plants contain ergosterol, which on irradiation with ultraviolet light is converted into another active form of the vitamin—ergocalciferol or vitamin D_2. The overirradiation of ergosterol may lead to the formation of some related compounds that have little or no antirachitic properties. Early in the history of vitamin D it was customary to irradiate a large number of foods, but now evaporated milk is the only food in which the vitamin D value is increased by irradiation. Others are enriched by the addition of vitamin D.

Toxicity

Since the demonstration over forty years ago that cod-liver oil was effective in preventing rickets, the disease has ceased to be a cause of concern to medical and public health authorities. Now the cause for concern lies at the other end of the continuum, with attention being directed toward the problem of overuse of vitamin D. In one of the earliest studies to assess the need for vitamin D, Jeans and Stearns showed that there was no extra benefit to be derived from levels above 400 I.U. per day and that levels of 1800 I.U. per day gave no extra benefits and actually retarded linear growth. Recently, reports of hypercalcemia in infants, in which practically all tissues of the body are adversely affected, have focused attention on the possibility that high levels of vitamin D are causative. The withdrawal of all sources of vitamin D alleviated the high blood calcium levels with its rapid onset of symptoms of loss of appetite, nausea, weight loss, and failure to thrive. The level of vitamin D intake that precipitates hypercalcemia varies greatly from one individual to another. Adults receiving 100,000 I.U. of vitamin D for weeks or months will develop symptoms. An intake of 1000 to 3000 I.U. per kilogram of body weight in infants (10,000 to 30,000 I.U. per day) are usually toxic. Apparently some infants experience a hypersensitivity to vitamin D and exhibit toxic symptoms on levels as low as 1000 I.U. per day, although the lower limit of toxicity is likely closer to 2000 to 3000 I.U. All forms of vitamin D are potentially dangerous, and the effects of an overdose resemble those of toxisterol or suprasterol.

The fact that there were no increases in benefits from vitamin D intakes in excess of 400 I.U. per day and a possibility of detrimental effects for sensitive individuals at levels above 2000 I.U. has led British authorities to persuade processors of vitamin D-enriched products to reduce the level of fortification so that a person consuming the recommended amount of the food would be protected against rickets and yet would not be in danger of excessive intake if he consumed all such fortified products. A report three years after the introduction of this policy, which reduced vitamin D intakes by one third to one half, indicated a decrease in the incidence of hypercalcemia and no increase in the incidence of rickets.

Large doses of vitamin A given concurrently with potentially toxic doses of vitamin D tend to reduce the incidence of toxic symptoms. Very little is known about the mechanisms of the toxicity, but it is suggested that the liver may fail to inactivate the excessive amounts ingested.

VITAMIN E

Vitamin E was first recognized as a dietary essential in 1922. At that time it was found to be necessary for normal reproduction in animals. Since a deficiency was shown to produce permanent sterility in male animals and a decrease in the ability of female animals to conceive or to carry a fetus to term if conception did occur, vitamin E became known as the antisterility factor. Although it is now known that a failure in normal reproduction in animals is only one of the results of a vitamin E deficiency and that human reproduction is not affected at all, the use of this term has persisted. Vitamin E deficiency states have been experimentally produced in many species and some theories of its biochemical role have been advanced, but its role in human nutrition is still very poorly understood.

Chemical forms

The term *vitamin E,* designating a fat-soluble vitamin, is applied to a group of chemical compounds known as the tocopherols (from Greek, *to bear child*). So far, seven related tocopherols, designated alpha, beta, gamma, delta, epsilon, zeta, and eta, have been identified as having vitamin E activity. Chemically they differ only slightly, but biochemically there are more marked differences in their effectiveness. Many researchers consider alpha-tocopherol as the biologically active form, but values on the vitamin E content of foods usually include all forms. The form predominating varies from one food to the next.

Functions

Since vitamin E deficiencies are rare in human beings but can be readily produced in experimental animals, most of our knowledge of vitamin E functions has come from experimentation on animals such as chicks, rats, rabbits, and guinea pigs, from which it becomes obvious that vitamin E affects different species in different ways. It has been possible, however, to postulate several functions for vitamin E.

Antioxidant in both animal and plant tissue. By being very readily oxidized itself, tocopherol reduces the amount of oxygen available to other substances that might otherwise be destroyed or changed by the uptake of oxygen. Thus, fats containing vitamin E are less susceptible to oxidation and the resulting rancidity than those devoid of vitamin E. Vitamin A, unsaturated fatty acids, and vitamin C in foods are similarly protected against destruction when vitamin E is present. Tissue lipids are likewise less susceptible to excessive oxidation (peroxidation), which may modify structure of the tissue and hence its function.

Oxidation of the fat in the membrane and the stroma of the erythrocyte or red blood cell occurs when the protection against oxidation is lost as blood levels of tocopherol drop. The resulting change in the structure of the membrane results in hemolysis or breakdown of the cell. Other evidence of the antioxidative role of vitamin E has been established. In fact some workers feel that its role as an antioxidant is the only biochemical function that can be attributed to vitamin E and that a loss of its antioxidant properties and the resultant lipid oxidation can provide an explanation for all manifestations of a vitamin E deficiency. Others dispute this on the basis that other antioxidants can substitute for or spare vitamin E in some but not all of its metabolic roles.

Cellular respiration. Vitamin E plays an essential role at the end of the respiration chain by which energy from glucose and fatty acids is finally released and water formed. This function has only recently been recognized and has not been completely clarified. The fact that it seems to be involved primarily in respiration in heart and skeletal muscles may provide a rationale for earlier but unsuccessful attempts to treat human heart diseases and muscular dystrophy with vitamin E.

Synthesis of essential body compounds. In species capable of synthesizing vitamin C, tocopherol acts as a necessary cofactor. It also stimulates the synthesis of coenzyme Q, a recently discovered essential in the respiratory chain by which energy stored in carbohydrate or fat is converted into the energy-rich compound ATP. It also plays a regulatory role in the incorporation of pyrimidines into the nucleic acid structure. This seems to be especially true in the bone marrow, where red blood cells are manufactured. In a vitamin E deficiency, abnormally large red blood cells (macrocytes) are formed when vitamin E fails to regulate the formation of nucleic acids.

Absorption and metabolism

As a fat-soluble substance, vitamin E requires the presence of bile for absorption, either from oil solutions or aqueous emulsions. It is apparently absorbed unchanged and is transported in the bloodstream as tocopherol. Tocopherol is stored in various tissues of the body, but the adipose tissue is the major site, with the uterus and testis also containing high amounts. Some metabolites of tocopherol similar to the products of oxidation of tocopherol in vitro appear in the liver—further evidence of its role as an antioxidant. The level of tocopherol in the blood is a sensitive indicator of vitamin E status with 0.4 to 0.8 μg. per 100 ml. considered a normal level. It is possible through the use of vitamin E supplements of 1 gm. per day to increase blood levels to 11 μg. and to double the amount present in adipose tissue.

A newborn infant has approximately 20 mg. of vitamin E stored in the body.

Requirements

The Food and Nutrition board of the National Research Council has agreed with the Food and Drug Administration that vitamin E is necessary in human nutrition but feels that there is insufficient evidence to establish a definite requirement. It assumes that since clinical symptoms that can be attributed to vitamin E inadequacy do not appear in a significant number of people that normal diets provide sufficient amounts. Estimates of requirement range from 10 to 30 mg., and it is agreed that the requirement increases as the level of polyunsaturated fatty acids in the diet increases. In one study in which tocopherol-depleted men were fed 30 gm. of the unsaturated fatty acid, linoleic acid, 30 mg. of alpha tocopherol acetate were required to maintain normal plasma levels and prevent erythrocyte hemolysis.

It appears that changes in dietary patterns in which liquid vegetable oils are substituted for animal fats may call for a reevaluation of human needs. The limited data available suggest that the average American ingests 2 to 16 mg. tocopherol per day, mostly from fats, oils, and butter, with from one fourth to one third being absorbed.

Studies in infants indicate their need to be less than 3 mg. per day even when the diet is high in polyunsaturated fatty acids. Serum tocopherol levels are low at birth (0.25 mg. per 100 ml.), although the mother's level increases to a high of 1.5 to 2 mg. per 100 ml. at the end of pregnancy, levels which are associated with preparation for lactation. Human milk, which provides approximately 0.5 mg. per kilogram of body weight of the infant, is higher in vitamin E than cow's milk and results in a faster increase in serum tocopherol levels of breast-fed babies. Infants with defective fat absorption may need supplementary vitamin E. Premature infants have low serum vitamin E values, which reflect the fact that most of the vitamin E is transferred to the fetus in the last two months of fetal life. After delivery these infants exhibit no other signs of vitamin E inadequacy regardless of dietary intake.

Food sources

Tocopherols occur in greatest concentration in vegetable oils, wheat germ oil being the source from which vitamin E was first obtained. The vitamin E value of this and other vegetable oils is given in Table 11-2. Generally speaking, the amount of vitamin E increases along with an increase in polyunsaturated fatty acids. The composition of the vitamin E activity varies from one oil to another, some being high in alpha tocopherol, others in some of the other forms. Tocopherols are also present in a wide variety of other plant and animal tissues as shown in Table 11-3.

A recent study of the vitamin E activity of typical meals showed that breakfasts ranged from 0.59 to 3.68 mg., lunches from 0.44 to 5.37 mg., and dinners from 1.61 to 6.38 mg. Only by choosing the meals highest in tocopherol from each group was it possible to obtain 15 mg., per day which is believed to be an adequate level of intake. They found a range for three meals of 2.6 to 15.4 mg. with an average intake of 7.4

Table 11-2. Tocopherol content of various oils*

Food	Milligrams per 100 gm.
Wheat germ oil	260
Corn oil	
Unhydrogenated	100
Hydrogenated	105
Cottonseed oil	
Unhydrogenated	91
Hydrogenated	80
Soybean oil	
Unhydrogenated	101
Hydrogenated	73
Sunflower oil, stabilized	59
Soybean oil	130
Coconut oil	8

*From Bunnell, R. H., Keating, T., Quaresimo, A., and Parmin, G. K.: Alpha-tocopherol content of foods, Am. J. Clin. Nutrition **17**:1, 1965.

mg., which they felt was low in light of the increased consumption of polyunsaturated fatty acids that increases the need for tocopherol. It is considerably lower than previously accepted values of 7.4 mg.

These same investigators found a 63% to 74% decrease in the tocopherol content during freezer storage of foods fried in oil. Since an increasing number of foods are being stored frozen, this may be additional cause for concern when coupled with the low intake. The heating of cooking oils destroys virtually all the tocopherol present, but esters of tocopherol such as tocopherol acetate are less than one fifth destroyed.

Fruits and vegetables are relatively poor sources of tocopherol, but fresh and frozen vegetables retain much more than canned products. Very little is lost in normal cooking procedures.

Deficiency

In animals. A lack of vitamin E in animals is manifest in a wide variety of ways, with symptoms involving the muscles, nervous system, reproductive organs, vascular system, and glandular system. Chicks show characteristic changes in the central nervous system known as *encephalomalacia.* These changes are greatest when the diet is low in vitamin E and high in polyunsaturated fatty acids that are susceptible to oxidation in absence of vitamin E. Ubichromenol will delay the onset of symptoms.

Rats show necrotic liver degeneration. These symptoms can be relieved or pre-

Table 11-3. Vitamin E content of 100 gm. of some representative foods*

Food	Milligrams per 100 gm.
Mayonnaise	50.0
Margarine (made with corn oil)	46.7
Yellow cornmeal	3.4
Whole-wheat bread	2.2
Beef liver, broiled	1.62
Egg	1.43
Fillet of haddock, broiled	1.20
Butter	1.0
Tomatoes, fresh	0.85
Green peas, frozen	0.65
Ground beef	0.63
Pork chops, pan-fried	0.60
Chicken breast	0.58
Cornflakes	0.43
Banana	0.42
White bread	0.23
Carrots	0.21
Orange juice, fresh	0.20
Potato, baked	0.085

*From Bunnell, R. H., Keating, J., Quaresimo, A., and Parmin, G. K.: Alpha-tocopherol content of foods, Am. J. Clin. Nutrition **17**:1, 1965.

vented by the amino acid cystine or the mineral element selenium, both of which can substitute for vitamin E in this instance. A condition known as *exudative diathesis,* in which there appear large patches of fluid accumulation beneath the skin on the breast, legs, abdomen, and neck, also occurs in rats and chicks. This condition is also relieved by selenium. Reproductive failure in rats, mice, and guinea pigs has been well established. Degeneration of the epithelium results in permanent sterility in males. Female rats which do conceive will resorb fetus by eighth day of 22 days' gestation period. Fetuses can be salvaged if vitamin E is given by fifth day, but if it is delayed until after the sixth day many congenital abnormalities appear.

The accumulation of a brown pigment (ceroid) in the uterus and kidney of rats has been attributed to vitamin E or selenium deficiency and is likely related to oxidative changes in unsaturated fatty acids. A similar pigment which occurs in nerve cells in human senility shows up in nerve cells when stress factors are superimposed on a vitamin E–deficient diet.

Muscular dystrophy, characterized by muscular weakness caused by fragmentation of muscle fibers, accumulation of fluid in interstitial spaces, and deterioration of hyaline membrane, occurs in vitamin E deficiency in guinea pigs, rabbits, and monkeys. The premature release of enzymes from the cell lysosome when the membrane becomes more susceptible to lipid peroxidation and accompanying breakdown has been suggested as a cause of muscular dystrophy. No relationship has been established between vitamin E nutrition and human muscular dystrophy believed to be an hereditary condition causing extensive wasting of certain voluntary muscles with an onset from birth to adulthood. Monkeys exhibit a characteristic anemic reaction to vitamin E inadequacy.

In human beings. Vitamin E deficiency is rarely seen in human beings. Certain biochemical changes have been associated with a low dietary intake coupled with either an increased need, as in a diet high in vegetable oils, with a high polyunsaturated fatty acid content, or with conditions that interfere with fat absorption. Increased susceptibility of the membrane of the erythrocytes to hemolysis is the most easily detected evidence of vitamin E deficiency. Other indications of vitamin E inadequacy are a drop in the level of tocopherol in blood, an increase in urinary excretion of creatine, and a decrease in creatinine excretion.

Work done on induced vitamin E deficiencies in mental patients in Illinois indicates that with low levels of tocopherol in the diet, plasma tocopherol levels drop below normal values of 1 mg. per 100 ml. of blood. This drop is accompanied by increased tendency to hemolysis in red blood cells, especially below 0.5 mg. tocopherol. When the lard in the diet (low in polyunsaturated fatty acids) was replaced by corn oil (high in polyunsaturated fatty acids) there was a further drop in serum tocopherol levels. An already high rate of erythrocyte hemolysis was not increased further. Larger amounts of vitamin E were required to maintain normal blood tocopherol levels when corn oil was substituted for lard.

Low serum levels of vitamin E have been associated wtih a macrocytic anemia in which the life-span of the red blood cells is decreased and the synthesis of both DNA and RNA is increased. Children with kwashiorkor and the vitamin A deficiency disease xerophthalmia have much lower serum tocopherol levels and a greatly reduced chance of responding to therapy than do children with kwashiorkor without xerophthalmia. There is also some evidence to suggest that the muscular changes that occur in infants suffering from cystic fibrosis of the pancreas resemble those of vitamin E deficiency in animals. Some have also shown an accumulation of the ceroid pigment in muscles.

Substitutes

Much of the confusion over the role of vitamin E has arisen because of ability of many other chemically unrelated substances to substitute for some or all of the many biochemical functions of the tocopherols. The mineral selenium either replaces vitamin E as an antioxidant or spares it so that several vitamin E deficiency symptoms do not develop. The distribution of selenium to certain tissues may be low, thereby offering an explanation of its failure to protect against all vitamin E deficiencies such as encephalomalacia and muscular dystrophy. Selenium does not have the same effect in maintaining coenzyme Q levels in tissues that vitamin E does. The distribution of selenium in the diet is unrelated to vitamin E in diet.

Ubichromenol has been shown to have vitamin E activity, especially in delaying onset of symptoms. The effect of selenium may be to enhance the ubichromenol activity in various tissues, which in turn may control the release of proteolytic enzymes from lysosomes.

A chemical antioxidant, DPPD (N-N' diphenyl p-phenylene), can replace all functions of vitamin E, at least for a considerable period of time. It is effective in preventing fetal resorptions.

The presence of the sulphur-containing amino acid cystine is also involved in influencing the antioxidative effectiveness of vitamin E and its substitutes.

Clinical uses

Because of the seemingly unrelated pathological changes in tocopherol deficiencies in animals there has been a temptation to use vitamin E in the treatment of a large number of conditions although no relationship between vitamin E nutrition and these conditions has been confirmed. Some 2000 papers have appeared on the therapeutic uses of vitamin E. Contradictory reports on their effectiveness continue to appear and in a few cases there is reasonable evidence of its therapeutic value. Perhaps most controversial is its use with women who have suffered repeated spontaneous abortions. Some evidence supports such therapy but much gives negative results. Some forms of ulcers have responded well to the use of vitamin E, but there is insufficient evidence to support claims for its effectiveness in heart disease, muscular dystrophy, male infertility, diabetes, menopause, or gangrene. Nor is vitamin E effective as an antifatigue or ergogenic substance for rats although it reportedly reduces the oxygen requirement of tissues.

There is good evidence to support the therapeutic use of vitamin E where there has been a depressed absorption of fat or where the intake of polyunsaturated fatty acids has increased or in severe protein deficiency.

VITAMIN K

Vitamin K was first discovered in 1934 by a Danish scientist who identified it as the fat-soluble factor necessary for the coagulation of the blood. Since the Danish word for the process is spelled *koagulation* he designated this factor as vitamin K.

Chemical forms

Several forms of vitamin K have now been identified, all belonging to a group of chemical compounds known as quinones. Vitamin K_1, which occurs only in plants, has been designated also as phytonodione or phylloquinone while vitamin K_2, which occurs primarily as the result of synthesis by microorganisms in the intestinal tract, is known as farnoquinone. These naturally occurring fat-soluble forms of the vitamin may be stored in the body, primarily in the liver. Vitamin K_1 is available commercially; vitamin K_2 is not, although two forms of it have been isolated from putrefied fish meal. Chemists have been able to produce synthetic forms of both vitamin K_1 and K_2, which are water-soluble and hence helpful in many therapeutic situations, especially those in which fat is poorly tolerated. These products, known as Hykinone and Synkayvite, can be given orally as well as intravenously and intramuscularly. A third fat-soluble synthetic form of K_1, menadione, can be given intravenously and intramuscularly but is not well tolerated orally.

Vitamin K is stable to heat and reducing agents but destroyed by light, acid, alkali, and oxidizing agents.

Functions

The ability of the blood to coagulate is dependent on the presence of many factors, among which are prothrombin and proconvertin. Vitamin K is necessary for the synthesis of prothrombin and proconvertin in the liver although it is not a part of either substance. Prothrombin levels in the blood determine the rate at which the blood will clot, high levels indicating good coagulability, low levels a depressed rate of coagulation. Proconvertin, also known as factor VII, is also required for the coagulation of the blood. There is some reason to believe that vitamin K is required for the synthesis of other factors involved in blood-clotting. It has also been suggested that vitamin K takes part in an oxidation reduction system in which the SH group in fibrinogen is oxidized to the S-S group of the clot, fibrin.

Recently evidence has accumulated indicating that vitamin K may be involved in a process called phosphorylation in which phosphate is added to glucose to facilitate its passage through cell membranes and its conversion into glycogen.

Coenzyme Q, which is a link in the respiratory chain of reactions involved in the ultimate release of energy from fatty acids and glucose, is similar to vitamin K chemically.

Absorption

Since vitamin K is fat-soluble its absorption is regulated by the same factors that govern fat absorption. An obstruction of the bile duct, limiting the secretion of fat-emulsifying bile salts, as occurs in obstructive jaundice, will reduce absorption, as will failure of the liver to secrete bile. The use of a nonutilizable oil such as mineral oil will cause the excretion of vitamin K in the feces.

Vitamin K is absorbed in the upper part of the gastrointestinal tract, as are other fat-related factors, which gives rise to the question of how much of the vitamin K synthesized in the lower part of the gastrointestinal tract will be absorbed.

An anticoagulant, dicumarol, which is very similar chemically to vitamin K, apparently replaces vitamin K in the liver where it not only is ineffective in promoting prothrombin synthesis but blocks a normal synthesis. It may also displace vitamin K from an enzyme system to block it. The widespread use of anticoagulant drugs to reduce undesirable blood-clotting, as in phlebitis or thrombosis, has made the use of vitamin K therapy more important to control hemorrhaging in these people.

Requirements

The National Research Council recognizes vitamin K as a dietary essential but has been unable to make any quantitative evaluation of needs because of its abundance in most diets. Only for newborn infants does there appear to be any need for special attention to vitamin K, and for them an intake of 1 to 5 mg. should be adequate.

Sources

For most individuals adequate levels of vitamin K are provided by green and yellow vegetables and from the synthesis of the vitamin by intestinal bacteria. The concentration of vitamin K in foods is highest in dark leafy green vegetables, with some being found in fruits, tubers, and seeds. It usually occurs in association with chlorophyll in the chloroplasts. Alfalfa is an especially rich source, but in spite of the efforts of food faddists is not an accepted item in average diets. There is no evidence of adult dietary inadequacies to warrant suggestions that the diet be supplemented with such a rich source.

Since much of the bacterial synthesis occurs in the lower intestine, only a small portion of that synthesized may actually be absorbed by the body. The amount synthesized will also be reduced when substances are taken that depress the growth of intestinal bacteria. Salicylic acid, an ingredient in most pain depressants of the aspirin type, and certain antibiotics and sulfonamides may act in this way. Young infants are the ones most likely to suffer from a subnormal level of intestinal synthesis, for during the first few days of life their relatively sterile intestinal tract does not contain the organisms that synthesize vitamin K. Very little vitamin K passes the placental barrier from the maternal circulation to be stored in fetal tissue, although if vitamin K is given to the mother at delivery a sufficient amount passes to stimulate prothrombin synthesis. Milk is very low in vitamin K so that even those who receive nourishment in the first few days of life do not receive an appreciable amount of vitamin K. Breast-fed infants are at an even greater disadvantage than bottle-fed infants because mother's milk is often not produced in significant amounts for several days and contains about one fourth the amount of vitamin K as cow's milk and there is less chance of vitamin K synthesizing bacteria developing in the lower intestine.

Deficiency

Because vitamin K can be synthesized and also is provided in adequate amounts in practically all diets, a deficiency in adults is invariably caused by a failure in absorption. Low prothrombin levels can also be due to failure of liver to synthesize it.

In infants, however, the lack of bacteria to synthesize vitamin K, the low stores of vitamin K in the infant at birth, and the small amount provided in milk characteristically lead to low prothrombin levels and a prolonged coagulation time. This occurs at a time when the incidence of hemorrhage is very high. The association between vitamin K and blood coagulation times led to the routine administration of vitamin K to the mother just prior to delivery or to the infant in the first days of life to reduce neonatal deaths caused by hemorrhage. After its use had become routine, however, an increase in a hemolytic type of anemia, an accumulation of bilirubin in the blood, and a condition known as kernicterus, in which there is an accumulation of bile pigment in the gray matter of the central nervous system, were attributed to vitamin K toxicity resulting from the uncontrolled use of synthetic vitamin K. An evaluation of vitamin K therapy in newborn infants has shown that it is desirable but that certain precautions should be observed to provide the greatest benefits and the greatest margin of safety. Several studies have shown that the normal incidence of hemorrhage of the newborn of one in four hundred infants is markedly reduced with vitamin K therapy and especially in babies who may get less than adequate oxygen at birth. Natural vitamin K_1 is considered the most desirable form, as there have been no reports of toxicity from oral administration of 1 to 2 mg. or from parenteral doses of 0.5 to 1 mg. of a water-miscible preparation to provide protection when given intravenously or intramuscularly to the infant, and the doses provided as much protection as 10 mg. Menadione, a synthetic vitamin K_1, cannot be given orally as it causes vomiting. A dose of 2 to 5 mg. given to the mother usually transfers adequate protection to the child, but larger doses that assure adequate levels for the infant may be hazardous to some infants. It is recommended that protection be provided by administering natural vitamin K to the child after birth rather than to the mother, with larger doses recommended for a child whose mother has been given anticoagulant therapy. It can be given orally, subcutaneously, intramuscularly, or intravenously.

SELECTED REFERENCES

Vitamin A

Dowling, J. E., and Wald, G.: Role of of vitamin A acid, Vitamins Hormones 18:515, 1960.

Editorial. Hypervitaminosis A: its broadening spectrum, Am. J. Clin. Nutrition 6:335, 1958.

Fell, H. B.: Effet of vitamin A on tissue structure, Proc. Nutrition Soc. 19:50, 1960.

Goodman, D. S., and Huang, H. S.: Biosynthesis of vitamin A with rat intestinal enzymes, Science 149:879, 1965.

McLaren, D. S., Tchalian, M., and Ajans, Z. A.: Biochemical and hematalogic changes in the vitamin A deficient rat, Am. J. Clin. Nutrition 17:131, 1965.

McLaren, D. S., Shirajan E., Tchalian, M., and Khoury, G.: Xerophthalmia in Jordan, Am. J. Clin. Nutrition 17:117, 1965.

McLaren, D. S.: Xerophthalmia, a neglected problem, Nutr. Rev. 22:289, 1964.

Olson, J. A.: The absorption of beta-carotene and its conversion into vitamin A, Am. J. Clin. Nutrition 9:1, 1961.

Owen, E. C.: Some aspects of the metabolism of vitamin A and carotene, World Rev. Nutr. Diet. 5:132, 1965.

Roels, O. A.: Present knowledge of vitamin A, Nutr. Rev. 24:129, 1966.

Symposium. Vitamin A, Proc. Nutrition Soc. 24:127-170, 1965.

Wolfe, G.: Some thoughts on metabolic role of vitamin A, Nutr. Rev. 20:161, 1962.

Vitamin D

Bransby, E. R., Berry, W. T. C., and Taylor, D. M.: Study of the vitamin D intake of infants in 1960, Brit. M. J. 1:1661, 1964.

Committee on Nutrition: The prophylactic requirement and toxicity of vitamin D, Pediatrics 31:512, 1963.

Committee on Nutrition: Vitamin D intake and the hypercalcemic syndrome, Pediatrics 35:1022, 1965.

Harris, F., Hoffenberg, R., and Bloch, E.: Calcium kinetics in vitamin D deficient rickets, Metabolism 14:1101, 1965.

Harrison, H. E.: Vitamin D and calcium and phosphate transport, Pediatrics 28:531, 1961.

Harrison, H. E.: Vitamin D and permeability of intestinal mucosa to calcium, Am. J. Physiol. 208:370, 1965.

Norman, A. W.: Actinomycin D and the response to vitamin D, Science 149:184, 1965.

Wasserman, R. H.: Vitamin D and the intestinal absorption of calcium, New York J. Med. 64:1329, 1964.

Vitamin E

Booth, V. H., and Bradford, M. P.: Tocopherol content of fruits and vegetables, Brit. J. Nutrition 17:575, 1963.

Bunnell, R. H., Keating, J., Quaresimo, A., and Parman, G. K.: Alpha tocopherol content of foods, Am. J. Clin. Nutrition 17:1, 1965.

Committee on Nutrition, American Academy of Pediatrics: Vitamin E in human nutrition, Pediatrics 31:324, 1963.

Herting, D. C., and Drury, E. E.: Plasma tocopherol levels in man, Am. J. Clin. Nutrition 17:351, 1965.

Horwitt, M. K.: Vitamin E in human nutrition—an interpretive review, Borden Rev. Nutr. Res. 22:1, 1961.

McMasters, V., Lewis, J. K., Kinsell, L. W., Van DerVern, J., and Olcott, H. S.: Effect of supplementing the diet of man with tocopherol on the tocopherol levels of adipose tissue and plasma, Am. J. Clin. Nutrition 17:357, 1965.

Vitamin K

Committee on Nutrition: Vitamin K compounds and the water soluble analogues, Pediatrics 28:501, 1961.

Wefring, K. W.: Hemorrhage in the newborn and vitamin K prophylaxis, J. Pediat. 63:663, 1963.

12

Water-soluble vitamins

ASCORBIC ACID

Vitamin C, cevitamic acid, hexuronic acid, and ascorbic acid are names that have all at one time or another been applied to the antiscorbutic or scurvy-preventative substance discovered in 1932 by King and Waugh, who isolated it from lemon juice, and Szent-Gyorgyi, who found it in the suprarenal gland, a gland located near the kidney, and in oranges and cabbage.

Descriptions of scurvy can be traced as far back as a papyrus from 500 B.C. found at Thebes, the writings of Hippocrates in 400 B.C., and other recurring references in recorded history. It had been known for 250 years that scurvy could be controlled by dietary means and since 1906 that it was a deficiency disease, but the search for the effective agent ended only with the isolation of the relatively simple white crystals of vitamin C in 1932.

The conquest of scurvy is of special historic interest because it was in an effort to cure this "scourge of the Navy" that the first carefully conceived nutrition experiment was conducted with human beings.

British seamen who embarked on long sea voyages without an opportunity to replenish supplies for long periods did so knowing that a large portion of the crew would die or be incapacitated by scurvy. For instance, Cook lost 100 of the 196 men who started around Cape Horn with him in 1774, and in 1497 Vasco da Gama lost 100 out of 150 men. In 1747, Dr. James Lind, a British physician, hypothesized that various "acidic principles" might have antiscorbutic properties. To test his theory he divided twelve sailors suffering from scurvy into six groups of two each and fed them the ship's basic diet plus one of six potential cures—oil of vitreol or sulphuric acid in water three times a day, two teaspoonfuls of vinegar three times a day, a half pint of sea water per day, and two oranges and one lemon per day. The results of his experiment are now legend—both oranges and lemons had miraculous curative powers, the sailors assigned to this treatment being restored to active duty within six days while those on other treatments showed no progress. Not only did he prove that scurvy could be cured, but he laid the foundation for the theory that lack of an essential food element could cause illness. Others had advanced similar theories even a century earlier, but their observations had gone virtually unnoticed.

It was fifty years later before the British Navy recognized his work to the point of requiring that all ships leaving British ports carry sufficient lime juice to have it available for its crew throughout the whole voyage. The routine use of lime juice led to the use of the term "limey" to refer to a British seaman, a term that now has been extended to all British servicemen.

Although the British navy was the first to take steps to prevent scurvy, many other groups had suffered from it and in some cases had found a cure. Crusaders felt that those who could survive the pain that attacked feet and legs and the changes in their gums until spring would usually be cured by warm temperatures. Carter's expedition, which was forced to spend a winter near Montreal in 1535, was spared when the Indians taught his group to use the bark of a pine tree, the ameda, to cure scurvy. French and Spanish sailors were spared because of the quantities of onions and leeks they carried. Sailors in the Mediterranean were seldom away long enough to deplete their tissue reserves of vitamin C. Scurvy had been known to occur in the late spring in European cities but not in rural areas. By this time, city dwellers had been reduced to a diet of meat and bread, while their counterparts in the country still had some cabbage, onions, and potatoes left in storage. Following failure of the potato crop, even rural populations experienced scurvy outbreaks. As late as 1846 Mormons making their way west to Utah were forced to winter in Nebraska on a diet of mush. Many of them succumbed to scurvy. Spaniards landing after long sea voyages in California in 1602, 1603, and again in 1769 lost many of their numbers and their first task after landing was the search for an herb or plant to cure scurvy.

Medical authorities who have considered scurvy a disease of the past have been appalled by some recent reports of infantile scurvy. Infantile scurvy was first reported in the late nineteenth century and paralleled the change from the use of wet nurses to preserved milk. It increased again when pasteurization of milk became mandatory. Again, it seems to be occurring among bottle-fed infants whose formula has been subjected to prolonged heat treatment and who receive no fruit juice or vitamin C con-

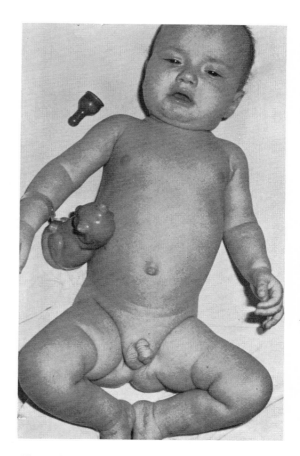

Fig. 12-1

Infant with scurvy. Note frog position of legs and apprehension of infant in anticipation of handling of tender limbs. (From Grewar, D.: Infantile scurvy, Clin. Pediat. 4:82, 1965.)

centrate. Canadian authorities, faced with a rapid increase in scurvy among 6- to 12-month-old babies, have suggested the enrichment of commercial formula preparations with ascorbic acid, the use of supplements, and the encouragement of breast-feeding, since human milk contains about six times as much vitamin C as pasteurized cow's milk. American nutritionists feel that education in the early use of orange juice or a vitamin preparation is a more reasonable approach to the problem. Australia, with the highest rate of infantile scurvy, has considered providing free orange juice or multivitamins rather than enriching milk. A typical case of infantile scurvy is shown in Fig. 12-1.

Chemical properties

Chemically, ascorbic acid is a very simple six-carbon compound closely related to the monosaccharides. The synthetic form of the vitamin, first produced in 1933, is derived from the monosaccharides—glucose of cane sugar or galactose of milk sugar. The body cannot discriminate between natural and synthetic forms so that they can be used interchangeably.

Vitamin C, with the formula $C_6H_8O_6$, is known as reduced ascorbic acid and is very susceptible to oxidation. It has now been established that the first product of the oxidation of this biologically active compound, dehydroascorbic acid, $C_6H_6O_6$, which has two less hydrogens, can be used equally as well by the body. It is apparently reduced again to the active form by the body before taking part in biological reactions. Further oxidation of dehydroascorbic acid produces a product with no antiscorbutic properties, and the oxidative process is irreversible. The changes are shown schematically in Fig. 12-2.

There is some evidence that reduced ascorbic acid is changed in kidney cells to dehydroascorbic acid, a form in which it is more readily transported to the tissues. It also penetrates into the cell more easily in this oxidized form.

Most animals have the ability to synthesize ascorbic acid and therefore need no dietary supply of it. So far, only five species have been found that lack the enzyme necessary to complete the conversion of glucose or galactose to ascorbic acid. This synthesis takes place primarily in the microsomes of the cell, especially liver cells. Man, monkey, guinea pig, the Indian fruit bat, and the red-vented bulbul bird are the only species that rely on a dietary source of

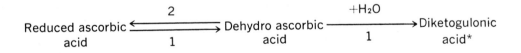

1 Oxidation

2 Reduction

* Biologically inactive

Fig. 12-2

Relationship of various chemical forms of ascorbic acid.

ascorbic acid. Of these, the guinea pig is used most extensively in research.

In plants, ascorbic acid is accumulated during the ripening process, presumably synthesized in the plant cells from the natural sugar in fruit.

D-ascorbic acid, structurally related to the biologically active L-ascorbic acid, is not utilized by the human being unless it is given in very small doses throughout the day. It is being used extensively as a preservative in processing meat. To avoid possible confusion and any implication that it is a vitamin, it has been recommended that the term erythrobic acid be applied to this compound.

Other reducing compounds have been found that can replace ascorbic acid in some of its biological roles, but none is effective in curing scurvy.

Functions

Although ascorbic acid is a relatively simple compound that has been available in a purified form at reasonable cost for over thirty years, biochemists, nutritionists, and physiologists have been unable to shed much light on its biochemical role. In contrast to most water-soluble vitamins it has no clear-cut role as a catalyst nor is it part of any enzyme or structure. Fragments of knowledge that will eventually form the total picture are elucidating some of its potential roles, but we still find the same general terms applied to ascorbic acid deficiency now as were used fifty years ago. The following are some of the more widely accepted roles.

Formation of collagen. The primary defect in scurvy is the failure of collagen in the fibroblasts in connective tissue. Collagen, the protein substance that binds the cells together in much the same way mortar binds bricks, is synthesized from many amino acids, one of which is hydroxyproline. Hydroxyproline must be made in the body from proline, and the conversion of proline to hydroxyproline depends on the presence of vitamin C. Thus, in an ascorbic acid deficiency, this change does not occur to provide the basic building material for collagen. A failure in collagen synthesis is observed primarily in tissues subjected to stress. Most collagen is quite inert metabolically and once laid down does not require vitamin C for maintenance, but certain fractions of collagen in some tissues are highly active and subject to rapid breakdown in ascorbic acid deficiency.

When the collagen is not formed or maintained in a scorbutic animal, the failure shows up in many ways. The need for ascorbic acid in healing of wounds is great. Here, new connective tissue, which is primarily collagen, must be formed. The high concentration of ascorbic acid found in scar tissue and the drops in blood level of the vitamin, which occur during healing, suggest that it is mobilized to the site of the healing. High levels are maintained after the scar tissue has been completely formed, indicating a need for maintenance of scar tissue. There is some controversy as to the need for increasing the dietary intake pre- and postoperatively for individuals whose tissues are apparently saturated with it. Some persons recommend intakes of 100 to 300 mg. per day to ensure rapid and complete healing while others feel this is unnecessary. However, since we have no evidence of adverse effects from higher levels, there is little reason to forego possible benefits from larger intakes.

Decrease in elasticity of the cell walls, which become fragile and frequently rupture to cause small pinpoint hemorrhages, is at least partially the result of failure of collagen in the muscle in which small blood vessels are embedded. These subcutaneous hemorrhages show up most often in areas subjected to mechanical stress, such as the gums, which often become soft, spongy, and hemorrhage easily, and the ends of the long bones. These changes occur when tissue saturation falls below 60% to 90% of normal levels.

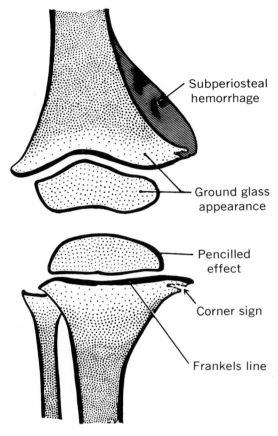

Fig. 12-3

Radiographic signs of scurvy. (Frim Grewar, D.: Infantile scurvy, Clin. Pediat. 4:82, 1965.)

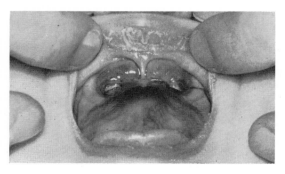

Fig. 12-4

Gum hemorrhage in scorbutic infant. Note occurrence only where teeth have erupted; it does not occur in edentulous gum. (From Grewar, D.: Infantile scurvy, Clin. Pediat. 4:82, 1965.)

The matrix of the bone shaft, which is primarily collagen, may be defective when collagen formation fails. It is less capable of holding calcium and phosphorus during bone calcification, resulting in weakened bone structure. Sometimes bones are displaced when supporting cartilage is weakened as a result of a lack of vitamin C for maintenance. Characteristic bone changes in scurvy are shown in Fig. 12-3 and gum changes in Fig. 12-4.

Dentin formation. Changes in tooth structure have been related to ascorbic acid status during a critical period in tooth formation. The dentin layer, arising from a group of cells known as odontoblasts, does not form normally in scorbutic animals, apparently because of the degeneration and death of the odontoblasts at the time calcification of the dentin layer should occur. This, of course, produces a tooth with a structural weakness that is less able to resist mechanical injury or to resist decay once it is initiated.

Tyrosine metabolism. The role of ascorbic acid in the utilization of the amino acid tyrosine is the one most clearly established by biochemists. It is necessary only when large amounts of tyrosine are being used. Under these circumstances vitamin C is needed in large amounts to protect one of the enzymes involved in the stepwise breakdown of tyrosine from destruction by the substrate on which it acts. When the enzyme is destroyed, intermediate products of tyrosine metabolism appear in the urine, indicating abnormal use of the amino acid and a failure of the body to oxidize it. Premature infants on high-protein diets often show a similar defect.

Utilization of iron and calcium. The absorption of iron from the intestinal tract is facilitated by the presence of vitamin C, which is effective as a reducing agent to keep ferrous iron in the reduced form in which it is most readily absorbed. The interrelationship with iron is also evident in that vitamin C activates some iron-containing enzymes. The role of ascorbic acid in facilitating calcium absorption may involve preventing its precipitation as an insoluble complex.

Utilization of folic acid. The conversion of the inactive form of the vitamin, folic acid, to the active form, the citrovorum factor, is catalyzed by ascorbic acid. It may be in this way that vitamin C is effective in preventing the megaloblastic anemia of infancy

Other functions. Many other functions have been attributed to ascorbic acid. In some cases the evidence is not clear-cut. In others, where the evidence indicates a strong possibility of a relationship, there has been no explanation of the biochemical role involved.

Ascorbic acid is believed to be involved in the production and secretion of hormones of the adrenal gland, but the mechanism is unclear since scorbutic subjects are able to produce normal levels of these steroids and adrenal glands respond normally to usual stimulation.

There is considerable evidence that blood cholesterol levels rise in an ascorbic acid deficiency and fall on the administration of the vitamin. This may indicate a role in lipid metabolism.

The conversion of the amino acid tryptophan to serotonin involved in maintaining blood pressure levels is dependent on ascorbic acid. Although only 1% of the tryptophan is used this way, it is a very essential compound.

Reports on the role of ascorbic acid in combating infection have been contradictory. When it has been found beneficial, the role has been obscure. No beneficial effects from high intakes of vitamin C could be demonstrated on the incidence and cure of the common cold, but tuberculosis patients experience a need for high intakes. The low blood levels of ascorbic acid reported in infections may be caused by a shift of the vitamin to the infected tissue. Much the same mechanism seems to

operate during stress with the mobilization of ascorbic acid from tissues of body to be concentrated in traumatized areas.

In the case of burns, skin grafts heal more quickly when ascorbic acid is present.

Large doses of ascorbic acid (525 mg. per day) have been demonstrated as beneficial in exposure to low environmental temperatures. The subjects maintained skin temperature more readily and experienced fewer and less severe symptoms of frostbitten feet. Here it is postulated that vitamin C accelerates the metabolism of the amino acids tyrosine and phenylalanine, precursors of the hormones adrenaline and thyroxine, which may stimulate basal metabolic rate and hence heat production.

Massive doses of ascorbic acid have been reported effective in treatment of such conditions as poisoning, hay fever, and arsenic sensitivity.

Biochemically there is evidence that ascorbic acid has a sparing action in relation to several vitamins of the B complex group. Such effects have been observed with thiamine, riboflavin, niacin, pantothenic acid, biotin, and folic acid. In some cases it appears to replace them; in others it appears to prevent their destruction.

Absorption and metabolism

Ascorbic acid is absorbed in humans in the upper part of the intestine, possibly by simple diffusion, and circulated in the blood. From the bloodstream it is picked up by the tissues, passing readily into such tissues as the adrenal tissue with 66 mg. per 100 gm. of tissue, kidney with 12 mg.%, liver with 32.8 mg.%, and spleen with 41.9 mg.%, most of which appears to be in equilibrium with serum. The eye, muscles, testes, and brain also accumulate some, but the concentration is markedly different from that in the blood serum. In the kidney some reduced ascorbic acid is changed to dehydroascorbic acid, in which form it more readily penetrates the cell barriers of erythrocytes, brain, and placenta, which it enters by active transport or an energy-requiring process. Although there are no extensive storage areas for vitamin C in the body some tissues, such as the adrenal tissue, especially the cortex, retain relatively large amounts that act as a buffer for other body tissues when dietary intake is low. Early estimates placed body stores at 5 gm., but more recent work studying the excretion of ascorbic acid through the respiratory tract suggests a figure as low as 1 gm. That this reserve is called upon in times of dietary deficit is evidenced by the fact that it takes as long as 17 weeks for the white blood cell level to drop to 0, which occurs before any detectable signs of scurvy are found in a diet devoid of vitamin C.

Isotopic studies with C^{14}-labeled ascorbic acid have provided a means of studying ascorbic acid catabolism in the body. Depending on the dose administered, between 20% and 66% of the dose has been exhaled as carbon dioxide within 24 hours. The larger the dose, the more is oxidized in this fashion. From 15% to 30% is excreted in the urine following a medium dose. This appears in the urine primarily as oxalic and threonic acid and some dehydroascorbic acid. A very small amount, usually less than 1%, is found in the feces. The remaining portion, between 30% and 50% of the dose, is usually retained in the body. The higher the previous diet, the less ascorbic acid is retained in the body. Since the body's capacity to store ascorbic acid is limited by the saturation level of various tissues, any excess is excreted in the urine or is oxidized and exhaled as carbon dioxide. There is no evidence of toxic effects from high levels of ascorbic acid.

Requirements

In the case of ascorbic acid there has been considerable controversy as to what criteria should be used in establishing recommended allowances.

Adults. Current standards are based on the assumption that an intake that leads to saturation of vitamin C reserves in the tissues is the most desirable. As a result, recommended levels are many times those known to prevent frank signs of scurvy. It has long been recognized that intakes as low as 10 mg. per day are sufficient to prevent scurvy. (Lind provided 20 to 30 mg. of ascorbic acid in the dose he prescribed for the British Navy.) Current research, taking into account the exhalation of CO_2 from the catabolism of ascorbic acid (in addition to the urinary excretion rate), suggests that minimum requirements may be even lower. In adults 10 mg. has been shown to prevent scurvy for 12 months and to cure it in 10 to 14 weeks, However, the level for maintenance of optimal health is undoubtedly higher.

Infants. Based on the amount of ascorbic acid found in mother's milk (average 4 to 8 mg. per 100 ml.), it is felt that a breast-fed infant receives 15 to 50 mg. per day. This leads to plasma ascorbic acid levels of 0.5 to 1.5 mg.%. Cow's milk provides only 4 to 6 mg.% and maintains much lower blood levels. It is recommended that 25 mg. be a minimum level of supplementation and that premature infants receive double the dose. Ascorbic acid supplementation should be started within the first ten days of life. Orange juice diluted with water has been satisfactory for most children, but the fact some developed allergic reactions when some of the oils from the rind were extracted along with the juice has resulted in more reliance on synthetic preparations, especially as provided in multivitamins for early feeding of vitamin C. Fruit juices other than orange juice do not provide enough vitamin C to make them effective in the diet of infants. For children, the National Research Council recommendations increase from 35 mg. for children one to three years of age to a high of 80 mg. for girls from 13 to 19 years and 100 mg. for boys 16 to 19 years. There is considerable discrepancy in research findings on which recommended allowances are based. Long-term studies show that children with an adequate supply of ascorbic acid have a better general condition in regard to growth and resistance to infection.

Adults. Recommended allowances for adults are 70 mg. for men and 75 mg. for women. These should allow for maintenance of an optimal level of health, optimal resistance to physiologic and pathologic stress, and maintenance of healthy gums. Saturation of adult tissues can be achieved at intakes of slightly over 80 mg. in five weeks. There is no increase in benefits with a large dose of 340 to 400 mg. There is no evidence to indicate that needs increase with age, although high levels may improve iron absorption in older persons whose level of hydrochloric acid secretion may be low.

Pregnancy. American standards for ascorbic acid intake in pregnancy are relatively high—100 mg. This is based on studies indicating a drop in blood serum levels and a decreased urinary excretion during pregnancy. It has been established that the developing fetus is parasitic on the mother in respect to vitamin C. Plasma levels in the fetus remain high (two to four times

as high as maternal levels), and a high concentration is also found in the placenta. The placenta may act as a barrier for the return of the vitamin to maternal circulation. Too high an intake by the mother during pregnancy may condition the infant to a rich supply so that he is much more susceptible to deficiency symptoms on restricted intakes.

Lactation. The ascorbic acid content of mother's milk reflects to a certain extent the dietary intake of the mother and usually varies from 4 to 8 mg. per 100 gm. of milk. An intake of 100 mg. per day by the mother should result in optimal levels in her milk.

The lack of agreement as to what constitutes a desirable level of intake of ascorbic acid is evident from Table 12-1, which compares recommendations prevailing in various countries. Even when the different philosophies on which the standards are based are considered, there are still some obvious discrepancies.

Food sources

Vitamin C is found almost exclusively in foods of plant origin. Aside from kidney, no other animal food is considered a sig-

Table 12-1. Comparison of dietary standards for ascorbic acid for selected age groups (in milligrams)*

		NRC	USSR	Canada	Japan	Great Britain	Australia	Norway
Children	1 to 2 years	40	40	20	30	15	—	30
	4 to 6 years	50	50	20	40	15	30	30
Boys	13 to 15 years	80	70	30	80	30	30	50
Men		70	70	30	65	20	30	30
Women		70	70	30	60	20	30	30
	Pregnancy	100	100	40	100	40	80	50
	Lactation	100	120	50	150	50	100	75

*Adapted from Young, E. G.: Dietary standards. In Beaton, G., and McHenry, E. W.: Nutrition II, New York, 1964, Academic Press Inc.

nificant source. The amount present in a plant tissue depends on many factors.

Part and type of the plant. The head of broccoli was shown to have 158 mg. of vitamin C per 100 gm. of vegetable compared to 115 mg. of vitamin C per 100 gm. of stem. But stems retained 82% during a 10-minute cooking period whereas heads retained only 60%. Counteracting some of the difference, thin-stemmed vegetables contained more vitamin C than thick-stemmed ones. Vegetables that wilt lose much more vitamin C than do those that do not wilt. Kale loses 1.5% of its total vitamin C per hour at room temperature while cabbage loses much less. Roots lose vitamin C slowly, but the loss is accelerated at higher temperatures.

Stage of maturity. Since the vitamin accumulates throughout the ripening process from the setting of the fruit, the longer the fruit remains on the vine or tree before harvesting the higher the ascorbic acid content.

In contrast, immature seeds such as peas and beans contain some ascorbic acid but lose it all at maturity.

Conditions of storage. Storing of vegetables at refrigerator temperatures at high humidity with a minimum of air movement will reduce ascorbic acid losses. The amount present in fresh vegetables bought in the temperate zone in the winter months is a function of the storage conditions during harvesting, shipping, and display in stores previous to selling. Losses are minimized at low temperatures and minimum exposure to air.

Season of year. A study of the ascorbic acid content of broccoli showed wide fluctuations with low values reported in May and peak values in December.

Method of processing. Any method of food processing that involves the application of heat is likely to result in a reduced ascorbic acid content. If processing is done in the absence of air, losses will be much lower. In frozen and canned foods that are picked at the peak of maturity and processed immediately under optimal conditions, the resulting product may have a higher vitamin C value than the fresh product, for which the period between harvesting and consumption may be long and characterized by poor storage facilities.

Blanching of vegetables prior to freezing is necessary in order to destroy certain enzymes that otherwise would catalyze the destruction of ascorbic acid. In home-frozen vegetables the vitamin C content is likely to be less than that in commercially frozen vegetables that have been picked at the peak of maturity and processed immediately.

Irradiation of potatoes results in no decrease in ascorbic acid values.

Method of cooking. Many of our best sources of ascorbic acid are normally consumed raw. For those characteristically cooked, however, the effect of cooking method assumes much importance.

In most cooking the greater part of the cooking losses occur in the early stages of cooking. For instance, broccoli heads lose 40% of their ascorbic acid values in the first 10 minutes. In the case of broccoli most of the loss is represented by leaching into the cooking water. On the other hand, cabbage with a lower initial amount loses more by destruction of ascorbic acid by heat than by leaching. The amount of water used has a greater effect on losses than does the total cooking time. Steaming was found to lead to higher retentions, 69% versus 45%, than boiling when tested on five vegetables. Steaming had no advantage over pressure-cooking.

Electronic cooking caused less destruction of ascorbic acid than did either pressure-cooking or boiling. In the case of broccoli, retentions of 85%, 80%, and 45% respectively were reported. For cabbage comparable values were 80%, 70%, and 38%.

Method of preparation. Any method that reduces the surface area exposed to air or water minimizes losses. Thus finely

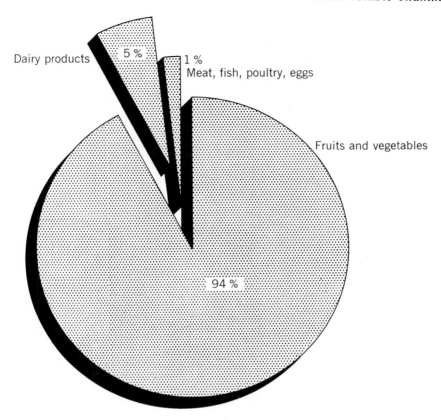

Dairy products — 5%

1% Meat, fish, poultry, eggs

Fruits and vegetables

94%

Fig. 12-5

Contribution of various food groups to ascorbic acid content of food supply. Based on Nutritive value of food available for consumption, United States, 1909-1964, Agricultural Research Service Publication 62-14, 1966.

shredded cabbage loses more ascorbic acid than do cabbage wedges. In the case of cabbage, however, the practice of serving it in vinegar, as in coleslaw, helps counteract the losses from exposure on the surface. Potatoes peeled, cut into smaller pieces, and cooked lose more than those cooked whole in their skins. The use of a dull knife in cutting fruit and vegetables may mash the cell, resulting in increased losses. The practice of crisping vegetables in cold water is undesirable since it results in the leaching of ascorbic acid into the water.

In Fig. 12-5, which shows the contribution of various food groups to the ascorbic acid in the American diet, it is seen that fruits and vegetables provide 92% of the ascorbic acid. The remaining 8% comes from meat, fish, and dairy products. Cereal products contribute none. Although one would have expected an increase in the total amount of vitamin C in the diet in recent years with the greater use of frozen vegetables and the increased availability of fresh produce the year round, dietary studies indicate that the ascorbic acid in the American diet was lower in 1959 than in either 1947 to 1949 or 1935 to 1939. There has been a shift from rich toward poorer sources in both vegetables and fruit juices.

The most recent tables of food com-

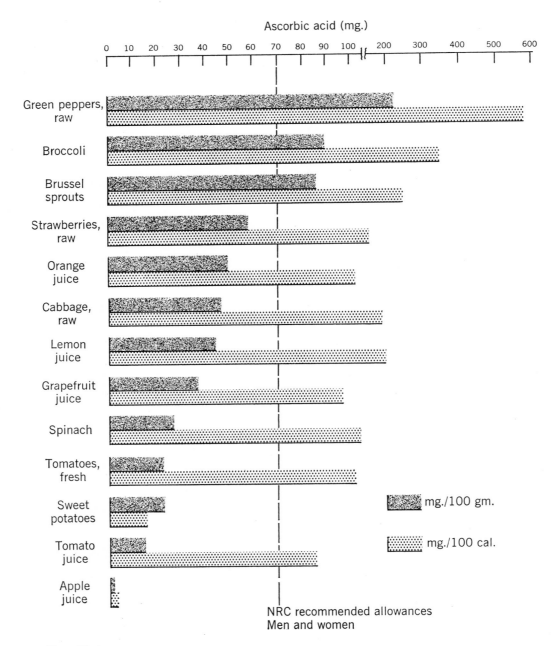

Fig. 12-6

Ascorbic acid content of 100-gm. and 100-kilocalorie portions of some representative foods. (Based on Watts, B., and Merrill, A.: Composition of foods—raw, processed and prepared, U. S. Department of Agriculture Handbook No. 8, Washington, D. C., 1963, U. S. Department of Agriculture.)

position have continued to record only the reduced ascorbic acid content of fruits and vegetables, although there is considerable evidence that the body utilizes both reduced and dehydroascorbic acid. In spite of the fact that values representing total ascorbic acid would be more meaningful, the food composition table in Appendix F is based on reduced ascorbic acid except for frozen fruits and vegetables, inadequate information being available on other foods. The ascorbic acid content of 100-gm. and 100-kilocalorie portions of some representative foods is presented graphically in Fig. 12-6. Table 12-2 gives both reduced, dehydroascorbic, and total ascorbic acid values for some representative foods for which data is available.

Aside from the more frequently used sources of vitamin C, such as citrus fruit and juices, broccoli, spinach, strawberries, and melon in season, there are several other rich sources. Parsley has a very high content (per 100 gm.) but is consumed in such small quantities that it is not an important source. Many of the early concen-

trates of vitamin C before synthetic vitamin C was readily available were made from rose tips gathered mostly by Indians in northern Alberta. Recently the acerola cherry, native to the tropics, has been identified as an extremely rich source (1500 mg. per 100 gm.), and while unpalatable alone, it is being used to fortify fruit juices less rich in ascorbic acid, especially for infant feeding. Camu-camu, a fruit native to South America, averages even more with 2000 mg. per 100 gm.

There is a trend in the food industry, especially among processors of fruit juices and fruit juice mixtures, to add vitamin C at a level of about 30 mg. per 4-ounce serving to give them a better chance of competing with citrus juices. For consumption by persons who do not recognize the difference in ascorbic acid values of various juices this is a commendable practice, although there is evidence that analyzed values many times vary considerably from value declared on the label, indicating a need for greater quality control. In keeping with the policy of recommending the en-

Table 12-2. Reduced, dehydroascorbic, and total ascorbic acid in 100 gm. of some representative foods (in milligrams)*

	Reduced ascorbic acid	Dehydroascorbic acid	Total ascorbic acid
Asparagus	7.9	26.9	34.8
Broccoli	48.2	9.8	58.0
Brussels sprouts	60.9	4.4	65.3
Cabbage, raw	54.4	22.3	76.7
Cantaloupe	15.5	18.2	33.7
Green pepper	41.0	4.8	45.8
Strawberries	53.8	12.9	66.7
Sweet potatoes	18.8	8.1	26.9
Tomato juice	15.2	2.3	17.5

*From Davey, B. L., Dodds, M. L., Fisher, K. H., Schuck, C., and Shih, D. C.: Utilization of ascorbic acid in fruits and vegetables. 1. Plan of study and ascorbic acid content of 24 foods, J. Am. Dietet. A. **32:**1064, 1956.

richment of food products only when there is evidence of a lack of the particular nutrient in a significant segment of the population, it is hard to rationalize such a practice. However, in Canada, the enrichment of apple juice with ascorbic acid has the approval of government agencies since it is conceivably puts a native product in a better place competitively with an imported one. The addition of ascorbic acid to dehydrated potatoes is a questionable practice because of the likelihood of its being destroyed by heat and oxidation in preparation and service. The enrichment of milk or carbonated beverages with ascorbic acid has not been endorsed in the United States. In the processing of frozen fruits, such as peaches and apples, ascorbic acid is frequently added because of its reducing properties that help prevent discoloration of the fruit.

Evaluation of nutritional status. In spite of the fact that the biochemistry of ascorbic acid in the cell is less well understood than is that of other nutrients, the assessment of nutritional status in regard to ascorbic acid is more satisfactory.

Several methods have been used to assess nutritional status for vitamin C in the body. It is now felt that no one method alone is completely satisfactory, but that a more accurate assessment is possible by a combination of several methods. By these methods it is possible to detect a difference between optimal and less than optimal nutrition.

Serum ascorbic acid levels have been widely used but do not bear a direct relationship to either dietary intake or white blood cell levels, which are felt to reflect state of tissue saturation. When serum values fall below 0.4 mg.%, they parallel white blood cell levels, but correlation for individuals is low. When tissues are less than 50% saturated, serum levels are too low to measure. This makes this determination virtually useless in discriminating between low and scorbutic levels of tissue saturation. When tissues are saturated, serum levels are close to 1 mg. per 100 gm. of blood.

The white blood cell or leukocyte level of ascorbic acid is a much more sensitive test of ascorbic acid nutrition. When tissues are completely saturated, leukocyte values are between 27 and 30 mg. per 100 gm. of blood. The fall in white blood cell level parallels the degree of saturation of the tissues so that a fall in these levels is indicative of depletion of body reserves. Scurvy does not develop until tissues are less than 20% saturated, indicated by a white blood cell level of less than 20 mg.%. This will not occur unless levels of intake fall below 10 mg. per day.

A measure of the amount of a test dose excreted in the urine within a short period following its administration has been the basis of the urinary excretion test for vitamin C status. The theory behind this test is that a depleted tissue will take up more of a test dose than will saturated tissues. Thus, where the intake has been adequate, the percentage of a test dose recovered in the urine will be high. When tissues are depleted, the amount appearing in the urine decreases, showing that more has been retained in the body. Table 12-3 shows the levels of these measurements under varying degrees of saturation.

Deficiency

Scurvy represents the most severe form of ascorbic acid deficiency but is relatively rare, especially in adults, now that its cause and cure are known. When it does develop, however, the early symptoms are relatively nonspecific, such as listlessness, fatigue, weakness, shortness of breath, aching bones, joints, and muscles, and loss of appetite. These are followed by more specific symptoms, such as swollen, sensitive gums, hardening and roughness around hair follicles, and small pinpoint or petecheal hemorrhages under the skin. The skin becomes dry, feverish, and rough and is

Table 12-3. Comparison of biochemical data on ascorbic acid at different levels of saturation in the tissues

Degree of saturation	Saturated	Less saturated	50% saturation	25% saturation
White blood cell levels of ascorbic acid	27 to 30 mg.%			20 mg.%
Serum levels of ascorbic acid	1 mg.%	0.4 to 1 mg.%	Too low to measure	
Urinary excretion; percent of test dose	60% to 80%	20% to 60%	Very low	
Dietary intake	> 100 mg.	40 to 100 mg.	10 to 15 mg.	5 to 7 mg.

covered by severe reddish blue spots. The hemorrhaging of the gums often predisposes to secondary infection.

Infantile scurvy, illustrated in Figs. 1-3 and 12-3, is most likely to occur in the period of rapid growth between 5 and 24 months of age. Breast-fed infants never have scurvy, but bottle-fed infants whose diets are not varied by 6 months of age develop symptoms of irritability, anorexia, growth failure, tenderness of lips, and anemia. The onset is very rapid and unless treated promptly the condition may result in rather rapid death. If treated, the recovery is equally as dramatic.

Delayed or incomplete wound healing is a very frequent manifestation of ascorbic acid deficiency, and anemia invariably occurs after 2 months of restricted intake. A drop in white blood cell levels is also frequent.

THIAMINE (THIAMIN)

The discovery of the chemical structure and the synthesis of thiamine by Williams in 1936 marked the end of a long and tedious search on the part of German, English, and American scientists to identify the substance in rice bran responsible for the cure of beriberi. As early as 1855 Takaki had

cured beriberi in the Japanese Navy by using the protein foods meat and milk to supplement the regular diet of the seamen.

In 1890 Eijkman, a Dutch physician, was able to cure the paralytic polyneuritis that had developed in chickens that had been fed scraps of polished rice from hospital wards by feeding unhusked rice or rice polishings. He also showed that he could cure human beriberi by similar treatment. His method of treatment worked although his explanation has since been shown to be erroneous. By 1910 Vedder in the Philippines had recognized that an active factor was present in a rice bran extract, tikitiki, and was capable of curing polyneuritis in chicks and beriberi in humans. By 1926 Dutch scientists had produced thiamine crystals, but another ten years elapsed, however, before they were chemically identified and synthesized. By the following year, 1937, both Swiss and American firms were producing thiamine commercially at a cost of approximately 450 dollars a pound, and Britain was formulating plans to use it to enrich bread.

Beriberi

Beriberi is a disease that was virtually unknown until the middle of the nineteenth century, although it had been described by the Chinese as early as 2600 B.C. With the trend toward the use of more highly refined cereals to improve storage conditions, beriberi became a major health problem. This was especially true in countries where a staple food item such as rice provided as much as 80% of the calories in the diet. The cause of beriberi was not identified at first as a dietary deficiency resulting from the removal of the outer layers of cereal grains. Instead, various other theories were advanced such as the presence of a toxic substance in the starch of rice for which there was an antidote in rice bran, the presence of a microbe, the absence of nitrogen in the diet, or the production of a toxic substance in the stomach from the use of rice. None of these theories stood scrutiny, and eventually the search narrowed to one for the active substance in a rice bran extract that had almost magical curative properties for beriberi, especially infantile beriberi. It was identified as a water-soluble substance easily destroyed by heat and alkali. After 25 years of constant experimentation Williams produced a few crystals of synthetic vitamin B or thiamine of known chemical composition which, without a doubt, possessed antiberiberi properties. Thiamine production is now commercially feasible, two hundred tons having been produced in the United States in 1961 at a cost of about nine dollars a pound—one fiftieth of the price prevailing 20 years previously. Japan, Switzerland, and France also produce appreciable amounts.

In spite of our knowledge of food sources of thiamine and the ready production of synthetic thiamine at reasonable prices, beriberi is still a problem in many parts of the world. The Philippines still reports an incidence of infantile beriberi deaths of 75 per 100,000 births. There, beriberi is listed as the fourth leading cause of death and led to 15,200 infant deaths and 6,130 adult deaths in the period of 1954

to 1958. In addition it is estimated that at least one and a half million persons suffer from some manifestation of the disease, either clinically or subclinically.

The incidence of beriberi can be attributed to the fact that the mills, which have taken over all but 5% of the rice milling in this country, are producing a very highly polished rice and with few exceptions are failing to comply with government regulations regarding enrichment even at a cost of less than one fifth of a cent per pound. The practice of repeated washings of the milled rice to remove the dust that accumulates during marketing in open bins causes a further loss of thiamine. It is estimated that after milling, washing, and cooking losses are considered that the average consumption of slightly less than 1 pound of rice per day provides only 0.27 mg. of thiamine. On the basis of the Food and Agricultural Organization criterion of 0.27 mg. of thiamine per 1000 nonfat calories in the diet, this level of intake will not protect against beriberi.

Infantile beriberi occurs most frequently from 2 to 5 months of age, is very rapid in onset, and unless treated within a matter of hours often results in death. Beriberi occurs more often in breast-fed than bottle-fed infants, reflecting the failure on the part of the lactating mother whose dietary thiamine is low to produce a milk with sufficient thiamine to protect her child. Human milk normally contains about half as much thiamine as cow's milk, but that of a woman on a thiamine-deficient diet is much lower. The situation may be complicated by the transfer of methyl glyoxal, a product of metabolism that accumulates in the body in thiamine deficiency, to the mother's milk. Milk from mothers suffering from beriberi has been found to contain about half as much thiamine as that from normal mothers. A child with beriberi develops very rapidly such symptoms as cyanosis (too much carbon dioxide in blood, giving child a bluish color), tachycardia (a very fast heartbeat), and a characteristic cry changing from a loud piercing one to a thin weak almost inaudible one, sometimes accompanied by vomiting and convulsions. Once thiamine is administered, symptoms are relieved within a matter of hours.

In adults, beriberi is quite a different condition and takes two very distinct forms. In wet beriberi the victim suffers from swelling of the limbs, usually starting at the feet and progressing upward throughout the body until the accumulation of fluid in heart muscle leads to eventual heart failure and death. Early signs of this edematous form are wristdrop and ankledrop.

In dry beriberi there is a gradual wasting away of body tissue, the patient becoming very thin and emaciated. In both forms there are symptoms of irritability, vague uneasiness, disorderly thinking, and nausea, all suggesting an involvement of the nervous system.

The disease continues to be a problem in areas of the world where polished rice is a staple in the diet and where the milling of rice has shifted from the home to the mill. In the United States, alcoholics are the only group in which the disease ever occurs. However, there is considerable evidence of subclinical thiamine deficiency, especially among persons who eliminate bread and cereal products, our most constant source of thiamine, from their diets in an effort to lose weight.

Early work in the study of thiamine was facilitated by the observation that chickens fed the beriberi-producing diet developed polyneuritis (inflammation of many nerves). These animals showed loss of neuromuscular coordination, had a poor sense of balance, and died within a short time of onset of the symptoms.

Chemical properties

Thiamine, which is usually available as the biologically active but more stable thiamine hydrochloride, is a white crystalline substance, soluble in water and very easily destroyed by heat or oxidation, especially in the presence of alkali. The term thiamine indicates that it is a sulphur-containing substance (thio) and it is also amine- or nitrogen-containing. It has also been known as aneurin, indicative of its role in preventing symptoms involving nerves. It is also referred to as the antineuritic factor.

Functions

Vitamin B_1 is known to be a part of the enzyme thiamine pyrophosphate (thiamine with two molecules of phosphate attached to it) or cocarboxylase, which is required in metabolism of carbohydrate, leading eventually to the release of energy and excretion of carbon dioxide and water. There are three stages in the metabolism of carbohydrates at which the absence of thiamine as part of a coenzyme leads to a slowing or complete blocking of the chemical changes. Although it has not been confirmed, it has been postulated that it is an accumulation of the intermediary products of metabolism blocked by the absence of the necessary thiamine-containing enzyme that causes typical thiamine deficiency symptoms. Since thiamine is part of cocarboxylase necessary for the decarboxylation (removal of carbon dioxide) from pyruvic acid as it is prepared to enter the citric acid cycle, pyruvic acid tends to accumlate when thiamine is lacking. A similar role for cocarboxylase exists at the stage in the metabolic cycle at which another intermediary product of both fat and carbohydrate metabolism, a-ketoglutaric acid, is decarboxylated to succinic acid. A third enzymatic role of thiamine is in activating transketolase, an enzyme involved in the direct oxidative pathway for glucose that occurs in all cells except skeletal cells. Even though less than 10% of all glucose is ordinarily used this way, this particular route is essential since it is the only way the body can produce both ribose, the sugar needed for the synthesis of RNA so essential in cell reproduction, and also an intermediary product needed for the synthesis of fatty acids. The level of transketolase found in the red blood cells has been found to be a very sensitive indicator of thiamine status. The level of transketolase in the red blood cells falls before there are any other manifestations of thiamine deficiency and tends to reflect dietary intake. Thus it has potential in detecting suboptimal nutritional status. In birds a decreased transketolase level depresses to about one seventh of normal the ability of the red blood cells to oxidize glucose directly, leading to the accumulation of methyl glyoxal, apparently because of failure to oxidize it.

Absorption

The absorption of thiamine occurs primarily in the duodenum and the small intestine. Absorption appears to be maximum at intakes of 2.5 to 5 mg. per day. Large intakes such as 10 mg. are absorbed three times as well in four divided dosages as in one single dose. Results from the use of sustained-release preparations of thiamine have yielded contradictory results.

Thiamine absorption is an active process requiring energy. Any thiamine synthesized in the lower gastrointestinal tract appears as cocarboxylase, which cannot be absorbed at this point, so that intestinal synthesis in humans appears to have no significance.

A substance in onion oil and garlic oil, alliin, combines with thiamine to form alliithiamine, a form in which the vitamin is more readily absorbed. The widespread use of onions and garlic in oriental diets with marginal amounts of thiamine may thus help to alleviate thiamine deficiencies. Another thiamine compound, thiamine bisulphide, is absorbed more freely than thiamine hydrochloride.

Since thiamine pyrophosphate (cocarboxylase) is too large a molecule to pass through the cell membrane, it becomes clear that this coenzyme is produced in the cell as needed and that the thiamine existing in either animal or plant foods as cocarboxylase must be split before being absorbed. It is then rejoined with the aid of enzymes to phosphates as needed in individual cells to produce cocarboxylase.

The decrease in gastric acidity that occurs in thiamine deficiency decreases the release of thiamine from thiamine complexes in the gastrointestinal tract, inhibiting the absorption of thiamine and accentuating the deficiency symptoms.

Metabolism

It is known that thiamine in excess of body needs is excreted in the urine. A measure of urinary thiamine in relation to dietary thiamine has been the basis for balance studies to assess the adequacy of intake. When thiamine excretion drops, a larger portion of the test dose is retained, indicating a tissue need for thiamine. On very low intakes excretion drops to zero. A radioactive test dose of thiamine appears in the urine as thiamine, thiamine disulphide, and about sixteen other degradation products.

The adult body contains from 30 to 70 mg. of thiamine. Although there is no storage site for the vitamin it has been observed that normal levels of 2 to 3 μg. per gram of heart muscle, 1 μg. per gram of brain, liver, and kidney, and 0.5 μg. per gram of skeletal muscle double following thiamine therapy and drop to half these values in thiamine depletion.

Requirements

Efforts to determine the minimum needs and optimal intakes for humans for thiamine have involved thiamine balance studies, in which the relationship between dietary intake and urinary excretion have been determined. A level of intake that leads to minimum but not zero excretion is believed to represent minimal needs but provides no protection against further reduction in thiamine intake.

Recommendations for all age groups assume a relationship between calorie intake and thiamine need. The assumption is based on the fact that thiamine is part of the coenzyme needed in at least three places in the metabolism of carbohydrate and one in the metabolism of fat. As calorie intake varies with age, size, physical activity, environmental temperature, or physical state of the animal, carbohydrate intake changes and an increased carbohydrate intake creates an increased need for thiamine. The current recommendations of the National Research Council based on a level of 0.4 mg. of thiamine per 1000 kilocalories are presented in Table 12-4. In keeping with their philosophy of setting recommendations at a level compatible with the potential of the nation's food supply and sufficiently high to provide a margin of safety to take into account practically all individual variations in need, efficiency of absorption, and normal losses in food preparation, these figures represent optimal intakes, for the most part about 100% above minimal requirements. These levels protect against deficiency symptoms and provide a buffer against zero intakes of thia-

mine. We have no evidence of benefits to be derived from intakes in excess of these levels. Since thiamine is water-soluble and the body has virtually no capacity to store it, excesses are excreted, and we have no indication of toxicity from its use.

Studies of older people show that their needs are relatively high, they excrete less at all levels of intake, experience a faster reaction to moderate depletion, and respond more slowly to the addition of thiamine to the diet.

The need for thiamine increases with an increased consumption of alcohol. This accounts for the reported incidence of beriberi among alcoholics in the United States. It appears that the vitamin is necessary for the metabolism of acetaldehyde, an intermediary product in alcohol metabolism, rather than directly for alcohol metabolism.

The amount of fat, especially moderate-chain fatty acids, in the diet influences the need for thiamine, and fat has frequently been referred to as a "thiamine sparer." Since only one of the reactions for which thiamine is needed is involved in the metabolism of fatty acids, it follows that

Table 12-4. Recommended daily intake for thiamine (in milligrams)

		United States*	Great Britain†	Canada‡
Children	1 to 3 years	0.5	0.6	0.4
	6 to 9 years	0.8	0.8	0.7
Boys	12 to 15 years	1.2	1.1	0.9
Girls	12 to 15 years	1.0	1.1	0.8
Men	18 to 35 years	1.2	1.1	1.1
	35 to 55 years	1.0	1.1	1.1
Women	18 to 35 years	0.8	0.8	0.9
	35 to 55 years	0.8	0.9	0.9

*Food and Nutrition Board: Recommended dietary allowance publication, National Research Council Publication No. 1146, 1963, National Academy of Science.
†British Medical Association: Report of the committee on nutrition, London, 1950, British Medical Association.
‡Dietary Standards for Canada, Canadian Bulletin on Nutrition 6, No. 1, 1964.

when fat calories replace carbohydrate calories, less thiamine will be required. Thus, thiamine intakes that are suboptimal in a high-carbohydrate diet prove adequate when fat replaces some of the carbohydrate. Others have suggested that there is a toxic product, presumably methyl glyoxal, that arises from carbohydrate metabolism but not from fat metabolism in the absence of thiamine. A third possibility is that fat protects thiamine from loss or destruction in the body.

There is considerable evidence that the need for thiamine decreases when some sulfonamides and other antibiotics are given. Several theories have been suggested to explain this effect, but there is no clearcut evidence to support any one of them.

Food sources

As shown in Fig. 12-7, cereal products provide about one third of the available thiamine; meat, fish, and poultry, one fourth; and dairy products, one eighth of that available to the American public.

Fig. 12-8 shows the thiamine content of 100-gm. and 100-kilocalorie portions of some of the more dependable sources of thiamine in the average American diet. Thiamine in vegetables is in nonphosphoryl-

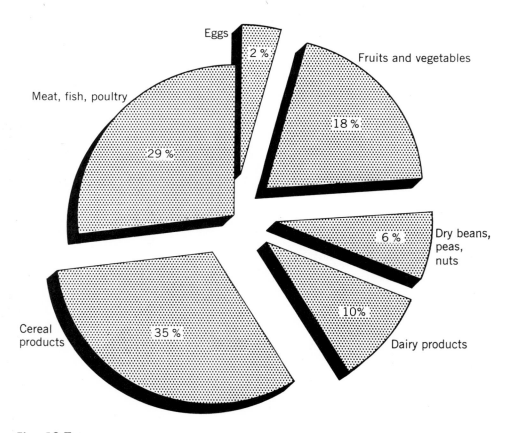

Fig. 12-7

Contribution of various food groups to the thiamine content of the food supply. (Based on Nutritive value of food available for consumption, United States, 1900-1964, Agricultural Research Service Publication 62-14, 1966.)

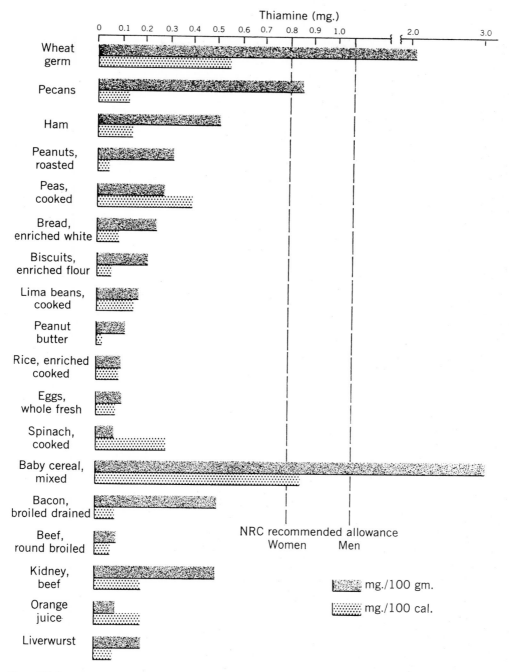

Fig. 12-8

Thiamine content of 100-gm. and 100-kilocalorie portions of some representative foods. (Based on Watts, B., and Merrill, A.: Composition of foods—raw, processed and prepared, U. S. Department of Agriculture Handbook No. 8, Washington, D. C., 1963, U. S. Department of Agriculture.)

ated form while that in meat occurs primarily as cocarboxylase or diphosphate, which must be broken before it is absorbed.

The richest sources of the vitamin are pork products. For that segment of the population who eat pork frequently, especially rural midwestern people, it represents a very dependable source of thiamine. Others whose religious beliefs prohibit consumption of pork must and do obtain adequate amounts from other sources.

Peas and other legumes are good sources. As will be noted from a comparison of fresh and dried peas there is an increase in the amount of thiamine with increasing maturity of the seed. The amount of the nutrient actually obtained from dried legumes will be reduced if they are soaked for a long period in water, which is discarded, or if baking soda is used to hasten the cooking time by softening the cellulose. The USDA now suggests that the use of minute amounts of baking soda (1/16 teaspoon per cup of beans) is satisfactory since reduced cooking time reduces thiamine losses sufficiently to compensate for increased losses resulting from the addition of an alkali.

Whole-grain cereals contain the greater part of their thiamine in their outer husks, the part that is removed in the milling process.

Enriched or whole-wheat bread may at first appear as an insignificant source, but in the amounts consumed, especially by low-income families, the use of bread products provides enough thiamine to ensure an adequate intake in diets that would otherwise be marginal. The use of enriched bread which has come with the mandatory enrichment laws in thirty states has been credited with decreasing the incidence of beriberi among alcoholics, many of whom eat bread or bread products—one of the cheaper sources of calories. Of bread and flour marketed in the United States 80% to 90% is now enriched at a cost of approximately 4 cents per 100 pounds.

Dried brewer's yeast and wheat germ,

both rich in thiamine, assume little importance in the American diet because of the infrequency of their use. Live yeast, found in compressed yeast cakes, is high in thiamine, but it has been established that these same yeast cells deprive the body of thiamine and may precipitate thiamine-deficiency symptoms. Cooking, of course, kills the yeast cells; thus it is only when live yeast is taken, as was once recommended as a therapeutic agent in certain skin conditions, that a problem occurs.

The enrichment of other cereal products, such as rice, macaroni, corn grits, and flour, assumes practical importance, depending on the extent to which these items are a staple food item in a diet.

The USDA reports that the American food supply provides about 1.8 mg. per person per day, which is not much above the daily adult requirement.

Certain fresh-water fish, a few salt-water fish, bracken ferns, and some shellfish, such as clams, shrimp, and mussels, contain a thiamine-splitting enzyme, thiaminase. Fortunately this enzyme is heat-labile (its co-enzyme is heat-stable), so that only in circumstances in which raw fish is regularly consumed is the presence of this enzyme detrimental in human nutrition.

Effect of cooking

The extent to which foods lose thiamine in preparation is determined by the physical and chemical properties of the vitamin.

Loss in solution. Since thiamine is water-soluble, it will leach out of a product in proportion to the amount of water available and the surface area of the food exposed to the water. Any method of preparation that minimizes the length of time a food is in contact with water and the amount of surface area will decrease thiamine losses. As much as 18% of the thiamine in rice is reportedly lost in the method used by Orientals of washing the rice several times before cooking. Modern marketing procedures, which protect the food from contamination from the air, eliminate the necessity for preliminary washing of rice. In fact, most packages warn the housewife not to wash rice and to cook it in a minimum of water to reduce cooking losses. This is especially important where the rice is enriched by coating it with an enrichment mixture.

Loss due to heat. Thiamine is destroyed by heat. The higher the temperature and more prolonged the exposure to heat, the greater the loss. Roasting pork at 325° F. allows a retention of 75% to 100% of the original thiamine while higher temperatures give lower yields. Destruction appears no greater in cooking in electronic ovens than in conventional ones. Thiamine in food is less susceptible to heat destruction than is the free form of thiamine. There is also a difference in rate of heat destruction between various foods, that in spinach, heart, liver, and lamb being more susceptible than that in peas, beans, pork, and carrots.

Loss due to oxidation. Cooking procedures that increase the amount of oxygen in contact with the food, especially under conditions of moist heat, speed up the destruction of thiamine. The use of rapid boiling water in cooking vegetables is an example of this.

Loss due to alkali. The destruction of thiamine is greatest in the presence of alkali. The addition of baking soda, an alkali, to cooking water is sometimes suggested as a means of preserving the bright green color of fresh vegetables. Its use for such purposes cannot be recommended because of the destructive effect it has on both thiamine and vitamin C.

Loss due to irradiation. The thiamine content of pork is virtually destroyed by the irradiation procedures sometimes used in food preservation.

Evaluation of thiamine status

The most sensitive test available for the determination of thiamine status is the red blood cell transketolase activity. These values reflect changes in dietary intake before any other signs of thiamine inadequacy are detectable. In animals, growth response is considered a fairly sensitive indicator of thiamine intake but is not as specific to thiamine as is transketolase activity, which was shown to drop 30% at one week and 51% at two weeks in rats who continued to grow during this period of thiamine deficiency.

Another promising indicator of thiamine status of an individual is the carbohydrate index, which is a function of pyruvic acid, lactic acid, and glucose in the blood after the administration of glucose and a standard exercise test. It, of course, is useful only for persons able to exercise.

The urinary excretion test for thiamine involves measuring the amount of thiamine excreted in the urine following a test dose. Persons with low levels of saturation in the tissues will retain more and excrete less than will persons whose intake has been more adequate.

Results of deficiency

Thiamine deficiency may result under several sets of circumstances aside from a low dietary intake, which frequently occurs when the diet is very low in calories or limited in variety. Failure of absorption, usually caused by some abnormality in the gastrointestinal tract, the inability of tissues to accumulate adequate stores of the vitamin, failure to utilize available thiamine, or an increased requirement such as occurs in a diet high in carbohydrate or alcohol, may lead to deficiency symptoms. At the moment we have no clear-cut indication of the relationship between clinical symptoms and biochemical changes that occur in a thiamine deficiency. Several explanations have been considered—first, that a lack of thiamine causes a failure to provide energy for the cell, second, that in thiamine deficiency some product essential for metabolism in heart or muscle cells is not formed, and alternatively, that some toxic product accumulates.

Since thiamine deficiency in humans usually occurs along with symptoms of deficiencies of other vitamins of the B complex it is difficult to attribute symptoms specifically to thiamine. It is often complicated by symptoms brought on by concurrent infection and varies with degree of deficiency and presence of stress situations such as pregnancy. However, in cases where thiamine has been effective in relieving particular symptoms, it is customary to consider them specific to thiamine. The following have been associated with a lack of thiamine although similar symptoms may occur as a result of other dietary inadequacies, especially those of B complex vitamins.

Loss of appetite. Loss of appetite or anorexia has been clearly demonstrated in experimental animals and has been related in many cases to thiamine inadequacy in humans. Anorexia accompanied by vomiting was the first sign of deficiency shown by a group of normal men subjected to an induced thiamine deficiency. Even at intakes of 0.2 mg. per 1000 kilocaries, which did not cause any other symptoms, there was loss of appetite, nausea, and constipation. While increased intake of thiamine will restore a depressed appetite to normal levels it is ineffective in stimulating the appetite beyond a normal level. The speed with which thiamine can stimulate the appetite has been dramatically demonstrated in the case of both dogs and rats. In both instances, deficient animals that have shown virtually no interest in food they would normally relish have returned to eat the same food in a matter of one or two hours after being given thiamine.

Decreased muscle tonus. The tonus or elasticity of the wall of the lower gastrointestinal tract is decreased in thiamine deficiency to the point that normal gastric motility is decreased, the colon becomes distended, and constipation results. Thiamine has been used with varying degrees

of success in treating constipation in older people in whom gastric motility is frequently subnormal.

Depression. Mental depression and confusion sometimes alleviated by the administration of thiamine has led to the somewhat misleading designation of thiamine as the "morale vitamin." Persons on low thiamine intakes show pronounced mood changes, vague feelings of uneasiness, fear, disorderly thinking, and other signs of mental depression. Mental changes associated with inadequate thiamine respond readily to thiamine supplements. This is well illustrated in a study of ten older women (aged 52 to 72 years) limited to 0.33 mg. of thiamine per day. They all showed increasing irritability, complained of fatigue and headache, and voluntarily restricted their social engagements. Urinary excretion of thiamine dropped progressively. Immediate improvement was observed when they were given 1.4 mg. for one day. Similarly, the restoration of thiamine to the diets of men who had been on a restricted thiamine intake led to the restoration of normal attitudes. Reports demonstrating that the use of thiamine supplements with children was effective in raising their I.Q. and intellectual performance have subsequently been discredited. In beriberi the most acute symptom is mental confusion leading to coma.

Neurological changes. Nystagmus caused by a weakness in the sixth nerve is known as Wernicke's syndrome. This symptom, a manifestation of changes occurring in the central nervous system, is most easily reversed by thiamine administration. Levels of thiamine in brain can be reduced by 50% without any noticeable clinical signs; further reduction to 30% of normal leads to slowness and unsteady gait, and at 20% there is severe disturbance of posture and equilibrium.

Peripheral neuritis, in which the nerves that control the extremities fail to function properly, shows up in a variety of ways in humans, usually affecting the legs first.

Neuromuscular coordination is affected in persons on low thiamine intake. Motor speed, eye-hand coordination, and body and manual steadiness reactions that had deteriorated on an intake of 0.05 mg. of thiamine per 1000 kilocalories were quickly restored with thiamine supplementation. Other signs of peripheral nervous system involvement are loss of ankle and knee jerk, painful calf muscles, and general atrophy of leg muscles manifest as difficulty in walking.

Beriberi. Beriberi, the final form of thiamine deficiency that manifests itself in either the wet (edematous) or dry (wasting) form, has been mentioned earlier.

Deficiencies in animals. In experimental thiamine deficiency in rats, complete deprivation leads to death in three to six weeks with no specific clinical symptoms, but when very small amounts are provided death is delayed to eight to twelve weeks. Rats develop spasticity of muscles and usually die in convulsive seizures complicated by heart lesions unless treated promptly.

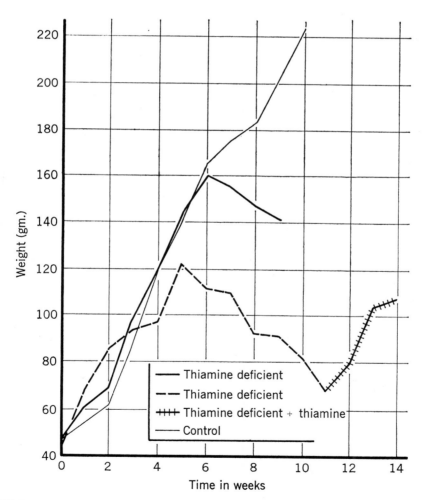

Fig. 12-9

Growth patterns of weanling albino rats with and without thiamine.

Growth retardation accompanying a dietary lack of thiamine is readily demonstrated in animals. Typical growth patterns of rats with and without thiamine are shown in Fig. 12-9. The growth response of thiamine-depleted animals to graded doses of thiamine is so specific that it has been used as the basis of a bioassay for the assessment of thiamine content of foods.

In birds a condition, polyneuritis (inflammation of many nerves), occurs upon thiamine deprivation. Birds quickly lose sense of balance and have depressed appetite and a chronic state of head retraction. All symptoms are quickly relieved with thiamine intake.

Therapeutic uses

Thiamine has been used in the medical treatment of a wide variety of conditions other than beriberi. A recent survey of the literature showed that it had been tried in 230 different conditions. In the period from 1936 to 1945 these ranged from neuritis, neuralgia, pains of various origins, diseases of the central nervous system, and cardiovascular symptoms. A renewed interest in thiamine therapy from 1951 to 1960 found it used in acidosis, diabetic coma, pyruvemia (accumulation of pyruvic acid in the blood), and toxemia of pregnancy. In addition, it is widely used as a supplement to stimulate a poor appetite. The possibility of observing beneficial results are greatest when malnutrition, nutritional imbalance, or impaired intestinal absorption have precipitated the symptoms.

RIBOFLAVIN

Riboflavin, which has also been known as vitamin B_2, vitamin G, and the yellow vitamin, was recognized in 1917 when it became clear that vitamin B retained some growth-promoting properties after its antiberiberi properties had been destroyed by heat. To differentiate the heat-labile component from this heat-stable fraction, the two components were designated vitamin B_1 and vitamin B_2 respectively.

At the time of the discovery of riboflavin, reports appeared almost simultaneously announcing the isolation of four substances necessary for growth—hepatoflavin, lactoflavin, ovoflavin, and verdoflavin. These discoverers, obviously isolating their factors from liver, milk, eggs, and grass respectively, had agreed on one aspect of its nature—it was a flavin compound, a substance that produces an intense yellow-green fluorescence in water. This substance had been concentrated from natural foods in 1925 and isolated in 1932, at which time it became evident that the active substance was composed of a protein plus a pigment, the flavin. With its synthesis in 1935 it soon became clear that the five-carbon sugar, ribose, was common to all forms, which were then designated riboflavine. Shortly afterward the final "e" was dropped but has been recently (1961) added in the official spelling in Britain.

Chemical properties

Riboflavin is a relatively stable vitamin; it is resistant to the effects of acid, heat, or oxidation. It is unstable in the presence of alkali and light. Since it is slightly soluble in water, some losses occur when riboflavin-containing vegetables cut in small pieces are cooked in large amounts of water for long periods of time. The major source of loss of riboflavin in food is that resulting from the action of either the ultraviolet or visible rays of sunlight on milk, a significant source of riboflavin in the American diet. Efforts of the dairy industry to reduce this loss have met with much popular resistance. The use of brown glass bottles that filter out the harmful rays of the sun are considered suitable only for less nutritional beverages! The flavor that housewives claim arises from the use of more opaque lined cardboard or plastic containers has limited their acceptance. The most successful efforts have been the provision of covered insulated boxes that protect the milk from exposure to sunlight after home deliveries.

Functions

Biochemically the most clearly established role of riboflavin is in carbohydrate, fat, and protein metabolism, where it is an essential part of the enzymes usually referred to as FMN (flavine mononucleotide) and FAD (flavine adenine dinucleotide). Both of these substances are essential for their capacity to transfer hydrogen atoms or positive charges from one compound to another, a necessary reaction in the liberation of energy from carbohydrates, fat, and protein within the cell mitochondrion. Riboflavin is also an integral part of other enzymes specifically involved in the transfer of hydrogen atoms in protein metabolism since these flavoproteins can be alternately oxidized and reduced. It is also necessary before the amino acid tryptophan, a source of the vitamin niacin in the body, can be converted into the active form of the vitamin.

The role of substances chemically related to riboflavin has been studied. Some can replace riboflavin completely; others are effective for a short time, apparently replacing the reserves of riboflavin but leading to death as soon as the original reserves are depleted; and others act as riboflavin antagonists. These replace riboflavin in enzyme systems where they cannot function as riboflavin does, so that they are of no more use than no riboflavin. In fact, they often prevent any available vitamin from functioning. In human beings, riboflavin deficiencies have been produced experimentally by the use of the riboflavin antagonist galactoflavin, in which the five-carbon ribose is replaced by a six-carbon sugar, galactose.

Absorption

Riboflavin is absorbed through the walls of the intestine by passive diffusion; that is,

it passes through the epithelial cells of the intestine without an expenditure of energy. The rate of absorption is proportional to the size of the dose. Within the intestinal wall it is phosphorylated (linked with a phosphate molecule), in which form it is carried to the tissues, where it occurs in this phosphate form or attached to a protein as a flavoprotein. There is relatively little storage of riboflavin in the body although the liver, with 16 μg. per gram, and kidney, with 25 μg. per gram, contain slightly higher concentrations than other tissues such as muscle with 2 to 3 μg. per gram. Some unabsorbed riboflavin appears in the feces, but most excretion occurs through the kidney in the urine. The amount of riboflavin excreted following a test dose of the vitamin reflects the extent to which tissues are saturated with the vitamin. The smaller the amount excreted, the greater the amount retained—presumably to bring the levels in the body tissues up to saturation levels. A loss of protein from the body is accompanied by a loss of riboflavin.

Requirements

Riboflavin requirements are directly related to caloric expenditures since riboflavin functions as an integral part of enzymes involved in tissue oxidation and respiration. An allowance of 0.6 mg. per 1000 kilocalories or a minimum of 1.1 mg. per day has been suggested by the National Research Council. As is true in all recommended allowances this value represents a substantial margin of safety over the 0.3 mg. per 1000 kilocalories required to prevent deficiency symptoms, maintain health, and provide adequate body stores and the 0.25 mg. per 1000 kilocalories on which experimental riboflavin deficiencies have been produced in human subjects.

During pregnancy the need for riboflavin increases from 0.6 to 0.7 mg. per 1000 kilocalories, which amounts to an increase of 0.3 mg. per day during the second and

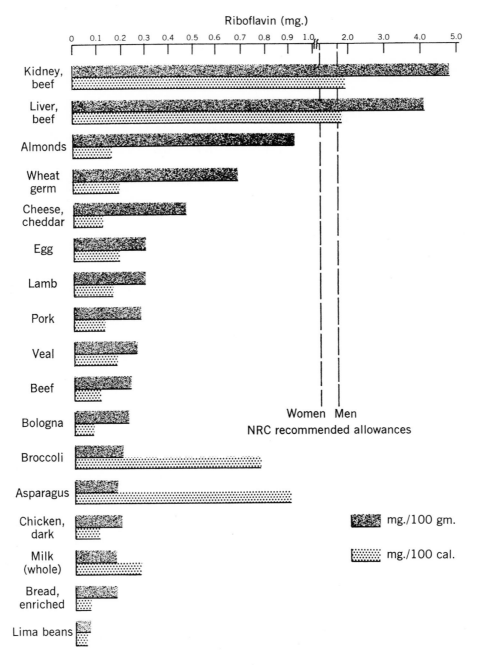

Fig. 12-10

Riboflavin content of 100-gm. and 100-kilocalorie portions of representative foods. (Based on Watts, B., and Merrill, A.: Composition of foods—raw, processed and prepared, U. S. Department of Agriculture Handbook No. 8, Washington, D. C., 1963, U. S. Department of Agriculture.)

third trimesters of pregnancy. During pregnancy the fetus and maternal tissues compete for the available riboflavin and in case of a dietary deficiency both suffer. To provide the 40 μg. (range of 37 to 60 μg.) of riboflavin per 100 ml. of mature human milk, an additional intake of 0.6 mg. above normal needs is recommended during lactation.

During infancy and early childhood the recommended intake of 0.5 mg. is readily provided by the milk consumption of human milk, containing 0.67 mg. per 1000 kilocalories, or cow's milk, with 2.3 mg. per 1000 kilocalories.

Dietary sources

Riboflavin is widely distributed in both animals and vegetable foods. The amount present in 100-gm. and 100-kilocalorie portions of representative foods is presented graphically in Fig. 12-10, while Fig. 12-11 shows the relative contributions of the major food groups.

Milk makes a very significant contribution, with 1 quart providing all of the recommended intake suggested for all ages and 2 cups providing a sufficient amount to take care of minimal needs. This assumes that adequate precautions are taken to minimize exposure to sunlight, which dras-

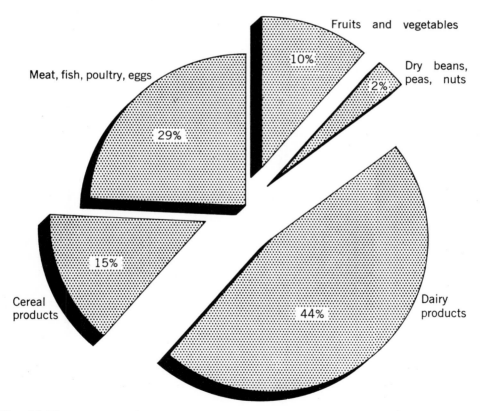

Fig. 12-11

Contribution of various food groups to the riboflavin content of the food supply. (Based on Nutritive value of food available for consumption, United States, 1909-1964, Agricultural Research Service Publication 62-14, 1966.

tically reduces the amount of riboflavin available.

Cereals are quite low except after germination. Enriched cereals have about twice as much riboflavin as whole-grain cereals.

There is evidence that riboflavin is synthesized by bacteria in the gastrointestinal tract, but there is little indication that a significant amount is absorbed in humans except when the diet is very high in starch. A diet high in starch, cellulose, and lactose stimulates riboflavin synthesis in the intestines while fat and protein have an inhibitory affect.

Deficiency symptoms

The lack of riboflavin for the production of a sufficient amount of the necessary enzymes manifests itself in a wide variety of ways.

In humans, an early form of ariboflavinosis (a lack of riboflavin) is a condition known as *cheilosis,* in which cracks appear at the corners of the mouth and the lips become inflamed. The tongue becomes smooth and takes on a characteristic purplish red color in a condition described as glossitis. These two signs are the ones used most frequently in nutrition surveys as indicative of and specific to low riboflavin intakes, although the intake must be low for several months before these symptoms manifest themselves. Changes in the skin, causing dryness and scaliness, have been associated with low riboflavin intakes but are not specific to this vitamin.

As is true in a deficiency of all vitamins, growth retardation occurs with a lack of riboflavin. Reproductive capacity is also reduced when riboflavin is lacking, and if conception does take place certain congenital malformations such as harelip and cataracts have been associated with a deficiency at a crucial stage in early (embryonic) development. This effect has been clearly demonstrated in animal experiments, but the relationship is much more difficult to establish in human pregnancy, partly because the relative rate of growth in human fetal development is much slower than in most animals. Thus a deficiency in humans must be much more prolonged than in animals to have the same severe consequences.

Other effects of a lack of riboflavin in the diet of animals for which no counterpart symptoms have been established in humans are loss of hair (alopecia) and the infiltration of blood vessels into the cornea of the eye (corneal vascularization), which may eventually form cataracts.

Toxicity

No reports of riboflavin toxicity have appeared even although amounts as high as 10 gm. per kilogram have been given to animals. Neither is there evidence of human toxicity.

NIACIN (NICOTINIC ACID)

Niacin, another water-soluble vitamin identified with the B complex, has been known as nicotinic acid and as the pellagra preventative (P-P) factor. It is a white crystalline substance first isolated from yeast and rice bran in 1912 but was not associated with pellagra until many years later.

History

The disease known as pellagra in Italy and mal de la rosa in Spain was first described in these countries in the eighteenth century where it occurred mainly among the poor, for whom corn was the dietary staple. Although there was evidence that the disease could be cured by changing the diet, it was not until 1917 that it was associated with the absence of a dietary factor.

The association of pellagra with diets monotonously high in highly refined maize or corn led to the theory that it was caused by a mold or a toxic or infectious substance in spoiled corn. A lack of nitrogen was implicated and later the absence of lysine, trypophan, or cysteine in conjunction with high leucine content in corn diets suggested an amino acid imbalance as a cause. The skin symptoms associated with pellagra were aggravated by exposure to sunlight, leading to the belief that the disease was caused by a sun poisoning. Since the pellagragenic corn diets, in which molasses and salt pork were often the only other foods, were consumed by persons on limited incomes often living in crowded unsanitary surroundings, the theories of the infectious or parasitic nature of the disease received further support. With several members of one family often developing pellagra there was an impetus for a search for an hereditary factor.

It was only in 1917 when Goldberger, a physician working with the U. S. Public Health Service, confirmed his theory that pellagra was associated with a dietary lack by producing pellagra by dietary restriction that progress was made in controlling the disease. His experiment with a group of prisoners who were promised reprieve if they would switch from the prison diet to one typical of the villages in which pellagra was prevalent is now classic. Since this diet was in many cases the one most familiar to the prisoners, they were willing subjects. After about five months, however, these men began to develop the classic symptoms of pellagra—dermatitis, diarrhea, and depression—while those on regular prison fare remained healthy. This fairly well refuted the infectious theory and established the relationship between a dietary factor and pellagra. It took an additional twenty years to identify the nutritional factor involved.

Pellagra, first reported in the state of New York in 1875, is the only vitamin deficiency disease that has ever been considered endemic to the United States and a major public health problem. Its incidence has been fairly well confined to the small mill villages of the southern states where the diet is predominately corn, mo-

lasses, and salt pork. In 1918 there were an estimated 10,000 deaths from the disease and another 100,000 cases, primarily in cotton-growing areas. At that time, when a dietary deficiency was suspected but the identity of the lacking nutrient had not been established, the most effective means of controlling the disease was to encourage the cultivation of home gardens for fresh produce and the increased use of meat and milk products.

Efforts to isolate the dietary factor responsible for preventing or curing pellagra were complicated by the fact that many other deficiencies produced similar skin symptoms. Thus it was not until 1937 when Elvehjem, working at the University of Wisconsin, showed that nicotinic acid, a substance that had previously been identified as part of two different enzymes, was effective in curing blacktongue, a condition in dogs analogous to human pellagra. The use of nicotinic acid in treating human pellagra brought very dramatic results and the census of pellagra victims in southern hospitals dropped precipitously.

Pellagra is still found in corn-eating countries such as Romania, Yugoslavia, and some parts of Egypt. The fact that it is not found in Central America, where corn provides 80% of the calories, can be attributed to the use of alkalis (usually soda lime) in its preparation, which helps liberate the niacin bound in the cereal.

Tryptophan-niacin relationship

A chemical analysis of some foods such as milk effective in curing or preventing pellagra indicated a very low niacin content. Also, diets low in niacin were not always pellagragenic. This apparent discrepancy was resolved in 1945 with the discovery that the amino acid tryptophan was also effective in curing pellagra. The relationship of tryptophan as a precursor of niacin has since been well established. Although for some time some investigators were convinced that niacin promoted the intestinal synthesis of niacin, it was only with the use of radioactive isotopes that it was unequivocally proved that tryptophan was converted to niacin in the cells. It has now been shown that 60 mg. of tryptophan is capable of producing 1 mg. of niacin. Although current food composition tables do not record the niacin equivalent values for foods, the sum of the preformed niacin and the niacin equivalent of the tryptophan more accurately reflects the pellagra-preventative value of the food, and dietary requirements are expressed as niacin equivalents. Tryptophan needed for synthesis of body protein will not be available for conversion to niacin, although it has not been clearly defined which need has priority. The conversion of the amino acid tryptophan to the vitamin niacin requires the presence of at least two other vitamins, thiamine and pyridoxine, and possibly riboflavin and biotin. Since vitamin B_6 is involved in the formation of niacin, it has not been surprising to find symptoms of pellagra appearing when INH, a vitamin B_6 antagonist used in the treatment of tuberculosis, is administered in high doses. Only the L form of tryptophan can be converted; D-isomers are biologically inactive.

Chemical properties

Niacin, a white crystalline substance that is extremely stable to heat, light, acid, alkali, and oxidation, was first isolated in 1912 from yeast and from rice bran many years before it was associated with pellagra. Because of its stability there is very little loss of the nutrient in normal procedures of food processing and preparation. It is active as either the acid or as the amide, nicotinamide. The amide is preferred for therapeutic doses since the use of large amounts of the acid, which acts as a vasodilator, may lead to flushing of the skin and tingling sensations.

Functions

Niacin is required by all living cells, where it plays a vital role in the release of energy from all three energy-building nutrients—carbohydrate, fat, and protein—and is involved in the synthesis of protein, fat, and pentoses. It acts as a coenzyme capable of accepting and releasing hydrogen atoms in at least forty of the places where these exchanges are involved in metabolism. The coenzymes of which niacin is an essential part are now identified as NAD (nicotinamide adenine dinucleotide) and NADP (nicotinamide adenine dinucleotide phosphate), both of which can accept or release hydrogen atoms at will. They have previously been known as coenzymes I and II and as DPN and TPN, and the use of these terms still persists in some literature. No other biochemical role has been established yet, but the central role it plays as a part of these coenzymes means that without it the body is unable to utilize carbohydrate, fat, or protein.

There is evidence that high intakes of 1 to 2 gm. three times a day of niacin but not nicotinamide may result in lowered blood cholesterol levels, apparently because of its interference with cholesterol synthesis from raw material available in the liver. Many other possible mechanisms by which it could possibly act as a hypocholesterolemic agent have been investigated but have been abandoned. The side effects of niacin are overcome as the treatment continues.

Absorption

Both niacin and tryptophan are readily absorbed, but the niacin is stored to a very limited extent. Any excess of niacin is methylated and excreted either as N-methyl nicotinamide or as the pyridine of N-methyl nicotinamide. The observation that animals excrete some radioactively labelled vitamin as carbon dioxide through the lungs has not been tested in human beings.

Requirements

Since niacin is so intimately involved in the release of energy from food it is not surprising to find that the National Research Council has based its recommended allowance for niacin on the caloric intake. The minimum need has been established at 4.4 mg. of niacin equivalent per 1000 kilocalories, to which a 50% margin of safety has been added in the recommended allowances of 6.6 mg. of niacin equivalent per 1000 kilocalories. It is also suggested that an absolute minimum intake of 8.8 mg. be maintained regardless of caloric intake since this appears to be the minimum level to prevent pellagra.

The amount required is influenced by factors other than calorie intake. In an amino acid imbalance the need for niacin increases. The type of carbohydrate may also have some effect, as there is data to show that carbohydrates containing fructose increase the need for niacin.

During the second and third trimesters of pregnancy an increase of 3 mg. over normal needs is indicated. For lactation, when human milk contains 0.5 to 0.7 mg. of niacin equivalent per 1000 kilocalories, the maternal diet should provide 7 mg. more than needed under normal circumstances. This will provide the breast-fed infant with 4 to 5 mg. per day, which apparently satisfies his needs.

Most American diets that are adequate in protein tend to supply sufficient niacin. Animal protein contains 1.4% tryptophan and vegetable protein, 1%. Thus a diet with 60 gm. of protein provides a minimum of 600 mg. of tryptophan, which can be converted into 10 mg. of niacin. Any tryptophan needed for the synthesis of body protein would not be available for niacin formation. However, once the growth process is completed, much more tryptophan can be diverted into niacin synthesis.

Most diets contain sufficient tryptophan to make 8 to 14 mg. of niacin and an additional 8 to 17 mg. of preformed niacin, making a total of 16 to 33 mg., an amount sufficient for practically all adult needs. It is only when the diet is low in protein and relatively high in a tryptophan-poor cereal that a deficiency is likely to occur. Gelatin is one protein completely devoid of tryptophan.

Dietary sources

The major sources of niacin are shown graphically in Table 12-5. Yeast, liver, meat, poultry, peanuts, and legumes are the richest sources. Milk and eggs, while low in performed niacin, contain high amounts of tryptophan and as such have a high niacin equivalent. Fig. 12-12 shows the relative contribution of different food groups to dietary niacin.

Recent evidence shows that much of the niacin in cereals such as rice and corn occurs as niacinogen. In this form it is closely bound to protein composed of at least seventeen different amino acids, from which it can be separated with great difficulty except by alkaline hydrolysis. For this reason the niacin in these foods has low biological value and does little to meet the body's requirement for the vitamin unless prepared with alkali.

As much as 80% to 90% of the niacin of cereals is in the outer husk and is removed in the milling process. The addition of niacin in enriched cereal products has done much to compensate for this loss.

Evaluation of niacin status

Since there is very little storage of this water-soluble vitamin in the body, we have learned much about it by studying the forms and the amounts in which it is excreted in the urine following a test dose. When the dietary intake is adequate a large percentage of the test dose is excreted, and most is in the form of a methylated end product of niacin metabolism known as N-methyl nicotinamide or the pyridone of N-methyl nicotinamide. In diets low in niacin, the excretion of the pyridone drops long before any clinical symptoms of pellagra are observable. The combined excretion drops to less than 2 mg., compared to normal excretion of 5 to 8 mg. of N-methyl nicotinamide and 7 to 10 mg. of the pyridone. When the die-

Table 12-5. Niacin, tryptophan, and niacin equivalents of some representative foods (milligrams per 100 gm. food)

Food	Niacin*	Tryptophan†	Niacin equivalent of trytophan‡	Total niacin
Beef liver	16.5	296	4.9	21.4
Peanut butter	15.7	330	5.5	21.2
Chicken, cooked	7.4	250	4.1	11.5
Beef, round	5.6	203	3.4	9.0
Bread, enriched	2.3	91	1.5	3.8
Orange juice	0.4	3	0.05	0.45
Spinach	0.3	37	0.6	0.9
Cottage cheese	0.2	179	2.9	3.1
Whole milk	0.1	49	0.8	0.9
Eggs	0.1	211	3.5	3.6

*From Watts, B., and Merrill, A.: Composition of foods—raw, processed and prepared, U. S. Department of Agriculture Handbook No. 8, Washington, D. C., 1963, U. S. Department of Agriculture.

†From Amino acid content of foods, Home Economics Research Report No. 4, Washington, D. C., 1957, U. S. Department of Agriculture.

‡Since 60 mg. of tryptophan can be converted into 1 mg. of niacin, niacin equivalent = $\dfrac{\text{milligrams tryptophan}}{60}$.

tary intake of both tryptophan and niacin has been low, less of the test dose is excreted, indicating that the body needs to retain more. Most of that excreted is in the form of N-methyl nicotinamide. Recently the use of a ratio of urinary excretion of pyridone to urinary excretion of N-methyl nicotinamide per gram of creatinine (indicative of muscle mass of the body) has provided a criterion on which to evaluate nutritional status of population groups with respect to niacin adequacy. A ratio of less than 1:1 is considered indicative of pellagra while a ratio between 1:1 and 1.3:1 is considered borderline.

Niacin deficiency

In pellagra, the skin, the gastrointestinal tract, and the central nervous system are affected. The symptoms progress through *dermatitis, diarrhea,* and *depression* preceding *death* in what has been characterized as the four D's of pellagra. The dermatitis of pellagra is often complicated by symptoms of other B vitamin deficiencies, but when a niacin deficiency occurs the character of the skin inflammation is very specific. It occurs almost exclusively on areas of the skin exposed to sunlight and in a symmetrical pattern on both sides of the body. There is a very clearly demarcated line between the afflicted and healthy areas of the skin. As the mucous linings of the gastrointestinal tract become involved, the patient suffers from diarrhea and other manifestations of infection. The hydrochloric acid secretion normally present in the gastric juice may be absent, and this may reduce the bactericidal function of the gastric juice and allow the growth

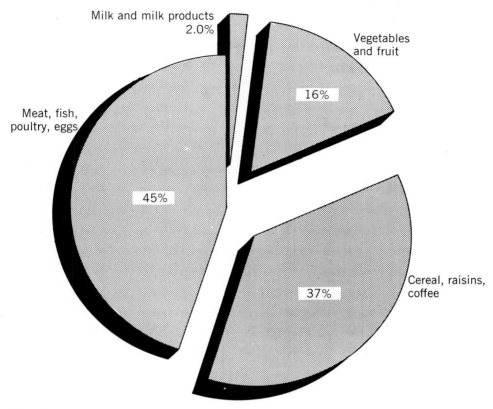

Fig. 12-12

Contribution of various food groups to the niacin content of the American food supply. (Based on Nutritive value of food available for consumption, United States, 1909-1964, Agricultural Research Service Publication 62-14, 1966.)

of infection-producing organisms. These changes in the gastrointestinal tract usually precede the degenerative changes that occur in the mental outlook of the patient. The irritability, headaches, and sleeplessness of early stages is soon followed by more severe mental symptoms such as loss of memory, hallucinations, delusions of persecution, and finally a severe depression that almost inevitably precedes death.

PYRIDOXINE (PYRIDOXOL)

Vitamin B_6 or pyridoxine, a vitamin required by all animals thus far studied, includes at least three chemically related substances—pyridoxol, pyridoxal, and pyridoxamine—all of which are biologically active as the vitamin in the body. Pyridoxine was first identified in 1934 as *adermin,* a substance capable of curing a characteristic dermatitis in rats that did not respond to any of the three factors then known in the B complex. This was followed by its isolation in 1938, the elucidation of its structure by Harris and Folkers one year later in 1939, and its synthesis the same year by Kuhn and Wendt. Since then many scientists have attempted to elucidate its role in body metabolism.

Pyridoxine is found widely distributed in nature. In plants it occurs as pyridoxol, the alcohol form bound to protein, a form in which it is not readily absorbed. Pyridoxamine and pyridoxal, the most prevalent forms in animal tissues, are readily available. Pyridoxine is a relatively stable compound, being slightly destroyed by oxidation and ultraviolet light. Pyridoxal is destroyed by alkali, but all three forms are stable to acid. The broad distribution of pyridoxine in food coupled with a relatively small need of the body for the vitamin makes it very difficult to induce a human deficiency sufficiently severe to produce characteristic symptoms by the use of a diet low in the vitamin. There is, however, reason to believe that certain biochemical changes do occur on a diet containing suboptimal amounts of pyridoxine, although no physical changes may be observed. The use of an antagonist, the chemically similar deoxypyridoxine, in conjunction with a diet low in vitamin B$_6$ has made it possible to produce deficiency states more rapidly in both animals and humans.

Functions

Pyridoxine functions as a coenzyme for many biological reactions in the form of pyridoxal phosphate. Zinc or magnesium catalyzes the formation of this active coenzyme. In contrast to thiamine, riboflavin, and niacin, which act as coenzymes for reactions involved in the release of energy from glucose and fatty acids, pyridoxine plays no direct role in energy metabolism. Instead it is involved primarily with reactions occurring in protein metabolism. Pyridoxine is necessary for the process of transamination, in which the characteristic amino (NH$_2$) group from an amino acid is transferred to another substance to produce a different amino acid needed for protein synthesis. Deamination, the removal of the amino group from some amino acids, is dependent on enzymes containing vitamin B$_6$—deaminases. This process must take place before protein in excess of the body's needs for growth can be used as a source of energy. The removal

of the carboxyl (COOH) group from certain amino acids in a process called decarboxylation also requires pyridoxal phosphate. This decarboxylation is necessary for the synthesis of the vital body regulators serotonin, norepinephrine, and histamine in the body, but in a vitamin B$_6$ deficiency only histamine synthesis is retarded. It also functions in the metabolism of sulphur-containing amino acids such as cysteine, from which it facilitates the removal of sulphur.

Pyridoxal phosphate is a cofactor necessary for the formation of a precursor of porphyrin, a substance that is an essential part of the hemoglobin molecule.

The most intensively studied role of vitamin B$_6$ in protein metabolism is in the conversion of the amino acid, tryptophan, into the vitamin, niacin. This conversion involves several biochemical steps, in one of which an intermediary product is converted to kynurenine in a reaction catalyzed by pyridoxal phosphate. Kynurenine in turn is changed to niacin. If large amounts of tryptophan are fed in what is known as a tryptophan load test, a person whose diet is low in pyridoxine does not produce enough pyridoxal phosphate to allow the conversion of all the kynurenine produced from tryptophan to niacin. Instead, a substance, xanthurenic acid, which is not utilized by the body, is produced from kynurenine. It is excreted in the urine, and a determination of xanthurenic acid in the urine is used as an indication of the extent to which pyridoxine is available. High urinary xanthurenic acid levels occur when available pyridoxine is limited, and low levels occur when there is sufficient to allow normal conversion of tryptophan to niacin. Serotonin, a body regulator, is also derived from tryptophan and pyridoxine is necessary for the decarboxylation reaction required in its synthesis.

Attempts to define a suggested relationship between vitamin B$_6$ and fatty acid metabolism have not succeeded in determining the site of the action. Efforts to confirm earlier beliefs that the conversion of the essential fatty acid linoleic acid to arachidonic acid was dependent on pyridoxine have been unsuccessful.

In carbohydrate metabolism, pyridoxine, as part of the enzyme phosphorylase, facilitates the release of glycogen from the liver and muscle as glucose-phosphate. This must occur before any stored carbohydrate can be available to the cells as glucose to be used as source of energy. Evidence is accumulating to indicate that pyridoxine may be needed for the formation of other enzymes involved in carbohydrate metabolism. Low blood glucose levels, low glucose tolerance tests, and a sensitivity to insulin in a pyridoxine deficiency provide some evidence of a relationship with carbohydrate metabolism.

The role of pyridoxine in the metabolism of the central nervous system is the concern of many workers. It is known that changes in electroencephalograms used to evaluate the functioning of the nervous system occur in pyridoxine deficiency and that in severe deficiency convulsive seizures takes place. It is thought that pyridoxine is necessary for the synthesis of a substance that controls the transmission of nerve impulses from one nerve ending to the next. The absence of this substance allows uncontrolled excitation of the central nervous system and eventual uncontrolled muscle seizures.

It has also been noted that in symptoms involving the brain there is a reduction in the enzymes dependent on pyridoxal phosphate as well as in the pyridoxal content of the brain. This suggests that pyridoxine may regulate the formation of these enzymes.

Vitamin B_6 is essential for the production of antibodies, as evidenced by the reduced production as available pyridoxine drops. Skin grafts take longer to heal in the absence of pyridoxine, apparently because of delayed hypersensitivity. This is important

in modern medical technology, where the success of tissue transplants in man depends on adequate pyridoxine.

A possible role for pyridoxine in cholesterol metabolism has been suggested from studies on monkeys which showed that pyridoxine-deficient animals developed arteriosclerotic changes similar to those found in man. However, efforts to identify the relationship have been unsuccessful. These animals had four times as much dental caries as animals with adequate pyridoxine and also showed changes in the fat in their liver.

A further relationship between pyridoxine and protein metabolism is reflected in the fact that D-methionine, normally not available to the body, is equally as available as L-methionine; D-tryptophan, 50% as available as L-tryptophan; and D-valine is 33% as available as L-valine when pyridoxine is increased.

Animal studies have suggested a relationship between pyridoxine and cobalamin metabolism as the levels of the latter drop with both an excess and a deficiency of pyridoxine.

Metabolism

Vitamin B_6 is active in the body as pyridoxal phosphate, which can be formed in the body from any one of the three forms found in food—pyridoxine, pyridoxal, and pyridoxamine. The pathways by which these substances can form pyridoxal phosphate is shown in Fig. 12-13. The maximum amount of pyridoxine that can be converted to the coenzyme form is 7 mg. per day.

Since pyridoxine is a water-soluble vitamin there is virtually no storage of it in the body. Any excess of the vitamin is oxidized to pyridoxic acid, which is metabolically inert and excreted in the urine. Most persons excrete 0.3 to 0.4 mg. per day, but levels as high as 0.7 to 0.8 mg. have been reported. Some pyridoxine (about 0.7 to 0.9 mg. per day) is excreted

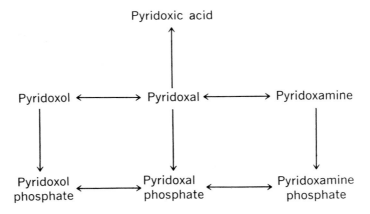

Fig. 12-13

Relationship of various chemical forms of pyridoxine.

in the feces, but it arises primarily from synthesis by intestinal microorganisms and does not indicate loss of ingested pyridoxine.

Practically half of the pyridoxine found in the body is in the form of the enzyme phosphorylase in the muscle mass. This enzyme, so essential to mobilize the body's carbohydrate reserves of glycogen in the muscle, represents the closest thing to storage of vitamin B_6 in the body.

Requirements

Since pyridoxine is necessary for practically all aspects of protein metabolism, the requirement for the vitamin varies directly with the protein content of the diet, the requirement of which in turn is a function of body size.

Although pyridoxine is involved to some extent in both carbohydrate and fat metabolism it is not concerned with aspects involved in the direct release of energy, so there is no basis on which to relate requirement to total calories. It is also possible that a high intake on a low-protein intake allows the body to use the amino acids on a low-protein diet more effectively than if the vitamin intake were also low.

Because of the small amounts needed in the body and its widespread distribution in foods it has been difficult to establish a recommended allowance for pyridoxine. The minimum requirement for an adult consuming 2600 to 2900 kilocalories is 0.67 to 0.75 mg. However, to allow a reasonable margin of safety and to allow for daily protein intakes as high as 100 gm. and stress conditions, a daily allowance of 1.5 to 2 mg. per day has been established for adults. On low-protein intakes 1.25 to 1.5 mg. may be adequate. If, however, the recommended allowance was set sufficiently high to meet the needs for virtually all healthy persons, as it is for most nutrients, the requirements would be much higher, ranging from 2.5 to 7 mg., which would be virtually impossible to obtain from dietary sources, especially under caloric restrictions.

Evidence indicates that the stress of pregnancy increases the need for pyridoxine, as the body is then less able to handle large amounts of tryptophan. It is suggested that supplemental vitamin B_6 be given during the third trimester of pregnancy. However, very large supplements should be avoided because of the danger of conditioning the infant to a higher requirement.

For infants it appears that 400 μg. of pyridoxine per day will be adequate to meet the needs of almost all infants who are not breast-fed.

Older people may have increased needs for the vitamin. Since pyridoxine needs are related to protein rather than caloric intakes, it is possible that older persons whose caloric intake drops while their protein remains high will find that their diet fails to provide adequate vitamin B$_6$. They have a lower level of the enzyme transaminase in the plasma, have less pyridoxal kinase in the brain, and excrete more xanthurenic acid after a tryptophan load test.

The requirement for the vitamin depends on interrelationships with other dietary factors. It tends to decrease as the amounts of choline, chlortetracycline, essential fatty acids, biotin, and pantothenic acid decrease.

Food sources

Very few foods can be considered poor sources of vitamin B$_6$. Among the richest, however, are muscle meats, liver, vegetables, whole-grain cereals, and egg yolks. The pyridoxine content of some representative foods is shown in Table 12-6.

Freezing of vegetables causes a 25% reduction in the amount present, and milling of cereals leads to losses as high as 80% to 90% of the original values.

Evaluation of vitamin B$_6$ status

Since vitamin B$_6$ is so widely distributed in foods and is needed in relatively small amounts, there is no specific nutritional deficiency disease that can be attributed to a lack of the vitamin. However, there is evidence that certain biochemical changes do occur when the intake is low or the needs of the individual are above normal.

A relative pyridoxine deficiency can be detected by measuring the amount of xanthurenic acid excreted following a test dose of 10 gm. of the amino acid tryptophan. High levels of xanthurenic acid indicate

Table 12-6. Pyridoxine content of average servings of food*

Representative foods	Micrograms per serving
Round steak	495.0
Canned salmon	450.0
Ham	440.0
Bananas	320.0
Potatoes	220.0
Lima beans	176.0
Cabbage	120.0
Spinach	114.0
Milk, whole	87.8
Strawberries	61.0
Orange juice, frozen	26.0
Grapefruit	25.0
Rice, converted	20.4

*From Hardinge, M. G., and Crooks, H.: Lesser known vitamins in foods, J. Am. Dietet. A. **38**:240, 1961.

lower vitamin B$_6$ status. The changes in blood urea levels after a test dose of the amino acid, alanine, also reflect vitamin B$_6$ status. Blood urea levels will rise and return to normal within six hours in a subject with adequate pyridoxine to facilitate deamination of alanine but will remain high if there is an inadequate amount of the vitamin available. In another test, requiring only one sample of blood, the amount of pyridoxal phosphate in the blood following an oral dose of 100 mg. of pyridoxine is determined. This indicates relative tissue saturation. Since pyridoxine is necessary for transaminase activity, the level of the enzyme transaminase in the blood is thought to reflect levels of vitamin B$_6$ available.

The fact that so many different methods of evaluating pyridoxine status are being used is evidence that none is completely satisfactory.

Deficiency symptoms

In 1951 it was first observed that infants who were inadvertently given a formula providing less than 0.1 mg. of pyridoxine showed signs of hyperirritability and convulsions. These symptoms disappeared on the administration of the vitamin. It has been postulated that these symptoms were the result of a low dietary intake by infants who had an increased need for the vitamin, possibly conditioned by high levels of supplementation of the maternal diet during pregnancy.

In adults the only symptom that has been attributed to lack of pyridoxine is a microcytic hypochromic anemia in association with high serum iron. Other less specific symptoms, such as weakness, nervousness, irritability, insomnia, and difficulty in walking, have been associated with inadequate intakes of vitamin B_6. Efforts to induce a deficiency state by dietary deficiency in humans produced only symptoms of irritability after fifty-four days. When the vitamin antagonist deoxypyridoxine was fed, skin changes such as glossitis, cheilosis, and stomatitis, different from those of a riboflavin or niacin deficiency, occurred.

Changes in urinary components occur in a pyridoxine deficiency. There is an increase in the amount of oxalate and a decrease in the amount of urinary citrate. Since citrate favors the solubility of oxalates, it is possible that the formation of urinary calculi or kidney stones, which occurs in pyridoxine deficiencies, reflects decreased solubility of the oxalate.

Clinical uses

Vitamin B_6 has been used in the treatment of many conditions. When isoniazid (isonicotinic acid hydrazide), which is chemically related to pyridoxine, is used in the treatment of tuberculosis, patients develop many of the symptoms of a pyridoxine deficiency, including an increase in xanthurenic acid in the urine. These symptoms are readily counteracted with the use of higher than normal amounts of pyridoxine. Apparently isoniazid combines with pyridoxal phosphate and inactivates the enzyme involved in decarboxylation of amino acids.

Pyridoxine has been used in doses of 50 mg. per day in the treatment of the nausea of pregnancy with at least some success. Pyridoxine-containing lozenges sucked three times a day during pregnancy significantly reduce the incidence of new cavities, possibly because of an inhibitory effect on the growth of microorganisms in the mouth that favor caries development. A similar reduction in tooth decay was observed in 10- to 15-year-old adolescents who were given lozenges with 3 mg. of B_6 three times a day. The observation that a pyridoxine-deficient person has a greater susceptibility to kidney stone formation has led to the use of the vitamin to prevent the development of stones. It has been observed that persons deficient in pyridoxine excrete more oxalate in the urine, which could account for the tendency to form kidney stones. This may be explained by the low levels of the transaminases necessary to convert oxalic acid to the nonessential amino acid glycine. However, when magnesium as well as pyridoxine is low, the appearance of urinary calculi is prevented.

Some types of anemia have responded to treatment with large (50-mg.) doses of pyridoxine, which may be necessary for the synthesis of the heme in iron-containing portions (protoporphyrin) of the hemoglobin molecule. The use of pyridoxine in treating acne, Parkinson's disease, and muscular dystrophy has met with no significant or consistent results.

PANTOTHENIC ACID
Discovery

Pantothenic acid, identified first as vitamin B_3, was so named to designate its widespread occurrence in foods (from the

Greek word *pantos,* everywhere). As knowledge of its role in biological reactions has developed it might have been so named for its universal and central role in the metabolism of carbohydrate, fat, and protein.

Pantothenate had been recognized as a growth factor for yeast and as a cure or prevention for dermatitis in chicks and graying of hair in rats before it was finally isolated in 1938 and synthesized in 1940. A yellow viscous oil, pantothenic acid has never been crystallized, although its synthetic calcium salt, calcium pantothenate, has been available in crystalline form for some time. It is in this form that it is incorporated into most nutritional supplements.

Chemical properties

Pantothenic acid is a water-soluble vitamin that is stable in moist heat in neutral solution but readily destroyed by dry heat. In acid or alkali it is relatively unstable.

There is little loss in cooking at normal temperature.

Chemically, pantothenic acid is a relatively simple compound containing the amino acid alanine. Before it participates in biological reactions, it unites with a sulphur-containing compound to form pantotheine, which in turn adds phosphate and an adenine molecule to form coenzyme A (also called CoA). Coenzyme A is the form in which most pantothenic acid is found in microorganisms and in animal tissues and in which it participates in a central role in most biological reactions. The activation of CoA involves the addition of the two-carbon acetate compound to form acetyl coenzyme A or acetyl CoA. These acetate molecules are readily accepted and transferred from the CoA molecule.

The relationship between pantothenic acid and activated CoA is shown in Fig. 12-14.

Since CoA appears within the cell but

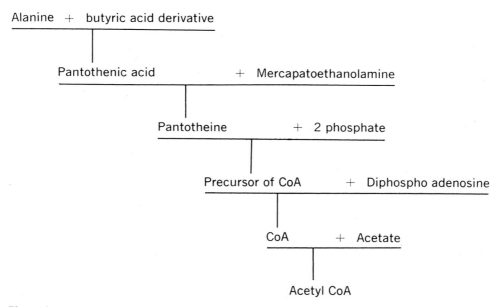

Fig. 12-14

Relationship between pantothenic acid and CoA.

not in the blood it must be synthesized within the cell and must pass the cell membrane with difficulty if at all. CoA appears in highest concentration in the liver, adrenal gland, kidney, brain, and heart, all of which are tissues characterized by high metabolic activity.

Functions

As part of coenzyme A, pantothenic acid participates in the release of energy from all three energy-yielding nutrients—carbohydrate, fat, and protein. Products in the oxidation of each of these eventually react with CoA in the Krebs cycle before all their energy is released. In addition CoA, and hence pantothenic acid, is necessary for the synthesis of fat. Besides functioning in the transfer of acetate groups to the Krebs cycle, CoA is involved as a source or acceptor of acetate groups for amino acids, vitamins, and sulfonamides. It is essential for the formation of porphyrin, a part of the hemoglobin molecule, and for the synthesis of cholesterol and some of the steroids produced by the adrenal glands. In essence, because of its central role in energy metabolism it can be considered vital to all energy-requiring processes within the body.

Requirements

It is well established that human beings as well as practically all other animals and microorganisms have a need for pantothenic acid. The amount needed has not been estimated with any certainty but is generally believed to be about 10 mg. or ten times the thiamine requirement. A 3000-kilocalorie diet will usually provide from 13 to 19 mg. of total pantothenic acid, of which 5 to 10 mg. will occur as free pantothenic acid. From 7 to 10 mg. is excreted daily in the urine. The wide range of intakes, blood values, and urinary excretion levels that appear in individuals with no evidence of deficiency make it very difficult to determine a minimum intake. Except

Table 12-7. Food sources of pantothenic acid*

Food	Milligrams per 100 gm.
Beef liver	9.34
Beef kidney	4.06
Egg yolk	4.22
Whole egg	1.58
Broccoli	1.29
Lima beans	1.30
Split peas	2.12
Wheat bran	2.90
Cornmeal	0.59
Sweet potato	0.94
Yellow corn	0.89
Whole milk	0.32
Nonfat milk	0.38
Almonds	0.58
Bananas	0.31

*From Agricultural Handbook No. 97, Washington, D. C., 1956, U. S. Department of Agriculture.

for periods of stress when needs may be relatively high, most diets will provide adequate amounts of pantothenic acid.

Food sources

The amount of pantothenic acid in foods representative of the main food groups is given in Table 12-7. Pantothenic acid is a component of all living matter. While organ meats and whole-grain cereals are the richest sources, all food groups make a significant contribution to the dietary intake. The richest sources so far determined have been royal jelly from the queen bee and fish ovaries prior to spawning.

Foods processed in dry heat are relatively poor sources of pantothenic acid.

Deficiency symptoms

The wide variety of reactions for which pantothenic acid is necessary is paralleled by an equally wide variety of deficiency symptoms. Chicks show a characteristic dermatitis around the eyes, a degeneration of the spinal cord, changes in the thymus gland, and fatty degeneration of the liver. Ducks experience anemia; rats experience growth failure, the accumulation of the reddish pigment porphyrin in their whiskers, and hemorrhaging in the adrenal gland; and pigs experience changes in the sensory nerves. Biochemically, an increase in copper in the skin has occurred in a panthothenic acid deficiency.

While humans apparently do not experience pantothenic acid deficiencies of sufficient magnitude to precipitate deficiency symptoms in most mixed diets, the low intakes may slow down many metabolic processes, resulting in a wide variety of subclinical symptoms. When human volunteers were fed a pantothenic acid antagonist along with a diet low in pantothenic acid the list of symptoms reportedly reversed by the vitamin was rather extensive. It included irritability, restlessness, burning feet, muscle cramps, impaired muscular coordination, sensitivity to insulin, decreased antibody formation, easy fatigue, mental depression, gastrointestinal disturbances, and upper respiratory infections. This list likely reflects impaired health of cells in many tissues. The site at which the symptoms first appear may be a function of some particular metabolic stress factors. High levels seem to improve the ability to withstand stress.

Pantothenic acid neither prevents nor cures graying of hair in humans in spite of any claims to the contrary by vendors of food supplements.

Therapeutic uses

Pantothenic acid has been used successfully in treating the paralysis of the gastrointestinal tract following surgery, which causes the accumulation of gas and severe abdominal pain. It appears to stimulate gastric mobility.

FOLACIN
Discovery

Folacin was discovered in the course of the search for the factor in liver responsible for its effectiveness in curing pernicious anemia, a condition characterized by large red blood cells and degeneration of nervous tissue and which was fatal unless treated with large quantities of liver. Although folacin (earlier known as folic acid) does not have the antipernicious anemia properties attributed to it in 1945 and for which medical scientists were searching, it has been established as a dietary essential for man, many animals, and microorganisms. It has been isolated from spinach, yeast, and liver, occurs in a wide variety of foods, and participates in many biological reactions.

The many names by which folacin has been known gives some indication of the various paths by which the substance was identified. As early as 1930, the Wills factor now believed to be folacin was identified in yeast and crude liver extracts and found to be effective in curing a tropical macrocytic anemia. In 1938, the term vitamin M was applied to a growth factor for monkeys, in 1939 factor U and vitamin B_c were used to identify growth factors for chicks and by 1940 the *Lactobacillus casei* factor or nor-eluate factor was found to be essential for the growth of that microorganism. As the chemical nature of all these substances became known, it was learned that the effectiveness of all these was due to the presence of pteroylglutamic acid (PGA). Since this substance could be extracted from green leafy vegetables such as spinach it was designated in 1941 as folic acid (from the Latin, *folium*) but the term has now been modified to *folacin* in keeping with current practices in nomenclature. Since many substances are now known to give rise to folacin in the body the use of the term has been restricted to pteroylmonoglutamate, the form from which the active coenzymes are directly derived, and the term *folate* is applied to the broader group of substances that give rise to folacin in the body. Substances with folic acid activity are synthesized by plants, in animal tissues, and by microorganisms in the intestinal tract. By 1945, scientists knew the chemical structure of pteroylglutamic acid and had succeeded in isolating and synthesizing it.

Chemical composition

Folate as it occurs in food is a combination of the chemical compounds pterin and para-aminobenzoic acid (PABA), which together are termed pteroic acid and to which are attached either one, three, or seven molecules of the amino acid, glutamic acid. It is interesting to note that earlier in the history of nutrition para-aminobenzoic acid was itself considered a vitamin. Before these complexes can be used in the body as a vitamin all but one of the glutamic acid molecules must be split off to form an unconjugated folic acid or folacin molecule, pteroylmonoglutamic acid (PGA). This release of the extra glutamic acid molecules is facilitated by specific enzymes and vitamin B_{12}. The folic acid is then reduced in the presence of ascorbic acid and the niacin-containing coenzyme NAD to tetrahydrofolic acid (THFA). This very unstable compound unites readily with a single carbon unit, which can be derived from many sources, to form a more stable substance known as the citrovorum factor or folinic acid, considered the biologically active form of the vitamin. This conversion of folic acid to folinic acid must occur before it can function, and anything that blocks this conversion renders ingested folate unavailable. The citrovorum factor undergoes very minor structural changes to become the coenzyme responsible for the many roles played by folacin in the body. The synthetic form of the citrovorum factor is known as leucovorin. In addition, the citrovorum factor occurs preformed in liver, either in the active form or combined with extra glutamic acid molecules that need only be removed to give a biologically active substance. Apparently the body stores folacin as the citrovorum factor in the liver. The relationship among the various forms of the vitamin is shown in Fig. 12-15.

Folic acid antagonists such as aminopterin and amethopterin, which are chemically related to folic acid, block the action of folacin by interfering with its conversion to THFA. This explains why the citrovorum factor has been effective in overcoming the effect of the antagonist while folate has not.

Absorption

Folic acid is absorbed in the upper part of the intestine by both active transport and diffusion. Its absorption is facilitated by ascorbic acid and by some antibiotics. It is believed that some of the glutamic acid molecules of the conjugates or complexes of three or seven glutamic acid units with folacin may be split by enzymes in the pancreatic juice and absorbed in both the upper and lower gastrointestinal tract.

The absorption of folic acid is reduced in nontropical sprue, a condition in which there are structural and functional abnormalities as a result of the degenerative changes in the jejunum portion of the small intestine. Consequently, symptoms of folacin deficiency occur in nontropical sprue.

Functions

It was determined shortly after the discovery of folacin in 1945 that although it cured macrocytic anemia by stimulating the regeneration of both red blood cells and hemoglobin, folacin was not the antipernicious anemia factor for which scientists were searching since it was ineffective in relieving the neurological symptoms. It did, however, play several essential roles in metabolism. Of the biochemical roles that have been clearly established, several are closely involved in blood formation.

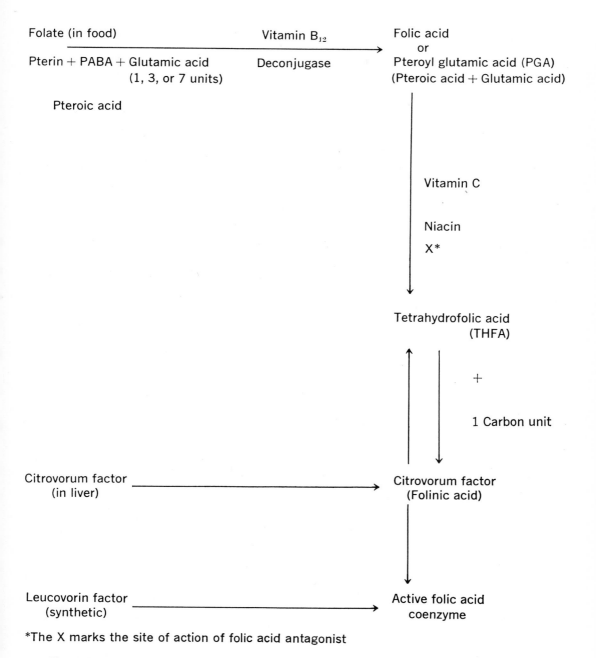

Folate (in food)   Vitamin B$_{12}$ Folic acid
                                               or

Pterin + PABA + Glutamic acid   Deconjugase   Pteroyl glutamic acid (PGA)
              (1, 3, or 7 units)   (Pteroic acid + Glutamic acid)

       Pteroic acid

                                                    Vitamin C

                                                    Niacin

                                                    X*

                                           Tetrahydrofolic acid
                                                     (THFA)

                                                     +

                                           1 Carbon unit

Citrovorum factor   Citrovorum factor
    (in liver)   (Folinic acid)

Leucovorin factor   Active folic acid
    (synthetic)   coenzyme

*The X marks the site of action of folic acid antagonist

Fig. 12-15

Relationship among various chemical forms of folacin.

Folacin functions in several biological reactions involving the transfer of single-carbon units, such as CH_3 or methyl groups, from one substance to another. In this role it appears to act as an intermediary, accepting the single-carbon group from one compound and passing it on to the next. Examples of this function are the formation of the amino acid methionine from one of its precursors, homocystine; the formation of the two-carbon amino acid, serine, from the single-carbon amino acid, glycine; the formation of the vitamin choline from its precursor, ethanolamine; and the synthesis of the amino acid, histidine. The conversion of nicotinic acid to N-methyl nicotinamide, the form in which it is excreted, depends on the addition of a methyl (single-carbon) unit obtained from folacin.

The synthesis of the purines adenine and guanine and the pyrimidine, thymine, all part of the nucleic acids, DNA (deoxyribonucleic acid) and RNA (ribonucleic acid), which are essential to reproduction of cells, enzymes, and body compounds, is dependent on folic acid coenzymes. A failure in the biosynthesis of purines in the absence of folate may be responsible for the megaloblastic anemia of folate deficiency.

The conversion or oxidation of the essential amino acid phenylalanine to tyrosine also requires folacin, as does the oxidation

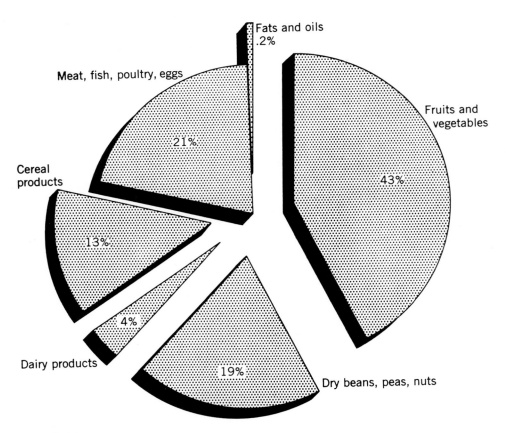

Fig. 12-16

Contribution of various food groups to total intake of folacin in the American food supply. (Based on Home Economics Report No. 76, 1965.)

and decarboxylation of tyrosine and the formation of part of the structure of hemoglobin, the porphyrin group.

Dietary requirements

The need for folate has not been clearly established. It is believed that the minimum need for adults lies between 0.025 and 0.250 mg. The National Research Council feels that an intake of 0.15 mg. of folic acid will provide protection against megaloblastic anemia and suggests that this amount should be increased during pregnancy.

Food sources

The usual dietary intake of folacin is unknown, although it is believed to be between 0.15 to 0.20 mg. per day. Although the content of the vitamin in many foods has not been established, current data rate liver, kidney, yeast, and mushrooms as the best sources. Among vegetables, asparagus, broccoli, lima beans, and spinach rank highest while lemons, bananas, strawberries, and cantaloupes are rich fruit sources. Milk contains very little folacin. Fig. 12-16 shows the contribution of various food groups to the total intake in the American diet. Table 12-8 gives values for the folic acid content of various foods.

Losses of folic acid in cooking and canning may range as high as 50% to 90%. Exposure to light also causes loss of folate.

The microbiological methods of assessing the folate activity of foods apparently do not give an accurate picture of the availability since persons consuming diets that may contain 500 to 1000 μg. of folate do not respond as well as they do to 25 to 50 μg. of synthetic folic acid.

Evaluation of folacin nutrition

Since folacin is involved in normal blood formation, an analysis of the blood of humans or animals has proven the best method of detecting an inadequacy of the nutrient. Folacin is necessary for the manu-

Table 12-8. Folic acid content of average servings of representative foods*

Food	Micrograms
Pork liver	126.0
Asparagus	109.0
Kidney beans (½ cup)	57.6
Carrots	22.0
Round steak	10.5
Potatoes	6.8
Cheddar cheese (1 ounce)	4.5
Peaches, canned	4.0
Bread (1 slice)	3.4
Chicken, light meat	2.8
Orange juice (½ cup)	2.6
Apple, medium	2.6
Egg, whole	2.5
Shrimp	1.8
Milk, whole	1.5

*From Hardinge, M. G., and Crooks, H.: Lesser known vitamins in foods, J. Am. Dietet. A. **38**:240, 1961.

facture of both red blood cells and white blood cells in the bone marrow and for the normal maturation of these.

In human folacin deficiency abnormally large red blood cells or erythrocytes, known as megabolasts, form when the newly formed immature red blood cells or reticulocytes fail to mature and lose their nuclei. Under these conditions, in which red blood cells grow larger, their number decreases but the amount of hemoglobin they contain does not decrease. These changes show up as high color index in which the percentage of normal hemoglobin level is compared to the percentage of normal red blood cell count. Normally the color index is approximately 1.

An analysis of the urine to determine the presence of the substance formiminoglutamic acid (FIGLU), which accumulates when there is a deficiency of folate, shows promise as a method of evaluating folacin status of an individual. This effect is accentuated when high levels of the amino acid histidine is fed since the formation of folacin coenzymes involves the conversion of histidine to glutamic acid and the use of a single-carbon unit left over in the formation of the coenzyme. If folacin is inadequate, coenzymes are not formed and the single-carbon unit (formimino) is not removed from the glutamic acid.

Deficiency symptoms

With increasing knowledge of folate metabolism have come increasing numbers of reports of folate deficiency. A deficiency of the vitamin has been implicated in conditions ranging from thalassemia to toxemia of pregnancy (20% of pregnant women found to be deficient) to rheumatoid arthritis. It has been suggested that as the relationship between folate deficiency and chemical disorders is clarified, it may be apparent that folate deficiency is the most prevalent of all vitamin deficiencies.

In experimental deficiency conditions it took adults about five months to develop symptoms of megaloblastic anemia. Infants with low reserves and higher needs for growth developed symptoms in eight weeks. Inadequate folate may reduce the production of leukocytes or white blood cells and hence the ability of the body to produce antibodies.

Although there is no clear reason for the relationship, it has been found that 90% of all alcoholics suffer from a folacin deficiency.

In folic acid deficiencies the blood picture is affected differently in different animals. In monkeys there is a reduced number of white blood cells (leukopenia) with a reduced resistance to intestinal infection and enlarged red blood cells (macrocytes). Chicks also show macrocytic anemia and slow growth. Pigs and rats manifest deficiency symptoms only when their ability

to synthesize folic acid is interfered with and when the diet is also devoid of folic acid.

Therapeutic uses

Folacin is effective in treating nutritional megaloblastic anemia caused by folate deficiency, the megaloblastic anemia of pregnancy and infancy, and some other anemias that fail to respond to vitamin B_{12}. In addition, it is effective in relieving some of the symptoms that occur in tropical sprue, such as anemia, glossitis, and gastrointestinal disturbances.

While folacin does relieve the anemia and glossitis associated with pernicious anemia, it not only fails to alleviate the degeneration of nervous tissue but accentuates the changes. Thus, in addition to failing to provide a complete cure for pernicious anemia the use of folic acid may be potentially dangerous in allowing the irreversible nervous system symptoms to develop.

Concern over the possibility that a dose of folacin, curing the megaloblastic anemia of pernicious anemia, may eliminate the most effective means of diagnosing the disease has led the Food and Drug Administration to set a limit of 0.1 mg. of folic acid as the amount that is permissible for use in vitamin supplements. This would be sufficient to protect against a folacin deficiency without curing megaloblastic symptoms of pernicious anemia. If the megaloblastic anemia has been primarily caused by vitamin B_{12} deficiency but has responded to folic acid therapy, the anemia is likely to recur.

The use of a folic acid antagonist such as aminopterin to interfere with the formation of the active coenzyme, which is necessary for the production of white blood cells (leukocytes), has been effective in decreasing the rate of leukocyte formation in leukemia, a fatal condition characterized by overproduction of white blood cells. Unfortunately, such a treatment also restricts the growth of other cells so it can be used only intermittently and provides only temporary relief.

COBALAMIN
Discovery

Until 1926, pernicious anemia, a condition characterized by an abnormal blood pattern in which red blood cells failed to mature and developed into abnormally large cells, by a degeneration of nervous tissue, and also characterized by glossitis, was a fatal disease of unknown origin with no known cure. In 1926 Castle established that the condition could be cured if the patient were fed large amounts of raw liver (at least three quarters of a pound per day). Noting that pernicious anemia patients had an abnormal gastric secretion, he postulated the theory that the antipernicious anemia substance was formed by the combination of an *extrinsic factor* in food, especially liver, and an *intrinsic factor* in the normal gastric secretion. Both the extrinsic and intrinsic factors were necessary for the prevention or cure of the disease. Castle's theory was held during succeeding years while scientists attempted to isolate and identify the active substance in food. The story of this search is the story of the discovery of the vitamin cobalamin or vitamin B_{12} now recognized as Castle's extrinsic factor.

The attempts to identify the active principle in liver were hampered by the fact that no animal or organism other than man had exhibited a need for the substance. Thus all clinical evaluations of new liver concentrates had to be made on human subjects suffering from pernicious anemia. Since persons were frequently in widely separated locations their usefulness as subjects was limited. Medical investigators were able to isolate progressively more concentrated extracts of liver that showed antipernicious anemia potency, but the progress was discouragingly slow in spite of the fact that with each advance pernicious anemia patients benefitted. It was

only with the discovery that the microorganism *Lactobacillus lactis* also needed the antipernicious anemia factor for growth that more extensive experimental work could be attempted, and the final isolation of the effective principle became possible. Clinical tests, which showed that an injected dose of the liver extract was much more effective than the same amount ingested, began to cast doubt on Castle's theory and eventually led to the conclusion that Castle's extrinsic factor in food was indeed the antipernicious anemia factor and that the intrinsic factor of the gastric mucosa was responsible and necessary for the active absorption of the substance. The favorable results that had been obtained when large amounts of liver were fed by mouth were explained on the basis that such large amounts of cobalamin were absorbed by diffusion rather than by active transport across the intestinal membrane, which required the intrinsic factor.

Chemical composition

By 1948, two years after folic acid had been discovered and determined *not* to be the sought-after antipernicious anemia factor, workers in Britain and the United States almost simultaneously succeeded in isolating small red crystals with high antipernicious anemia potency from the liver extracts. This substance was soon identified chemically as one containing about 4% of its weight as the mineral cobalt, previously known to be essential only in the diets of sheep and cattle. The cobalt was present in the center of a chemical molecule resembling hemoglobin or chlorophyll, in which iron and magnesium are the characteristic mineral elements. In addition to containing cobalt, one active form of the vitamin was found to possess a cyano- group closely bound in the molecule. The antipernicious anemia factor was first identified as vitamin B_{12}, but the term cobalamin is now the accepted name.

Once cobalamin was isolated and chemically identified, its role in biological reactions was more easily studied. In contrast to other vitamins, a deficiency of cobalamin is primarily the result of a defect in the mechanism by which it is absorbed rather than a dietary deficit.

The term cobalamin is now used to designate all of the many forms in which the vitamin may appear in animal tissues as an active coenzyme. Hydroxycobalamin, cyanocobalamin, nitritocobalamin, and thiocyanate cobalamin are among the forms known to exhibit vitamin effects, although others have been identified. Of these forms, cyanocobalamin is the most active, although hydroxycobalamin appears to be retained longer by the body.

The animal protein factor (APF) that was known to stimulate growth in animals was found to be identical with vitamin B_{12}. It appears to promote the retention of nitrogen and hence to raise the biological value of the protein of the diet, leading to more rapid growth per unit of food. The apparent beneficial effects of the antibiotics aureomycin and penicillin in stimulating growth in animals is now attributed to the fact that they inhibit the growth of organisms that destroy vitamin B_{12}. Their use, then, essentially increases the vitamin B_{12} available and indirectly enhances growth. The usefulness of cobalamin as a growth factor for children has been investigated, but results are inconclusive and suggest that it is effective only in underweight children and only if the general nature of the diet improves.

Absorption

The absorption of vitamin B_{12} is governed by a heat-labile mucoprotein secreted from the glands of the wall of the stomach and found in normal gastric juice. As it mixes with food in its passage through the digestive tract, this intrinsic factor, which is different in each species, releases vitamin B_{12} from the protein complex in which it occurs in food. It then helps attach the

vitamin to a receptor in the intestinal mucosa in a reaction catalyzed by the mineral, calcium. Cobalamin is released to the mucosa or absorbing cells in the intestinal wall by the action of intestinal enzymes, which also are different in each species. A failure in any stage in the absorption can render dietary cobalamin unavailable.

The percentage of the intake that is absorbed decreases as the actual amount in the diet increases. On an average intake of 16 μg., from 3 to 5 μg. are absorbed. However, in minimal intakes of 0.5 μg. as much as 70% is absorbed.

If the gastric juice of a person lacks this intrinsic factor necessary for absorption of cobalamin, there is no uptake of the vitamin at all from the amounts normally provided in food. However, if amounts about one thousand times the normal dosage are given, as in oral doses of liver extract, sufficient amounts to meet the needs of an individual may pass through the intestinal wall by diffusion. Since the intrinsic factor in the hog's stomach is similar to that from the human gastric mucosa, it has been possible to administer a concentrate of hog's stomach to facilitate the absorption of cobalamin from either food or therapeutic preparations.

Experimentally it has been demonstrated that the vitamin may be taken in by inhalation. It is poorly absorbed, however, if administered rectally. It is most effective if injected intramuscularly so as to bypass the defective absorptive mechanism.

The efficiency of absorption appears to diminish with increase in age, with a pyridoxine deficiency, with an iron inadequacy, and in hypothyroidism but increases during pregnancy and when an intrinsic factor concentrate is fed along with it. The use of sorbitol, an alcohol derivative of carbohydrate, has also improved cobalamin absorption, especially among older people with depressed gastric secretions.

The administration of a radioactive dose of cobalamin and measurement of its excretion gives an indication of the effectiveness of absorption. In feces of normal subjects 30% is found while pernicious anemia patients excrete 70%.

Metabolism

Once cobalamin is absorbed it passes into the bloodstream, where it is bound again to a protein, the form in which it circulates to various tissues. Any vitamin absorbed in excess of the capacity of the blood to bind it is rapidly excreted in the urine, and there is evidence that in some cases a vitamin B_{12} deficiency may be caused by limitations in the cobalamin-binding capacity of the blood. The body holds on to any absorbed protein-bound vitamin very tenaciously, storing any excess beyond immediate needs in the form of a cobamide enzyme in combination with protein, primarily in the liver, which has 1 to 2 μg. per gram. The uptake in the liver is facilitated by ascorbic acid. The average storage amounts to 2000 μg., an amount sufficient to last about six years.

Functions

Cobalamin is necessary for normal growth, for maintenance of healthy nervous tissue, and for normal blood formation. The exact biochemical role of the vitamin in maintaining all these functions has not been determined, but some aspects have been identified. In many respects there is a complex interrelationship between the roles of cobalamin and folacin.

The functional form of the vitamin is a coenzyme that exists in many forms but is generally referred to as a cobamide coenzyme. The conversion of the vitamin to this active form involves many nutrients including niacin, riboflavin, and manganese.

In the bone marrow cells where erythroblasts, the forerunners of red blood cells, are formed, cobalamin coenzymes are necessary for the synthesis of thymine, which is an essential part of the genetic material DNA. If DNA is not produced the cells cannot divide but instead continue to produce RNA and to synthesize protein, increasing in size to become very large cells called megaloblasts. The red blood cells that are produced by these megaloblasts are large and immature macrocytes that are characteristic of the blood of pernicious anemia patients and differ from the mature erythrocytes in a normal blood. Once cobalamin is available, the megaloblasts are no longer formed, and the erythroblasts produce normal mature red blood cells, the erythrocytes. The role of cobalamin in nucleic acid synthesis, which may include the formation of deoxyribose from ribose as well as thymine synthesis from methyl groups, is important in all body cells, but its effect is more pronounced in erythrocytes, which develop very rapidly at a rate of at least 200 million per minute.

The way in which cobalamin affects the nervous system is not clear. However, it is known that vitamin B_{12} keeps glutathione, an integral part of several enzymes involved in carbohydrate metabolism, in the reduced state in which it is biologically active. Since the nervous system relies entirely on carbohydrate as its source of fuel, anything that disrupts carbohydrate metabolism will deprive nervous tissue of its energy source and hence interfere with its normal functioning. Since the nervous system has a limited range of pathways by which it can handle carbohydrate, it may be dependent on vitamin B_{12}. Levels of pyruvic acid and lactic acid, intermediary products in carbohydrate metabolism, increase from 50% to 100% in a cobalamin deficiency, suggesting a block in glucose metabolism.

Like folate, cobalamin is concerned with metabolism that involves single-carbon units such as methyl groups. Unlike folate, which aids the transfer of these single-carbon units from one substance to another, cobalamin is necessary for the synthesis or formation of these units, which in turn are vital in the formation of many essential body compounds.

In the metabolism of folic acid, vitamin B_{12} catalyzes the release of folic acid with one glutamic acid molecule from folic acid conjugates of three or seven glutamic acid molecules that occur in foods. In addition, it facilitates the formation of the folic acid coenzymes from the citrovorum factor or folinic acid.

Besides its direct role in folic acid and nucleic acid metabolism and its more indirect role in carbohydrate metabolism, the vitamin appears to play a role in fat and protein metabolism, but the mechanisms have not been clarified.

Food sources

Vitamin B_{12} is found only in foods of animal origin. Animals absorb the vitamin after it has been synthesized by bacteria in their rumen from the plant foods they eat, provided sufficient cobalt is available. Microorganisms in the gastrointestinal tract of human beings are also able to synthesize the vitamin, but the site of synthesis is too far down in the colon to permit absorption.

The best sources of cobalamin are the animal foods—liver, which contains about one part per million, kidney, milk, and meat, in all of which it occurs in a protein complex. In diets of everyone except strict vegetarians, who make absolutely no use of animal products, the diet is always adequate. Deficiency symptoms result from failure in the absorptive mechanisms rather than any lack of the nutrient.

Commercially, cobalamin is obtained as an inexpensive fermentation by-product of the production of the organism used in production of the antibiotic penicillin. If it is obtained from liver, one ton of liver is required to yield 20 mg. of the vitamin. It is sometimes advertised as the red vitamin because of the bright red crystals it forms.

Cyanocobalamin is stable to acid and oxidation but is destroyed by alkali. About 70% is normally retained in cooking.

Dietary requirements

The need for cobalamin is extremely small and has been very difficult to determine, but there is some evidence that a diet containing 3 to 5 μg. per day, from which 1 to 1.5 μg. is absorbed, satisfies the need of most adults. Body stores normally range from 800 to 11,000 μg. Pernicious anemia patients will experience relief on as little as 0.1 μg. by intramuscular injection or 5 to 15 μg. taken orally with the intrinsic factor.

Deficiency symptoms

As indicated earlier, there is virtually no evidence of a deficiency state from a lack of dietary source of the nutrient except among strict vegetarians who develop neurologic symptoms but not changes in their blood pattern. Pernicious anemia, the major manifestation of an inadequate amount of the nutrient, results from a lack of the intrinsic factor secreted by the glands of the stomach from partial or complete removal of the stomach, from a lack of the protein in the blood that binds absorbed cobalamin, or from lack of the substance that releases it from the mucosal cells to the blood. Intestinal infestation with a fish tapeworm that avidly absorbs any available vitamin also produces an induced deficiency state. Diagnosis of vitamin B_{12} deficiency can be made on the basis of blood levels of the vitamins, which are determined by microbiological techniques. Normal levels of 100 to 1000 μg. per milliliter fall below 100 in pernicious anemia, and changes in the nature of blood cells from small nonnucleated cells to larger nucleated ones help confirm the diagnosis.

Pernicious anemia can now be readily controlled by injections of cobalamin. About 1000 μg. are given twice in the first week, followed by 250 μg. per week until the blood pattern has returned to normal. A dose of 250 μg. every three weeks is usually sufficient to protect against recurrence of the condition. The most crucial aspect of pernicious anemia therapy is a sufficently early diagnosis that treatment can be begun before neural degeneration has become irreversible. In contrast to the victim of pernicious anemia prior to 1925, who faced almost certain death, or after 1926, who was forced to eat large amounts of liver daily, today's patient has at his disposal a relatively simple and inexpensive form of treatment.

BIOTIN
Discovery

Recognition of biotin as a dietary essential occurred in 1924 when it was identified as bios II, one of three factors necessary for the growth of microorganisms. Between this time and the time of its synthesis in 1943, various scientists had sought the nature of substances they had named vitamin H and coenzyme R. Once the chemical nature of this sulphur-containing nutrient was determined it was clear, as had been the case in the study of many other nutrients, that all three were the same substance, now identified as biotin.

Symptoms of biotin deficiency occur in animals only after the ingestion of a diet low in biotin and high in raw egg white. Raw egg white contains a carbohydrate-containing protein, *avidin*, which binds biotin in a complex too big to be absorbed but which the body cannot break to release biotin. Experimentally it was found that in humans the diet had to provide 30% of its calories from raw egg white in order to induce a biotin deficiency. Since this represents approximately 27 egg whites in a 3000-calorie diet it is obvious that the ingestion of the occasional raw egg white is not going to precipitate a deficiency state. Cooking denatures avidin so that it no longer has the ability to bind protein.

Chemical properties

Biotin has been isolated in at least five active forms from food. One of these, biocytin, is a combination of biotin and the amino acid lysine. Other forms are biotin sulfone, which is a potent antagonist, and biotinal, which can be oxidized to an active form.

In animal tissues the protein-bound biotin is fat-soluble while the free biotin found in plants and excreted in the urine is water-soluble.

In addition to the biotin provided by the diet, the body is able to absorb a considerable amount, which is synthesized by intestinal bacteria. Conditions that reduce the number of microorganisms in the intestine may reduce the amount of biotin synthesized. Sulfonamides and oxytetracycline are known to reduce the number of biotin-synthesizing organisms. Some of the symptoms that develop with the use of sulfonamides may be evidence of biotin deficiency since biotin administration seems to counteract them.

Functions

Biotin is a very active substance participating in many biological reactions. In animal cells it occurs bound to protein where it acts as an enzyme.

The best established role of biotin enzymes is in the addition (carboxylation) or removal (decarboxylation) of carbon dioxide in various reactions. Since these two reactions are quite common in nature we find biotin involved in both the synthesis and oxidation of fatty acids and the oxidation of carbohydrate. Its role in deamination, which must occur before amino acids can be used as a source of energy, has been established for at least three amino acids, aspartic acid, threonine, and serine. It is necessary for the synthesis of nicotinic acid but the mode of action is not clear. The synthesis of the digestive enzyme, pancreatic amylase, is another biotin-dependent reaction.

Failure of some of these functions shows up in an impaired utilization of glucose, a decrease in the incorporation of amino acids into protein, and up to 30% reduction in fat in the cell mitochondria caused by failure in the synthesis of fatty acids.

Dietary requirements

So far it has been impossible to establish whether or not humans need a dietary source of biotin and, if so, the magnitude of the need. It is thought that the body uses approximately 150 μg. per day, an amount adequately provided by the diet even without that provided by intestinal synthesis.

Food sources

Most of the biotin in food occurs bound to protein from which the body can readily liberate it. Liver, kidney, egg yolk, and yeast have been shown by biological assay to be the richest food sources, followed by some vegetables such as cauliflower, nuts, and legumes. In general, all other meats, dairy products, and cereals are considered poor sources.

Most diets contain between 150 and 300 μg. of biotin, which is supplemented by some from the intestinal synthesis by bacteria that is stimulated on a sucrose-containing diet. There is no evidence on which to justify the inclusion of biotin in the formula for a multivitamin supplement.

Deficiency symptoms

The effects of a biotin-deficient diet in animals are many and varied but seem to be characterized by early changes in the skin. Dermatitis, characterized by either scaliness or hardening, which frequently starts in the region of the eye, is common. This is often followed by loss of hair and evidence of muscular atrophy.

In a study in which four human subjects became deficient on a diet devoid of biotin and high in avidin, the symptoms observed were very similar to those of a thiamine deficiency and included dermatitis, loss of appetite, nausea, muscle pains, and high blood cholesterol levels, among many other symptoms. In both cases there is a derangement of the metabolic enzyme systems.

Although there is no evidence of a nat-ural biotin deficiency in human adults, recent evidence has suggested that two types of dermatitis, Leiner's disease and seborrheic dermatitis, which occur in infants, may be caused by a biotin lack. They respond rather dramatically to biotin therapy, although similar conditions in adults are not responsive.

SELECTED REFERENCES

Ascorbic acid

Abt, A. F., von Schuching, S., and Roe, J. H.: The effects of vitamin C deficiency on healed wounds, Bull. Johns Hopkins Hosp. **105**:67-76, 1959.

Abt, A. F., von Schuching, S., and Enns, T.: Vitamin C requirements of man re-examined, Am. J. Clin Nutrition **12**:21-29, 1963.

Davey, B. L., Fisher, K. H., and Chen, S. D.: Utilization of ascorbic acid in fruits and vegetables, J. Am. Dietet. A. **32**:1069, 1956.

Grewar, D.: Infantile scurvy, Clin. Pediat. **4**:82, 1965.

Lorenz, A. J.: The conquest of scurvy, J. Am. Dietet. A. **30**:665, 1954.

Ossofsky, H. J.: Infantile scurvy, Am. J. Dis. Child. **109**:173, 1965.

Rivers, J. M.: Ascorbic acid metabolism of connective tissue, New York J. Med. **65**:1235, 1965.

Szent-Gyorgyi, A.: Lost in the twentieth century, Ann. Rev. Biochem. **32**:1, 1963.

Uhl, E.: Ascorbic acid requirements of adults: 30 mg. or 75 mg.?, Am. J. Clin. Nutrition **6**:146-150, 1958.

Whitacre, J., McLaughlin, L., Futriel, M. F., and Grimes, E. T.: Human utilization of vitamin C, J. Am. Dietet. A. **35**:139, 1959.

Thiamine

Bradley, W. B.: Thiamine enrichment in the United States, Ann. New York Acad. Sc. **98**:602, 1962.

Brin, M.: Thiamine deficiency and erythrocyte metabolism, Am. J. Clin. Nutrition **12**:107, 1963.

Brin, M.: Erythrocyte as a biopsy tissue for functional evaluation of thiamine adequacy, J.A.M.A. **187**:762, 1964.

Dreyfus, R. M., and Victor, M.: Effects of thiamine deficiency on the central nervous system, Am. J. Clin. Nutrition **9**:414, 1961.

Brozek, J.: Psychologic effects of thiamine restriction and deprivation in normal young men, Am. J. Clin. Nutrition **5**:109, 1957.

Salcedo, J.: Experience in the etiology and prevention of thiamine deficiency in the Philippine Islands, Ann. New York Acad. Sc. **98**:568, 1962.

Sebrell, W. H.: A clinical evaluation of thiamine deficiency, Ann. New York Acad. Sc. **98**:563, 1962.

Wurst, H. M.: The history of thiamine, Ann. New York Acad. Sc. **98**:385, 1962.

Riboflavin

Lane, M., Alfrey, C. P., Mengel, C. E., Doherty, M. A., and Doherty, J.: The rapid induction of human riboflavin deficiency with galactoflavin, J. Clin. Invest. **43**:357, 1964.

Windmueller, H. G., Anderson, A. A., and Mickelson, O.: Elevated riboflavin levels in urine of fasting subjects, Am. J. Clin. Nutrition **15**:73, 1964.

Niacin

De Lange, D. J.: Assessment of nicotinic acid status of population groups, Am. J. Clin. Nutrition **15**:169, 1964.

Goldsmith, G. A.: Niacin-tryptophane relationship in man and niacin requirement, Am. J. Clin. Nutrition **6**:479, 1958.

Goldsmith, G. A., Miller, O. N., and Unglaub, W. G.: Efficiency of tryptophane as a niacin precursor in man, J. Nutrition **73**:172, 1961.

Goldsmith, G. A.: Niacin, antipellagra factor; hypocholesteremic agent, J.A.M.A. **194**:167, 1965.

Sydenstricker, V. P.: History of pellagra; its recognition as a disorder of nutrition and its conquest, Am. J. Clin. Nutrition **6**:409, 1958.

Pyridoxine

Baker, E. M., Canham, J. E., Nunes, W. T., Sauberlich, H. E., and McDowell, M. E.: Vitamin B_6 requirement for adult men, Am. J. Clin. Nutrition **15**:59, 1964.

Bunnell, R. H.: Vitamin B_6, Science **146**:674, 1964.

Coursin, D. B.: Present status of vitamin B_6 metabolism, Am. J. Clin. Nutrition **9**:304, 1963.

Coursin, D. B.: Vitamin B_6 requirements, J.A.M.A. **189**:27, 1964.

Polansky, M. M., and Murphy, E. W.: Vitamin B_6 in fruits and nuts, J. Am. Dietet. A. **48**:109, 1966.

Polansky, M. M., Murphy, E. W., and Toepfer,

E. W.: Components of vitamin B_6 in grains and cereal products, J. A. Of. Agr. Chem. **47**:750, 1964.

Review. Pyridoxine and dental caries; human studies, Nutr. Rev. **21**:143, 1963.

Shriver, C. R., and Hutchison, J. H.: The vitamin B_6 deficiency syndrome in human infancy: biochemical and clinical observations, Pediatrics **31**:240-250, 1963.

Pantothenic acid

Zook, E. G., MacArthur, M. S., and Toepper, E. W.: Pantothenic acid in foods, Agricultural Handbook No. 97, Washington, D. C., 1956, United States Department of Agriculture.

Folacin

Metz, J., Festenstein, H., and Welsh, P.: Effect of folic acid and vitamin B_{12} supplementation on tests of folate and vitamin B_{12} nutrition in pregnancy, Am. J. Clin. Nutrition **16**:472, 1965.

Santini, R., Brewster, C., and Butterworth, C. E.: The distribution of folic acid active compounds in individual foods, Am. J. Clin. Nutrition **14**:205-210, 1964.

Vilter, R. W., Will, J. J., Wright, T., and Rullman, D.: Interrelationships of vitamin B_{12}, folic acid and ascorbic acid in the megaloblastic anemias, Am. J. Clin. Nutrition **12**:130-144, 1963.

Cobalamin

Chow, B. F.: Nutritional significance of vitamin B_{12}, World Rev. Nutr. Diet. **1**:127, 1960.

Chung, A. S. M., Pearson, W. N., Darby, W. J., Miller, O. N., and Goldsmith, G. A.: Folic acid, vitamin B_6, pantothenic acid, and vitamin B_{12} in human dietaries, Am. J. Clin. Nutrition **9**:573, 1961.

Schweigert, B. S.: The role of vitamin B_{12} in nucleic acid synthesis, Borden Rev. Nutr. Res. **22**:19, 1961.

Sullivan, L. W., and Victor, H.: Studies on the minimum daily requirement for vitamin B_{12}, New England J. Med. **272**:340, 1965.

Wilson, T. H.: Intrinsic factor and B_{12} absorption —a problem in cell physiology, Nutr. Rev. **23**:33, 1965.

13

Other nutrient factors

In addition to the nutrients that have already been definitely established as vitamins, there are several other vitamin-like substances that, on the basis of current information, fail to meet all the criteria necessary to be classed as vitamins but still have some properties of vitamins. In some cases they are present in larger amounts than vitamins; in others the body can synthesize sufficient amounts to meet body needs if precursors are present; and for others it has been impossible to determine any essential biological role.

Because these dietary factors are sometimes given vitamin status, it is felt that a brief discussion of present knowledge of their status is warranted here. Undoubtedly, some will in the future be established definitely as vitamins while others will definitely be dropped from this classification.

MYOINOSITOL

Myoinositol, which is also known as muscle sugar and mesoinositol, is one of nine six-carbon compounds closely related chemically to glucose. Of these nine, only myoinositol is biologically active. It was first recognized in 1928 as a growth-promoting factor for yeast and as a cure for alopecia in mice.

It is present in practically all plant and animal tissues in concentrations higher than those normally associated with vitamins. In animal cells it occurs primarily as a phospholipid, which is sometimes referred to as lipositol. In grains it is present as a more complex water-soluble compound, phytic acid, the organic acid that binds both calcium and iron in an insoluble complex and prevents their absorption. It also occurs in nucleated erythrocytes. In soybeans it occurs in a free form, and in other plant and animal tissues it occurs as an unidentified complex. There is some evidence that sharks and certain other fishes store carbohydrate as inositol rather than as glycogen.

Methods of analyzing for inositol are tedious and relatively inaccurate, but from available data it appears that heart muscle, brain, and skeletal muscle contain more inositol than other tissues.

The biological significance of inositol is unknown, although several roles have been attributed to it. It may act as an intermediary product between carbohydrate and aromatic compounds, or it may retard the loss of vitamin C in scorbutic guinea pigs. It is believed to lead to a decrease in ribonucleic acid (RNA) synthesis, but none of its possible roles has been clearly established. It has, however, been found essential for the growth of liver and bone marrow cells.

Human beings apparently consume about 1 gm. of inositol a day in food. In addition, the body is able to synthesize sufficient amounts to meet its needs from glucose. Synthesis occurs within the individual cell rather than by intestinal organisms. The amount excreted in the urine is small and variable, averaging 37 mg. per day with a range from 8 to 144 mg., although diabetics excrete much more. Normal blood levels range from 0.37 to 0.67 mg. per 100 ml.

CHOLINE

Choline was identified in 1937 as a dietary factor that prevented the accumulation of fat in the liver of dogs. Since then, it has been determined that the effectiveness of choline is due to three methyl (CH_3) groups present in its molecule, which are available to other biological compounds, many of which have a need for it. As a methyl donor, choline provides one of the substances necessary to mobilize fat from the liver to be transported in the bloodstream to other cells of the body. Methyl groups are exchanged in a wide variety of biological reactions, and as a source of these choline facilitates many reactions.

Choline can be readily synthesized in the body from the amino acid glycine, providing another source of methyl group is available. These methyl groups may be provided by another amino acid, methionine; they can be synthesized in the presence of adequate folic acid or cobalamin; or they

may be obtained from a variety of other sources. Thus it appears that choline cannot be considered a vitamin since the body is not solely dependent on a dietary source of either choline or a direct precursor.

In the body choline occurs as a constituent of the fat-related substance lecithin, a form in which much fat is transported, and sphingomyelin, which occurs in nerve tissue. As such, it is a structural part of fat and nerve tissue and does not catalyze any reactions or act as part of a coenzyme. In addition, choline reacts with acetyl CoA to form an acetylcholine that is responsible for transmitting nerve impulses from one nerve ending to the next.

Choline is widely distributed in food, being present in relatively large amounts in all foods that contain fat, as shown in Table 13-1. With the exception of legumes, fruits and vegetables contain virtually no choline.

The need for dietary choline has not been established since it is very small or nonexistent when the diet contains sufficient methionine to provide methyl groups for the synthesis of choline or adequate amounts of folacin and cobalamin to stimulate the synthesis of methyl groups.

Choline is not associated with any specific deficiency disease in human beings. It does, however, exert a protective action in cirrhosis of the liver among alcoholics. In rats and dogs the symptoms associated

Table 13-1. Choline content of representative foods

Food	Choline content (grams per 100 gm.)
Egg yolk	1.7
Meat	0.6
Fish	0.2
Cereal	0.1

with choline deficiency are aggravated by a pyridoxine deficiency, while in chickens and turkeys the perosis induced by choline deficiency can be cured by folic acid, manganese, or choline.

COENZYME Q

The most recently discovered (1961) nutritional factor is coenzyme Q, a lipidlike substance that is somewhat similar in its chemical makeup to vitamin K. It belongs to a group of compounds known as ubiquinones, and the forms that appear to be biologically important have from thirty to fifty carbon atoms in a side chain attached to the basic quinone structure. The fifty-carbon side chain occurs exclusively in higher animals.

Coenzyme Q is found in practically all living cells and appears to be concentrated in the mitochondria. Here it apparently operates as an essential link in the respiratory chain in which energy is released from energy-yielding nutrients as the high-energy compound ATP. It appears to be reversibly oxidized and reduced readily. Without this substance one would anticipate incomplete release of energy.

The ubiquinones are likely to be synthesized readily in the body, the ring structure from amino acids such as phenylalanine and the side chain from acetate available as an intermediary in carbohydrate and fat metabolism. A pantothenic acid deficiency has been shown to depress coenzyme Q synthesis by 50%, likely because of decreased availability of acetate. Ubiquinones, therefore, are of little dietary significance and cannot be truly classed as vitamins. In contrast to other fat-soluble vitamins, they can be excreted in the urine.

Ubichromenol, which is similar to vitamin E in structure and biological activity, can be formed from ubiquinone. Both vitamin E and selenium operate to maintain high tissue concentration to coenzyme Q.

BIOFLAVONOIDS

The bioflavonoids were first suggested as dietary factors in 1936 when it was observed that extracts of both red pepper and lemon increased the antiscorbutic effect of ascorbic acid. A wide range of chemical substances, mostly belonging to the flavine and flavonoid compounds, were believed to exert a favorable influence in reducing capillary bleeding caused by the increased permeability of the cell membrane. For a while these compounds, of which *hesperidin* was one of the most active, was designated vitamin P, but the use of this term was dropped in 1950.

So far, scientists have been unable to ascertain any specific biological role for this group of compounds, although they agree that they may have some pharmacologic effects. In addition there is no proof of clinical usefulness of the compounds that have been advocated at various times as therapeutic agents in the treatment of a range of unrelated conditions such as cerebral accidents, arthritis, abortions, common colds, and retinal hemorrhages. There have been many suggestions as to the mode of action of the bioflavonoids but none have been substantiated.

Bioflavonoids occur in highest concentration in the peel and juice of citrus fruit, in tobacco leaves, in buckwheat, and in some other fruits and vegetables. There is no evidence at the present time of a dietary need for bioflavonoids and certainly no justification for their inclusion in nutritional supplements; nor is there a justification in the promotion of certain foods on the basis of a high concentration of the substance.

LIPOIC ACID

Lipoic acid is a fat-soluble factor known to be essential for growth of several microorganisms. It has been isolated from liver and yeast, and several aspects of its biochemical role have been elucidated. At the present time there is some question as to whether it should be considered a vitamin for humans since there is no evidence yet that humans or other mammals require a dietary source of the substance. Although it does participate in biochemical reactions in mammalian tissues, the amounts needed to meet these needs are likely synthesized in the body.

Lipoic acid is now identified in five distinct forms; three forms are fat-soluble; one is a water-soluble complex; and one, which is bound to protein, has been known as factor 11 and 11A, pyruvic oxidation factor, thioctic acid, and protogen. Lipoic acid, the official name, and thioctic acid, indicative of the sulphur found in the molecule, are the names most frequently used now. The fat-soluble lipoic acid can be reversibly oxidized to the water-soluble β-lipoic acid.

Function

Lipoic acid is essential along with the thiamine-containing e n z y m e, pyrophosphatase, for the reactions in carbohydrate metabolism that convert pyruvic acid to acetyl coenzyme A. This is the point at which it joins the intermediary products of protein and fat metabolism in the Krebs cycle for the reactions involved in liberating energy from these nutrients. In its active form lipoic acid is bound to a protein in a reaction requiring energy in the form of ATP and a metal ion such as calcium or magnesium. In plant cells it may be involved in catalyzing some of the reactions of photosynthesis.

There have been several attempts to relate lipoic acid nutrition to metabolic disorders in animals and humans but most of the results have been contradictory. Some evidence showed that lipoic acid limited the plasma lipid formation on cholesterogenic diets in rabbits; other evidence showed that it stimulated tumor growth; and still other evidence showed that it led to a reduction in voluntary alcohol consumption. But none of the evidence is clearcut. In humans lipoic acid has been beneficial in the human liver disease, hepatic coma.

14

Selection of an adequate diet, dietary standards, and tables of food composition

The recommended dietary allowances (RDA) provide a very useful guide for nutritionists, dietitians, and agricultural experts in planning and evaluating diets of population groups and in planning food production programs. They are, however, of little value to the average individual or homemaker who may become confused by the many units—milligrams, grams, international units, and kilocalories—in which requirements are expressed. In addition, she seldom has access to tables of food composition or the inclination or ability to make the involved calculations necessary to evaluate a particular diet pattern in relation to recommended allowances.

If we believe that the standards set forth in the RDA are desirable and worthwhile goals, they must be expressed in terms of the foods or food groups around which a homemaker plans her family's meals. This food guide must be sufficiently simple to make it practical for use by the average homemaker and yet sufficiently detailed to make it consistent with scientific facts and to accomplish its purpose within

the framework of accepted food patterns of the country. The members of the Food and Nutrition Board, which developed the first dietary standards, emphasized that it was possible to achieve the level of nutrition they advocated through a well-chosen diet of natural foods. They also pointed out that it was possible to achieve this optimal nutrition through an unlimited number of combinations of foods—the choice of which might be determined by the availability of foods in a local market, socioeconomic status of the family, the cultural background, and the physical condition and food preferences of the individual.

A sound nutrition program involves ascertaining the nutritive value of available foods, their contribution to meeting nutritional needs, and educating the public in a wise choice of foods.

FOOD SELECTION GUIDES
Basic seven food groups

To translate the recommended allowances into familiar diet patterns the Bureau of Home Economics of the U. S. Department of Agriculture recommended that certain types of foods be included in the diet in specified amounts. By using their plan a person with no scientific knowledge of nutrition could select an adequate diet. Their recommendations became the basis of the *Basic Seven* developed as part of the National Wartime Nutrition Program of the Research Administration of the U. S. Department of Agriculture in 1943. This familiar guide, presented in Table 14-1, was the basis of practically all nutrition education programs from 1943 until its revision in 1956. Other similar plans have been promoted by special trade groups, but the basic seven has remained the standard. It served a major purpose in providing a guide which would lead to the consumption of a diet adequate in most nutritional factors provided by the so-called protective foods—foods which provided a larger proportion of the needs for two more nutrients than of calories. However, the complexity of a seven-group plan coupled with the lack of specificity as to what constituted a

serving limited its effectiveness in many nutrition education situations.

While the United States was promoting the seven-group plan, many other countries were developing plans designed to accomplish the same educational objective and which involved three, four, or five groups based on their particular needs.

Basic four food groups

In 1956 the United States Department of Agriculture recommended that the complex seven-group plan be replaced by a simpler, less detailed four-group plan which they termed *Essentials of an Adequate Diet*. This plan, shown in Table 14-1, differed from the basic seven only in that the three fruit and vegetable categories were grouped as one and the fat group was eliminated entirely. The elimination of the fat group was justified on the grounds that the consumption of foods from the other groups usually led to the use of fat to improve the flavor and palatability of the

Table 14-1. Comparison of food guides—*Basic Seven* (1943) and *Essentials of an Adequate Diet* (1958)

Food group	Basic seven	Essentials of an adequate diet
Milk and milk products	Children, 3 to 4 cups	Children, 3 to 4 cups
	Adults, 2 cups	Adults, 2 or more cups
Fruits and vegetables		4 servings
Green and yellow vegetables	1 serving	
Citrus fruits or raw		
cabbage	1 serving	
Potatoes, other vegetables,		
and fruits	2 servings	
Meat, poultry, fish, and eggs	1 serving	2 or more servings
	1 egg (at least 4 per week)	
Bread, flour, cereal	3 servings	4 or more servings
(enriched or whole-grain)		
Butter or fortified margarine	Equivalent of	
	2 tablespoons	

food. In addition, the change was made at a time when there was increasing concern about the increase in fat consumption by the American public, especially in light of its possible role in the development of atherosclerosis. The U. S. Department of Agriculture did not want to find itself encouraging the consumption of a food that might later be proved to be the villain in a degenerative disease.

Food plans

As an aid to persons with a limited amount of money to spend on food, the U. S. Department of Agriculture publishes food plans that indicate the amounts of various types of foods to purchase per week for each member of the family to ensure the availability of an adequate level of nutrients. There are three plans based on different income levels—low cost, moderate cost, and liberal cost. When followed, they ensure a satisfactory level of nutrition for the whole family, assuming reasonably good practices in food preparation. The distribution of food to various family members is, however, the responsibility of the homemaker.

NUTRITIVE CONTRIBUTION OF FOOD GROUPS

Each of the four food groups is chosen because of a unique contribution it makes to the nutritive value of the diet. The contribution of each of the groups is shown graphically in Figs. 14-1 to 14-4. The values shown in the graphs represent a composite of a typical selection of foods within each category. It must be recognized that by differing the choices within the framework of the guide there may be wide variations in the nutritive quality of the diet. For instance, the choice of foods represented in the graph represents approximately 1400 kilocalories. It is quite possible to stay within the framework of the plan and choose foods ranging in calorie value from 800 to 1800. Likewise, the choice of vege-

tables may yield less than 1000 or more than 10,000 I.U. of vitamin A.

Milk and milk products

The recommendation that the equivalent of 2 cups of milk be used by an adult can be met in many ways, as may be seen by the list of equivalents in Table 14-2. The use of nonfat milk in place of whole milk will reduce the energy value by half and eliminate the vitamin A altogether. Neither of these is necessarily undesirable. Most persons have no difficulty in obtaining sufficient calories, and the vitamin A in one serving of a vegetable such as carrots will make up for the loss of vitamin A in 20 cups of nonfat milk. Thus, if it is desirable to restrict caloric intake the use of nonfat milk is justified. The use of chocolate milk increases the calorie value but in no way reduces the nutritive value of whole milk.

Cottage cheese may be a poor substitute for whole milk if one is concerned about the calcium values since calcium will be reduced if the cheese has been prepared by acid coagulation rather than rennin coagulation.

As shown in Fig. 14-1, the major contributions of the milk group are high-quality protein containing all eight essential amino acids, calcium, which is very difficult to obtain in sufficient amounts from other sources alone, and riboflavin. The riboflavin available from milk depends on the conditions under which it is stored. Since exposure to sunlight may reduce the riboflavin content by as much as 50%, many dairies have taken some responsibility in helping to reduce this loss by selling milk in brown glass bottles or paper cartons or providing insulated boxes to cut down light exposure. Many times this has been done in the face of consumer opposition.

The limited nutritional factors in milk are iron and ascorbic acid. Both of these are present in small amounts in a form which is very available, but it has been well established that a milk diet alone is incapable of providing adequate iron to regenerate hemoglobin in infants after 6 months of age. The small amount of ascorbic acid normally found in milk is reduced still further by the process of pasteurization so that it is an undependable source of the vitamin.

Ice cream is a good substitute for milk as a source of calcium on the basis of weight but contains only half as much calcium on the basis of calories.

Milk is available to the consumer in many forms at widely varying prices determined primarily by the perishability of the product rather than the nutritive considerations. The relative costs of various forms of milk of essentially equal nutritive value are presented in Table 14-3. By choosing the least expensive form that meets a particular need it is possible to reduce the cost of milk in the diet by an appreciable sum.

Fruit and vegetables

The U. S. Department of Agriculture in *Essentials of an Adequate Diet* recommends that the diet contain four servings

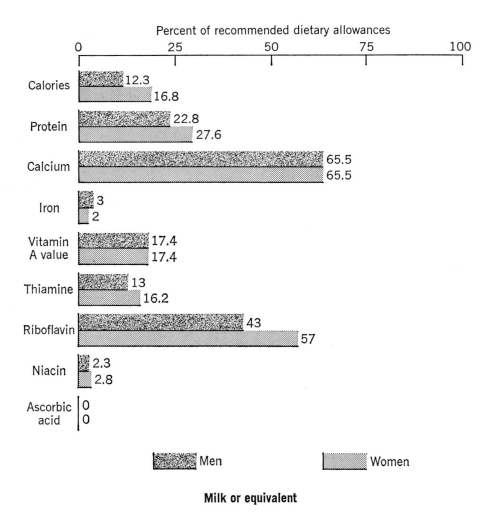

Milk or equivalent

Fig. 14-1

Nutritive contribution of two cups of milk to diet of an adult.

Table 14-2. Amount of milk substitutes needed to provide the amounts of calcium and protein in 1 cup of whole milk

	Amount required to provide 280 mg. calcium		Amount required to provide 9 gm. protein	
	Grams	Measure	Grams	Measure
Nonfat milk	231	1 cup	250	1 cup
Cheddar cheese	37	1⅓ ounces	36	1⅓ ounces
Cottage cheese	298	1⅓ cups	66	⅓ cup
Ice cream (10% fat)	192	⅙ quart	200	⅙ quart
Cream cheese	451	30 table-spoons	113	9 table-spoons

of fruits and vegetables, but in order to keep the plan simple makes no suggestion as to the choice to be made within this group. Since foods in this group represent such diversity in physical structure and nutritional value, persons who use this guide as a basis for a nutrition education program urge people to consume one serving of a citrus fruit or another fruit or vegetable high in ascorbic acid every day and a serving of dark green or yellow vegetable as a source of vitamin A every other day. In this way the major contribution of this group in providing vitamins C and A will be satisfied, as shown in Fig. 14-2.

A 4-ounce serving of fruit juice is considered an average serving. Citrus juices are generally rich sources, but other fruit juices vary considerably in their ascorbic acid content, as shown in Table 14-4. In using the guide emphasis should be placed on those juices that provide at least 30 mg. of vitamin C in a 4-ounce portion, especially if the diet contains no other rich source. An analysis of samples of fruit juices enriched with ascorbic acid shows a wide variation in the amount present regardless of the declaration on the label.

In other fruits and vegetables the amount of vitamin C present varies with the va-

Table 14-3. Relative costs of other forms of milk compared to fresh whole milk

Form	Relative cost*
Fresh whole milk	100
Fresh homogenized whole milk	104
Fresh homogenized chocolate milk	108
Fresh nonfat milk	76
Evaporated whole milk	56
Evaporated nonfat milk	52
Dried whole milk	112
Dried nonfat milk	20 to 40

*Based on prices in northeastern United States, Spring, 1966.

riety, the degree of maturity, the season, climatic conditions, and the length and conditions of storage. In apples, for instance, there is a range of ascorbic acid values from 5 to 19 mg. per 100 gm., depending on the variety, and these values fall to almost half after several months of storage. The loss of nutrients that occurs in fruits and vegetables begins right after harvest

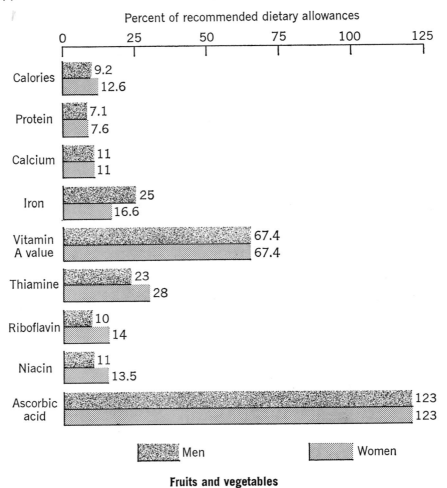

Percent of recommended dietary allowances

Fruits and vegetables

Fig. 14-2
Nutritive contribution of four servings of fruit or vegetables to diet of adult.

and may be very rapid in the first few hours. In addition to chemical losses there is the loss attributable to the removal of parts of the plant during preparation to make the product more palatable. The wilted outer leaves of lettuce, the leaves of broccoli, the skin on potatoes, and the bitter dark green leaves of endive, all of which are parts often discarded in preparation, have higher concentrations of some nutrients than the parts consumed. The fact that ascorbic acid is a relatively unstable nutri-ent, being readily destroyed by heat, oxida-tion, and alkali, suggests that people be urged to use methods of preparation and harvesting that minimize the loss of nu-trients such as limiting exposure to air, especially at high temperatures, cooking in a minimum amount of water for the short-est period of time, keeping the period of storage to a minimum, and serving imme-diately after cooking. Other seasonal fruits rich in ascorbic acid are strawberries, can-taloupe, and cherries; among vegetables, broccoli, asparagus, spinach, and cabbage are important sources, especially when they are prepared in a way that minimizes losses during preparation.

Since relatively few of the dark green or yellow fruits and vegetables that are very rich sources of vitamin A are popular items in the diet, it was thought that a more realistic approach to a food guide would be to suggest the use of these every other day. This was additionally justified because of the stability of vitamin A and the fact that those foods that are rich sources usually provide more than the day's allowance in one serving, which means that the excess will be stored for future use. Thus a daily intake of foods rich in vitamin A is not absolutely necessary although it may be desirable. The amount of vitamin A in some typical dark green and yellow vegetables is given in Table 14-5, where the relationship between degree of pigmentation and vitamin A values become apparent.

Aside from the unique contributions of vitamin A and ascorbic acid the fruit and vegetable group contributes about 25% of the day's intake of iron; this could conceivably be much higher. The amount varies with the foods chosen, iron content being higher in leaves than in stems, fruit, or underground portions. Calcium intake from this group is small compared to that from the milk group but will assume more importance if milk intake is low. If peas or beans are chosen a rich source of thiamine is provided and riboflavin will be high if dark green leafy vegetables such as spinach are used.

Generally speaking, fruits and vegetables are poor sources of protein and that present is of low biological value because of a lack of some essential amino acids. Roots and tubers contain 2% protein and 20% carbohydrate while legumes such as peas and beans have 4% protein and 13% carbohydrate. Of the latter group, soybeans have a high biological value, and while they

Table 14-4. Comparison of ascorbic acid content of different fruit juices*

Juice	Milligrams of ascorbic acid per 100 gm.
Orange, fresh	50
Orange, frozen	45
Grapefruit	38
Tomato	16
Pineapple	9
Apple	1
Prune	1
Grape	Trace
Commercially enriched juices	25

*Based on Watts, B., and Merrill, A.: Composition of foods—raw, processed and prepared, U. S. Department of Agriculture Handbook No. 8, Washington, D. C., 1963, U. S. Department of Agriculture.

Table 14-5. Vitamin A content of representative vegetables*

Vegetable	Vitamin A per 100 gm. (I.U.)
Carrots, cooked	10,500
Kale	8,900
Spinach, cooked	8,100
Sweet potatoes, cooked	8,100
Mustard greens	7,000
Winter squash, baked	4,200
Endive	3,300
Asparagus, cooked	900
Green beans, cooked	540
Peas, cooked	540
Yellow corn, cooked	400
Lima beans, cooked	280
Leaf lettuce	264
Celery, raw	240
Head lettuce	175

*Ibid.

have been promoted extensively in under-developed countries as a source of protein, the production of soybean oil is the major use of the product in the United States. The energy contribution of the fruit and vegetable group is generally low because of the high proportion of cellulose and water and virtually no fat content. Immature seeds such as peas and beans and starchy tubers such as potatoes contribute two to four times as many calories as do celery, carrots, spinach, and cabbage, which are high in cellulose and water but low in starch. One must remember, however, that the caloric contribution of a fruit or vegetable may double or triple, depending on the way it is served or the type of product in which it is incorporated, as shown in Table 5-4.

Table 14-6, based on data from an Agricultural Research Service study, shows the percentage of the total intake of each nutrient provided by fruits and vegetables. Because they contribute a higher percent-age of the intake of the seven nutrients than they do of calories, fruits and vegetables can truly be called protective foods.

Another important nutritional benefit from the use of fruits and vegetables can be attributed to the bulk provided by cellulose. This promotes normal gastric motility and greatly facilitates the passage of food through the digestive tract, thus aiding in the prevention of constipation.

One should not overlook the value of many fruits in stimulating the appetite, as sources of an organic acid in the stomach to facilitate calcium and iron absorption in persons with a reduced secretion of hydrochloric acid, and the beneficial effect on dental health if fruits, sometimes described as "detergent food," are eaten at the end of a meal. In this capacity they help remove carbohydrate that may have adhered to the tooth surface.

Meat, fish, and poultry

The inclusion of meat and meat substitutes as a separate group is justified on the basis of the amount of high-quality protein it provides. As shown in Fig. 14-3, the meat group contributes about 50% of the protein in the diet as well as 43% of the iron and 50% of the niacin. One average 3- to 4-ounce serving should contribute about 20 gm. of protein, but the amount will vary slightly with the type of meat. Table 14-7 expresses the approximate composition of different meats, and Table 14-8 shows the amount needed to provide 20 gm. of protein. Meat substitutes such as eggs, cheese, peas, beans, or peanut butter may contain somewhat less, but since they are usually consumed in combination with cereal protein, as in cheese or peanut butter sandwiches, cereal and milk, or eggs on toast, the combined protein values will approach that of a meat and will usually cost less.

The lipid contribution of meat is quite variable, ranging from 1% to 40%; it depends on the type of animal, its condition at

Table 14-6. Percentages of various nutrients provided by fruits and vegetables*

Nutrient	Percentage
Energy	8.6
Protein	7.1
Calcium	8.7
Iron	19.7
Vitamin A value	52.4
Thiamine	20.2
Riboflavin	9.0
Niacin	18.1
Ascorbic acid	92.4

*From Stiebeling, H.: Foods of the vegetable-fruit group—their contributions to nutritionally adequate diets, Borden Rev. Nutr. Res. **25:**51, 1964.

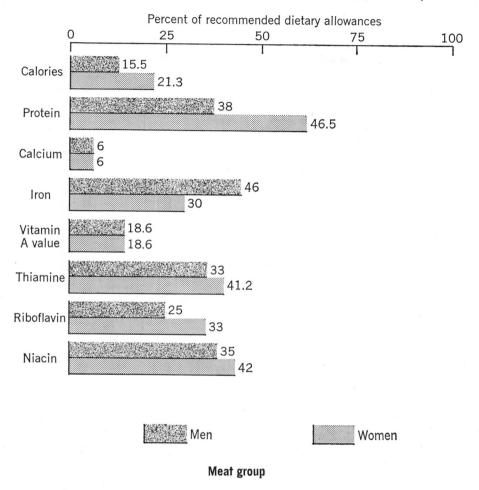

Percent of recommended dietary allowances

Calories	Men	15.5
	Women	21.3
Protein	Men	38
	Women	46.5
Calcium	Men	6
	Women	6
Iron	Men	46
	Women	30
Vitamin A value	Men	18.6
	Women	18.6
Thiamine	Men	33
	Women	41.2
Riboflavin	Men	25
	Women	33
Niacin	Men	35
	Women	42

Men   Women

Meat group

Fig. 14-3

Nutritive contribution of two servings of meat or meat substitute to the diet of an adult.

time of slaughter, the cut, the extent to which the meat is trimmed, and the method of preparation. The higher the grade of meat, the more fat marbled throughout the muscle fiber and the higher the caloric value. Prime grade beef may have 25% lipid compared to 16% in standard grade and even less in utility grade. Fish and shellfish contain high-quality protein that is easily digested; and at the same time they are relatively low in lipid content.

Dried peas and beans, with a protein content ranging as high as 35%, and nuts,

with 15% protein, are frequent substitutes in the meat group. Two to three eggs, with 6 gm. of protein each, are also a good substitute for meat.

The amount of iron depends on the meat chosen, being low in chicken and fish but very high in glandular organs. Pork liver is the richest source of iron and also one of the least expensive. Muscle meats high in both hemoglobin and myoglobin plus liberal amounts of iron-containing enzymes are good iron sources.

Since phosphorus is a component of most

Table 14-7. Approximate composition of meat and meat substitutes

Food	Moisture (percent)	Protein (percent)	Fat (percent)	Calories per 100 gm.
Beef	60.3	18.5	21.0	263
Pork (medium fat)	48.5	12.7	38.5	401
Veal	68.0	19.1	12.0	190
Lamb	56.0	13.4	27.1	310
Chicken	63.8	31.6	3.4	166
Egg (whole)	73.7	12.9	11.5	163
Salmon	63.4	27.0	7.4	182
Cod	64.6	28.5	5.3	170
Lobster	76.8	18.5	1.5	95
Scallops	73.1	23.2	1.4	112
Sardines	70.7	19.2	8.6	160

proteins, meat is one of the best sources of phosphorus in the diet.

The vitamin content of the general classes of meat is shown in Table 14-9. If pork is chosen, the meat group becomes the major source of thiamine.

Table 14-8. Amount of meat or meat substitutes needed to provide 20 gm. of protein

Food	Grams
Chicken	67
Cod	70
Veal	74
Beef liver	77
Peanut butter	80
Lamb	90
Dried peas	90
Pork	90
Salmon (pink)	100
Luncheon meat	105
Frankfurters	160
Eggs	160

Because of its high protein and hence tryptophan content, the meat group becomes a major contributor of niacin in the diet, two servings providing about 50% of the recommended allowance; veal and poultry are the richest sources.

The vitamin A, calcium, and ascorbic acid contents of meat are very low. Liver is a rich source of vitamin A and kidney a good source of ascorbic acid, but since neither is a consistent item in the diet, meat makes a limited contribution of these nutrients in the diet.

Meat is often the most expensive single item on the menu; thus we have come to plan our meal around the meat or protein dish. The cost of a serving of meat may range from a low of eight cents for pork liver to a high of sixty cents for filet mignon for a 3- to 4-ounce serving.

Cereal and cereal products

Four servings of enriched or whole-grain cereal products are recommended primarily for their contribution to the day's intake of thiamine, riboflavin, niacin, and iron (Fig. 14-4). The contribution of this group to the protein intake may be significant.

Table 14-9. Content of B complex vitamins in 100 gm. of meat and eggs*

Food	Thiamine (mg.)	Riboflavin (mg.)	Nicotinic acid (mg.)	Vitamin B_6 (mg.)	Pantothenic acid (mg.)	Folic acid (μg.)	Vitamin B_{12} (μg.)
Beef	0.08	0.15	4.5	0.35	0.7	14	2.5
Veal	0.17	0.35	7.0	0.35	0.7	20	1.2
Pork	0.8	0.18	4.1	0.45	0.7	7	1.0
Lamb	0.15	0.20	4.6	0.35	0.7	7	2.8
Poultry	0.08	0.16	7.0	0.50	0.8	3	3.2
Eggs	0.1	0.35	0.1	0.25	1.3	8	0.7

*From Siedler, A. J.: Nutritional contributions of the meat group to an adequate diet, Borden Rev. Nutr. Res. **24:**29, 1963.

Although most cereal products, with 7% to 14% protein, contain incomplete or low-quality protein, they are so frequently served in conjunction with a complete protein that will provide the essential amino acid lacking that the quality of the cereal protein is improved. Examples are macaroni and cheese, rice with chicken, poached egg on toast, or cereal and milk. In addition, two vegetable or cereal products served at the same time can supplement each other. The current practice of using dried milk solids in commercially prepared bakery products enhances the protein quality.

The early concept that only such products as bread, rice, macaroni, and dry or cooked cereal would fulfill the recommendation for the cereal group has been modified so that any product made primarily of flour will be considered in the group. Although only 30 states have compulsory enrichment of bread and flour, over 80% of the flour now sold in the United States is enriched, and it is felt that most products made from flour contain appreciable amounts of the B vitamins and iron. Thus, waffles, muffins, pancakes, pastry, cakes, and cookies can all be considered part of the cereal group. The use of milk or non-fat milk solids in many of these products increases the calcium to significant levels and supplements the cereal protein. One of the major justifications for the inclusion of cereal products is the contribution of relatively significant amounts of many nutrients at minimum cost.

One ounce of cereal, dry weight, is considered as one serving. Thus one ounce of a prepared cereal such as bran flakes or one ounce of cooked oatmeal will provide an average serving. The volume of one ounce of puffed cereal is usually so large that only half an ounce will be used as a serving.

Recently there has been a trend in the highly competitive breakfast cereal business to promote a cereal product enriched with any number of nutrients in addition to thiamine, riboflavin, niacin, and iron (which must be added to enriched cereals) and vitamin D and calcium (which are optional nutrients). There seems little justification for adding lysine to provide the limiting amino acid in most cereals or for adding ascorbic acid or vitamin A and D to cereal products. None of these are nutrients normally present in whole-grain cereal nor

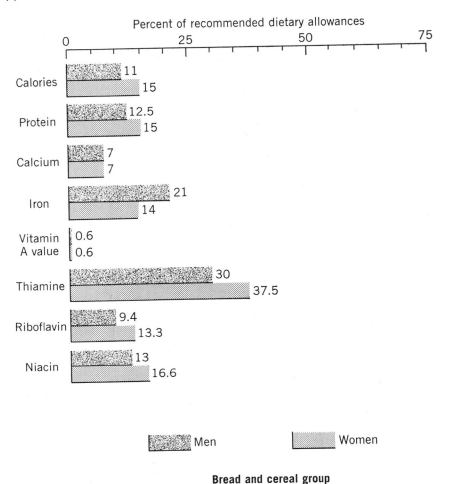

Percent of recommended dietary allowances

Bread and cereal group

Fig. 14-4
Nutritive contribution of four servings of whole-grain or enriched cereal to the diet of an adult.

are they generally lacking in the western diet; therefore their addition seems only to raise the cereal to the status of a glorified vitamin pill, which apparently gives it some trade advantage.

Converted rice is an interesting item in the cereal group. It is prepared by parboiling the rice kernels prior to polishing. During this process the nutrients normally concentrated in the outer husk are driven into the kernel, where they remain when the husk is removed. Thus, we have a refined cereal that has been enriched with its own

nutrients. This process has been used in India for many years.

FOUNDATION OF AN ADEQUATE DIET

As can be seen from Fig. 14-5, the inclusion of 2 cups of milk or its equivalent, two servings of meat or meat substitutes, four servings of fruit and vegetables, and four servings of enriched or whole-grain cereals will ensure an intake of over 75% of the NRC recommended daily allowances of all nutrients except calories for the adult male. With this foundation there is little

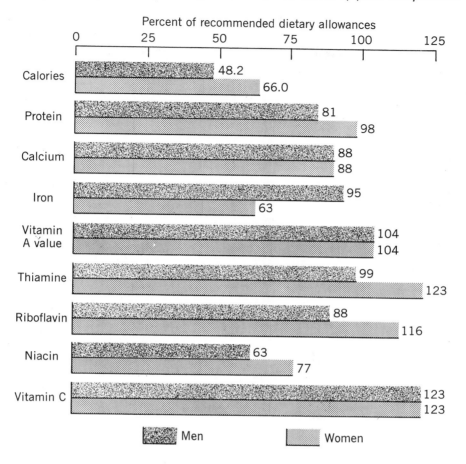

Four food group essentials of adequate diet

Fig. 14-5

Contribution of all four food groups of the essentials of an adequate diet to the nutritive intake of the adult.

need for guidance in the selection of additional foods to provide the calories needed to meet individual requirements. In many cases it will be met at least partially through additional servings of the four food groups. The use of the visible fats and oils, which are natural accompaniments to the cereals and vegetables and which constitute about one third of the total fat intake, will provide upwards of 15% of the total calories. The use of carbohydrate-rich foods, which is advocated by some trade

groups as the least expensive way of obtaining the additional calories, does not receive the wholehearted endorsement of nutritionists because of the adverse effect that sugar, especially in the form of icings or sticky candies, has on dental health.

For women, prior to the menopause there is need to stress the use of foods high in iron as sources of the additional calories since these women are the group most likely to have an intake inadequate in iron.

The number of calories provided by the

Table 14-10. Caloric value of two diet patterns meeting requirements of essentials of an adequate diet*

Food group	Diet I foods	Kilocalories	Diet II foods	Kilocalories
Milk	Nonfat milk (2 cups)	160	Whole milk (1½ cups)	290
			Ice cream (½ cup)	145
Meat	Chicken, broiled (3 ounces)	185	Chicken, fried (3 ounces)	245
	Salmon, canned (3 ounces)	120	Ham (3 ounces)	340
Fruit and	Tomato juice (½ cup)	25	Sweet potatoes, baked	155
vegetable	Carrots (½ cup)	22	Lima beans	75
	Apple (1 medium)	70	Grape juice (½ cup)	82
	Green beans (½ cup)	12	Figs (4)	120
Cereal	Puffed wheat (1 cup)	50	1 waffle	240
	Bread, thin-sliced (3 slices)	135	2 cookies (3-inch diameter)	220
			Oatmeal (1 ounce)	115
			Muffin	135
Total		879		2162

*Calculations are based only on energy value of the food prepared and served without any flavor adjunct such as butter, sugar, syrup, sauces, etc. Based on Nutritive value of foods, Home and Garden Bulletin No. 72, Washington, D. C., 1960, U. S. Department of Agriculture.

four basic food groups will depend on the selection of foods made within each category. To illustrate the range possible within the specifications of the four-group plan, the caloric value of two extremes is calculated in Table 14-10. Admittedly there will be differences in the level of other nutrients also, but the selection was made within the framework of the plan.

As the Food and Nutrition Board of the National Research Council emphasized with the publication of its first dietary standards, the level of nutrition they advocated as a goal in planning the food supplies of the nations could be met in innumerable ways by an unlimited combination of foods. The suggestions made in the basic four groups represent but one pattern that follows dietary practices acceptable to a large number of people living in the United States. Although adherence to such a plan will usually ensure at least a minimal level of nutritional adequacy, failure

to follow such a plan must never be construed as evidence of dietary inadequacy, but it should prompt a more careful evaluation of its nutritive content. Such a guide does provide a quick and easy basis for evaluating the adequacy of a prescribed or popular diet. If the minimum recommendations are met one can be reasonably confident that the diet has a sound nutritional basis.

That the food supply available to the American public has the potential for meeting the nutritional needs of all citizens is evident in Table 14-11, in which estimates of the amount of each nutrient available per person at the retail level are tabulated.

DIETARY STANDARDS

Although the concept that food contained more than the energy-yielding nutrients was well established by 1920 and a knowledge of the role and need for many

Table 14-11. Estimate of nutrients available per person per day on the retail markets in the United States compared to NRC recommended allowances for the adult male*

Allowances for adult male	Amount available	Recommended allowances
Energy (kilocalories)	3170	2900
Protein (grams)	97	70
Fat (grams)	147	
Carbohydrate (grams)	371	
Calcium (grams)	0.96	0.8
Phosphorus (grams)	1.51	
Iron (milligrams)	16.6	10.0
Vitamin A (I.U.)	7700	5000
Thiamine (milligrams)	1.83	1.20
Riboflavin (milligrams)	2.26	1.70
Niacin (milligrams)	21.5	19
Ascorbic acid (milligrams)	99	75

*From Nutritive value of food available for consumption, United States, 1909-1964, Agricultural Research Service Publication 62-14, 1966.

other nutrients had been ascertained by 1935, it was not until 1940 that any formal effort was made in the United States to evaluate existing knowledge and establish dietary standards. Previous efforts on the part of individuals and groups had attracted very little attention. The economic depression of the 1930's focused attention on some nutritional deficiencies, and some effort was made to incorporate the then-current knowledge of nutrition in programs of food subsidization. It was only in the face of threat of war in 1940, however, that there was any strong feeling that nutritional science could make a contribution to the national security. The country had been appalled at the very high rejection rate among young service recruits for reasons that could be attributed to suboptimal nutrition. It was against this background that 25 scientists met in 1940 as the first Food and Nutrition Board of the National Research Council, charged with the respon-

sibility of establishing dietary standards that could be used to evaluate the dietary intake of large population groups and to provide a rational guide for practical nutrition and for the planning of agricultural production schedules. It was recognized that there was insufficient evidence of the nutritional needs of humans to propose exact requirements but that there was a need for a standard that reflected more than minimum needs. It was felt that even if the standards based on the available information should later prove to be inaccurate they were very necessary. Indeed, it was with the belief and hope that they would soon be revised that the first standards were proposed.

National Research Council recommended allowances

The task of determining dietary standards was not an easy one. In the case of some nutrients there was very little information available, for others there was little agreement among the fifty or more scientists consulted, and for others it was recognized that there seemed to be such a wide range of requirements for the individual that it was difficult to arrive at an acceptable figure. The data on which judgments were made was derived from surveys of large groups of individuals to determine presence or absence of disease in relation to nutritive intake, from controlled feeding experiments with limited numbers of individuals, and from critical metabolic studies on several species of animals. The group did, however, agree in 1941 on the first National Research Council recommended dietary allowances (RDA), which were published in 1943. These allowances were numerical expressions of the quantities of certain nutrients believed to be needed by individuals who were classified into several age and sex categories for essentially all healthy persons in the United States under the existing conditions. They did not represent average requirements, which would be adequate for only half the population, but figures that would include the whole range of requirements of all normal healthy persons. As such they became goals to be used in planning national food supplies and meals for large groups. The term *allowance* was purposely chosen to avoid any implication of finality and to encourage a reevaluation of the figures as more information on which to base judgments became available. In order to allow for nutrient losses that might occur in cooking and storage of food, to cover the wide range of requirements in the population, and to provide a buffer under stress conditions, a margin of safety of from 10% to 50% was added to the minimum requirements for each nutrient. The amount added varied from one nutrient to another, depending on the body's ability to store the nutrient, the range of observed requirements, the availability of the nutrient in the American diet, the possible hazards from an excessive intake, and the difficulties involved in establishing precise requirements.

It was emphasized that the allowances did not provide a criterion for judging the nutritional status of an individual but were a valuable guide for persons involved in feeding a population group. For individuals they served as a point of reference for judging nutritional adequacy; but only when an individual showed clinical, physical, or biochemical evidence of a dietary lack in addition to the suboptimal intake could he be considered deficient in the nutrient.

The original recommended dietary allowances have undergone five revisions, the latest being published in 1964. These are presented in Appendix C. The philosophy on which the allowances are based has remained essentially the same, but improved analytical techniques and increased knowledge of the biological importance of most nutrients has led to some change and to an increasing level of confidence in the recommended allowances, although the figures do not represent the opinions of all nutritionists. It is still believed that they provide sufficient buffer in cases of nutritional stress but will not meet the additional requirements of persons depleted by disease. The major goal of the allowances is to permit and encourage the development of food practices by the population of the United States that will provide the greatest dividends in health and resistance to disease.

Although the RDA have never been assumed to be either a minimal or optimal level of intake they have served several useful purposes. They have provided a yardstick for groups like the Quartermaster Corps in planning diets. They have been widely accepted as a basis for evaluating diets, as an official guide for practically all nutrition projects, such as the school lunch program and cereal enrichment, and a basis for formulating regulations governing the composition of foods, dietary supplements, and drugs. They are admittedly high for use under conditions of economic stringency or national emergencies but under normal conditions are a worthwhile goal.

In addition to the ten nutrients for which discrete recommendations are made many other nutrients are discussed in light of our current knowledge of their requirements and major biological roles. Among those discussed are carbohydrate, fat, alcohol, water, several micronutrient elements, cobalamin, folacin, pyridoxine, pantothenic acid, biotin, vitamin E, and vitamin K. It is hoped that the lack of information on requirements for these nutrients will stimulate research.

Other dietary standards

Many other countries have established dietary standards for their populations. However, comparison or evaluation of these is not valid until one recognizes the philosophy behind them. Care must be taken to distinguish among terms such as standards, requirements, and allowances,

which must be defined before an interpretation of proposed nutrient intake can be made.

The British Medical Association had a slightly different philosophy in establishing the British dietary standards. They chose levels they felt represented the needs of the average healthy individual that were never intended, as were the American standards, to cover the needs of all persons. British standards tend to be lower for some nutrients than American standards, although in a few instances they are the same in spite of the differences in philosophy behind them. The Canadian standard of 1964 is based on a sufficient excess above minimum requirements for the maintenance of health among the marjority of Canadians. Previously they had considered their standards a nutritional floor below which adequate nutrition cannot be assumed but one well above the level required to prevent clinical deficiency symptoms.

The Food and Agricultural Organization (FAO), charged with devising a standard to

Table 14-12. Comparison of United States, British, Canadian, and FAO dietary standards for the adult male and adult female

Classification	Kilo-calories	Protein (gm.)	Calcium (gm.)	Iron (mg.)	Vitamin A (I.U.)	Thiamine (mg.)	Riboflavin (mg.)	Ascorbic acid (mg.)
United States								
Female (128 pounds, 64 inches)	2100	58	0.8	15	5000	0.8	1.3	70
Male (154 pounds, 69 inches)	2900	70	0.8	10	5000	1.2	1.7	70
Britain								
Female	2250	66	0.8	12	5000	0.9	1.4	20
Male	2750	80	0.8	12	5000	1.1	1.6	20
Canada								
Female (124 pounds)	2400	40	0.5	10	3700	0.70	1.2	30
Male (158 pounds)	2850	50	0.5	6	3700	0.90	1.4	30
FAO		34	0.4 to 0.5					

meet the needs of fully active, healthy individuals that is equally applicable in all cultures under vastly different agricultural and climatic conditions, has thus far proposed practical allowances for three nutrients—calories, calcium, and protein. A comparison of the American, Canadian, British, and FAO standards is given in Table 14-12.

Minimum daily requirements

A second set of dietary standards is used in the United States by the Food and Drug Administration for labelling purposes. These are known as minimum daily requirements (MDR) and provide a standard legally acceptable for use by food processors in making claims for the nutritive content of their product in advertising. They do not bear a consistent relationship to RDA but are invariably lower. This is frequently a source of confusion to consumers who do not recognize the difference in the two standards. Thus one finds the distributor of a fruit juice containing 30 mg. of ascorbic acid per 4-ounce serving advertising that one serving will provide 100% of the adult MDR. This is not, however, 100% but only 43% of the RDA of 70 mg. for an adult. A comparison of minimum

daily requirements (MDR) and recommended dietary allowances (RDA) is given in Table 14-13.

FOOD COMPOSITION TABLES

While the use of food composition tables as applied to food intake records provide our least expensive and most widely used tool in estimating the nutrient intake of an individual or group, it is only with an understanding of the method by which the tables were developed that one can recognize their limitations and make an intelligent interpretation of the results. The food composition tables in Appendix F are based on values in the standard publication for food composition in the United States, U. S. Department of Agriculture Handbook No. 8—*Composition of foods— Raw, Processed and Prepared*. Originally published in 1950 and revised in 1964, this publication presents food values in terms of 100-gm. edible portion (E.P.) and one pound as purchased (A.P.) of the foods. Information is given about the energy value and contribution of 16 different nutrients for 2483 food items in the 1964 edition, which represents an expansion from values on energy and 11 nutrients for 751 foods in 1950. In Appendix F, as in the U. S. De-

Table 14-13. Comparison of minimum daily requirements (MDR) and recommended daily allowances (RDA) for several nutrients

Nutrient	MDR (adults)	RDA (adult man)	MDR (children 6-11 years)	RDA (boys 9-12 years)
Vitamin A (I.U.)	4000	5000	3000	4500
Thiamine (mg.)	1.0	1.2	0.75	1.0
Riboflavin (mg.)	1.2	1.7	0.9	1.4
Ascorbic acid (mg.)	30	70	20	70
Vitamin D (I.U.)	400	—	400	400
Calcium (gm.)	0.75	0.80	0.75	
Iron (mg.)	10	10	10	

partment of Agriculture Home and Garden Bulletin No. 72 (1964), food values are expressed in terms of average servings or common household units. Differences in values for the same foods in these two editions may reflect changes in marketing and processing techniques as well as improved analytical techniques. For instance, breeding of poultry has produced a product with a reduced fat content, the use of dried milk solids in bread has led to an increase in its calcium content, and the use of cooking oils with higher percentages of unsaturated fatty acids has changed the character of fat in many food products.

While the details of the biological and chemical techniques by which the values are derived are beyond the scope of this discussion, some mention of the methods by which the data were compiled should provide a rational basis on which to evaluate the values obtained in dietary calculations.

There is great variation in the amount and specificity of data available for different foods and different nutrients. Much data that was potentially useful could not be used because of a lack of an adequate description of the product, the source of the product, the method of processing, or the basis on which data were presented. Most of the data was obtained from published and unpublished analyses made by laboratories of government agencies, colleges, universities, and private industry. Only data on food samples adequately identified was usable. In some cases very few or only a single analytical report were available. In other cases data was available on several varieties of the same food at several seasons of the year and from various geographic areas. An example of such is the ascorbic acid in oranges. The single value appearing in the table represents a weighted average obtained by making use of marketing information on the extent to which each variety was consumed, percentage of the domestic production coming from

each geographic area, and the size of the crop in each season. Thus, while the value may not be accurate for any one specific orange it does provide a value representative of all oranges consumed in the United States.

Similarly, values for other foods and nutrients take into account varietal, seasonal, and geographic differences in the nutrient content of foods, loss or gain of nutrients through harvesting, handling, commercial processing, packaging, storage, home practices of preparation, cooking, serving, and consumption statistics. The factors that result in changes in the content of important nutrients vary with both the food and the nutrient. The vitamin A value of sweet potatoes varies with the variety, the ascorbic acid in potatoes with the maturity and conditions of storage, vitamin A in butter with the season, and ascorbic acid in oranges with the site of production and the time of harvesting.

In addition to Handbook No. 8, there are many other food composition tables in wide use today that are based on sound analytical data. The beginning student is cautioned not to be concerned over differences between values from different tables since they often merely represent slightly different interpretations of the same analytical data. Usually the differences are small when one considers the errors in the methods of collecting data. To be concerned over minor differences is to attribute an unwarranted degree of accuracy to the tables.

The nutrients for which values are presented in the table are those for which data was available for a sufficient number of foods to justify their inclusion. For nutrients such as pantothenic acid, folic acid, amino acids, vitamin B_{12} and magnesium, tables have been published separately. As more precise analytical methods become available tables for other nutrients will undoubtedly be published.

For those nutrients currently tabulated

a brief explanation of the derivation of the values follows.

Energy value expressed as kilocalories is calculated by a modification of a method used by Atwater in 1899 when the first table of chemical composition of food was published. In this, an energy equivalent is determined for each gram of carbohydrate, fat, and protein in a range of separate food groups such as eggs, milk, meat, fruits and vegetables, and cereals. These are based on the heat of combustion (as measured in the bomb calorimeter) for each of these energy-yielding nutrients and the coefficients of digestibility for each of these in each general class of food. From data on the carbohydrate, fat, and protein in a food, it is then possible to calculate the energy value of a food.

The values of 4, 9, and 4 kilocalories per gram of carbohydrate, fat, and protein respectively are widely used to represent their physiologic fuel values. Their use is justified when applied to whole diets but because these values vary from one food to another they must be used with reservation for individual foods. For instance, the physiologic fuel value of protein for which the widest variation is found is 4.35, 4.25, 2.70, 3.20, 3.15, and 2.90 kilocalories from eggs, meat, cereals, legumes, fruits, and vegetables respectively. The calculations shown in Table 14-14 illustrate variations in heat of combustion, coefficients of digestibility, and hence physiologic fuel values observed with different foods.

Protein is determined by measuring the nitrogen in a food, and from knowledge of the percentage of nitrogen in a specific protein, which is constant, it is possible to calculate the amount of protein. Many proteins such as eggs, meat, corn, and beans contain 16% nitrogen, but others such as milk contain less and nuts and many cereals slightly more. Assuming an average of 16% nitrogen in protein, a factor of 6.25 has been widely used to convert nitrogen values to protein values, especially in mixed diets, but if a more precise figure is needed factors of 6.38 for milk, 5.7 for refined flour, 5.8 for whole-wheat flour, and 5.3 for nuts give more accurate estimates. The fact that all foods, especially vegetables, contain some nonprotein nitrogen is a source of error in protein calculations.

Fat values are admittedly difficult to determine and have been obtained largely by simple solvent extraction methods. This method may overestimate by including nonfat material and underestimate by fail-

Table 14-14. Calculations of physiologic fuel value of energy-yielding nutrients in two classes of foods

Food	Heat of combustion	Coefficient of digestibility	Physiologic food value
Eggs			
Protein	4.50	97	4.36
Fat	9.50	95	9.02
Carbohydrate	3.75	98	3.68
Potatoes			
Carbohydrate	4.20	96	4.03
Fat	9.30	90	8.37
Protein	3.75	74	2.78

ing to separate the fat from a protein-fat or carbohydrate-fat complex in which it frequently occurs in food.

Carbohydrate values are obtained by subtracting the total percentage of water, mineral, protein, and fat from 100. This is known as *carbohydrate by difference* and is used because there is no satisfactory method of determining carbohydrate by direct analysis. The values for carbohydrate include sugars, starches, fiber, and other complex forms of carbohydrate, some of which are not available to the human as a source of energy. The values reported for indigestible fiber or cellulose are based on methods which now appear to yield low values as new procedures suggest values three to four times as high.

The food composition tables record values for vitamin A in food and the potential vitamin A from the precursor carotenoids. In foods such as oranges and corn where cryptoxanthine, a biologically active precursor of vitamin A, is present in large amounts, the vitamin A values may be underestimated since methods for determining carotenes do not include cryptoxanthine. On the other hand, some yellow- and red-pigmented foods have carotenoids that are not physiologically available but which will be measured. Even when it is accurately measured the extent to which carotene is utilized varies from 33% to 100%. Some vitamin A values are obtained by biological assay and others by physiochemical means.

Thiamine values are determined by chemical or microbiological methods but make no allowances for the losses which may occur through solution or destruction by heat or alkali during home preparation and storage. Riboflavin is generally determined by fluorometric and microbiological methods, but no method has been developed to assess the increase in riboflavin which occurs with cooking which may reflect the liberation of bound riboflavin not measured by current methods. Methods of

determining niacin involve the conversion of the amide form that occurs in many foods to the acid form. Although it has been well established that tryptophan in excess of the body's needs for protein synthesis can be converted into niacin (60 mg. tryptophan yielding 1 mg. niacin) the values in the tables report only niacin content and not niacin equivalents (niacin content plus niacin that could be formed from tryptophan). It is suggested that niacin equivalents will be about 50% higher than the niacin values recorded in the tables even after subtracting about 500 mg. of tryptophan to meet the needs for protein synthesis.

The National Research Council, on the other hand, has recognized that the body does not discriminate between niacin which is preformed in food and niacin obtained from tryptophan and has established its allowance in terms of niacin equivalents. It is very possible then that the calculated niacin values for a diet may be considerably lower than the actual niacin available so that failure of a calculated diet to meet an established standard cannot be considered evidence of an inadequate intake of the nutrient.

One interesting aspect of the niacin content of foods is the presence of a biologically inactive form of the vitamin trigonelline in many seeds and nuts. The roasting process for coffee beans tends to convert it into an active form so that coffee beverage provides some niacin in the diet.

A similar situation exists in regard to the data for ascorbic acid in food composition tables. We know that the body uses both reduced ascorbic acid and dehydroascorbic acid. However, the limited data available on dehydroascorbic acid and total ascorbic acid values had led to the inclusion of only reduced ascorbic acid values in the current food composition tables for raw, canned, and dehydrated fruit and vegetables. For some foods this may lead to markedly low values while for others the differences may be insignificant. It is highly possible that for such a labile nutrient as ascorbic acid that any underestimate caused by failure to include the variable dehydroascorbic acid values will merely compensate for losses during storage and preparation or for the measurement of other reducing substances as ascorbic acid. It is also possible that some dehydroascorbic acid undergoes further oxidation to an inactive form. The data for frozen foods includes the total for dehydroascorbic acid and reduced ascorbic acid and were obtained on foods under rather ideal conditions permitting almost complete retention of the vitamin. These values may be high since much storage of frozen foods is under less than ideal conditions and treatment of the food during thawing and serving may cause considerable loss.

In spite of their recognized limitations, the food composition tables allow estimates of the nutritive content of diets that approximate those determined by direct chemical analysis but at a much lower cost in time, equipment, and money. These tables represent an indispensable tool for people concerned with evaluating national food supplies, developing programs of food distribution, planning and evaluating food consumption surveys, and in estimating the nutritive intake of individuals. The availability of the information from food composition tables on cards and magnetic tapes for use in computers has greatly facilitated the use of this information in menu planning and the analysis of dietary intake and has increased tremendously the scope of calculations that can be reasonably made with this information.

SELECTED REFERENCES

Selection of an adequate diet

Maynard, L. A.: An adequate diet, J.A.M.A. **170**:457, 1959.
Phipard, E. F., and Page, L.: Meeting nutritional needs through foods, Borden Rev. Nutr. Res. **23**:31, 1962.
Siedler, A. J.: Nutritional contributions of the meat group to an adequate diet, Borden Rev. Nutr. Res. **24**:29, 1963.

Stiebeling H. K.: Foods of the vegetable-fruit group—their contributions to nutritionally adequate diets, Borden Rev. Nutr. Res. **25**:51, 1964.

Dietary standards

Dietary standards for Canada, Canad. Bull. Nutrition **6**:1, 1964.
Engel, R. W.: 1963 recommended dietary allowances, J. Am. Dietet. A. **44**:91, 1964.
Food and Nutrition Board, National Research Council: Recommended dietary allowances, Publication No. 1146, Washington, D. C., 1964, National Research Council.
Food and Agricultural Organization: Protein requirements, FAO Nutr. Stud., No. 16, 1957.
Food and Agricultural Organization: Calorie requirements, FAO Nutr. Stud., No. 15, 1957.
Food and Agricultural Organization: Calcium requirements, FAO Nutrition Meeting Report Series No. 30, 1962.
Hegsted, D. M.: Establishment of nutritional requirements in man, Borden Rev. Nutr. Res. **20**:13, 1959.
Report of Committee on Nutrition, London, 1950, British Medical Association.
Roberts, L. J.: Beginnings of the recommended dietary allowances, J. Am. Dietet. A. **34**:903, 1958.

Food composition

Amino acid content of foods, Home Economics Research Report No. 4, Washington, D. C., 1957, U. S. Department of Agriculture.
Fatty acid content of foods, Home Economics Research Report No. 7, Washington, D. C., 1959, U. S. Department of Agriculture.
Folic acid content of foods, U. S. Department of Agriculture Handbook No. 29, Washington, D. C., 1951, U. S. Department of Agriculture.
Hardinge, M. G., and Crooks, H.: Lesser known vitamin in foods, J. Am. Dietet. A. **38**:240, 1961.
Harris, R. S.: Reliability of nutrient analyses and food tables, Am. J. Clin. Nutrition **11**:377, 1962.
Leung, W. T. W.: Problems in compiling food composition data, J. Am. Dietet. A. **40**:19, 1962.
Mayer, J.: Food composition tables: Basis, uses, and limitations, Postgrad. Med. **28**:295, 1960.
Pantothenic acid food, U. S. Department of Agriculture Handbook No. 97, Washington, D. C., 1956, U. S. Department of Agriculture.
Watts, B.: Concepts in developing a food composition table, J. Am. Dietet. A. **40**:297, 1962.
Watts, B., and Merrill, A.: Composition of foods—raw, processed and prepared, U. S. Department of Agriculture Handbook No. 8, Washington, D. C., 1963, U. S. Department of Agriculture.

15

Evaluation of nutritional status

Just as it is relatively easy to identify individuals who are markedly obese or markedly undernourished from superficial observations, it is a simple matter to diagnose severe nutritional deficiency states such as beriberi, pellagra, or scurvy without the aid of any sensitive biochemical assessment technique. However, these deficiency diseases are encountered relatively infrequently, especially in developed countries, and the nutritionist has become concerned with developing techniques of evaluating nutritional status sufficiently sensitive to identify individuals who have a marginal nutritive intake, which fosters a low level of vitality and health and which may eventually result in subclinical nutritional deficiency symptoms. It is important to identify these conditions in the early stages before the tissue changes have advanced to a point where they cause irreversible damage. Often the severe deficiency states will become obvious only when they have prevailed for a long period of time or when a person experiences a severe stress such as surgery or a prolonged fever or infection.

While primary and secondary causes of nutritional deficiencies lead to the same results, the cause and hence the treatment will be different. For instance, the symptoms developing when the diet is devoid of vitamin B_{12}, as it is on a strict vegetarian diet, and those resulting from a genetic defect in the gastric mucosa, which prevents the formation of the intrinsic factor needed for B_{12} absorption, will be the same, but the conditions will be treated quite differently.

The ways in which nutritional deficiencies develop are outlined in Fig. 15-1. The techniques for detecting the changes are shown in boxes.

Because of the multiple causes of nutritional deficiencies and the diverse ways in which deficiencies of various nutrients manifest themselves, no one method of assessing nutritional status has proven completely satisfactory. As a result, several techniques are used to identify individuals whose limited nutritive intake or inability to absorb or utilize a nutrient have resulted in biochemical changes in tissues, which, **295**

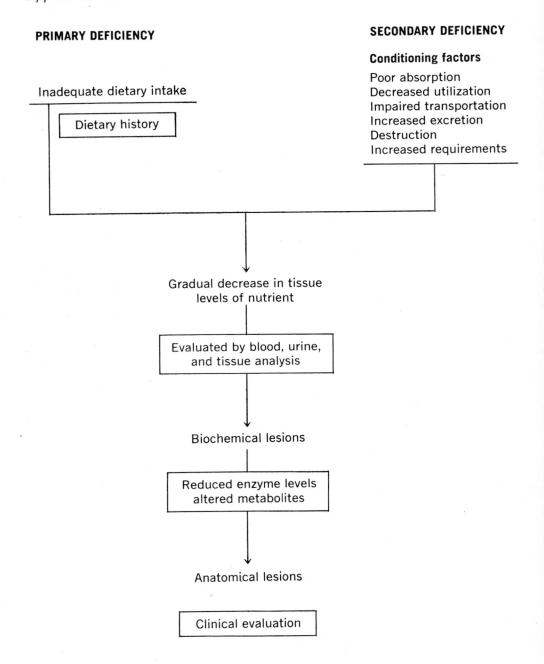

PRIMARY DEFICIENCY

SECONDARY DEFICIENCY

Conditioning factors

Poor absorption
Decreased utilization
Impaired transportation
Increased excretion
Destruction
Increased requirements

Inadequate dietary intake

Dietary history

Gradual decrease in tissue
levels of nutrient

Evaluated by blood, urine,
and tissue analysis

Biochemical lesions

Reduced enzyme levels
altered metabolites

Anatomical lesions

Clinical evaluation

Method of evaluation

Fig. 15-1

Development and evaluation of deficiency deficiencies. (Adapted from Krehl, W. A.: The evaluation of nutritional status, M. Clin. North America **48:**1129, 1964.)

if continued sufficiently long, will produce clinically observable symptoms. The techniques by which attempts are made to assess nutritional status of an individual include clinical observations, biochemical analyses, physical or anthropological measurements, and dietary evaluations. In addition, some information of nutritional adequacy of population groups can be elucidated from the vital statistics of a country. The general features and unique advantages and limitations of each of these methods will be discussed.

CLINICAL OBSERVATIONS

Clinical observations lend themselves to use in nutritional surveys of population groups because they involve an assessment of the health of those parts of the body that can be observed in a relatively short period of time in a routine physical examination and do not involve obtaining blood, urine, or tissue samples. The most commonly observed tissues are the eye, skin, hair, mouth, teeth, tongue, mucous membranes, thyroid gland, and lower extremities. Many of the changes in these tissues, while often specific for a single nutrient, do not occur until the deficiency is well advanced. In other cases they may be caused by the lack of several nutrients. While clinical observations are of limited value in the early diagnosis of a deficiency state or in identifying marginal intakes that prevail for short periods, they are widely used to confirm biochemical and dietary data. Because of the subjective nature of the judgment in a clinical evaluation, it is extremely unreliable even when used by highly skilled observers.

In the eye, the most commonly observed symptom is a dryness of the cornea and conjunctiva usually associated with a lack of vitamin A. An increase in severity of vitamin A deficiency shows up as Bitot's spots or foamy white spots in the cornea, followed by a complete opacity in the cornea in a condition known as xerophthalmia.

Infiltration of the cornea by blood vessels is associated with a low intake of riboflavin.

The color of the mucous membranes in which the blood supply is close to the surface provides an opportunity to observe the pigmentation of the blood. A pale mucous membrane is suggestive of anemia whereas a more highly colored membrane usually occurs in persons with adequate hemoglobin levels.

The condition of the skin is often a reflection of the nutritional state of the individual, although all skin changes are by no means of nutritional origin. Deficiencies of some of the vitamins manifest themselves in varying forms and degrees of dermatitis. Skin lesions on areas of the skin exposed to sunlight occur in niacin deficiency, cracks at the corners of the mouth or cheilosis reflect a lack of riboflavin, pyridoxine, or iron, and a roughness and hardness of the papillae at the base of the hair follicle is associated with a lack of vitamin A. The latter occur primarily on the arm, chest, back, and thighs. Pyridoxine deficiency sometimes causes a dermatitis in the area surrounding the nose (nasolabial area). In infants eczema may indicate an essential fatty acid deficiency. A dry inelastic skin is most frequently observed following dehydration.

The presence of small pinpoint hemorrhages under the skin following the application of either positive or negative pressure is indicative of fragility in the capillary wall, often a manifestation of ascorbic acid deficiency.

One of the first clinical observations to be correlated with a nutritional factor was the enlargement of the thyroid gland associated with a deficiency of the mineral iodine. Other clinical observations that may be significant are soft, spongy, bleeding gums, indicative of lack of ascorbic acid, edema, especially of the lower extremities, which accompanies thiamine deficiency and protein inadequacies, and inflammatory changes in the surface of the tongue, reflecting thiamine and riboflavin inadequacies. Beading of the ribs, especially at the junction with the breastbone, occurs with a lack of vitamin D.

Although tooth decay is seldom the result of current dietary inadequacies, especially in adults, an observation of the extent and nature of dental caries is usually recorded in a clinical examination.

BIOCHEMICAL EVALUATIONS

The biochemical evaluation of nutritional status involves quantitative determinations of nutrients or related metabolites in such tissues as the blood and urine. Occasionally analysis will be made of a biopsy sample of liver or bone, but the use of this rather hazardous and involved technique is not justified in routine nutritional evaluations. Variations in the composition of the blood and other body fluids often reflect changes in the quantity and composition of the diet, but an understanding of the metabolism of the nutrient is necessary to interpret the findings since in many instances the homeostatic mechanisms of the body will mask changes that would otherwise reflect nutritional status. Biochemical data often confirms findings from clinical observations and dietary studies or may identify subclinical deficiencies even when no clinical symptoms are evident. They can be used for some nutrients to assess the range from frank deficiency levels through adequate, optimal, and excessive levels of nutritive intake.

The interpretation of findings from biochemical data is hampered by the fact that the levels of many nutrients and metabolites in the blood and urine vary sufficiently throughout the day that the use of values from a single determination may be misleading. In addition, the body has many homeostatic mechanisms that operate to compensate for dietary inadequacies, such as an increased level of calcium absorption or mobilization of bone calcium when intakes are low, a decrease in energy expenditure when calories are restricted, or an increased uptake of iodine from the blood in deficiency status. It is only when the body's ability to handle these changes is overwhelmed that diagnostic changes will occur in the nutrient or metabolite levels in the blood and urine. The causes of the observed deviations—whether dietary, genetic, environmental, or physiologic—cannot always be clearly defined or separated from one another.

Many of the analytical techniques for evaluating the constituents of the blood and urine have been adapted for use on very small samples. These microtechniques enable biochemists to be able to make determinations for as many as 15 or 20 nutritional factors or metabolites with a sample of blood as small as 5 ml., which may be collected in capillary tubes from a fingertip puncture.

A discussion of all the information that can be obtained from a biochemical analysis of blood and urine is well beyond the scope of this presentation, but general types of information will be discussed.

Blood levels of nutrients

The determination of either blood serum or blood plasma nutrient level may reflect the most recent intake of a nutrient or may be indicative of the body's reserves. For instance, levels of ascorbic acid in the blood are a measure of the ascorbic acid in transit from one tissue to another, and as such reflect recent intake. After about 6 weeks of a deficient diet, however, normal vitamin C serum levels of 0.5 mg. will drop to zero when reserves are only 50% depleted. The level of the vitamin in the white blood cells, however, will drop only when tissue saturation is down to 20% of normal, which will occur only at the time other symptoms of scurvy are about to appear. Blood levels of calcium are of little value in assessing nutritional status because the body has so many mechanisms that operate to maintain normal blood levels that only when these mechanisms fail or body reserves are depleted will any change occur in blood calcium levels. The large reserves of vitamin A maintained in the liver similarly make blood vitamin A levels rather meaningless as an indicator of current intakes. Recently, increased use has been made of serum lipid values, especially cholesterol and triglycerides, to screen persons who may be potential victims of coronary heart disease.

Blood levels of metabolites

In many cases, the absence of a vitamin leads to a block in the normal series of reactions in the metabolism of carbohydrate, fat, or protein. An accumulation of one of the intermediary products in the blood often indicates a lack of the nutrient required for metabolism to proceed beyond that point. For instance, an increase in the pyruvic acid in the blood occurs when there is insufficient thiamine available to form the enzyme necessary to decarboxylate pyruvic acid formed in carbohydrate metabolism.

Tissue enzyme levels

Since many vitamins act as parts of enzymes or as coenzymes, it is frequently possible to determine the level of enzyme in a tissue as a measure of the amount of the nutrient available. For instance, the level of the enzyme transketolase in the red blood cells is a sensitive indicator of the available thiamine, which is part of a coenzyme that works in conjunction with transketolase in the metabolism of glucose. Transketolase values are easily determined, and a drop in the level may precede any other signs of a deficiency. As such, they are a valuable diagnostic tool in detecting subclinical thiamine deficiency.

An increase in the amount of another enzyme, alkaline phosphatase, occurs in a vitamin D deficiency. On the other hand, a drop in the level of this enzyme has also been reported in protein deficiency so that

these two forces in some instances may counteract one another. Since all enzymes are protein in nature, a drop in all enzyme levels could be expected when labile protein reserves are depleted.

Urine analysis

Biochemical determinations of the nutrients or metabolites in the urine often give valuable information about the nutritional status of an individual. Not only is the amount of a nutrient found in the urine significant, but the presence of substances not normally found in the urine is also informative. In a saturation test the urine is analyzed to determine the proportion of a large test dose of a water-soluble vitamin that is excreted. It is assumed that an individual whose tissues are saturated with the nutrient will retain little and excrete most of the dose while a person who has had low intakes will retain more in an effort to raise tissue levels to normal. This test has been widely used in efforts to assess the ascorbic acid status. Test doses of 200 to 1000 mg. are used.

A variation of this is a load test such as the tryptophan load test. This amino acid requires the vitamin pyridoxine if it is to be metabolized and excreted in a normal manner as an N-methylnicotinamide. If insufficient pyridoxine is available, an abnormal urinary constituent, xanthurenic acid, appears. The level of xanthurenic acid in the urine is low when pyridoxine reserves are high and high when little pyridoxine is available for tryptophan metabolism. Similarly, histidine load tests are used to evaluate folic acid nutriture. In the absence of folic acid, formiminoglutamic acid (FIGLU), an intermediary product of histidine metabolism, accumulates and appears in increased amounts in the urine.

The amount of creatinine in the urine is a direct reflection of the muscle mass of an individual. Such information is helpful in determinations of body composition, where it is desirable to know the percentage of body weight represented by fat or muscle tissue. Some other urinary data are more meaningful when expressed in terms of the amount of creatinine excreted at the same time. This is especially true where data are obtained from a single urinary sample rather than from a complete 24-hour specimen. For instance, urinary nitrogen in relation to creatinine excretion in a four-hour specimen is considered one of the best indicators of protein nutrition as well as the level of protein metabolism. The excretion of several vitamins is routinely recorded as a function of creatinine excretion.

The excretion of riboflavin reflects fairly accurately the daily intake of the vitamin. An excretion of 50 μg. or less per day is usually associated with other riboflavin deficiency symptoms. Since about 10% of the intake under 1 mg. is excreted, an excretion as low as 50 μg. would result from an intake of less than 0.5 mg., which on the basis of recommended allowances would be regarded as a suboptimal intake.

Other biochemical tests

The rate of hemolysis or breakdown of the red blood cell membrane is sufficiently influenced by the amount of vitamin E available that it has become an adequate test for vitamin E status.

The routine determinations of hemoglobin and hematocrit (blood solids or packed cell level) are useful in assessing red blood cell formation, which is dependent on the amount of available iron and protein in the diet. Plasma albumin levels are maintained by synthesis of protein within the body and will be normal when adequate amounts of amino acids are available. However, the serum levels usually fall only after other signs of protein deficiency are evident.

Anthropological data

Scientists have attempted for years to establish a criterion of nutritional adequacy that involves the use of simple body measurements such as height, weight, chest circumference, ankle circumference, and skinfold thickness. So far, their efforts have met with only limited success. This is partly because of the difficulties of standardizing the techniques by which the measurements are obtained. Height and weight measurements can be obtained fairly readily, but the others involve a high degree of skill if they are going to be useful when compared to established standards. Techniques for using calipers to measure bone structure are very difficult to master, especially if measurements are made on persons with an appreciable amount of fat covering to obscure the bony framework. A second problem is that improved medical and nutritional knowledge is creating a situation where larger and healthier mothers are giving birth to larger and healthier babies whose growth is accelerated. The question raised, then, is whether or not the standards developed twenty to thirty years previously are still valid.

Height and weight tables, long used as a growth standard, have many limitations. If they fail to recognize differences in body build for persons of the same age and sex they are assuming too high a degree of hereditary homogeneity in the population. On the other hand, the use of tables based on different body builds with no basis on which to choose the proper category—small, medium, or large frame—requires a subjective evaluation and allows the user to categorize himself in whichever category he feels fits in with his predetermined opinion.

Two general types of tables have been used. The first type merely records the average weight for height and age based on insurance statistics. The most recent table of this type was released in 1959 by the Society of Actuaries in a publication entitled *Build and Blood Pressure Study* and was based on measurements of nearly 5 million insured persons in ordinary indoor clothing and shoes, from ages 15 to 69. Values in this table tended to be lower for women and higher for men than earlier tables published in 1912 and 1952.

The second type of table, which is more useful in evaluating nutritional status, is one giving "ideal" or desired weights for height. These tables ignore age and use three classifications of body build—small, medium, and large frame. In each of these is presented the range of weights that is associated with the lowest mortality. These weights are essentially the average weights at age 27 for men and age 23 for women. Unfortunately, again no criterion is given on which to base a judgment of body size. The original tables of ideal weights published in 1942 were replaced in 1960 by tables designating desirable weights based on the 1959 *Build and Blood Pressure Study* in which the same classifications of body frame types were used but in which the desirable weights were believed compatible with lowest mortality, about 4 pounds lower for men and 1 to 2 pounds less for women. It is these tables that are presented in Appendix E. Desirable weights were generally 15 to 25 pounds below average weights for both sexes. All of these standards have been criticized because they represent only people who buy insurance, who may be a distinct population group, and also because they imply that overweight is a cause of early mortality whereas their data show only the relationship.

In adults the body chest breadth as measured on roentgenograms of the thoracic area provide a good measure of stature. A weight of 3.4 kg. per centimeter of body chest breadth is an acceptable standard for weight, but the cost of such a procedure limits its usefulness to research studies rather than to use in large populations.

For evaluating the growth of children Faulkner has developed a chart summarizing the best available data giving the fifth, fiftieth, and ninety-fifth percentile heights and weights for children from birth to 18 years. He suggested that children following outside the range from the fifth to the ninety-fifth percentile should be evaluated further to determine if their deviation in growth was cause for concern. His standards are presented in Appendix D.

The use of a parental midpoint scale has recently been advocated by Garn for use with children. In this he proposes that the most acceptable standard for growth of a child is one that recognizes the role of hereditary factors and reflects in the stature of the parents. He has developed tables, one for boys and one for girls, in which he establishes height standards for children of known parentage from birth to age 18 based on the average height of both parents. He feels that his parent-specific scales are much more individualized than are tables based on height for age, irrespective of the hereditary growth capacity of the child. The Fels parent-specific standards for boys and girls are reproduced in Table 15-1.

A very widely used growth standard based on successive height and weight measurements for a child is the Wetzel grid. In this the child serves as his own control and his progress is assessed on the basis of his own standard. A typical grid is reproduced in Fig. 15-2. The child's weight in relation to height is plotted and falls in one of the nine developmental channels ranging from channel B4 for a tall, thin person to channel A4 for an obese individual. In subsequent measurements the growth progress is determined by his advancement within a developmental channel. Deviations on successive measurements into channels away from the median channel are often diagnostic of some medical or nutritional abnormality. A trend in the direction of channel A4, which is indicative of excess weight for height, may serve as a warning to initiate caloric restriction and to try to determine the underlying cause of the developing obesity. Trends in the other direction toward channel B4, on the other hand, may signal infection or other conditions leading

Table 15-1. Fels parent-specific standards for height: children's stature by age and midparent stature in inches*

| Age | Midparent stature† | | | | | |
| | 64.0 inches | | 66.5 inches | | 69.0 inches | |
	Boys	Girls	Boys	Girls	Boys	Girls
1-0	29.0	29.0	29.5	29.0	30.5	29.5
2-0	33.6	33.0	34.5	33.5	35.0	34.5
3-0	36.5	35.5	37.5	37.0	39.0	38.0
4-0	39.0	38.0	40.5	41.0	42.0	41.0
5-0	41.5	40.5	43.5	43.0	44.5	43.5
6-0	43.5	43.5	45.5	45.5	47.0	46.0
7-0	45.7	46.0	48.0	47.5	49.0	49.0
8-0	48.0	48.0	50.0	49.5	51.5	51.0
9-0	50.0	50.5	52.0	52.0	53.5	54.0
10-0	52.0	53.0	54.0	54.0	55.5	56.5
11-0	54.5	55.5	56.0	56.5	58.0	59.0
12-0	57.0	58.0	58.5	59.0	60.0	61.5
13-0	59.5	60.5	61.0	62.0	63.0	63.5
14-0	62.5	62.5	63.5	63.0	66.0	65.5
15-0	65.5	63.0	66.0	64.0	69.0	66.5
16-0	66.5	63.0	68.0	64.0	69.5	67.0
17-0	67.5	63.5	69.0	64.5	70.0	67.5

*Age-size tables for Ohio white children whose midparent stature (or parental midpoint) is the average of the stature of the two parents. All values rounded off to the nearest half inch. (From Garn, S. M.: The applicability of North American growth standards in developing countries, Canad. M. A. J. **93**:914, 1965.)
†Average of maternal and paternal statures.

to loss of appetite and weight. Again the value of the grid is in presenting a visual record of a growth trend.

With the increasing incidence of obesity in the population and a realization of the necessity of recognizing those individuals with excess body fat rather than those with just above average body weights, attempts have been made to find a method of assessing body fatness. Determination of body density, which involves a comparison of the weight of the body under water with that in air and correcting for the air in the lungs, is the most precise way of estimating body fat but is impractical for use on large groups. Special skinfold calipers that exert a specific pressure on a specific area of skinfold have been developed to measure the thickness of a skinfold in various parts of the body as an indication of the amount of subcutaneous fat. The most satisfactory sites are the upper arm over the triceps, midway between the tip of the scapula and the elbow, and a skinfold below the tip of the right scapula. It has generally been felt that this device is useful only for normal or moderately fat persons and is not equally useful in all parts of the body. However, Selzer has postulated that the single skinfold measurement of the triceps is useful in diagnosing obesity.

X-ray plates have also been used to as-

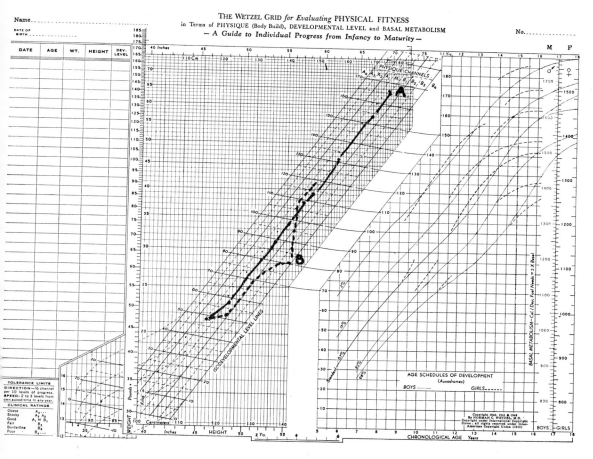

Fig. 15-2

The Wetzel grid. The grid is used to assess growth and physical fitness on the basis of successive weight measurements. Growth curve **A** represents a normal growth pattern. Growth curve **B** represents simple growth failure with subsequent recovery. (Courtesy Dr. Norman Wetzel and National Education Association, Cleveland Heights, Ohio.)

sess the amount of subcutaneous fat in various areas of the body. By this technique it has been possible to measure body fat in such areas as the hips, where caliper measurements of skinfold thickness are of little value. This technique has been standardized to the extent that each millimeter of outer fat is believed to represent 1 to 2 kg. of total body fat.

The difficulties of making accurate anthropometric measurements of body structure in very obese people impose limita-

tions on the usefulness of some of the anthropometric indices. In addition to wishing to know something of body composition for purposes of identifying obese persons, doctors use fat-free weight estimates to determine drug dosages.

Recently a formula using four anthropometric measurements has been devised for estimating body fat, which reportedly correlates very well with other methods of estimating body fat. It involves measurement of arm and thigh circumferences, abdomi-

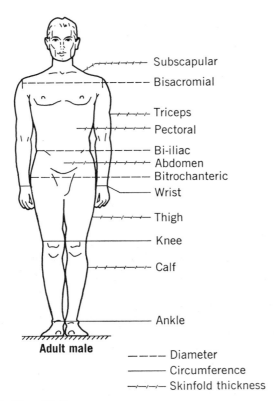

Subscapular

Bisacromial

Triceps

Pectoral

Bi-iliac
Abdomen
Bitrochanteric

Wrist

Thigh

Knee

Calf

Ankle

Adult male

– – – – Diameter

———— Circumference

–╱–╱– Skinfold thickness

Fig. 15-3

Anthropometric measurements used in various formulas for evaluating nutritional status.

nal skinfold, and weight. The formula for calculating body fat in Caucasian females between 25 and 34 years of age, for example, has been established as follows:

Kilograms of body fat = arm circumference (cm.) × 0.354 + thigh circumference (cm.) × 0.403 + abdomen skinfold (mm.) × 0.159 × weight (pounds) × 0.083 − 26.189.

Although it uses measurements readily attainable, the formula involves rather extensive calculations.

Willowby's standards are based on six measurements shown in Fig. 15-3—knee, ankle, and wrist circumferences and the bisacromial, bi-iliac, and bitrochanteric diameters. These provide a basis for assessing the optimal weight of an individual based on body build after a series of rather complex calculations developed by Mc-Gavack. Values from this method provide a goal that many obese people can achieve and maintain more readily than using the values from the SAT (Standard Actuarial Tables), which are based on age, sex, and body frame without any criterion for assessing frame type. Numerous other anthropological indices have been proposed from time to time, but the limitations of these methods have precluded their acceptance for general use. This is especially true in obese persons, whose body build imposes more severe limitations on the accuracy of measurements of bony structures.

DIETARY EVALUATION

An evaluation of nutritional status by an assessment of nutritive intake determined by a variety of means in relation to a variety of available standards is not in itself sufficient evidence to suggest that a person is well or poorly nourished. However, when low dietary intakes of a specific nutrient are found in conjunction with biochemical and clinical signs of a deficiency, the dietary data serves to confirm the diagnosis and provides a basis on which to build a dietary treatment. An apparently adequate diet may be taken by a person exhibiting deficiency symptoms, and, conversely, persons with apparently suboptimal intakes may show no evidence of deficiency symptoms. In these cases the discrepancy can often be explained on the basis of the wide individual variability in nutritive needs resulting from differences in ability to absorb a nutrient or efficiency of utilization. In addition, a dietary evaluation reflects only the immediate intake while much of the biochemical and clinical evidence reflects long-term nutritive intake. A recently improved diet would not immediately result in relief of the symptoms so that a discrepancy between dietary and clinical findings can be explained on the basis of the continuation of deficiency symptoms after the initiation of a better diet.

Dietary evaluations are carried out in a number of ways, each with its own merits and limitations. In a general way they can be categorized as *indirect* and *direct*.

Indirect methods of dietary evaluation

Food balance sheet. The most common of the indirect methods is the national food balance sheet. In this, the records of agricultural productivity and of the export and import of food products of a country and estimates of food wastage are used to obtain a measure of the kinds and amounts of food and hence of nutrients available to a country. Adjustment must be made for food directed to animal feeding. Since no information is provided on the distribution of food within a country, this is in no way an assessment of the nutritive intake of individuals nor does it provide information of the variation of intake that occurs within socioeconomic status, cultural background, age, occupation, or sex. It is, however, useful in detecting year-to-year trends in nutritive intake, in providing a basis for planning the emphasis that should prevail in agricultural production and processing, and in pinpointing possible nutritional shortages.

Vital statistics. The vital statistics of a country provide a second indirect method of assessing nutritional adequacy. Records of the ages and cause of death in a country provide a measure of the extent and nature of morbidity and mortality of a population. Where the death rate from nutritionally related conditions such as beriberi or kwashiorkor is high, malnutrition is undoubtedly present. When the incidence is low, it may reflect adequate nutrition in regard to these nutrients, but it is equally possible that the recording of mortality and morbidity statistics has not been sufficiently accurate to reflect these less well known causes of death. Instead they may only reflect the ultimate cause of death such as heart dis-

ease or tuberculosis. The incidence and death rate from infectious diseases such as measles or tuberculosis is often higher in a malnourished population that lacks the ability to combat the infection. In these cases, however, it is difficult to distinguish the role played by nutrition from that of environmental hygiene and medical practices. When used with a recognition of their limitations, vital statistics or public health indices provide a useful tool in evaluating current trends on the nutritional status of a population.

Direct methods

Direct methods involve an evaluation of the dietary intake of a much smaller unit, such as an institution, a family, or an individual. These methods will be discussed in increasing order of specificity of data obtained.

Food inventory. The food inventory method is used with either a socially homogeneous group such as residents in an institution or members of a family who are fed from a common kitchen. A record is made of all the foods in the institution at the beginning of the study, all food purchased or grown for consumption during the period of the study (usually two weeks to a month), the food remaining in the inventory at the end, and an estimate of the waste of food occurring during the course of the study. From this information an approximation of the nutritive value of the food available to those eating in the group during the period is calculated. There are several limitations to this method. With no indication of who consumes the food it is quite possible to have some members of the group adequately nourished or even overnourished while others may lack one or more nutrients even though the amount consumed by the group would have been adequate for all had it been properly distributed.

Second, studies on small family units have shown that the homemaker modifies her habits of purchasing food during a time when she is made more conscious of her buying habits. One study showed an increase in the purchase of nonperishable staples such as flour and sugar when records were kept for short periods of time. The mere presence of a person recording the food inventory creates a situation in which food habits may vary from normal. It may also increase the reluctance of families, especially in higher income groups, to participate.

Individual food intake. No matter what standard of evaluating an individual's dietary habits is used, whether it be a dietary score or nutritive value calculated from tables of food composition, it is necessary to have as complete a record as possible of the food intake for a specified period of time or to have typical food patterns. These are obtained in several ways.

Twenty-four hour recall. The subject is interviewed by a trained interviewer who asks him to recall and describe the kinds and amounts of food consumed in the previous 24 hours. The subject is often given food models, measuring cups, or a ruler to help him describe the amounts of food consumed. This method has two major advantages. Since it is a retrospective account taken at an unannounced time, it reduces the possibility of the subject modifying his food habits during a time when he knows they are being assessed. The use of the immediately past 24 hours does not involve an appreciable memory span, thus increasing the likelihood of obtaining a complete record. Since it does not require written records, it is suitable for use in illiterate populations. By asking appropriate questions, the trained interviewer is able to probe further and elicit information that might otherwise have been forgotten. However, individual interviews are a rather costly method of obtaining dietary information. If data is desired on a group such as school children, 24-hour diet records are sometimes obtained as written records.

Comparison between diet records from 24-hour recall and seven-day written records show the 24-hour recall tends to be higher, which has been interpreted to reflect a desire of the subject to make a good impression on the interviewer.

Dietary history. A dietary history is an effort to obtain qualitative rather than quantitative information on long-standing food habits that influence the appearance of clinical signs and symptoms. Used in conjunction with the 24-hour recall of food intake, it is considered by many as a very effective method of assessing nutritive adequacy. The subject is asked for information on his past dietary habits—the number and type of meals he normally eats, the frequency and extent to which he uses the various food groups (green and yellow vegetables, milk or milk substitutes, meat, eggs, cereals, etc.), his food likes and dislikes, food allergies, and seasonal variations in intake. From this data it is possible to establish whether the pattern observed in the 24-hour record represents a typical or an atypical food intake. Much of the success of this method depends on the cooperation of the subject and the effectiveness of the interviewer. It is relatively costly in time and money, a typical interview requiring at least 45 minutes. Estimates of dietary intake from dietary history tend to be low compared to those from other means.

Food intake records. When evaluating the diets of large groups of literate subjects the use of written food intake records has proven an inexpensive and relatively satisfactory method of obtaining data. The question not yet answered satisfactorily is how many and which days should be used. In a country such as the United States, with a varied food supply and a tradition for consuming a varied diet, a one-day food record is considerably less representative of usual dietary patterns than in a country where the diet seldom varies. It is recognized that for many people dietary patterns on weekends differ from those on week-days. Yet experience has shown that persons asked to keep a seven-day food record lose interest in the task as the period progresses and keep progressively less satisfactory records or stop entirely. Some investigators have found three weekdays and one weekend day provide a more accurate picture. If no provision is made to see that records are kept daily, there is always the possibility that the task will be put off until the end of the period, leading to errors from incomplete or inaccurate recall. Many investigators have chosen to use the three-day written food record as the one giving sufficiently useful information within a period of time in which one could expect to maintain the cooperation of subjects. Some studies in a highly selected group have made use of 28-day records at four seasons of the year, but this involves a strong commitment and high degree of cooperation on the part of the subjects.

Weighed food records. When a precise individual dietary analysis is required, the weighed food record provides the most accurate means of obtaining it. All food taken by the subject must be accurately weighed and corrected for any plate waste. This involves training the subject to keep accurate records or assigning an investigator to be present at all times to help. In either case there is the problem that the work involved in record keeping and/or the presence of a stranger may lead to a modified eating pattern.

Evaluation of food intake records

Dietary score. Several dietary scores similar to the one in Table 15-2, proposed by the U.S. Department of Agriculture, are used to give a rapid evaluation of the adequacy of the diet. Most are based on the essentials of an adequate diet or other dietary guides. A maximum score of 100 indicates that the diet is based on a sufficient variety of protective foods that it will provide an adequate foundation of most of the

nutrients. Scores less than 100 represent diets that lack one or more food groups with the increased possibility of an inadequacy of one or more nutrients. This scoring system is one that can be readily used by a homemaker to evaluate the quality of the meals she serves.

Calculations from tables of food composition. Many tables based on chemical analyses of food composition are available. The standard reference is the United States Department of Agriculture Handbook No. 8, which has been compiled after a careful analysis of data available from many research laboratories. Consideration was given to variety, method of preparation, sources in terms of climates and soil environment, degree of maturity, and many other factors that influence the nutritive value of foods as consumed by the American public. An abbreviated version of this table published as Home and Garden Bulletin No. 72, *Nutritive Value of Foods in Common Portions* is reproduced in Appendix F. With an accurate description of the kind and amount of food eaten, it is possible to use these or similar tables to calculate the amount of various nutrients present in a diet. This method assumes that the food consumed can be represented by the food described in the table. One of the major limitations to the analysis of diets from food records is the variations and limitations in an individual's estimate of the amount of food eaten and his failure to describe the food in sufficient detail. Tables for a short method of dietary calculation have been developed in which similar foods are grouped in broad categories and one figure given for the nutritive value of the whole group. Estimates of nutritive content using the short method agree rather closely with those obtained from the long method and may be quite satisfactory for the analysis of diets in which the amount of food has been estimated in the first place. Persons using data derived from calculations from diet records should be cau-

Table 15-2. Food selection check sheet

Food	Credits	Daily score						
Milk								
One cup of milk	10							
Second cup of milk	10							
Third cup of milk or more	10							
	30							
Fruits and vegetables								
One serving of green or yellow vegetables	10							
One serving of citrus fruit, tomato, or cabbage	10							
Two or more servings of other fruits and vegetables, including potato	10							
	30							
Breads and cereals								
At least two servings of whole-grain or enriched cereals or breads	15							
Meats								
One serving of egg, meat, fish, poultry, or cheese (or dried beans or peas)	15							
One or more additional servings of egg, meat, fish, poultry, or cheese	10							
	25							
	100							

tioned against reporting the values as precise figures (i.e., protein to 0.1 gm. or thiamine to 0.01 mg.) since this represents a degree of accuracy not justified within the limitations of the method of collecting the data.

Chemical analysis. In research situations, where it is essential to know as exactly as possible the intake of a nutrient, the food intake is weighed accurately and a representative or aliquot sample is saved for chemical analysis in the laboratory. The cost of such a means of determining nutritive value of a diet and the fact that the intake of the subject may be regulated preclude its use in routine dietary studies. It is useful when a carefully prescribed diet is being consumed but has many limitations on a freely selected diet.

Standards for evaluating dietary intake. Knowledge of the nutritive content of a diet is meaningless unless it can be compared to some standard. In the United States the most commonly used standard is the daily recommended allowances prepared by the Food and Nutrition Board of the National Research Council. These standards, shown in Appendix C, were established as the result of careful evaluation of evidence of nutritional needs for various

Table 15-3. Suggested guide to interpretation of nutrient intake data*

	Deficient	Low	Acceptable	High
Protein, grams per kilogram	<0.5	0.5–0.9	1.0–1.4	>1.5
Iron, milligrams per day	<6.0	6–8	9–11	>12
Calcium, grams per day	<0.3	0.30–0.39	0.4–0.7	>0.8
Vitamin A, I.U. per day	<2000	2000–3499	3500–4999	>5000
Ascorbic acid, milligrams per day	<10	10–29	30–49	>50
Thiamine, milligrams per 1000 calories	<0.2	0.20–0.29	0.3–0.4	>0.5
Riboflavin, milligrams per day	<0.7	0.7–1.1	1.2–1.4	>1.5
Niacin, milligrams per day	<5	5–9	10–14	>15

*From Manual for nutrition surveys, ed. 2, Washington, D. C., 1963, Interdepartmental Committee on Nutrition for National Defense.

nutrients by various population groups and an evaluation of figures on agricultural productivity, imports, and exports to determine the availability of nutrients in the food supply. In addition to meeting minimum requirements, the standards provide an additional intake to cover individual variations in requirements and other potential benefits to health. As such, these standards do not represent minimum requirements and any failure to consume the recommended amounts must *not* necessarily be interpreted as evidence of dietary deficiencies. In fact, a large segment of the population can maintain a high level of health on intakes at below half the recommended amounts, although a small group may require the full amounts. In most studies of dietary adequacy, intakes of two thirds the recommended allowances have been considered adequate and those below this level as indicative of a possible but not necessarily a suboptimal state of nutrition. Because of the wide individual variation in need for a specific nutrient a great deal of caution must be observed in comparing the intake of an individual to that of the recommended allowances.

The Interdepartmental Committee on Nutrition for National Defense has developed a *Suggested Guide to Interpretation of Nutrient Intake Data* to apply to 25-year-old physically active males 67 inches tall and 143 pounds in weight. It is reproduced in Table 15-3.

Unless low dietary intakes are accompanied by some clinical or biochemical abnormalities associated with a lack of the nutrient it is dangerous to assume that the intake is below the need of that individual. However, low intakes should prompt an evaluation of nutritional status.

SELECTED REFERENCES

Arroyave, G.: Biochemical evaluation of nutritional status on man, Fed. Proc. **20**:39, 1960.

Bridgforth, E. B.: Statistics in clinical appraisal of nutritional status, Am. J. Clin. Nutrition **11**:433, 1962.

Brin, M.: Erythrocyte as a biopsy tissue for functional evaluation of thiamine adequacy, J.A.M.A. **187**:762, 1964.

Byron, A. H., and Anderson, E.: Retrospective dietary interviewing, J. Am. Dietet. A. **37**:558, 1960.

Garn, S. M.: The applicability of North American growth standards in developing countries, Canad. M. A. J. **93**:914, 1965.

Harris, R. S. (editor): Symposium on recent advances in appraisal of nutritional intake and nutritional status in man, Am. J. Clin. Nutrition 11:331, 1962.

Hollingsworth, D.: Dietary determination of nutritional status, Fed. Proc. 20:50, 1960.

Hunscher, H. A.: Pertinent factors in interpreting metabolic data, J. Am. Dietet. A. 39:209, 1961.

Hutson, E. M., Cohen, N. L., Kunkel, N. D., Steinkamp, R. C., Rourke, M. H., and Walsh, H. E.: Measures of body fat and related factors in normal adults, J. Am. Dietet. A. 47:179, 1965.

Krehl, W. A.: The evaluation of nutritional status, M. Clin. North America 48:1129-40, 1964.

McGavack, T. H.: Optimal weight determination —experiences with a method of Willoughby as a guide to reduction, Metabolism 14:150, 1965.

Pearson, W. N.: Biochemical appraisal of the vitamin nutritional status in man, J.A.M.A. 180:49-55, 1962.

Phipard, E. P.: The recommended allowances in assessing diets, J. Am. Dietet. A. 36:37, 1960.

Plough, I. C., and Bridgforth, E. B.: Relations of clinical and dietary findings in nutrition surveys, Pub. Health Rep. 75:699, 1960.

Rao, M. V. R.: Clinical evaluation of vitamin and mineral status in man, Fed. Proc. 20:32-38, 1960.

Selzer, C. C., Goldman, R. F., and Mayer, J.: The triceps skinfold as a predictive measure of body density and body fat in obese adolescent girls, Pediatrics 36:212, 1965.

Wadsworth, G. R.: Nutritional surveys—clinical signs and biochemical measurements, Proc. Nutrition Soc. 22:72, 1963.

Wilson, C. S., et al.: A review of methods used in nutrition surveys conducted by the Interdepartmental Committee on Nutrition for National Defense (ICNND), Am. J. Clin. Nutrition 15:29, 1964.

Young, C. M.: Body composition and body weight: criteria of overnutrition, Canad. M. A. J. 93:900, 1965.

16

Nutrition in pregnancy and lactation

PREGNANCY

From a nutritional point of view the nine months of pregnancy must be considered as a period of stress during which the demands of the developing fetus are superimposed on those for normal maintenance of the adult woman. For the teen-aged mother the demands are even greater, as maternal tissue is also experiencing a period of rapid growth with high nutritional requirements. The needs of the growing fetus require an increased dietary intake on the part of the mother but one considerably less than the combined needs of the mother and fetus during pregnancy. The mother experiences a series of physiologic adaptations, some of which result in an increased efficiency in the absorption of some nutrients, a decrease in the excretion or loss of nutrients, and, in many cases, alterations in metabolism that result in conservation of nutrients. The capacity of the mother to adapt to the nutritional demands of pregnancy is so extensive that a mother whose diet has been reasonably adequate prior to pregnancy is usually able to bear a full-term viable infant without any extensive modification in her diet. However, it is strongly recommended that the mother's food intake be of sufficiently good quality that the fetus will be able to grow without causing depletion of the mother's reserves of nutrients. The extent of the recommended increase over the normal nutrient needs of the mother to meet the demands of pregnancy varies from one nutrient to another, as shown graphically in Fig. 16-1. Since the question of the pregnant teenager is one of more recent concern, we have practically no evidence on which to determine the level of nutrient intake that will be adequate to meet the stress of both maternal growth and reproduction. For some nutrients such as iron and vitamin A the infant accumulates sufficient amounts to establish a storage supply to last through the early stages of infancy. For others, such as vitamin D, ascorbic acid, and calcium, there is virtually no storage in the infant's body at birth so that the mother

311

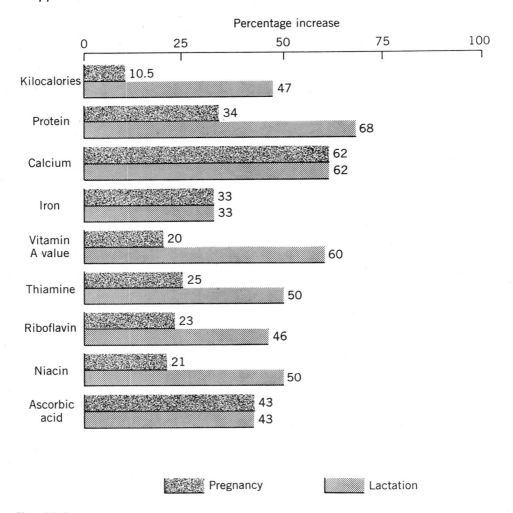

Fig. 16-1

Increase in nutritive needs of mother during pregnancy and lactation above normal needs. (Based on Recommended dietary allowances, National Academy of Sciences Publication No. 1146, Washington, D. C., 1963, National Academy of Science.)

need provide only enough to maintain normal fetal growth.

Rate of growth

The rate of fetal growth, which determines the quantitative but not the qualitative nutritive needs, is very slow in the first half of pregnancy, after which it accelerates rapidly until close to term when it slows down again. At a gestational age of 25 weeks the growth increment is only 6 gm. per day while at 34 weeks it is estimated at 40 gm. per day and by term has dropped to 13 gm. The fetal weights of a group of Colorado infants at various stages of gestation are shown in Table 16-1. The relatively slow development of the human fetus means that nutritional deficiencies must prevail over a long period of time if they are to have a marked effect on fetal de-

Table 16-1. Fetal weight at different ages in gestation*

Age (weeks)	Total weight (grams)
24	900
28	1240
30	1484
32	1750
34	2278
36	2750
38	3052
40	3230
42	3310

*From Lubchenko, L. O., Hansman, C., Dressler, M., and Boyd, E.: Intrauterine growth as estimated from liveborn birth weight data at 24 to 42 weeks of gestation, Pediatrics **32**:793, 1963.

velopment. In contrast, many animals that are used in nutrition investigations develop at a very rapid rate, produce litters of larger size relative to maternal size, and thus are much more responsive to short-term dietary deviations. A comparison of the rate of development and the relationship of litter size of mice, rats, and humans is shown in Fig. 16-2. It will be observed that mice produce a litter weighing 30% of maternal weight in three weeks while the human mother takes nine months to develop a fetus representing 5% of her weight.

Physiologic stages of pregnancy

Implantation. Pregnancy can be divided into three main phases, each with specific nutrient needs, from a physiologic point of view. The first two weeks of gestation is a period of *implantation* during which the fertilized ovum becomes imbedded in the wall of the uterus and the placenta develops. The placenta, which weighs from 325 to 1000 grams at birth, is the tissue through which the nutrients and oxygen needed for fetal growth are transferred from the maternal tissue to the fetus and through which fetal waste is excreted. There is no direct circulatory connection between the fetus and the mother, but in the placenta the two independent circulatory systems come in sufficiently close contact with one another that nutrients are able to pass from one to another. In the placenta, which regulates the flow of nutrients to the fetus, there is approximately 13 square meters of contact between the two circulations. For some nutrients, such as iron, cobalamin, and vitamin C, the placenta allows the passage of sufficient amounts to meet the demands of the growing fetus even at the expense of maternal reserves. For others, such as thiamine, riboflavin, and vitamin D, it allows the maternal and fetal tissue to compete while vitamin A and vitamin E will cross the placental barrier to nourish the infant only after the maternal needs are met. Thus the placenta that develops during this early stage becomes the regulator of fetal nutrition, the success of which depends not only on the nutrients available in the bloodstream of the mother but also on the way in which the placenta governs their transfer. In addition to promoting the active transfer of nutrients, the placenta is capable of synthesizing some body compounds.

Organogenesis. The next six weeks (from two to eight weeks of age) are known as the period of organogenesis, during which the developing fetal tissue undergoes differentiation. The beginnings of the various individual organs such as the heart, lungs, liver, and kidney and the various aspects of skeletal formation are established during this period, and the presence or absence of many nutrients may be crucial for the continued growth of a normal fetus. There is considerable evidence in animal studies linking the absence of certain nutrients during organogenesis with specific congenital abnormalities in the newborn. For instance, riboflavin deficiency has been

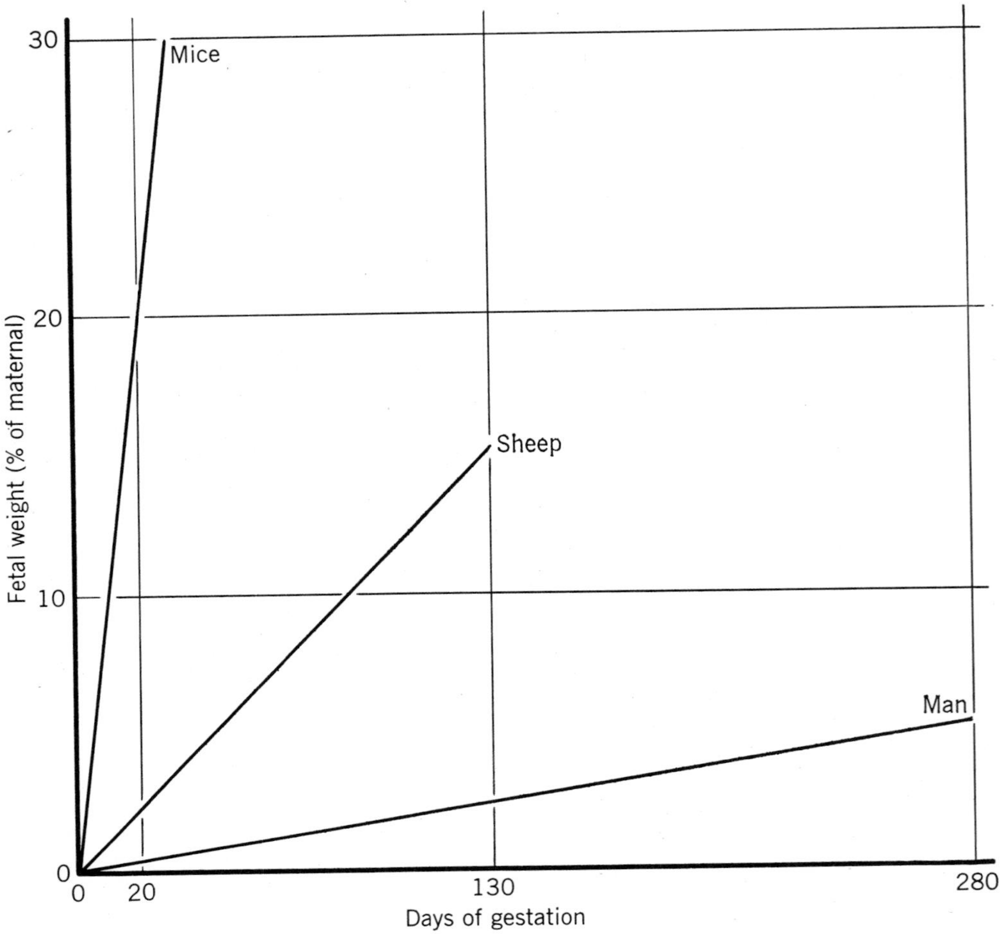

Fig. 16-2

Products of conception of three mammalian species in percentage of maternal weight. (From Smith, C. A.: Prenatal and neonatal nutrition, Pediatrics **30**:145, 1962. [From data of McCance, R. A., and Widdowson, E.: The chemistry of growth and development, Brit. M. Bull. 7:297, 1951.])

associated with poor skeletal formation and vitamin A deficiency with cleft palate. It has been difficult to prove such a relationship in human nutrition because any dietary information must come from retrospective accounts of the nutrient intake and not from experimental manipulation of the diet. Once the abnormality is observed, however, it is sometimes possible to implicate nutritional factors. It is quite possible that the effects of dietary deprivation will

not be as pronounced in humans as in animals because the human experiences a relatively long period of gestation and produces a relatively small offspring in relation to maternal size. Thus, a dietary lack would have to prevail over a fairly long period to bring about the same effect in humans that a short-term deficit will produce in animals. The likelihood of a nutritional inadequacy with its potential hazards to the fetus during organogenesis is increased since this rather critical period occurs at an earlier stage in pregnancy than it is customary for a pregnant woman to seek medical advice, which, it is assumed, includes some guidance in selecting an adequate diet. In addition, many women experience nausea of pregnancy that depresses appetite and food intake and in many cases reduces the amount of food available for absorption to a critically low level. It is under such conditions that the mother who has had good dietary habits prior to conception has an advantage over her less well-fed counterpart who may not have entered pregnancy with such good reserves.

Growth. The remaining seven months of pregancy are known as the growth period. During this time the differentiated tissues continue to grow until they reach a functional size capable of supporting extra-uterine life of the infant. The needs for nutrients at this time are high both quantitatively and qualitatively, although a deficiency will usually result only in a premature birth or smaller infant rather than the serious deficiency symptoms observed in a dietary lack during organogenesis.

The more severe abnormalities of pregnancy have been atttributed to either a deficiency or an excess of vitamins. From studies on animals it is evident that the stage in pregnancy at which the deficiency occurs determines susceptibility to the deficiency and the way in which it is manifest. If the inadequacy occurs in the very early stages the result may be a failure in pregnancy reflected in a spontaneous abortion; at certain stages during differentiation it may show up in a variety of forms of congenital abnormalities such as cleft palate, harelip, malocclusion, or defective tooth formation; and again, there are stages, especially after differentiation is complete, at which a vitamin deficiency will have virtually no effect on the developing fetus. Different animals will vary in their susceptibility to deficiencies depending on their genetic makeup. In human

studies it has not been possible to implicate vitamin deficiencies in the formation of congenital abnormalities since in severe deprivation mothers either become sterile or abort or deliver stillborn, premature, or smaller but normal children.

Physiologic adaptations

During pregnancy there are many changes that occur in the body physiologically, biochemically, and hormonally, all of which influence the need for nutrients and the efficiency with which the body uses them. Only those that have a direct bearing on nutrition will be discussed.

Blood volume is known to increase about 25% above normal levels, undoubtedly, partially at least, in response to the need to carry nutrients to the fetus and metabolic waste such as carbon dioxide and nitrogenous end products away. This hemodilution results in a lowered per unit volume concentration of many nutrients, an observation that is often erroneously interpreted as evidence of a deficiency. Frequently the total amount may have increased although the per unit measurement will have dropped.

The decrease in gastric motility common in pregnancy has the advantage of slowing the passage of food through the gastrointestinal tract, thus increasing the length of the time the digestive mass is in contact with the villi in the lining of the tract and enhancing the possibility of greater absorption of nutrients. On the other hand, it may lead to considerable discomfort because of inability to empty the gastrointestinal tract, especially true in the latter part of pregnancy.

The observed decrease in the secretion of hydrochloric acid reduces gastric acidity, which could have a depressing effect on calcium and iron absorption in which the ionization of the element from its complex depends on acid. However, this negative effect is counterbalanced by other factors that lead to an increased absorption of these two elements in the last trimester of pregnancy.

During the early part of pregnancy there is a decline in basal metabolic rate that gradually increases to a high point of 13% above normal in the last trimester.

Nutritive needs

The change of nutrient intake recommended to meet the nutritional stresses of pregnancy varies with the nutrient, depending on many factors, such as the body's mechanism for adapting to increased demands for the nutrient, the nature of the metabolic demands of pregnancy, and the nutrient reserves of the mother. The National Research Council recommended dietary allowances are based on rather scanty information as to quantitative needs during pregnancy. To better understand the kind of dietary adjustment that may be necessary during pregnancy the needs for each nutrient will be discussed separately.

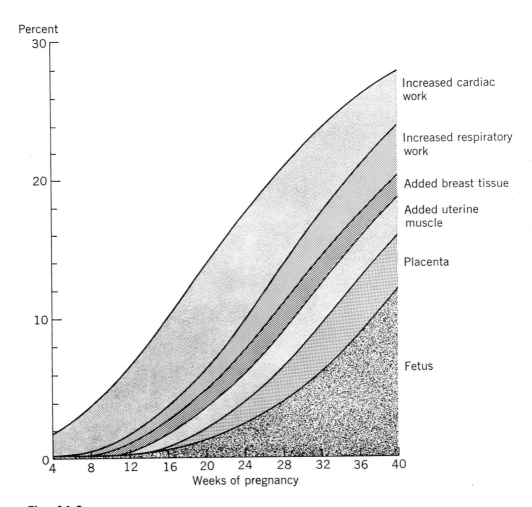

Fig. 16-3

The components of increased oxygen consumption in pregnancy. (From Hytten, F. E., and Leitch, I.: The physiology of human pregnancy, Philadelphia, 1963, F. A. Davis Co.)

Energy. During pregnancy, caloric needs are influenced by two opposing sets of forces. On one side, the growth of the fetus, although very slow at first, calls for additional energy, as does the growth of the placenta, the increase in maternal body size that is normal during pregnancy, and the additional work of carrying the growing infant. On the other hand, the early drop in basal metabolism and the decreased activity frequently experienced by the mother depresses the calorie requirement. It is estimated that the growth of the fetus and maternal tissue calls for approximately 80,000 kilocalories but the normal energy requirements are reduced by 40,000 kilocalories through decreased activity and the early decline in basal metabolic needs, which results in a net increased requirement of 40,000 kilocalories. This can be met by increasing the energy intake by 200 kilocalories a day during the second half of pregnancy when two thirds of fetal growth occurs. This is illustrated in Fig. 16-3, showing the components of the increased energy need of pregnancy. For some mothers who greatly reduce their activity there may never be a demand for an increase in energy in spite of the increased basal energy requirement and fetal growth needs of the last trimester. Along with the growth of the developing infant itself, a concurrent increase in the size of supporting maternal tissues occurs. The nature of the weight gain experienced in pregnancy is shown in Table 16-2, which shows that a normal pregnancy calls for considerable weight gain over and above that represented by the size of the fetus. Thus if the net gain in maternal weight is less than 20 to 25 pounds one must assume that the growth of the child as a parasite on the mother has caused a depletion of the mother's tissue reserves. A failure in the development of mammary structures during pregnancy may preclude a normal and successful lactation period.

In Indian mothers in a poor community

Table 16-2. Nature of maternal weight gain in pregnancy*

Tissue		Weight in pounds
Fetus	7	(Range 5 to 10 pounds)
Placenta	1	
Amniotic fluid	3	
Uterus	2	
Breasts	3	
Increase in blood volume	2	Relatively constant
Tissue fluids	3	
Fat	3	
Total	24	

*From Rhodes, P.: Significance of weight gain in pregnancy, Lancet **1**:663, 1962.

an increase in body water from 56.1% in first 12 weeks of gestation to 70.9% after 28 weeks was observed. Since the maternal weight gain was not great enough to account for this gain and the women were in positive nitrogen balance, there must have been a loss of body fat concurrent with gain in body water.

There has been much conflict in the literature as to what constitutes a desirable gain in weight for a pregnant woman. The practice of allowing the mother unrestricted weight gain on the theory that she was "eating for two" was widely accepted in the early part of the century. The undesirable consequences of this regime, such as toxemia, difficulties of labor with increased risk to the mother, and the birth of large babies who suffered many complications in early life, soon became evident. The proponents of unlimited weight gain were replaced by a group recommending calorie restriction sufficiently severe to limit weight gain to 10 to 12 pounds, a regime that resulted in equally undesirable consequences.

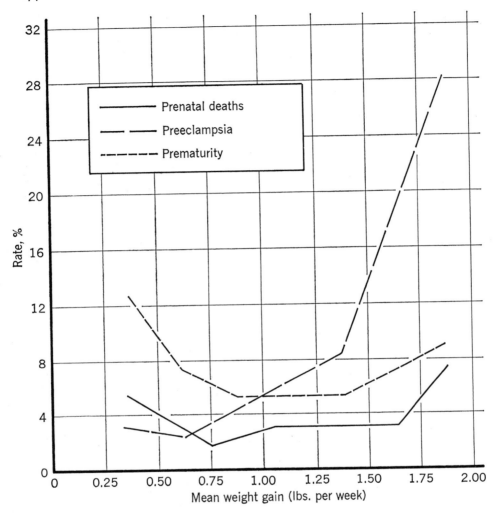

Fig. 16-4

Incidence of three major obstetrical complications by mean weight gain between 20 weeks and delivery. (From Hytten, F. E., and Leitch, I.: The physiology of human pregnancy, Philadelphia, 1963, F. A. Davis Co.)

Mothers who failed to gain weight in the second trimester were very likely to have premature deliveries with increased risk to the health of the baby and to experience toxemia or eclampsia with its symptoms of proteinuria, high blood pressure, headache, blurred vision, and edema, especially in the extremities. The relationship between weight gain and complications of pregnancy is shown in Fig. 16-4.

One study on the relationship of weight gain to the incidence of toxemia showed that the mothers who experienced eclampsia were the ones who gained less than 15 pounds or over 29 pounds during gestation. Research data showed that women consuming less than 1800 kilocalories per day were unable to maintain a positive nitrogen balance, which means that if the fetus continued to grow, it did so at the expense of maternal tissue that would not be replaced as fast as it was depleted. In addition, the restriction in energy intake seldom led to the birth of a smaller baby with less strain on the mother during labor. In fact, it is believed that the birth weight of the infant is more closely correlated with the weight of the mother at conception than to the weight gain of the mother during pregnancy. It would appear, then, that caloric restriction prior to pregnancy so that the mother enters the reproductive period at normal body weight will do more to assure the birth of a child of average weight than will caloric restriction during pregnancy.

Many women restrict their weight gain in fear that a gain may remain a permanent weight increment. Studies show that about eight pounds of weight gained during pregnancy remains immediately after birth and only four pounds at six weeks postpartum. All of the gained weight is usually lost in six to eight months.

While some workers maintain the woman who is obese at the onset of pregnancy can successfully reduce her own body size without jeopardizing the health of the infant or herself if the qualitative aspects of the diet are guarded carefully, the preponderance of the evidence suggests that any major adjustments in the mother's weight should be undertaken under normal circumstances rather than during a period of nutritional stress such as pregnancy. Women who gained less than 15 pounds have been demonstrated to have double the incidence of preeclampsia of those who gained more. Aside from the physiologic stress produced by caloric restriction, the emotional tension accompanying it, especially in the face of a stimulated appetite, may have even more adverse effects. If weight gain is to be controlled, however, the only effective way to do it is through calorie restriction rather than by a restriction of salt or water intake.

Jackson, studying the effect of weight reduction in obese pregnant women on pregnancy, labor, delivery, and the condition of the infant at birth, concluded that a carefully controlled weight gain offers protection from the complications of pregnancy and is safe if the carefully planned diet is used after the first 16 weeks, the critical period of development. Only 4% of 48 women who had successfully lost an average of 11.3 pounds during pregnancy experienced toxemia of pregnancy while 39% of 44 who were unsuccessful had toxemia symptoms. Unfortunately, once the motivation of pregnancy was removed 80% of the subjects returned to their old eating habits and prepregnancy weight.

After a careful evaluation of all relevant data the Food and Nutrition Board of the National Research Council has suggested that an additional 200 kilocalories per day in the last half of pregnancy will take care of the energy demands of pregnancy and lead to desirable weight gain of 22 to 30 pounds.

Protein. The growth of the infant makes heavy demands for protein of high biological value. If two thirds of the protein comes from animal sources, 1.5 gm. of protein per kilogram of body weight will be adequate to meet the needs for the increase in maternal tissue and also to support the growth of the fetus. The National Research Council suggests an additional 20 gm. per day. Protein intake of the mother influences the birth length of the fetus, taller babies being born to mothers with high-protein diets than to those with limited protein intake within the limits determined by heredity. The smaller babies born to mothers on diets inadequate in protein are more susceptible to the hazards of early life and have a decreased chance of survival.

A 7½-pound infant whose body contains the normal 2% nitrogen will have 412 gm., or almost a pound, of protein. The greater part of this protein has been deposited in the fetal tissue at a rate of 1.5 gm. per day during the last half of pregnancy when the growth hormone produced during pregnancy stimulates the retention of nitrogen.

The increase in protein in the mother's body is accounted for by the development of the mammary glands, the growth of the accessory tissue supporting the fetus, and the reserves to meet the needs for lactation. Failure to obtain sufficient protein may be caused by poverty, ignorance, food idiosyncrasies, and fear of developing a large baby.

Toxemia of pregnancy, which alternately has been associated with an excess and a lack of dietary protein, appears to be the result of a complex of poorly defined factors and there is no clear-cut evidence to implicate protein.

Calcium. Although the infant's bones are poorly calcified at the time of birth there is still a demand for an appreciable amount of calcium for fetal development during pregnancy. The demand of approximately 50 mg. a day for the first trimester increases to 120 mg. per day in the second trimester and jumps to 450 mg. in the last trimester. This leads to the deposition of approximately 22 gm. of calcium in the body of the newborn infant. To help meet this need, the mother becomes more efficient in absorbing calcium. The decrease in absorption that occurs under conditions of emotional stress, such as may prevail among unwilling mothers, may counterbalance this increased absorption, a normal response to the demands of pregnancy. If the dietary intake is still not adequate to meet these needs, calcium will be withdrawn from maternal reserves to fulfill the needs of the developing fetus. It is estimated that about 30% of fetal calcium has been obtained from maternal stores. The amount of dietary calcium needed is reduced if vitamin D is available and increased if it is not. Ideally, there should be a storage rather than a depletion of calcium in the mother's tissue during pregnancy to help anticipate the demands for calcium,

which are particularly high during lactation.

Iron. Since infants are born normally with high hemoglobin levels (18 to 22 gm. per 100 ml. of blood) and with a supply of iron in the liver to last three to six months after birth, the maternal organism is called upon to transfer large amounts of iron to the fetus during pregnancy. It has been estimated that the daily requirement of iron for the growth of the fetus, the formation of the new maternal tissue necessary to nourish the fetus, and the formation of new hemoglobin because of the increase in maternal blood volume amounts to 1.5 mg. a day. The absence of menstrual losses effects a saving of 200 to 300 mg. of iron during the nine-month period, but there is still a net increase of 0.5 mg. per day over normal requirements. Assuming that the normal rate of absorption of 10% of dietary iron improves in response to the increased demands of pregnancy, the National Research Council believes that an intake of 15 mg. per day is adequate to meet the fetal needs and maintain maternal stores. An increase in the level of transferrin, the protein in the blood responsible for the transport of iron which increases the capacity of the body to absorb iron, has been observed in pregnancy. The absorption of iron is three times as high during the last trimester, the period when the reserves are established, as during the first trimester of pregnancy.

There are many conflicting reports in the literature on the incidence of anemia during pregnancy. The normal 25% increase in blood volume leads to a dilution of the amount of hemoglobin found in the blood. Thus a drop in hemoglobin level measured in terms of 100 ml. of blood may reflect an actual increase rather than a decrease in the total amount of hemoglobin available to transport oxygen to the tissues and carbon dioxide away from the tissues. Women with relatively high hemoglobin levels may exhibit typical iron-deficiency symptoms such as fatigue, lassitude, and loss of appetite. These are usually relieved by iron therapy. Some workers maintain that if a hemoglobin level below 10 gm. per 100 ml. of blood is considered a criterion of anemia, then iron-deficiency anemia occurs during pregnancy only when there is a severe blood loss.

There is some evidence that hemoglobin levels do not necessarily reflect the adequacy of the iron supply and that the maintenance of normal bone marrow levels of iron and iron-containing enzymes in the liver and kidneys are more sensitive criteria.

Macrocytic (large-cell) anemia, which frequently occurs in pregnancy, is believed to be caused by a relatively inadequate intake of dietary folate. Recent studies indicate that iron deficiency puts additional stress on folate metabolism and may convert a subclinical folate deficiency into a megaloblastic anemia.

Iodine. Pregnancy increases the need for dietary iodine. Levels of iodine that will prevent goiter under normal circumstances frequently prove inadequate in pregnancy, leading to goiter in the mother, especially an adolescent mother. When the mother has goiter, the chances that the child will develop goiter are increased ten times. In addition, the incidence of cretinism, the severe form of iodine deficiency, among infants rises to 1% when the incidence of goiter in mothers reaches 55%.

In many parts of the country diets are adequate in iodine only when iodized salt is used in cooking. Should salt intake be restricted in an attempt to control toxemia of pregnancy, the woman is deprived of her only reliable source of iodine and should be encouraged to use some other supplementary source as a protection against goiter.

Other mineral elements. Little work has been done to determine quantitative needs for other mineral elements during pregnancy, but it seems reasonable to suggest that the body's ability to adapt to a state of stress by improved absorption and decreased excretion will take care of some but not all of the additional needs for mineral elements. We do have evidence that infants develop teeth with increased resistance to dental caries when the mother's diet contains adequate fluorine. There is now considerable evidence accumulating that, contrary to early opinion, the pregnant animal's need for sodium is increased above those for normal maintenance and that sodium restriction may have many adverse effects. This has been borne out by the successful use of diets high in salt rather than the usual salt-restricted diet in the treatment of toxemia of pregnancy in a group of 1000 pregnant women. Evidence from animal studies has also shown need for increased intakes of sodium during reproduction.

Fat-soluble vitamins. While it is fairly well established that the pregnant animal has a series of adaptive mechanisms to cope with increased demands for minerals during pregnancy there is no evidence that such a system of adaptation exists for vitamins.

Vitamin A. Aside from the fact that animals on vitamin A–deficient diets have a poor reproductive performance, very little is known about the need for vitamin A during pregnancy. The National Research Council, however, has suggested that a small increase to 6000 I.U. per day should be adequate, especially if some is preformed vitamin A. A lack of vitamin A during the early stages of fetal development in animals has been implicated in cleft palate and skeletal and eye defects. Similar relationships in humans have not been established.

Vitamin D. The need for vitamin D is set at 400 I.U. per day to promote the absorption and utilization of calcium and phosphorus that are so essential in bone formation. Unless milk fortified with vitamin D or a combination of other foods to which vitamin D has been added are used, a normal diet cannot be relied upon to provide adequate amounts for women living in the temperate zone. Supplements providing 400 I.U. per day are recommended. However, recent evidence linking mental retardation in infants with excessive intakes by the mother during pregnancy has given rise to a great deal of caution in the use of supplements along with fortified foods to avoid overdoses and the resultant toxic effects. If milk fortified with 400 I.U. of vitamin D per quart is used there is no need for an additional source of the nutrient; in fact it should be avoided.

Vitamin E. The observation of a role of vitamin E in promoting normal reproduction and reducing the number of abortions and stillbirths in animals led to many studies to elucidate a similar role in humans. So far scientists have been unable to determine any unique role of the tocopherols in human reproduction in spite of some evidence that they may be beneficial to women who have experienced repeated abortions or a failure to conceive. There is no evidence of any increased need for vitamin E in pregnancy and, as under normal conditions, the requirement appears to be adequately met by a normal diet with little likelihood of a deficiency unless the diet contains abnormally high amounts of polyunsaturated fatty acids.

Vitamin K. As the vitamin concerned with the synthesis of prothrombin necessary for normal coagulation of the blood, vitamin K has long been considered to play a role in preventing neonatal hemorrhaging, which was often fatal to either the mother or the fetus. It became routine practice to give vitamin K orally to the mother in the last several weeks of pregnancy or even by injection during labor to prevent hemorrhage. Evidence of some adverse effects such as hyperbilirubinemia and hemolytic anemia from the use of large doses of the synthetic form have led to the recommendation that a synthetic analogue be given in a controlled dose to the mother at a level sufficiently high to prevent hemorrhage but low enough to preclude adverse reactions. Similar protection is afforded by giving the natural form of the vitamin, either by injection or orally to the infant.

Thiamine. The relationship between thiamine needs and calorie intake remains the same during pregnancy as under normal circumstances, thus calling for a slight increase in intake. The normal urinary excretion of thiamine drops in pregnancy, indicating that more thiamine is being retained and used by the tissues. Some investigations have shown that thiamine helps relieve nausea of pregnancy.

Riboflavin. Based on studies showing increased urinary excretion of riboflavin in pregnancy it has been suggested that a minimum of 0.7 mg. per 1000 kilocalories, or 1.6 mg., is needed to meet the demands of the growing fetus and the mother.

Animal studies have shown that a lack of riboflavin in the thirteenth and fourteenth embryonic days interferes with cartilage formation, resulting in skeletal malformations such as shortening of the long bones and a fusion of the ribs.

Pyridoxine. Women under normal stress of pregnancy exhibit an altered tryptophan metabolism that can be corrected by additional pyridoxine. The ability to handle sodium is also impaired in pregnancy unless adequate pyridoxine is available.

Pyridoxine has been used experimentally to help control nausea of pregnancy, but the results, while encouraging for some individuals, have not been conclusive and there is no satisfactory theory to explain this phenomenon.

Folic acid. Folate intake during pregnancy has been associated primarily with the promotion of normal fetal growth and the prevention of a macrocytic anemia of pregnancy. Although the need for folic acid in pregnancy is known to increase, the amount required is yet unknown. In iron deficiency there is a further increase in need, but even when iron is adequate the need exceeds 20 μg. per day.

The importance of folic acid in promoting a normal pregnancy is emphasized by the fact that the use of a folic acid antagonist, aminopterin, induces the resorption of fetuses in animals. Its use in human beings does not lead to resorption or abortion of a fetus but rather to the birth of a child with congenital malformations such as harelip, cleft palate, or hydrocephalus.

Cobalamin. It has been confirmed that the infant is parasitic on the mother for cobalamin, as evidenced by the higher vitamin B_{12} levels found in fetal blood than maternal blood even when maternal levels are depleted. The capacity to absorb cobalamin is increased in pregnancy, but a large amount is transferred to the fetus. A daily intake of 100 μg. of cobalamin or 25 μg. of cobalamin plus 5 mg. of folic acid is necessary to maintain constant serum cobalamin levels. If these amounts are not supplied, the serum vitamin B_{12} levels drop but return to normal without supplementation after pregnancy.

Ascorbic acid. The NRC recommended allowances for ascorbic acid are increased by 30 mg. during pregnancy, although there is little evidence on which to base these figures. Ascorbic acid does pass the placental barrier very freely, and serum values of a child have been established at two to four times that of the mother. There is some evidence to indicate that the placenta is capable of synthesizing ascorbic acid, which could account for the higher levels in fetal tissues.

Role of nutritional supplements during pregnancy

The reproductive period is one in which heavy demands are made on the mother to provide the nutrients needed for normal fetal development. It has been shown that the increase in need varies from one nutrient to another, the smallest increase being for calories. To provide the amounts of protein, minerals, and vitamins recommended without exceeding the caloric allowance a woman must choose her food very carefully and almost exclusively from protective foods (i.e., those that provide as high a percentage of the day's requirements of at least two nutrients as they do of calories). The selection of a diet adequate for pregnancy is relatively easy if one is concerned with an isolated day or two, but the pregnant woman must maintain this high level of nutritive intake for the 280 days of the normal gestation period. To do this she must constantly be conscious of her food choices. The woman who takes such a responsibility seriously is subjecting herself to a constant stress during a period that is frequently characterized by at least some degree of emotional stress. To allow her a little more freedom in the selection of food and an occasional indulgence in a favorite food, it may be reasonable to suggest that she use a supplement that provides a balanced formula at protective levels—possibly 25% of the day's recommended allowance. Because of the competitive nature of the drug market most manufacturers find it necessary to market supplements providing an excessive amount of the nutrients needed and to include many for which there is little likelihood of a deficiency occurring even in pregnancy or to include ineffectual amounts of others. The use of such supplements is not only an economic waste and unnecessary from a nutritional point of view but a practice that could produce nutritional imbalances, especially if the product contains mineral elements, and could adversely affect the fetus if the fat-soluble vitamins reached toxic levels. The Food and Drug Administration maintains that there is justification for the inclusion of only twelve nutrients in dietary supplements—vitamins A and D, ascorbic acid, thiamine, riboflavin, niacin, vitamins B_6 and B_{12}, calcium, iron, iodine, and phosphorus.

Table 16-3 gives the composition and

Table 16-3. The nutritive content and cost of several nutritional supplements used during pregnancy

Brand		A	B	C	D	E	F	G
Vitamin A	(I.U.)	5000	4000	6000	4400	4000	6000	2500
Vitamin D	(I.U.)	400	400	400	500	400	400	1000
Thiamine	(mg.)	2	1.5	3	10	3	1.5	1
Riboflavin	(mg.)	1	2	3	10	2	2.5	1.5
Niacin	(mg.)	6	12	20	100	10	15	6
Pyridoxine	(mg.)		1	2	2	1	3	
Calcium pantothenate	(mg.)		2.5	0.5	20		0.5	
Ascorbic acid	(mg.)	100	60	75	300	50	100	25
Cobalamin	(µg.)		3	12	4		2	2
Calcium	(mg.)	125		100	50	230	250	
Iodine	(mg.)			0.15	0.15	0.01		
Iron	(mg.)			45	10	30	40	30
Magnesium	(mg.)			6	6			
Zinc	(mg.)			1.5	1.5	0.085		
Manganese	(mg.)				1	0.05		
Copper	(mg.)			1	1	0.15		
Potassium	(mg.)				5	0.835		
Cost per day	(cents)			4.0	7.0	4.6	4.8	

cost of some supplements promoted in the retail trade in the spring of 1966. From this it is obvious that the supplement contains amounts of some in excess of total needs of pregnancy while making insignificant contributions of others. The money spent on some of these might do much more toward promoting a satisfying pregnancy if it were spent on some form of recreation, an additional dress, or domestic help!

Supplements may be especially useful for a woman experiencing nausea of pregnancy whose dietary pattern may be disturbed, but again they should be restricted to protective levels.

Iron supplements, often not incorporated in the multivitamin-mineral preparations, are recommended for women whose hemoglobin drops below 10.5 gm. per 100 ml. Therapeutic iron in doses of 100 to 110 mg. of iron as ferrous sulphate or ferrous gluconate are most frequently recommended. Calcium to meet the needs of the growing fetus can be provided in calcium supplements, but the amounts in routine vitamin-mineral preparations are seldom significant.

One additional basis for caution in the use of high-level nutritional supplementation during pregnancy has been brought to light recently with the observation that the animals may become conditioned to a high intake during fetal life if the intake of the maternal organism is high and reflect this in an increased need in the postnatal period. This has been advanced as a possible explanation for the increase in infantile scurvy among infants in technically advanced countries. The toxic effects of too much of the fat-soluble vitamins A and D has been well documented.

Research workers at Vanderbilt University believe that the mother can adapt to such a wide range of nutrient intake during the stress of pregnancy that there is no need for supplementation.

Dietary modifications in pregnancy

In addition to a need to modify the normal diet pattern to take care of the quantitative needs for nutrients, there may be value in other modifications. During the early part of pregnancy when appetite may be disturbed, the consumption of smaller and more frequent meals has been helpful to many women. The same pattern is helpful in the latter part of pregnancy when the problem is one of discomfort following large meals because of crowding of the abdominal cavity.

Between the fourth and seventh months, particularly, many women experience an insatiable appetite. To control this to help limit weight gain to a desirable level, the practice of eating a small meal slightly before the time when hunger sensations become most severe has been found a useful method of controlling the total intake.

The use of a diet relatively high in bulk may be helpful in maintaining normal gastric motility at a time when there is a tendency toward constipation.

The way in which the nutritive needs of pregnancy are met will vary with the preferred food habits or likes and dislikes of the women. Usually a diet containing three cups of milk or its equivalent, two servings of meat, fish, or poultry, one egg, a dark green or yellow vegetable, and a generous serving of a citrus fruit will provide a foundation for a nutritionally adequate diet.

EFFECT OF NUTRITION ON PREGNANCY

It has been fairly well established that the nutritional status of the mother at the time of conception is as important for the outcome of pregnancy as is the diet during the period of gestation. The nutritional status of the mother at conception is generally a reflection of long-standing food habits that change in relatively few people during pregnancy in spite of the motivation one would expect to prevail at this time. Because of the influence of many factors, such as the maternal age, birth rate, birth interval, and metabolic interrelationships, it is difficult to delineate specific dietary effects.

The impact of the nutrition of the mother on the course of pregnancy and the condition of the infant at birth has been the subject of many investigations, but not all have led to the same conclusions. The now classic study of Burke, which has been described in the introductory chapter, points most conclusively to a relationship between maternal diet and well-being of the infants, the chances of a child with a high pediatric rating being born to a mother with a good or excellent diet being much better than when the maternal diet is rated as poor or very poor. Studying Canadian women, Ebbs found a similar relationship, with mothers on good diets experiencing few complications during pregnancy and giving birth to infants with a greater chance of surviving the neonatal period. More recently, however, a group of investigators at Vanderbilt University failed to demonstrate a relationship between the quality of maternal diet and the course and outcome of pregnancy. They felt that complications of pregnancy led to suboptimal intakes rather than the converse. Although they found a relationship between diet and the course of pregnancy only at dietary intakes of less than 1500 kilocalories and 50 gm. of protein, they emphasized that these findings should not be interpreted to mean that good nutritional practices should not be encouraged. None of the subjects in their study had markedly suboptimal diets so that they may have entered pregnancy in sufficiently good nutritional status to provide a buffer against the stress of pregnancy.

Thomson in England in 1959 was unable to demonstrate any difference in the diet of mothers who had a normal clinical history during pregnancy and those who experienced some clinical abnormality. There was no relationship between diet and the duration of gestation, the birth weight of the infant, fetal malformation, perinatal deaths, or failure of lactation. In this study one can conclude that the abnormalities of reproduction were not caused by dietary deficiencies. However, this must not be interpreted to mean that dietary inadequacies could not cause abnormalities of pregnancy.

In 1963, after reviewing 4300 obstetrical cases, Thomson and Billewicz found that the incidence of prematurity, cesarean section, and perinatal deaths increased as the dietary rating of the maternal diet fell. Their results are shown in Table 16-4.

Other investigators have indicated a relationship between specific dietary factors and specific complications of pregnancy. Toxemia of pregnancy is often associated with diets low in protein, failure to gain enough weight, or too large a weight gain. The incidence of abortion in early pregnancy among women with low-protein diets is almost twice as high as it is in women with high-protein diets.

The effect of diet prior to pregnancy can be illustrated from data on babies born during a period of wartime starvation in two different countries—Holland and Russia. In Holland the children born during a hunger period had been conceived prior to the period by mothers whose previous diet had been good. The babies were shorter and lighter than babies born to mothers whose diets were adequate throughout pregnancy but there was no increase in stillbirths, prematurity, and congenital malformation, all indications of the protective effect that a good diet prior to pregnancy may exert during the course of pregnancy. In contrast, mothers whose babies were born during the siege of Leningrad and whose diets had been poor prior to pregnancy experienced a stillbirth rate double the normal rate, a 41% incidence of prematurity among live births, and a high rate of neonatal deaths. A reduced rate of conception also occurred.

Table 16-4. Incidence of obstetric abnormalities in Aberdeen primigravidae by maternal health and physique as assessed at the first antenatal examination (twin pregnancies have been excluded)*

| | Maternal health and physique | | | |
	Very good	Good	Fair	Poor; very poor
Prematurity† (percent)	5.1	6.4	10.4	12.1
Cesarean section (percent)	2.7	3.5	4.2	5.4
Perinatal deaths per 1000 births	26.9	29.2	44.8	62.8
Number of subjects	707	2088	1294	223
Percentage tall (5 feet 4 inches or more)	42	29	18	13
Percentage short (under 5 feet 1 inch)	10	20	30	48

*From Thomson, A. M., and Billewicz, W. Z.: Nutritional status, maternal physique and reproductive efficiency, Proc. Nutrition Soc. **22:**55, 1963.
†Birth weight of baby 2500 gm. or less.

Additional evidence suggesting that the lifetime diet habits of the mother influence the outcome of pregnancy is advanced by Thomson, who found a prematurity rate of 32 per 1000 births and a neonatal death rate of 19 per 1000 births in children born to mothers over 64 inches tall. These, he assumed, represented women who had been relatively well nourished throughout their lives. Similar statistics on women under 61 inches tall who may have been less well nourished during their own growth period showed a threefold increase in prematurity, with 91 per 1000 infants weighing less than 2500 gm. and a doubled incidence of neonatal deaths. Many other studies have suggested that the better the state of nutrition of the mother prior to or at the time of conception, the greater the chance of normal pregnancy leading to the birth of a healthy child.

LACTATION

The decision to breast- or bottle-feed an infant is one often surrounded with much emotion. The advantages of breast-feeding will be discussed in greater detail in Chapter 17, but some of the more cogent considerations are that it represents a very satisfying emotional experience for the mother, provides a source of nourishment uniquely suited to the growth demands and physiologic capacity of the human infant, is a foolproof method that can be duplicated only by intelligent, constant, carefully guarded, artificial feeding, and is one that, seldom, if ever, causes allergic reactions—an especially important consideration for parents with a family history of allergy. The decision to breast-feed is generally made very early in pregnancy or even before conception. Once the decision has been made the likelihood of success depends to a large extent on the genetic makeup of the mother, her attitude toward breast-feeding, her understanding of the process of lactation, and the support and encouragement she receives from medical personnel in her efforts to initiate a successful experience.

NUTRITIVE NEEDS

The nutritive demands on the mother during lactation far exceed those of pregnancy, although she may actively cease to feel the responsibility of "eating for two." The fact that the output of milk in the first month of lactation exceeds the increase in mass during the full nine months of pregnancy coupled with the fact that a normally developing infant doubles the birth weight accumulated in nine months of pregnancy in five months of life emphasizes the extent of the demands which the breast-fed infant makes on the mother. Milk secreted in one month represents more kilocalories than the net energy costs of pregnancy. This same milk contains 240 gm. of protein. The infant synthesizes more tissue each day in postuterine life than during fetal life and in addition must provide for its own temperature regulation, more extensive body movements, and take care of many more intermediate steps in the utilization of food.

The health of the mother who is lactating successfully can be ensured only if her own nutritive intake is satisfactory. In most cases a severe deficiency of a nutrient in the maternal diet will be reflected in a decreased secretion of milk, but in a few instances a milk of inferior quality will be produced. The recommendations for dietary intakes during lactation are based on even fewer data on the quantitative needs than are those for pregnancy. It is fairly well established that these levels will support the average production of 850 ml. of milk, but it is entirely possible that satisfactory lactation can be maintained on somewhat lower levels of intake. Indeed, observations among poorly nourished lactating women in developing countries is testimony to this. There is also evidence that many women produce much more than 850 ml. of milk. For instance, one study among Budapest mothers of 19 to 23 years of age showed an average secretion of 1029 ml. at three weeks, 1263 at seven weeks, and 1492 at 14 weeks, with some mothers secreting over 2500 ml.

Recommended allowances

An <u>adequate diet during pregnancy is</u> one of the best bases for the initiation of <u>breast-feeding</u>, but the nutritional goals for successful continuation of lactation are less obvious. Lack of clear-cut information on the nutritive composition of milk, the volume of milk produced, and the efficiency of milk production has complicated the task of arriving at recommended levels of nutrients in the maternal diet to allow adequate milk production. There is lack of agreement as to what constitutes a normal composition of either colostrum, transitional, or mature milk, but just as cows of different genetic makeup secrete milks of different nutritive composition, human mothers with still greater heterogeneity of heredity can be expected to produce milks of varying compositions. The fact that many mothers, especially in developing countries, are able to maintain a prolonged and satisfactory lactation period in diets well below currently accepted standards suggests a reappraisal of nutritional goals for lactating women. Since it is quite possible that in these cases lactation has been carried on at the expense of maternal reserves, which may be depleted to the point of endangering the maternal health, high standards are likely justified for the maintenance of a satisfactory level of milk production. The basis for current standards will be discussed for individual nutrients. Fig. 16-1 shows the suggested increase in nutritive intake for lactation over those required under normal conditions. The increase suggested can be met by the equivalent of an additional meal of approximately 1000 kilocalories of protective foods each day.

Energy. The production of 850 ml. of milk, representing 600 kilocalories, requires an additional 400 kilocalories, indicating that the conversion of energy in milk is 60% efficient. Thus, it is recommended that energy intake be increased 1000 kilocalories above normal requirements.

In addition to the large demands of the growing fetus the mother must provide energy to meet the demands created by her own return to an active physical routine.

Protein. The synthesis of 1 gm. of milk protein requires that 2 gm. be available from the maternal tissues. This calls for a dietary intake of approximately 1.5 gm. per kilogram of body weight. Studies in poor Indian women showed that increase in the protein content of the mother's diet from 60 to 69 gm. resulted in no change in the protein content of the milk.

Calcium. The production of milk with its characteristically high calcium content, even though human milk contains only one fourth as much calcium as cow's milk, calls for an intake of 1.5 gm.—almost double the normal adult requirement—to prevent a severe depletion of maternal calcium reserves.

Iron. Since relatively little iron is transferred to the infant through milk, the need for iron in the maternal diet does not increase above that for pregnancy. The amount that does occur in human milk is very well utilized and may delay the normal drop in hemoglobin levels in early infancy.

Vitamin A. Although most infants have a fair reserve of vitamin A stored in their liver at the time of birth, human milk provides both vitamin A and carotenoids. An intake of 8000 I.U., easily achieved by the regular use of green and yellow vegetables, allows the production of milk with sufficient vitamin A to meet the needs of the infant. In one study of vitamin A supplementation of the diet of poor Indian women no increase in the vitamin A in the milk was observed. The investigators hypothesized that once the mother's reserves have been restored that the levels in the milk would increase.

Thiamine. Thiamine is one nutrient for which a deficiency in the mother's diet is reflected in the production of a milk low in the nutrient rather than in a diminished output of milk. In addition, a mother whose diet is very low in thiamine may secrete a substance, glyoxal, which accumulates in thiamine deficiency. The presence of this potentially toxic substance along with a low thiamine content in milk is associated with infantile beriberi. An intake of 1.6 mg. should allow the production of a milk with adequate thiamine levels. While cow's milk may have a higher thiamine content than human milk, the fact that this heat-labile vitamin is destroyed during pasteurization and sterilization of the formula makes human milk a more dependable source.

Riboflavin. Milk is one of the most dependable sources of riboflavin in the adult diet, and human milk provides high levels for the infant.

Ascorbic acid. The amount of ascorbic acid in human milk is higher than that in cow's milk, which, because of losses during heat processing, is incapable of meeting the needs of the infant after the first two weeks. The transfer of ascorbic acid to human milk calls for an intake of 150 to 200 mg., which is easily obtained from two servings of citrus fruits. An analysis of human milk has revealed a seasonal variation in its ascorbic acid content, reflecting changes in maternal intake.

Vitamin D. Vitamin D is transferred to a limited extent to the milk so that even breast-fed infants require a supplementary source of the vitamin for maximum utilization of calcium and phosphorus for bone formation.

Other nutrients. The transfer of the micronutrient elements, iodine and fluorine, through the mother's milk to the infant is quite efficient and contributes appreciably to the intake of the child when the mother's intake is adequate, protecting against goiter and reducing tooth decay.

These relatively high nutritional requirements of lactation require a significant increase in the quantity of food consumed and also dictate that the qualitative aspects of the food be carefully controlled. The use of an extra serving of meat, green and yellow fruits or vegetables, citrus fruit, and the equivalent of two cups of milk over and above a normal adequate diet will take care of the additional nutrients required. Obviously this quantity of food cannot be incorporated into three regular meals without taxing the capacity of the stomach. Since most lactating women have very good appetites it is quite feasible to suggest an eating pattern that includes five or six meals a day. If between-meal snacks are kept relatively low in satiety value, there is little decrease in the appetite for regular meals. While an increased intake of fluids does not increase milk production, it is desirable to help prevent overtaxing the kidney's ability to concentrate the urine to get rid of metabolic waste.

DIETARY SUPPLEMENTS

In light of the very high level of nutritional intake prescribed for normal lactation it is likely sound practice to recommend the use of a dietary supplement that provides protective levels of the nutrients for which there is the possibility of a dietary lack. This does not imply the endorsement of a supplement providing therapeutic levels of some nutrients and insignificant amounts of others.

Stimulation of lactation

Many techniques have been suggested to stimulate satisfactory level of lactation. Likely none are as effective as a constant stimulation of the mammary gland by the vigorous sucking of an infant and the presence of adequate nutritive reserves in the mother's tissues as a result of an adequate diet before conception and during pregnancy to initiate milk production. The first fluid secreted by the human breast, colostrum, is a thin, yellowish, watery fluid that bears little physical resemblance to milk and has its own unique nutritional compo-

Table 16-5. The composition of colostrum; immature and mature human milk and cow's milk per 100 ml. of milk*

Nutrient	Colostrum (1 to 5 days)	Human Transitional (6 to 10 days)	Mature	Mature cow milk
Energy, kilocalories	58.0	74.0	71.0	69.0
Fat, gm.	2.9	3.6	3.8	3.7
Lactose, gm.	5.3	6.6	7.0	4.8
Protein, gm.	2.7	1.6	1.2	3.3
Casein, gm.	1.2	0.7	0.4	2.8
Lactalbumin, gm.		0.8	0.3	0.4
Calcium, mg.	31.0	34.0	33.0	125.0
Phosphorus, mg.	14.0	17.0	15.0	96.0
Iron, mg.	0.09	0.04	0.15	0.10
Vitamins				
A, I.U.	296	283	176	113
Carotene, I.U.	186	63	45	63
D, I.U.			0.42	2.36
E, mg.	1.28	1.32	0.56	0.06
Ascorbic acid, mg.	4.4	5.4	4.3	1.6
Folic acid, μg.	0.05	0.02	0.18	0.23
Niacin, mg.	0.075	0.175	0.172	0.085
Pantothenic acid, mg.	0.183	0.288	0.196	0.350
Pyridoxine, mg.			0.011	0.048
Riboflavin, mg.	0.029	0.033	0.042	0.157
Thiamine, mg.	0.015	0.006	0.016	0.042

*Based on Food and Nutrition Board, National Academy of Sciences: The composition of milks, National Research Council Publication No. 254, Washington, D. C., 1953, National Research Council.

sition as shown in Table 16-5. The flow of colostrum may not begin for two to four days postpartum—a delay that is often erroneously interpreted as a failure of lactation.

Oxytocin, a hormone of the pituitary gland, has been effective in stimulating lactation through stimulation of the letdown reflex in which there is a contraction of the smooth muscles surrounding the alveoli of the nipple to allow the release of milk. It helps counteract the inhibition of the reflex, which is often caused by pain, emotional conflict, and embarrassment. While large amounts of estrogens suppress lactation, small amounts appear to have a stimulating effect by preventing an abnormal engorgement of the breast. Almost every culture has its own medicinal or food galactogogues, which are effective to varying degrees. These include garlic, cottonseed, candy, beer, ale, and large quantities of milk.

The relationship between fluid intake and volume of mammary secretion has not been established. Even when fluid intake is low, the volume secreted remains constant while urine volume drops, indicating that the mother has had to concentrate her urinary excretions. So while low intakes do not suppress milk volume and high intakes do not stimulate milk production, liberal fluid intake is suggested to preclude the necessity of the formation of a highly concentrated urine.

Duration of lactation

The period of time for which lactation is continued varies with a great many factors, both social and physiologic. In many cultures breast-feeding is carried on for two to three years with milk being the sole source of food for a year or more. In other cultures breast milk may be supplemented with other foods as early as three or four weeks. The latter case is believed to lead to less vigorous sucking, which in turn leads to a reduction in milk output and usually early weaning. There is some evidence that this same group experiences an earlier return to a regular pattern of ovulation with subsequent pregnancies occurring sooner. The observed trend for a longer lactation period in lower socioeconomic groups now appears to be reversing itself, with mothers of higher socioeconomic and educational status breast-feeding their infants for six months or more.

For some mothers lactation is terminated when the amount of milk produced declines to a point where such extensive supplementary feeding is required that it is no longer feasible to continue breast-feeding.

SELECTED REFERENCES

Pregnancy

Beaton, G.: Nutritional and physiological adaptations in pregnancy, Fed. Proc. (No. 1, Part III) 20:196, 1961.

Burke, B. S., Stevenson, S. S., Worcester, J., and Stuart, H. C.: Nutrition studies during pregnancy. V. Relation of maternal nutrition to condition of infant at birth: study of siblings, J. Nutrition 38:453, 1949.

Clements, F. W.: Nutrition in maternal and infant feeding, Fed. Proc. (No. 1, Part III) 20:165, 1961.

Ebbs, J. F., Tisdall, F. F., and Scott, W. A.: Influence of prenatal diet on mother and child, J. Nutrition 22:515, 1941.

Hellman, R. W.: Nutrition in pregnancy and lactation, M. Clin. North America, 48:1141, 1964.

Holly, R. G.: Dynamics of iron metabolism in pregnancy, Am. J. Obst. & Gynec. 93:370, 1965.

Jackson, H. N., Burke, B. S., Smith, C. A., and Reed, D. E.: Effect of weight reduction in obese pregnant women on pregnancy, labor, and delivery and on the condition of the infant at birth, Am. J. Obst. & Gynec. 83:1609, 1962.

Larson, R. H.: Effect of prenatal nutrition on oral structures, J. Am. Dietet. A. 44:368, 1964.

Lubchenco, L. O., Hansman, C., Dressler, M., and Boyd, E.: Intrauterine growth as estimated from liveborn birth-weight data at 24 to 42 weeks of gestation, Pediatrics 32:793, 1963.

McCollum, E. B.: Symposium on prenatal nutrition, J. Am. Dietet. A. 36:236, 1960.

McGanity, W. J., Bridgforth, E. B., and Darby, W. J.: Vanderbilt cooperative study of maternal and infant nutrition; Effect of reproductive cycle on nutritional status and requirements, J.A.M.A. 168:2138, 1958.

Macy, I. G.: Metabolic and biochemical changes in normal pregnancy, J.A.M.A. 168:2265, 1958.

Pike, R. L.: Sodium intake during pregnancy, J. Am. Dietet. A. 44:176, 1964.

Rhodes, P.: The significance of weight gain in pregnancy, Lancet 1:663, 1962.

Seifert, E.: Changes in beliefs and food practices in pregnancy, J. Am. Dietet. A. 39:455, 1961.

Smith, C. A.: Prenatal and neonatal nutrition, Pediatrics 30:145, 1962.

Stearns, G.: Nutrition status of mother prior to conception, J.A.M.A. 168:1655, 1958.

Thomson, A. M.: Diet in pregnancy. 3. Diet in relation to the course and outcome of pregnancy, Brit. J. Nutrition 13:509, 1959.

Thomson, A. M., and Billewicz, W. Z.: Nutritional status, maternal physique and reproductive efficiency, Proc. Nutrition Soc. 22:55, 1963.

Wishik, S.: Nutrition in pregnancy and lactation, Fed. Proc. 18:4, 1959.

Lactation

Bigwood, E. J.: Nitrogenous constituents and nutritive value of human and cow's milk, World Rev. Nutr. Diet. 4:95, 1963.

Gopalan, C., and Belavady, B.: Nutrition and lactation, Fed. Proc. (Part 2) 20:177, 1960.

Macy, I. G., Kelly, H. J., and Sloan, R. E.: The composition of milks, National Research Council Publication No. 254, Washington, D. C., 1953, National Research Council.

Mayer, J.: Nutrition and lactation, Postgrad. Med. 33:380, 1963.

Woody, D. C., and Woody, H. B.: Management of breast feeding, J. Pediat. 68:344, 1966.

17

Infant nutrition

The adequacy of nutrition in infancy is crucial to the well-being of the individual throughout life. The infant who is adequately nourished undergoes a normal rate of physical and mental development. On the other hand, one who is inadequately nourished in respect to one or more nutrients will experience a stunted growth and other biochemical changes associated with undernutrition, which may be reversed if the inadequacy is corrected while the growth reponse is still present. Mental and neurological development may be more seriously affected, and there is some evidence that a depressed brain development caused by severe dietary restriction at a critical period in infancy may result in a permanent mental retardation. Thus, in the light of future development, both mental and physical, the importance of an adequate nutritive intake in early infancy cannot be overemphasized.

BREAST-FEEDING

The incidence of breast-feeding in the United States, which underwent a decline from an almost universal practice at the turn of the century to 38% incidence in 1946, declined still further to 21% in 1958. In some regions the incidence was as low as 12% of all babies leaving the hospital and in others as high as 47%. Studies since that time have indicated increased interest in breast-feeding among the more educated higher socioeconomic groups. A recent report shows that 50% of mothers in a college town are breast-feeding successfully. Similarly, a study of 2233 mothers in the Boston area showed that while only 22% of the total group were breast-feeding, 69.3% of those married to students breast-fed and that 39.8% of the upper social class and only 13.6% of the lower social class breast-fed. College education was an important factor in the decision to breast-feed. There was no relationship between a daughter's decision and her mother's. The pattern of feeding used by the better-educated group is frequently followed several years later by less educated mothers and those of lower socioeconomic status in a wavelike sequence with the lower socioeconomic group emulating the higher. Whether the current trend prevails will not be ascertained for several years.

In a few cases the decision regarding the initial type of feeding is often based ·on very special circumstances such as tuberculosis or breast cancer, which preclude breast-feeding. But in most cases the decision will be made after a consideration of the relative merits of the two types since, for all intents and purposes, either should be possible and successful in a Western culture. In developing countries, on the other hand, breast-feeding is essential if the child is to survive the neonatal period.

Considerations favoring breast-feeding

Nutritional. In general, it is felt that the nutrient composition of the milk of each species is the one best suited to the growth needs of its offspring and where possible it should be used, but if this is not possible then the milk of another species should be modified to approximate the composition of the maternal milk.

The difference in nutritive composition of human and cow's milk is well documented and is presented in Fig. 17-1, which indicates the relative amounts in each type of milk, showing that breast milk contains more of some nutrients and less of others. The absolute amounts for some nutrients are given in Table 16-5, which includes a comparison of colostrum and mature milk with data from several laboratories. The lower concentration of some nutrients such as calcium and protein in breast milk is believed to reflect the differing growth needs between the human infant and the calf. The latter doubles its birth weight in two months, compared to the human infant, which takes five months. Not only does the total amount of some nutrients differ but also the physicochemical properties of the form in which they exist. For instance, human milk, in which the protein is predominately lactalbumin, contains only half as much protein as cow's milk, in which most of the protein is in the form of casein. Casein forms a hard curd when subjected to the action of rennin in the stomach whereas lactalbumin forms a soft flocculent curd on which digestive enzymes act freely. Fatty acids in human milk are less saturated and have longer carbon chains and are utilized more effectively than the short-chain, more saturated fatty acids in cow's milk. The calorie value of the two milks is very similar, as is the total fat content, but reduction in protein is compensated for by a higher amount of lactose in human milk. Fat provides 50%, protein 7%, and carbohydrate 43% of the calories in human milk, compared to 50%, 20%, and 30% respectively in cow's milk.

The disaccharide lactose found in both human and cow's milk is present at twice the level in human milk. Lactose has several advantages in infant feeding over other carbohydrates in that it facilitates the absorption of calcium and magnesium, leading to a higher mineral content available for growth in bones, and it favors amino acid absorption and nitrogen retention. Since the digestion of lactose is incomplete in the upper gastrointestinal tract, some of it reaches the lower gastrointestinal tract where the *Lactobacillus* organisms convert it into lactic acid and other organic acids. This acid medium is conducive to the growth of fermentative rather than undesirable putrefactive organisms, thus decreasing the likelihood of infection. The benefit is especially great when the lactose-protein ratio is high, as is true in breast milk. The addition of lactose to modified cow's milk formulas is generally not practical because of its high cost and low solubility and the problems of inducing diarrhea if the amount is too high. There is some evidence also that lactose favors riboflavin and pyridoxine synthesis, although it may be of little benefit to the infant if it occurs in the lower gastrointestinal tract. The mechanism by which lactose facilitates calcium absorption likely involves its role

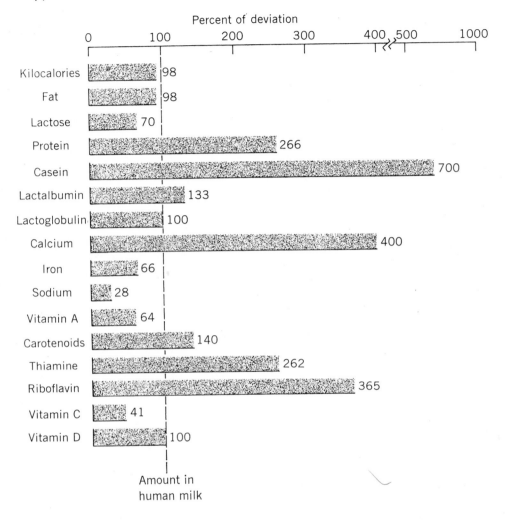

Comparison of nutritive value of cow's
and human milk

Fig. 17-1

Relative amounts of various nutrients in human and cow's milk. (Based on data from Composition of human milk, National Research Council Publication No. 254, Washington, D. C., 1953, National Research Council.)

in a chelating agent either as the disaccharide or monosaccharide galactose or in preventing the precipitation of calcium.

The amount of the heat-labile vitamins, thiamine and ascorbic acid, found in human milk is almost completely available to the infant whereas the amount available from cow's milk may be substantially reduced from the application of heat in the pasterization of milk and sterilization of the formula.

One unidentified factor in human milk has been designated as the *Lactobacillus bifidus* factor since it creates a medium in the gastrointestinal tract conducive to the growth of the microorganism *Lactobacillus bifidus.* This microorganism, by producing acetic or lactic acid from lactose, depresses the growth of pathogenic organisms and decreases the susceptibility to infection. It is postulated that the factor in human milk is lactulose, a derivative of lactose known to occur in large amounts in breast milk and in higher amounts in heat-treated than untreated cow's milk. The growth of *L. bifidus* is enhanced on a high-lactose, low-protein diet with a lactose-protein ratio of 7:1 to 4:1. The presence of a protein-splitting enzyme in breast milk reduces complete proteins to the less complex peptone stage, on which digestive enzymes act more effectively. These enzymes in cow's milk are destroyed by the heat of pasteurization.

Colostrum, the secretion of the breast that precedes the secretion of mature milk, differs from milk in appearance and nutritional properties. This watery yellowish fluid is believed to contribute a high degree of *passive immunity* to the infant consuming it because its antibodies are absorbed intact during the first few days of life. Considerable evidence indicates that it contains a poliomyelitis antibody. There is not universal agreement as to the nutritive value of colostrum. Between the fifth and tenth day colostrum undergoes changes in chemical and physical composition until by the tenth day it has usually assumed the characteristics of mature milk.

Psychological. The psychological advantages of breast-feeding have been freely discussed but are poorly documented. The consensus of opinion is that the infant derives a sense of security and belonging in the early mother-child relationship from the warmth of the mother's body and from the comfort of being held rather than from the feeding process per se. Harlow, in a classic study with monkeys, showed that those fed by a surrogate mother (a bottle inserted in a wire screen covered with warm terry cloth) were equally as well adjusted as those fed by the real mother. Monkeys fed by a bottle alone showed more evidence of emotional instability. Research with dogs and ducks has identified a critical period during the first few days of life when imprinting or learning, which is remarkably resistant to modification, occurs. It may be that the impact of the mother on the child in this critical period will have implications for breast-feeding. Although psychologists so far have been unable to elucidate consistent differences in personality between bottle-fed and breast-fed infants, if it can be demonstrated that breast-feeding increases a mother's feeling of competence in dealing with her child. It is conceivable that more carefully controlled studies may show effects on personality that have so far largely evaded detection. There is some feeling that the greatest psychological advantages accrue to the mother who feels that she is involved in a unique relationship with the child and is fulfilling her true maternal role.

Other factors. Various other advantages have been attributed to breast-feeding. Since the work of obtaining milk from the breast is much more difficult than from most bottles it is felt that the use required of muscles of the mouth leads to the development of the jaw and reduces the incidence of crowded dentition in later years. Others maintain that the hormonal balance that exists in lactation favors the contraction of the uterus, thus speeding the return of the mother's abdomen to normal size. The reduced likelihood of contamination, the elimination of the possibility of mistakes in mixing the formula, or the necessity of finding a satisfactory formula are more salient factors favoring breast-feeding among the less well-educated segment of the population and in developing countries than they are for the intelligent middle-class mother. However, a mistake in the preparation of infant formula in a hospital when salt was used instead of sugar became a tragic example of the possibility of human error in preparing a formula.

The incidence of infection is generally lower in breast-fed than in bottle-fed infants, as reflected in lower morbidity rates.

The growth rate of breast-fed infants exceeds that of bottle-fed infants for the first four to five months of life, after which bottle-fed infants experience a more rapid growth rate. No differences between the two groups can be ascertained at two years of age. The use of breast milk virtually eliminates the possibility of a milk allergy whereas reports on the incidence of cow's milk allergy range from 0.3% to 7% of artificially fed infants. The increased incidence of "cot deaths" among infants has been explained as an allergic reaction after the aspiration of cow's milk protein which has been spit up in sleep by a bottle-fed infant who apparently was sensitized to cow's milk protein at an early age.

Considerations favoring bottle-feeding

Available substitute. The availability of safe and satisfactory preparations in which cow's milk has been modified to provide a satisfactory substitute for human milk leads many mothers to choose bottle-feeding. To be most satisfactory, cow's milk must be modified so that it resembles human milk as closely as possible in composition and in physicochemical properties. The dilution of cow's milk to provide a concentration of protein similar to that of human milk also causes a reduction in curd tension and leads to the formation of a softer, more flocculent curd that can be more readily handled by the proteolytic enzymes in the gastrointestinal tract of the infant. Other methods of modifying the character of the curd that are sometimes used in place of or in addition to dilution include the use of pancreatic enzymes, heat treatment, the addition of an acid such as citric acid or acid-producing microorganisms, or the addition of alkali in the preparation of infant formulas. There seems to

be little advantage of one method over another. The dilution of milk has the advantage of creating a calcium concentration more nearly approximating human milk and the disadvantage of reducing the caloric value from a normal level of 67 kilocalories per ounce. The addition of a readily utilizable carbohydrate such as dextromaltose or sucrose can raise the caloric value to that of human milk. The lower level of sodium deemed desirable to reduce the burden on the kidney through which sodium is excreted in the urine can be achieved by removing much of the electrolyte by dialysis, a method sometimes employed in commercial formula preparations. Other processors have attempted to simulate the higher linoleic content of human milk by replacing the butterfat with its short-chain saturated fatty acid by corn oil with long-chain unsaturated fatty acids. Fat in this form is tolerated better by the infant and provides more adequate levels of the essential fatty acid, linoleic acid. The use of too high a level of polyunsaturated fatty acids may, however, increase the need for vitamin E. No satisfactory substitute for the colostrum provided by the human breast has been found.

The safety of bottle-feeding has increased with increasing awareness of the importance of aseptic techniques in the preparation of infant formula. Sterilization of feeding equipment and formula has reduced the transmission of pathogenic organisms and the resulting disease. Prior to the discovery of microorganisms as the cause of disease, the hazards of bottle-feeding were so great that they led to a marked increase in infant mortality and morbidity rates over breast-feeding. Some reports still indicate a markedly higher mortality and morbidity rate in bottle-fed infants than in breast-fed infants, but, among the infants born to middle-class mothers in technically developed countries there generally is no significant difference.

Psychological. For many mothers bottle-feeding represents the only alternative to breast-feeding. They may have many psychological blocks concerning breast-feeding, ranging from considering it a bovine function to considering it a form of "uneating." Others are unwilling to risk breast-feeding for fear that their figures may become permanently distorted and that it will take longer to return to a prepregnancy weight. Neither belief has been adequately documented. If the mother lacks the desire to breast-feed the chances of it succeeding are greatly reduced.

Economic. According to a study conducted by the Maternal and Child Health section of the American Public Health Association, the cost of the increased amount of food required by the mother to provide the recommended 1000 kilocalories, 0.5 gm. of calcium, and 40 gm. of high-quality protein needed over and above that suggested for the nonpregnant, nonlactating woman is higher than the cost of the one quart of milk needed by the infant. On a moderate-cost diet they felt that the addition of a quart of milk, 6 ounces of orange juice, 2 slices of whole-wheat bread, a half ounce of butter, and an egg would provide the added nutrients at a cost of 41 cents. On a low-cost food budget they considered the use of one fourth pound of nonfat milk solids, 2 ounces of cooking oil, an ounce of enriched cornmeal, one third pound of turnip greens, and a vitamin supplement every other day at a total cost of 15 cents. The cost of these relatively simple additions to the diet is about equal to the 15 cents suggested by the same committee as the cost of a modified evaporated milk formula. Commercially prepared formulas in which the milk has been adequately modified to simulate human milk cost approximately 25 cents per day. The cost of equipment such as bottles and sterilizers has not been included.

Social. For many mothers the freedom and flexibility of social life that bottle-feeding affords is an overriding consideration in the choice of bottle-feeding. In fact, among fifty-five mothers who had had a satisfying breast-feeding experience, the loss of freedom and restricting of their social life were considered disadvantages by twenty-nine mothers. Most of these mothers had found, however, that an occasional bottle could be substituted for a breast-feeding with no adverse reaction from the child, although the mother might have experienced physical discomfort. Some studies found that mothers chose bottle-feeding because they needed to see the amount of milk the child was consuming.

Disadvantages of breast-feeding

Since a fairly high percentage of mothers choose not to breast-feed there must be some objections or disadvantages to it. Among these are failure of the mother to secrete adequate milk, constant fatigue reported by many mothers, the lack of freedom, the impossibility of turning the responsibility over to someone else, the possibility of breast infection, and a desire to quickly restore the mother's figure to normal.

From a physiologic point of view there are reports of the transmission of the hormone pregnanediol through the mother's milk, resulting in hyperbilirubinemia in the infant.

For some mothers a failure to recognize that the onset of lactation may be delayed until three to five days after birth and that the physical appearance of colostrum is quite different from milk and that their milk has not "turned to water" may explain their decision to abandon attempts at breast-feeding. The desire of mothers for either economic or psychological reasons to leave the hospital as soon as possible after birth can mean that if lactation is not established shortly after birth the mother will give up her plans in the interest of taking the infant home on a functioning feeding routine, that is, bottle-feeding.

Table 17-1. Recommended dietary allowances for infants[*]

Nutrient	0 to 1 year	1 to 3 years
Kilocalories	45 to 60 per pound	1300
Protein (gm.)	0.9 to 1.3 per pound of body weight	32
Calcium (mg.)	700	800
Iron (mg.)	0.5 per pound of body weight	8
Vitamin A (I.U.)	1500	2000
Thiamine (mg.)	0.4	0.5
Riboflavin (mg.)	0.6	0.8
Niacin (mg.)	6	9
Ascorbic acid (mg.)	30	30
Vitamin D (I.U.)	400	400

[*]From Recommended dietary allowances, National Academy of Sciences, National Research Council Publication 1146, 1964.

Adequacy of milk diet

The NRC recommended allowances for infants are shown in Table 17-1. A diet composed solely of human or cow's milk consumed at a level of approximately 800 ml. per day will provide recommended amounts of all the nutrients needed, except ascorbic acid, and vitamin D up to three months of age. At three to six months when fetal iron reserves are depleted, milk is incapable of providing sufficient iron to maintain hemoglobin level.

Ascorbic acid is a limiting factor only for bottle-fed infants whose formula is subjected to high heat during processing. These infants should receive a supplementary source of ascorbic acid by the tenth day of life. After the discovery of antiscorbutic properties of oranges, orange juice was fed as a source of vitamin C, starting with 1 teaspoon of juice diluted with an equal amount of water and building up to about 2 tablespoons of juice. With an increasing number of reports of allergic reactions, apparently from the oil of the orange rind which was extracted with the juice, there was a trend toward the use of a synthetic source of ascorbic acid that minimized any sensitizing reaction. This is a very general practice in the first few months of life, after which the child can be given a fruit juice high in ascorbic acid. There is some evidence that infants born to mothers who had an extremely high ascorbic acid intake during pregnancy have a conditioned need for a high level of the vitamin.

The amount of vitamin D in either human or cow's milk is a function of the diet of the mother or cow, but even under ideal conditions does not approach the 400 I.U. recommended by the Food and Nutrition Board of the National Research Council. Thus, unless a child has regular exposure to sunlight, it is necessary to provide a vitamin D supplement, preferably by five days of age. Cod-liver oil, the most popular source after the discovery of its antirachitic properties in promoting normal calcification of bones and teeth, has been replaced by water-miscible preparations to avoid the danger of lipoid pneumonia from the aspiration of the oily particles of cod-liver oil into the lungs. If, however, a bottle-fed infant is given a formula made with evaporated or homogenized milk, which is normally fortified with 400 I.U. of vitamin D per quart, no supplementation is necessary. In light of current reports of toxic reactions caused by the use of diets high in vitamin D it is likely undesirable.

The low level of iron in milk is not a cause of concern since infants are born with a reserve of iron in the liver to meet their needs for three to six months. It thus seems appropriate to add some source of iron to the diet by three to six months of age to prevent a drop in hemoglobin levels to a level of less than 10 gm. per 100 ml. of blood—a level considered indicative of anemia. Many commercial formula preparations are now fortified with iron. Since a drop in hemoglobin level from the 18 gm. characteristic of birth levels is normal and the body absorbs virtually no iron until there is a need for it, the supplementation of formula in the early weeks of life appears unnecessary. One study of the use of a formula supplemented with vitamins and iron (12 mg. per 32 ounces) produced no differences in growth and development, number of illnesses, or in hemoglobin, hematocrit, or serum iron levels up to three to three and a half months of age. The blood values were higher after this time when the iron-fortified formula was used. Another extensive study of the use of iron-enriched formula from birth suggests that its use does provide a protection against subsequent drop in hemoglobin levels by maintaining hemoglobin levels 1 to 1.5 gm. higher at nine months of age. Whether the infant's mechanism for regulating iron absorption is sufficiently sensitive to prevent the uptake of excess iron, leading to iron overload when it is fed prior to a time of need, has not been investigated.

Temperature of milk

The question of the temperature of a milk feeding has been raised recently with the contention of several investigators that formula from the refrigerator is well tolerated by 50% of very young infants and 75% of older infants and gives as good a growth response as that which has been warmed to body temperature. Peters found that feeding ice-cold milk lowered gastric temperature for at least an hour, decreased the activity of proteolytic enzymes, and hence delayed digestion.

Nutritive needs of infants

Precise information on the nutritive needs of infants is available for only a few nutrients, but the National Research Council has suggested levels of intake that appear to support growth in healthy infants.

Energy. An intake of 110 kilocalories per kilogram of body weight or 43 kilocalories per pound appears to be adequate to meet the needs for maintaining body temperature, for growth, and for activity. A very placid infant is reported to need as few as 70 kilocalories per kilogram while a crying infant may need as many as 130 kilocalories. Since the body surface area of infants per unit of body weight is twice as great as in adults the insensible heat loss from the surface is twice as great.

An excessive intake of calories leading to a rapid gain in weight is equally as undesirable in infants as in adults. MacKeith, in discussing the question "Is a big baby a healthy baby?", suggested that a baby who weighs 27 pounds at one year of age is more likely to grow up to be an obese adolescent or adult than one weighing less. Bakwin has raised the question of a relationship between early feeding of solids, calorie intake, and subsequent obesity.

For a newborn infant milk provides all the calories. Filer reports that by six months of age 70% of the energy is still provided by milk, with meat providing 10%, and cereal, fruit, and vegetables each 5%.

Protein. The needs for protein during the period of very rapid skeletal and muscular growth of early infancy are relatively high. An intake of 2.5 to 3 gm. of protein of high biological value per kilogram of body weight supports a level of nitrogen retention sufficiently great to allow normal growth. There was no difference in nitrogen retention in a group of infants receiving 10% of their calories from protein and a group receiving 15%. Nor were there any differences in the composition of fat-free tissues on low- or high-protein intakes. There is no evidence of advantages of protein intakes above this level and some evidence of disadvantages. Infants receiving whole unmodified cow's milk have suffered from a hypochromic macrocytic anemia caused by gastric bleeding leading to large blood losses in the feces, apparently the result of an allergy to the cow's milk protein. The frequency with which other manifestations of a cow's milk allergy are also reported indicates that the high protein content of cow's milk may cause the development of a protein sensitivity. Protein in excess of the body's need for growth and repair of tissue must undergo deamination in the liver so that the nonamino portion of the amino acids can be used as a source of energy. The nitrogenous NH_2 group must be converted to urea and excreted through the kidney. Since the infant has a limited capacity to concentrate metabolites in the urine, the excretion of more wastes requires a larger volume of water. If the necessary water is not available, urea will accumulate and the infant ironically suffers from protein edema. In addition, the need for the liver to produce the enzymes, deaminases, which are necessary to remove the amino group, may lead to an undesirable hypertrophy or increase in size of the liver.

It is also postulated that the higher rate of infection in infants fed cow's milk may occur because mechanisms that might normally be concerned with the formation of antibodies are used to combat foreign milk protein.

In rats it was found that the animals on a high-protein diet who had had hypertrophy of the liver were less able to adjust to a low-protein diet than those that had previously been on a moderate- or low-protein diet.

Studies to evaluate the relative biological value of meat and milk proteins have shown similar protein efficiency ratios (gain per unit of protein). Both meat and milk protein are well tolerated in the digestive tract, and infants appear to have adequate proteolytic enzymes to handle meat protein and milk protein if the curd tension is adequately reduced.

The amino acid requirements of infants are proportionately higher than in adults. In addition to the eight amino acids needed by adults, histidine is required by infants at < 35 mg. per kilogram of body weight per day, a level surpassed in both breast- and bottle-feeding.

In one study of six-month-old infants it was found that 70% of the protein in the diet came from milk, 15% from meat, and 3% each from egg, cereal, and vegetables.

Thiamine. The recommended allowance of thiamine for infants is 0.4 mg., again reflecting a relationship between caloric intake and thiamine requirements. Breast milk is usually adequate if the mother's diet is adequate, but it is one nutrient for which the mother does not reduce the quantity of milk rather than produce a milk of lower nutritional quality. This has been observed primarily in developing countries where cereals and starchy roots are eaten, the diet of the mother is high in carbohydrate and very low in thiamine, and infants are solely breast-fed for a year or more. These infants failed to gain weight, were constipated, and vomited frequently. In bottle-fed infants the possibility of a deficiency of heat-labile thiamine occurs when the formula is subjected to high heat.

Attempts to show that thiamine is beneficial as an appetite stimulant have failed to reveal any value in infant feeding; nor have scientists been able to demonstrate any benefit from thiamine supplementation on height, weight, manual dexterity, or retentive memory. It is conceded that once the metabolic defect caused by a thiamine deficiency has been corrected that the appetite improves.

In infants from six months to two years of age, diet records showed that those infants whose diets were adequate in thiamine were receiving enriched cereal while those who did not receive adequate thiamine were not using enriched cereals.

Riboflavin and niacin. Since riboflavin and niacin are involved primarily in the enzyme systems necessary for the release of energy from carbohydrate, fat, and protein the requirement increases with increased caloric intake. Because of the high proportion of milk in the infant's diet both riboflavin and niacin precursors are usually found in adequate amounts.

Pyridoxine. The need for pyridoxine in humans has not been established, but all of the few available reports of a deficiency in the human dietary have involved infants fed a commercial formula that had been subjected to high temperature. Most such preparations are not fortified with pyridoxine to provide the levels normally found in human milk. Infants on deficient pyridoxine diets experience convulsive seizures.

Cobalamin. There have been several reports and many claims in advertising that cobalamin acts as a growth stimulant. The Academy of Pediatrics, in reviewing the literature on the subject, found that in thirteen studies involving 546 "normal children" only two studies involving 69 children reported a significant and stimulating effect on growth with either oral or intramuscular doses of cobalamin. In all of these the children were underweight at the beginning. Since infants carry a reserve of vitamin B_{12} from the prenatal period there is little likelihood of a dietary deficiency.

Ascorbic acid. Infant needs for ascorbic acid have been set at 30 mg. per day, although many studies suggest that a much lower level will provide protection against scurvy and others suggest that the infant may be conditioned to even higher levels. Breast-fed infants usually receive adequate

amounts, but because of the destruction of heat-labile ascorbic acid during pasteurization, infants fed cow's milk usually rely on a dietary supplement during the first few months.

Calcium. Because of the rapid rate of calcification of bone to provide the rigidity and strength needed to support the weight of the body by the time the baby walks, a very rich dietary source of calcium is needed in early infancy. Milk, the staple item in the diet at this time, is capable of providing the infant's needs but the efficiency with which it is used is greatly enhanced when vitamin D is available simultaneously. Although some calcification of teeth has begun in the prenatal period, the availability and utilization of calcium in the postnatal period is a crucial factor in adequate tooth formation.

Iron. The infant's need for iron is determined to a large extent by his gestational age. Normally a full-term infant has benefitted from the transfer of a significant amount of iron from the mother to the fetus. If such reserves from fetal life are present the infant will need virtually no dietary iron for at least three months. In fact, if it is added to the milk very little will be absorbed before three to four months of age, when a drop in hemoglobin level reflects depletion of reserves in the liver. By that time, an intake of 6 mg. per day is recommended. This may be obtained from enriched cereal or egg yolk and later on from meat.

The premature infant with a shorter gestational period is deprived of these fetal reserves and will need a dietary source earlier. The same is true of twins, who must compete for maternal reserves and share that available.

Phosphorus. Studies by Widdowson have shown beneficial effects on the absorption of calcium and magnesium when breast-fed infants were given supplements of 120 mg. of phosphorus per day, suggesting that the amount of phosphorus in breast milk may limit the calcification of bone and the growth of soft tissue at an early age. Strontium uptake was unaffected.

Fluorine. Although fluorine has not been established as a dietary essential it is mentioned in a discussion of infant feeding because of the beneficial effects in providing resistance to tooth decay that accrue when fluorine is present during the period of calcification of dental tissues. If the mother is using fluoridated water, it will be reflected in the level of fluorine in the breast milk. Bottle-fed babies whose formulas are diluted with fluoridated water will also receive protection. Since infants normally consume very little water in the first few months it is likely desirable to provide it in some supplement, although if mothers' supplies have been adequate the infant will carry some fluorine reserve at birth.

Water or fluid. While the intake of water is crucial at all stages in the life cycle it receives a little more attention in infancy than at other times because the demands are relatively greater then. The surface area per unit of body weight is twice that of the adult, which leads to a heat and water loss through the skin at a rate almost double that of the adult. Because of the high basal metabolic rate (two times that of an adult) there are proportionately more metabolic wastes, which calls for more water so that the kidney can adequately excrete them. This, coupled with the fact that the kidney of an infant does not have the ability to concentrate urine to the extent that a mature kidney does, means that relatively more water is required in the elimination of the same amount of metabolites. The metabolic waste is higher on a diet high in protein when the nitrogen from the deamination of amino acids in excess of needs for growth must be eliminated. More water is also required if the diet contains excess electrolytes such as sodium and potassium. An infant receiving a diet of human milk requires 20 ml. of water per kilogram of body weight to provide a sufficient amount for the kidney to handle excretory products.

If undiluted cow's milk is used, 87 ml. is required and if cow's milk, with one third of the calories coming from added carbohydrate, is used, 61 ml. At a normal room temperature of 70° F., any one of these formulas would provide enough water, but at 93° F. the cow's milk would not provide enough since proportionately more water is lost through the skin. If normal excretion of metabolic waste is to occur, additional water should be given. Even with a formula providing the normal 20 kilocalories per ounce, parents should offer the child additional water when the environmental temperature is high. Body water will be reduced to 70% of normal before influencing the renal excretion of water.

Vitamin A. The recommended allowance for vitamin A can be adequately met in a diet containing one quart of whole milk. If nonfat milk is substituted, however, the major source of vitamin A is withdrawn and does not seem to be replaced by the provitamin A in green and yellow vegetables. Most of the nutritional supplements used as a source of ascorbic acid and vitamin D also contain vitamin A.

Vitamin D. The necessity of a dietary supplement of vitamin D for infants born in the temperate zone or those born in the tropics who are denied any exposure to sunlight is well documented. An intake of 400 I.U. per day promotes normal calcification of bones and teeth, and there seems to be no increase in benefits beyond this level. In fact, more concern is being expressed now for the infant who consistently receives in excess of 2000 I.U. per day than for those receiving less than the recommended amounts. An excess intake leads to such symptoms as depressed appetite, vague aches and pains, and retarded growth.

INTRODUCTION OF SOLID FOODS

At the turn of the century pediatricians were recommending that the milk diet of infants be supplemented with a food such as meat or cereal after one year of age. By 1917, Dr. Emmett Holt was suggesting that a meat broth could safely be introduced at eight or nine months of age but that solid foods should be withheld until one year. By 1956, the pendulum had swung so far in the opposite direction that some pediatricians were recommending that an infant could be put on solid foods and be expected to adhere to three meals a day by two or three weeks of age. The Academy of Pediatrics, recognizing a trend in infant feeding practices toward progressively earlier introduction of solid foods in the absence of any evidence of a nutritional or physiologic need, surveyed practicing pediatricians to determine their recommendations and the bases for them. It found that the physicians were indeed suggesting the use of cereal by three to six weeks of age, followed by other foods so that by four or five months the child had received a full diet of meat, eggs, fruit, vegetables, and cereal. Their reasons for this practice reflected their response to the demands of mothers that they follow this "progressive" procedure rather than to any indication that the infant needed the solid food. The pressure exerted by commercial companies marketing special infant foods is also a contributing factor to the mother's anxiety to conform to what she believes to be sound eating habits.

A rational approach to the question of the timing and sequence of additions to the infant's diet should involve a consideration of the nutritional needs of the infant, his physiologic readiness to use foods other than milk, his physical capacity to handle them, and the relative advantages and disadvantages of adding semisolid or solid foods.

Nutrition. From a nutritional standpoint it has been established that the nutritive needs of an infant can be readily met for the first three months by a milk diet supplemented with sources of ascorbic acid and vitamin D. Since these are normally provided by the use of a therapeutic vitamin preparation or by the addition of cod-liver oil and orange juice, the provision of these nutrients involves only the use of liquids. By three months of age it is desirable to provide some rich source of iron since milk is a very poor source and fetal reserves begin to be depleted at this age. This may be provided in several foods. The most usual method is to use an iron-enriched cereal, which contributes 12 mg. per ounce or 0.92 mg. per tablespoon. If fed as a single-grain cereal, these cereals are minimally allergenic and the consistency can be readily adjusted to the infant's ability to handle it. Egg yolk, a rich source of iron (1 mg.), vitamin A, protein, and riboflavin, is recommended by many investigators although there is no consistent evidence that it promotes hematopoiesis more effectively than cereal. It is likely unwise to use egg for infants with a family history of allergy since the high protein may cause a reaction in sensitive individuals. Meat, providing 0.23 mg. per tablespoon, has also been recommended, but again in the absence of any evidence of unique benefits it is generally conceded that meat should be added later. Fruits and vegetables (0.05 to 0.32 mg. per tablespoon) may be used as a source of iron although the concentration is lower than in meat, cereal, or egg yolk. There are some efforts to promote the iron enrichment of milk on the theory that the iron should be provided by the major source of calories, especially among poor families who may be able to provide only a limited variety of foods.

With the increase in size of the infant it becomes increasingly difficult to meet the protein needs for growth on a diet of milk alone. By six months of age most infants are able to tolerate whole milk with its protein content of 3.2%. In addition to this, other dietary sources of complete protein are recommended; egg yolk with 33% protein, meat with 20%, and cottage cheese with 17% are considered suitable additions to the diet by six months of age.

Foods that provide the additional iron and protein needed by the growing child usually meet any additional needs for thiamine and niacin.

Physical development. Infants vary in the rate at which the normal routing, sucking, and extrusion reflexes inherent at the time of birth are replaced by the ability to swallow; and as these changes occur, an infant must learn to use them in the eating process just as he learns to walk or talk. The lower jaw is very poorly developed at birth to facilitate sucking, but as the child matures it becomes better developed and prepared for chewing functions. This swallowing reflex involves sufficient ennervation of the tongue to enable it to form any solid food placed at the tip of the tongue into a ball and throw it to the back of the mouth where first gravity and then the peristaltic action of the esophagus takes over to convey it to the stomach. This usually occurs at three months of age, but before this the extrusion reflex that causes the infant to forcibly reject food or objects placed at the front of the tongue must diminish in strength. Since the ability to move food from the tip of the tongue to the throat normally develops at two and a half to three months of age, any effort to feed solid or semisolid foods prior to that time means that some other way must be employed to convey the food to the esophagus. Either it must be placed sufficiently far back in the mouth that it can reach the esophagus by gravity or the consistency of the product must be so thin that it is merely a semisolid food and the infant is able to suck it from the spoon as a liquid rather than using a swallowing mechanism. Many times the infant who cannot manipulate the tongue to swallow cannot use it to reject objects or food placed in his mouth either. Thus it is not uncommon to have mothers report that infants who had apparently accepted solid food at three to six weeks of age appear to reject it at 10 to 12 weeks. Developmentally, few infants are ready to handle anything but liquid food until 10 to 12 weeks of age. Any effort to force them earlier may result in a frustrating and unhappy feeding experience for both the mother and the child.

Physiologic development. The ability to handle foods other than milk also depends on the physiologic development of the infant. All the secretions of the digestive tract contain enzymes especially suited to the digestion of the complex nutrients of milk but few needed for other foods.

For instance, the secretion of the salivary glands is minimal at birth but increases in volume until it becomes sufficiently copious to cause drooling by two or three months in the infant who has not developed the ennervation of the outer part of the lips necessary to prevent it. Since salivary enzymes are involved only in the digestion of the complex starches, they are unnecessary as long as the child is receiving only milk with the disaccharide lactose as the only carbohydrate. The appearance of salivary amylase in the saliva between two and three months of age marks the time when the infant is first ready to handle more complex carbohydrates such as the starch in cereals.

The proteolytic enzymes are present in adequate amounts to digest milk protein as long as it is sufficiently dilute to produce a soft flocculent curd on which the enzymes can act. As the child matures the secretion of proteolytic enzymes in the intestinal juice increases this capacity of the infant to digest nonmilk proteins. By four to six months of age most infants are able to handle most proteins.

The kidney function of the full-term infant is not completely mature. The well-developed glomeruli filter the blood presented to the kidney quite satisfactorily, but the tubules, which are functionally less mature, are unable to resorb water and some solutes adequately. The tubules become efficient by six to eight weeks, after which there is less concern over the use of a high-protein, high-sodium diet.

Other considerations. Many reasons have been advanced to either support or reject the introduction of solid foods from two to eight weeks of age. The belief of many mothers that they can hasten the time at which the infant sleeps through the night has not been corroborated by experimental data where the criterion of eight consecutive hours of sleep was considered "sleeping through the night."

One must also consider that if the infant does sleep through the night at an early age, he must either experience a reduction in total food intake or consume larger amounts at each of the remaining feedings, thus taxing the capacity of the stomach. Some scientists have expressed fear that such a pattern of overeating at an early age may persist throughout life and be a possible factor in obesity of children and adolescents. Such obesity of early onset is one of the most difficult types to treat.

One study to determine the effect of the addition of solid foods on the nutritive intake of infants showed that in the first two months solid foods were consumed in such small amounts that they had little influence on the nutritive adequacy of the diet. Later when more food was eaten it tended to replace milk rather than be used in addition to it. This corresponds with the findings of Thomson, who showed that the volume of milk increased with body weight from 3 to 5 kg. but remained stationary as weight increased from 5 to 7 kg. after three months of age.

Since the nutritive value of the solid food consumed in the first few months is usually of minimum significance, the major argument in favor of its use is that the child becomes accustomed to a wider variety of flavors and textures of food early and continues to accept these as he matures. Beal found that the age at which a child accepted solid foods did not parallel an advancement in the age at which the food was offered. As a result she reported a period during which the child and mother experienced an unpleasant feeding relationship with the mother trying to feed an infant who was not yet ready for the food. She felt that the forcible feeding of semisolids before the ninth to twelfth weeks tended to increase the incidence of feeding problems and food dislikes in the infant. The relationship between the age of introduction of solid foods and their acceptance is shown in Fig. 17-2.

Although there is not unanimous agreement in the literature, there are many studies reporting an increased incidence of food allergy among infants who are introduced to a variety of foods at an early age. This is an especially important consideration among infants with a family history of allergy. For these infants, allergists suggest delaying the time of initial introduction of solid foods and choosing foods that are minimally allergenic, such as vegetables, fruits, and rice cereal. They also advise feeding each food for a relatively short time and then switching to another to avoid the sensitization that may arise from prolonged exposure to one food.

As discussed earlier, if the added food is high in protein, there is the necessity of deaminating the protein in excess of needs and excreting the urea, which calls for an increase in urine volume. This can be a problem, especially at high environmental temperatures. Failing this the electrolytes will be retained with resulting edema.

György recognizes that the extrusion or "thrust" reflex is innate to normal infants but that it may be suppressed by prolonged spoon-feeding. He suggests that the inhibition of this natural defense mechanism might lead to frustration and mental insult, finally manifesting itself in a neurotic reaction.

In addition to an immaturity of secretion of digestive enzymes, the young infant has

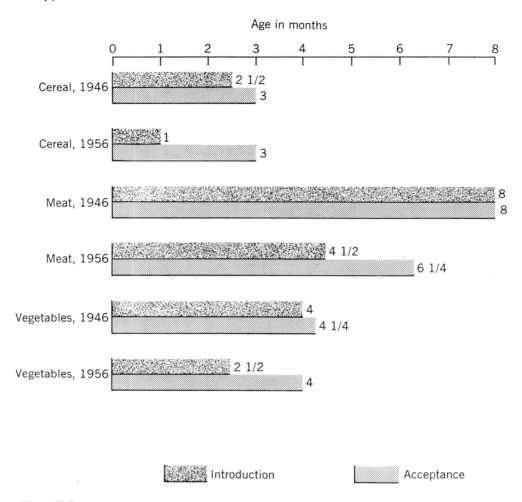

Fig. 17-2

Comparison age of introduction of solid food and acceptance between 1946 and 1956. (Based on Beal, V. A.: On the acceptance of solid foods and other food proteins of infants and children, Pediatrics **20**:448, 1957.)

low levels of many cellular enzymes. One which has been known for some time is phenylalanine hydroxylase, which is required for the metabolism of phenylalanine. A diet high in protein in the neonatal period will tax the infant's ability to tolerate the amino acid phenylalanine.

Additions to the diet. In spite of current trends in infant feeding practices which show that 90% of infants in the United States are fed solid food before three months of age, the Academy of Pediatrics,

after a careful consideration of all of the factors involved, recommends that the optimal time for introducing solid foods into the infant's diet is two and a half to three months of age. They agree that there is no nutritional superiority or psychological benefit from any earlier introduction.

Once the child is physically and physiologically capable of handling solid foods, the sequence and timing with which they are introduced should be determined by the nutritional needs of the child. Single-grain cereals are frequently used first because of their iron content, their ease of preparation and storage, and relatively low cost. This is usually followed by a variety of strained fruits and vegetables, with care being taken to avoid those that may be irritating to the gastrointestinal tract either through roughage or the production of gas. Egg yolk, which provides vitamin A, iron, and riboflavin, is frequently used as an early source of protein. By six months of age most infants will also be receiving meat. The order of use of foods is not crucial, as is evidenced by the number of patterns on which children thrive. More important is the provision of the nutrients needed to supplement a milk diet in a form suited to the digestive capacities of the child and the formation of a set of eating habits that will lead to good nutrition throughout childhood.

In most infants the eruption of the first teeth and the physical readiness to chew both occur at approximately five to six months of age. It is very important that the infant be given an opportunity to chew at this critical time in order that this capacity be developed. Dry bread is the most acceptable food to stimulate chewing. Caution should be exerted to avoid the use of hard flintlike materials such as crisp bacon and certain commercial biscuits, which may irritate the throat.

As the infant's digestive capacities develop, the strained foods of early infancy can be replaced by less finely chopped foods with a final transition to table foods. There is a wide range in the age at which this transition is made in a normal child, and failure of a child to keep up with the neighbor's child in this regard must not be considered prognostic of success in college or on the gridiron.

SELECTED REFERENCES

Andelman, M. B., and Sered, B. R.: Utilization of dietary iron by term infants, Am. J. Dis. Child. **111**:45, 1966.

Athreya, B. H., Coriell, L. L., and Charney, J.: Poliomyelitis antibodies in human colostrum and milk, J. Pediat. **64**:79, 1964.

Bakwin, H.: Feeding programs for infants, Fed. Proc. **23**:66, 1964.

Beal, V. A.: An acceptance of solid foods and other food patterns of infants and children, Pediatrics **20**:448, 1957.

Beal, V. A., Myers, A. J., and McCammon, R. N.: Iron intake hemoglobin and physical growth during the first two years of life, Pediatrics **30**:518, 1962.

Butler, A. M., and Wolman, I. J.: Trends in the early feeding of supplementary foods to infants, Quart. Rev. Pediat. **9**:63, 1954.

Call, J. D.: Emotional factors favoring successful breast feeding of infants, J. Pediat. **55**:485, 1959.

Committee on Nutrition, American Academy of Pediatrics: On the feeding of solid foods to infants, Pediatrics **21**:685, 1958; Trace elements in infant nutrition, Pediatrics **26**:715, 1960; Infantile scurvy and nutritional rickets, Pediatrics **29**:646, 1962; The prophylactic requirement and toxicity of Vitamin D, Pediatrics **31**:512, 1963.

Dahl, L. K.: High salt content of western infants' diets, Nature **198**:1204, 1963.

Farquhar, J. D.: Iron supplementation during first year of life, Am. J. Dis. Child. **106**:201, 1963.

Filer, L. J., and Martinez, G. A.: Caloric and iron intake by infants in the United States: an evaluation of 4,000 representative six-month olds, Clin. Pediat. **2**:470, 1963.

Foman, S. J., Owen, G. M., and Thomas, L. N.: Milk or formula volume ingested by infants fed ad libitum, Am. J. Dis. Child. **108**:601, 1964.

Forbes, G. B.: Do we need a new perspective in infant nutrition?, J. Pediat. **52**:496, 1958.

Grunwaldt, E., Bates, T., and Guthrie, D.: The onset of sleeping through the night in infancy, Pediatrics **26**:667, 1960.

Gryboski, J. D.: The swallowing mechanism of the neonate, Pediatrics **35**:445, 1965.

Guthrie, H. A.: Effect of early feeding of solid foods on nutritive intake of infants, Pediatrics **38**:879, 1966.

Guthrie, H. A.: Nutritional intake of infants, J. Am. Dietet. A. **43**:120, 1963.

György, P.: Orientation in infant feeding, Fed. Proc. **20**:169, 1960.

György, P.: The late effects of early nutrition, Am. J. Clin. Nutrition **8**:344, 1960.

Hansen, A. E., Wiese, H. F., Boelsche, A. N., Hoggard, M. E., Adam, D. J., and Davis, H.: Role of linoleic acid in infant nutrition, Pediatrics **31**:171, 1963.

Heiner, D. C., Wilson, J. F., and Lahey, M. E.: Sensitivity to cow's milk, J.A.M.A. **189**:563, 1964.

Heseltine, M. M., and Pitts, J. L.: Economy in nutrition and feeding of infants, Am. J. Pub. Health **56:**1756, 1966.

Holt, L. E., and Snyderman, S. E.: Protein and amino acid requirements of infants and children, Nutr. Abstr. & Rev. **35:**1, 1965.

Illingworth, R. S., and Lister, J.: The critical or sensitive period, with special reference to certain feeding problems in infants and children, J. Pediat. **65:**839, 1964.

MacKeith, R. C.: Is a big baby healthy?, Proc. Nutrition Soc. **22:**128, 1963.

Mott, G. A., Ross, R. H., and Smith, D. J.: A study of vitamin C and D intake of infants in the metropolitan Vancouver area, Canad. J. Pub. Health **55:**341, 1964.

Rueda-Williamson, R., and Rose, H. E.: Growth and nutrition in infants; the influence of diet and other factors on growth, Pediatrics **30:**639, 1962.

Salber, E. J., and Feinlieb, M.: Breast feeding in Boston, Pediatrics **37:**299, 1966.

Snyderman, S. E., Boyer, A., Roitman, E., Holt, L. E., and Prose, P. H.: The histidine requirement of the infant, Pediatrics **31:**786, 1963.

Stitt, G., and Heseltine, M. M.: Some practical considerations of economy and efficiency in infant feeding, Am. J. Pub. Health **52:**125, 1962.

Widdowson, E. M.: Effect of giving phosphate supplements on the absorption and excretion of calcium, strontium, magnesium and phosphorus to breast-fed babies, Lancet **2:**1250, 1963.

Widdowson, E. M.: The experimental approach to some pediatric problems, Proc. Nutrition Soc. **22:**121, 1963.

Williams, H. H.: Differences between cow's and human milk, J.A.M.A. **175:**104, 1961.

18

Nutrition from infancy to adulthood

In discussing the nutritive needs during infancy in Chapter 17, we dealt with the character of the diet and the gradual change in both variety and quality of the dietary intake that occurs as the child's nutritive needs increase and as his ability to handle a greater variety and complexity of foods improves during the first year of life. The age at which an infant makes the transition from bottle- or breast-feeding and from pureed or chopped baby foods to drinking from a cup and eating selected items from the regular family diet varies greatly from one child to another. Some make the adjustment as early as eight months of age while others may not reach this stage of maturity until two years of age or later. Aside from encouraging the child to chew when the ability to chew is established and to feed himself when he has the manual dexterity to manipulate a spoon, there is little · reason to push the change. Indeed there is some evidence to suggest that the infant should not be denied the work of sucking from either the breast or bottle at too early an age, as this may predispose to poorly developed jaws with attendant problems of crowded dentition or thumb-sucking in early childhood. The present chapter will deal with the nutritive needs and special considerations in adapting food to the child's needs after the pattern of feeding of early infancy has been modified to include the use of table foods.

CHILDREN'S NUTRITIVE NEEDS

As one would expect, the rapid and constant increase in body size that occurs during the growth period is unique and calls for an increase in the intake of practically all nutrients. The dietary standards proposed by the Food and Nutrition Board of the National Research Council represent the level of intake they feel will provide optimal health benefits to practically all children in each age group. The recognition that growth of children occurs in spurts—with a period of rapid increase in skeletal height followed by a slow increase in height but a more rapid increase in weight—should suggest that these values may represent an excessive margin of safety at one time and **349**

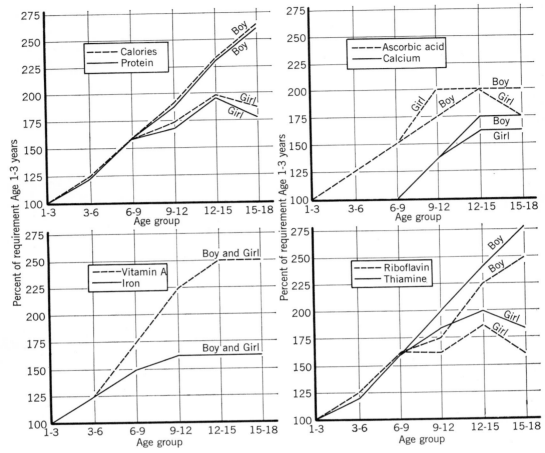

Fig. 18-1

Increase in nutritive needs during growth from age 1-3 years to 18 years. (Based on Recommended dietary allowances, National Academy of Sciences Publication 1146, Washington, D. C., 1964, National Academy of Sciences.)

a very realistic goal at another. They do remain, however, the standard against which to assess dietary adequacy and the nutritional goal used in planning food intakes. Although the total nutritional need increases with age the requirement on the basis of body weight declines.

Fig. 18-1 represents the percentage change in nutritive needs over a base of 1 to 3 years that occurs with increasing age. It is obvious that the suggested increment varies from one nutrient to another. As one would expect, the increase in energy

needs represents the amount of energy needed for basal metabolism, activity, and the amount stored as new muscle or adipose tissue. Requirements for basal metabolism and activity will increase proportionately with body size while that for growth will vary with the rate of growth and deposition of new tissue. Since many of the water-soluble vitamins, such as thiamine, riboflavin, niacin, and pantothenic acid, are involved primarily in energy metabolism, it is not surprising to find their requirements increasing in proportion to total energy needs. Pyridoxine, involved in the utilization of dietary protein and in the synthesis of tissue protein, will be required in greater amounts during periods of rapid muscle growth. Any increase in muscle mass that must accompany bone growth requires a positive nitrogen balance that is met by protein intakes of 1.5 to 2 gm. per kilogram of body weight. The increase in total body size necessitates a larger vascular system to transport nutrients to the tissues and waste products away, thus making demands for nutrients needed in blood formation—iron, protein, and folacin. Bone growth increases the need for protein, calcium, phosphorus, and vitamin D. Although the biological roles of vitamin A and ascorbic acid have not been elucidated there is adequate evidence that the amount needed increases with body size. While we know that the overall need for nutrients increases throughout the growth period there will be periods when growth is slow, with needs for certain nutrients reduced proportionately. Children frequently reflect these fluctuations in need by fluctuations in appetite, a phenomenon that may be the cause of much anxiety to the parents. It is quite common and quite natural for a child who has a hearty appetite to go through a period in which both the appetite and food intake are noticeably reduced. Unless such a period is very prolonged and accompanied by signs of undernutrition such as lethargy, fatigue, and increased susceptibility to infection, it should be no basis for concern. The unnecessary concern of some mothers over their children's food habits is exemplified in a study in Minnesota that showed that several mothers rated their children's food habits as poor when they met all criteria for nutritionally adequate meals. Figure 18-2 represents the fluctuations in appetite with age as reported by mothers of Colorado children.

In response to concern over appetite variations, promoters of dietary supplements have recommended both thiamine and co-balamin to stimulate appetite and growth in children, but experimental evidence indicates that thiamine is of value for only the most severely deprived human and that cobalamin is of no value as an appetite stimulant, although both play significant roles in metabolism.

Transitional foods

In supervising the change from an infant diet to regular adult-type diet there are several factors about a child's reaction to food that should be kept in mind to facilitate the transition and minimize the trauma of the experience for both the mother and the child. Lowenberg, who has made extensive observations of the reaction of children to food, suggests that their acceptance of food represents a favorable reaction to the color, flavor, texture, and temperature of the food as well as to the size of the servings and the attitude and atmosphere in which it is presented. A rejection of food may be attributed to an unfavorable reaction to one of these. She advises that the wise mother will try to analyze the reactions and determine their cause.

Children favor foods that are soft in texture and are less accepting of foods that are dry or flintlike, have tough or stringy parts, or are too thick. For instance, they prefer thin to thick puddings, celery with the strings removed, stewed tomatoes with the fibers cut, soft mashed potatoes to baked potatoes, moist ground meats to dry fish, and soft bread to coarse bread. This preference for moist foods may reflect the absence of a copious supply of saliva to provide a natural lubricant for the food. In terms of temperature they prefer foods that are lukewarm to those that are very cold or very hot. By serving a child's food first, one finds that it is at the right temperature by the time others at the table are served. Removing milk from the refrigerator sufficiently long before serving to warm it slightly increases its acceptance. The tendency of a child to dawdle over ice cream

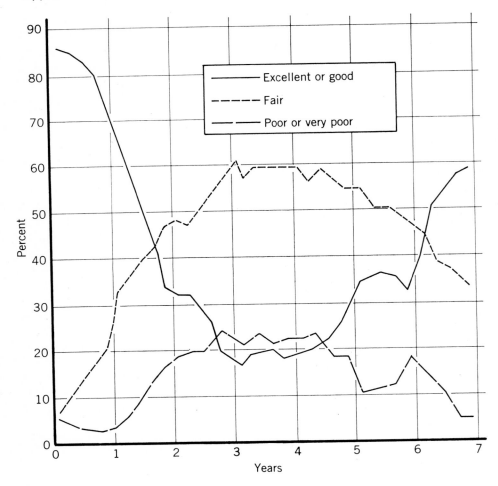

Fig. 18-2

Percentage of children 6 months to 7 years whose appetites were rated excellent, fair, or poor by their mothers. (From Beal, V. A.: On acceptance of solid foods and other protein foods of infants and children, Pediatrics **20**:448, 1957.)

until it is semisolid reflects his distaste for very cold foods. Children are very sensitive to flavors, reacting to off-flavors that may go undetected by adults, although experimental evidence does not support the notion that children are more sensitive to flavor variations than their parents are. Their sensitivity to flavor has been observed when they reject milk with a slight taint or recognize when food has been only slightly scorched. In the case of vegetables, children will often refuse vegetables of the cabbage or onion families when they are cooked in such a way as to maximize the retention of nutrients and the flavor but will accept them when cooked in a larger amount of water or when served with a cream sauce to modify the flavor. Once the mild flavor of the vegetable has been accepted it can be presented gradually in a more intensified form until it approaches normal flavor concentration, which also maximizes the retention of nutrients.

The quantity of food offered a child at

one time influences his reaction to it. It is more satisfactory from a psychological point of view to offer a child less than you anticipate he will eat and have him return for more than to present him with such a large quantity that he is defeated before he begins to eat it. The use of small 6-ounce glasses that can be easily grasped in the child's chubby hands is preferable to a large 8- to 10-ounce glass that overtaxes his manual dexterity and the capacity of his stomach. Allowing the child to serve himself so that he can determine the amount of food on his plate or the preparation of food in bite-size pieces may produce greater acceptance of the meal.

Visually the child is responsive to a colorful meal whether the color is provided by the plate and setting, the combination of foods, or the judicious use of edible garnishes. Care should be exercised to avoid unnatural food shapes, inedible material, or colors not normally found in food, such as blue or purple, in an attempt to give the meal eye appeal.

Young children in their curiosity about their environment like to experience the feel of food. They also find that many foods are more easily manipulated with the hands than with utensils. Thus the preparation of foods such as strips of meat, wedges of lettuce, or raw vegetables as finger foods allows the child to experience the feel of foods and is certainly justified if it encourages their use. The age at which a child develops sufficient manual dexterity to handle the utensils to manipulate food is again an individual matter, but until the child reaches the stage of motor development where he is skilled in their use, food should be presented in a way that requires a minimum of manipulation for its enjoyment.

Snacks. Snacks in the diet of young children have been encouraged by some and condemned by others. During periods of high nutritive needs the small child may be unable to take in sufficient food to satisfy his needs in three meals without overtaxing the capacity of his stomach. On the other hand, if snacks of high satiety value are taken too near regular meal hours, they may reduce the food intake at mealtimes. Munro found that snacks given 2½ hours before lunchtime had no effect on the appetite for lunch but did reduce the calorie intake at lunch, although the combined intake from lunch and snacks was greater than from lunch alone. A very cogent argument in favor of well-chosen snacks is provided by research showing that smaller, more frequent meals are utilized in such a way that depresses the formation of adipose tissue while stimulating muscle formation, as desirable during growth as in the prevention of obesity.

Food jags. While it is deemed desirable to educate children to accept a wide variety of foods and to develop an accepting attitude toward new foods, it is recognized that it is very common for young children to go on food jags in which they accept a very limited number of foods and reject all others. Should the accepted foods represent a nutritionally adequate, albeit monotonous, diet, as is often observed, there is little evidence that these preferences should provoke undue concern since they seldom persist for prolonged periods nor is there evidence that they lead to bizarre food habits in adulthood. It has been observed, however, that the quality of the diet of 12- to 14-year-old girls was highly correlated with the number of different food items eaten during the day, thus emphasizing the importance of encouraging the use of a variety of foods during the years when food habits are forming.

Food preferences. Several studies to determine food preferences of children which represent their reaction to the taste, texture, and temperature of food, have all led to similar conclusions. Only 37% to 41% of the children studied liked vegetables while over two thirds liked fruits. The fact that vegetables are generally unpopular may reflect the many and possibly unsatisfactory ways in which they are prepared. Meat, milk, and bread ranked next in popularity with from two thirds to nine tenths of the children accepting them. The food likes of young children appear to be related to those of other members of the family, especially the father, whose food preferences influence the frequency with which specific foods are served and hence the extent to which the child is familiar with them.

Adequacy of diets of infants and children. The findings on dietary adequacy of nine-month-old to 2-year-old infants is illustrated in Fig. 18-3, which shows clearly that iron, ascorbic acid, and vitamin A are the nutrients most likely to be provided in less than recommended amounts.

Relatively few studies have been concerned with the nutritive intake of young children, but in practically all studies the results have shown that the most common nutrient deficiencies are calcium, iron, and vitamin C with vitamin A, protein, and riboflavin the ones most likely to be present at recommended levels. A relatively small number of children, about 20%, have intakes of one or more nutrients of less than two thirds of recommended amounts, but an equally small number have intakes for all nutrients that either meet or exceed these levels. Since the standards involve such a wide margin of safety, these deficiencies are not a major concern unless there is some evidence of impaired physiologic function.

EVALUATION OF NUTRITIONAL STATUS

Since childhood is a period of active growth and a well-nourished child can be

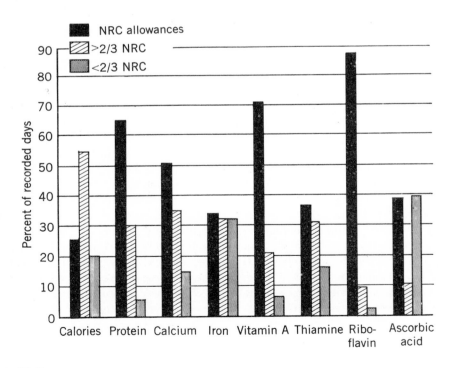

Fig. 18-3

Nutritive adequacy of diets of forty 9-month-old to 2-year-old infants. (Based on data of Guthrie, H. A.: Nutritional intake of infants, J. Am. Dietet. A. 43:120, 1963.)

expected to have a growth pattern characterized by regular increments in both height and weight, physical growth has become a readily available standard on which to assess nutritional status. Children in this generation are achieving a more rapid rate of growth and reaching maturity at an earlier age than those a few decades ago. This is a function not only of improved nutrition but also of favorable environmental factors and the advances in medical science that have reduced or elimated many of the diseases that depressed growth in the earlier period. It is important that any growth standard used in evaluating nutritional status be one derived from recent data. Falkner has developed such a standard (Appendix D), in which he presents height and weight data for the fifth, fiftieth, and ninety-fifth percentile for boys and girls of different ages on the theory that a range of values is more valuable than norms. He emphasizes that while data from standards will give a smooth curve, those from individuals will be characterized by peaks and valleys. He also presents data on yearly growth increments in both height and weight as a guide for assessing growth rates and stresses the importance of assessing pubertal stage as child approaches this age. These standards are not as genetically specific as those of Garn, shown in Chapter 15, which are based on the parental midpoint size.

Nutritional inadequacies in childhood

Severe malnutrition in childhood in the United States is seldom encountered now because of the availability of medical services to practically everyone and the improvement of techniques for identifying abnormalities before they develop into full-fledged deficiency syndrome. Rickets, pellagra, and beriberi are virtually unknown, and only an occasional case of scurvy is recorded. Of all forms of malnutrition, anemia and obesity are the most common

in addition to varying degrees of subclinical deficiency states.

Anemia, primarily the result of a lack of dietary iron, is encountered most often among children in lower socioeconomic groups, where the reported incidence of hemoglobin levels below 10 gm. per 100 ml. of blood ranges from 20% to 40%. In most cases the lack of dietary iron reflects parental ignorance of the importance and sources of iron or poverty, which restricts the amount and variety of foods available. In some cases the situation is aggravated by the presence of intestinal parasites. A few instances are recorded of anemia resulting from the exclusive use of a milk diet after the first six months of life. Treatment of anemia of childhood usually involves the therapeutic use of iron salts at levels providing 30 to 100 mg. of iron per day, often in conjunction with ascorbic acid, until the hemoglobin levels have been restored to normal levels. This is followed by the use of a diet high in iron-rich foods such as meat, green leafy vegetables, and enriched cereals. The child who suffers from anemia is usually lethargic, fatigues easily, and is highly susceptible to infection.

Obesity, a form of overnutrition, represents the other end of the nutritional spectrum. Childhood or juvenile obesity is a particular problem because it is very refractory to treatment and tends to persist into adulthood. This increasing problem may be attributed to several factors. Many mothers, in their concern over the child's food habits, unwittingly establish a pattern of overeating when they introduce solid foods at a very early age, equate weight gain with good health, or use food as a reward for good behavior. The situation is further complicated by inactivity, as discussed in Chapter 20. The syndrome of the pale flabby child who spends his summers in an air-conditioned house, immobilized in front of a television set and drinking calorie-laden carbonated beverages to keep cool, is frequently observed and is a cause for concern. The importance of preventing obesity in childhood through an education program involving both sound food selection and exercise cannot be overstressed.

ADOLESCENCE

The period of transition from childhood to adulthood, commonly called adolescence, is a very eventful, if relatively short, stage in the life cycle characterized by accelerated physical, biological, and emotional development. Adolescence influences both nutritional needs and the absorption and utilization of nutritive intake. This period witnesses a rapid enlargement of organs and tissues and changes in physiologic functions in response to hormonal changes. As reflected in the National Research Council recommended dietary allowances, this phase of the life cycle is the one of highest nutritive needs in the life of a male and for girls is surpassed only during pregnancy and lactation. These allowances represent the needs for the increase in body size and the maturation of organs. Since the 13- to 19-year-olds numbered 24 million in the United States in 1965 and since they are at a vulnerable age when the dietary patterns and attitudes they develop toward food are going to influence the health of their children and dictate the food patterns of the next generation, they are a prime and challenging target for nutrition education programs.

Adequacy of diets

Evaluations of the nutritive adequacy of the diets of young adults between 12 and 18 years of age in various regions in the United States have all yielded essentially the same results, although there are differences in degree. In all instances it was observed that the diets of boys were more adequate and less variable than those of the girls. This can be explained in part by the fact that the extra quantity of food required to meet the energy needs of boys (1100 kilocalories) dictates at least a mini-

Table 18-1. Percentage of boys and girls with nutrient intakes below NRC recommended dietary allowances*

	Boys (percent)	Girls (percent)
Calcium	10–42	15–70
Iron	0–18	10–45
Ascorbic acid	10–65	20–60
Thiamine	3–30	8–50
Vitamin A	3–38	5–45
Riboflavin	2–25	10–45
Niacin	2–30	5–22

*Based on Morgan, A. F.: Nutritional status U.S.A., California Agricultural Experiment Station Bulletin 769, 1959.

mal level of other nutrients whereas girls, with lower caloric intakes, are forced to make more judicious choices of foods to meet the needs for all other nutrients. In general, the diets of girls provide a higher proportion of their needs for ascorbic acid and calories than do those of boys, although ascorbic acid was often low for both. Girls' diets are generally low in iron, but this is not accompanied by a higher incidence of anemia. Calcium is more frequently low in the diet of girls than boys, and vitamin A is low in both, a reflection of a general rejection of vegetables. Protein and niacin intakes, which parallel the use of meat, were most often adequate. Table 18-1 presents data on the percentage of adolescents in various studies in the United States whose intake of different nutrients fell below two thirds of the NRC recommended dietary allowances. In general, the subjects with the poorest diets are those who skipped more meals, ate smaller quantities of food at meals, and ate fewer snacks.

Factors influencing food habits

Few attempts have been made to determine the attitudes that influence the selection of a diet. Young girls who were concerned about their health, who were emotionally stable and conforming, and who came from a home characterized by good family relationships chose better diets than those motivated by considerations of group status, sociability, independence from parental control, or enjoyment of eating. Criticism of their eating patterns led girls to skip meals more frequently, and skipping breakfast was found to be very common. Better meals were selected in winter than summer because of the regularity of schedules. The more meals eaten away from home the less likely an adolescent is to consume meals of adequate nutritional content, which no doubt represents a response to the habits of the peer groups. This is especially true when lunch money is used to buy lunches outside the school, a practice that is becoming less frequent with the trend toward short lunch periods in high schools and lack of freedom to leave the school building. School lunches that qualify for federal and state subsidies are selected to provide one fourth to one third of the nutritive needs of the schoolchild. Packed lunches are found to be somewhat less adequate, and those purchased outside the school are very poor. It is obvious that many factors contribute to the poor food habits observed during the teen years, but the most frequently observed causes are failure to eat breakfast (or less frequently some other meal of the day), lack of time or companionship for regular meals, drinking no milk (which may be a rebellion against parental influence), lack of supervision in the selection of meals eaten away from home, and an overriding fear of obesity, especially among girls.

Obesity

Studies indicate that 30% to 35% of teenagers are overweight although not necessarily obese, but practically all teen-agers, especially girls, are either fat or fearful of becoming fat. Because of their image of the fashion model in a size-six dress, girls often adopt an unrealistic and unhealthy standard of body size to which they aspire. Hence they embark on a self-directed program of weight reduction that can easily be hazardous to health because of inadequate levels of nutrients at a time when there are still high nutrient demands for growth. The problem is even greater when weight reduction is carried out spasmodically with a period of weight loss followed by one of weight gain.

As will be discussed in Chapter 21, the major cause of caloric imbalance among adolescents is a depressed level of activity rather than an excessive food intake. Whether the cause of this inactivity is physiologic or psychological or both has not been determined. It has been observed that obese youngsters have significantly lower serum iron with normal hemoglobin levels than nonobese youngsters. The low serum iron levels could be indicative of low levels of myoglobin and other iron-containing pigments that might cause an unconscious reduction in activity when the oxygen available to the cells was reduced. This situation, characterized by reduced activity, can be better handled by a program of consistent moderate exercise than by one of spasmodic and vigorous activity. The nature of activity patterns that are developed in late adolescence often prevails throughout adulthood, so it becomes important in terms of preventing obesity in adulthood to develop habits of active exercise at an early age. Equally important is the observation that the earlier a person learns to respond to satiety signals, the more likely he is to be able to adjust his food intake to correspond to his needs in response to a sensitive satiety mechanism.

Breakfast

The importance of breakfast in any group is well documented, and there is likely no nutritional substitute for a good breakfast.

Since adolescence is a time when skipping breakfast hits a peak and a time during which dietary habits that may persist for life are formulated, this is a period when attention should be directed toward the problem. Studies show that the calcium and ascorbic acid intake of persons who omit breakfast are reduced by about 40% and the intake of iron and thiamine by 10%. Leverton also found that 17- to 19-year-old college women who skipped breakfast obtained 18% of their energy intake from snacks while those who ate breakfast snacked less frequently and obtained only 7% of their energy intake from snacks. Since the snacks chosen were characteristically high in calories relative to other nutrients, those who snacked more had diets that were less adequate nutritionally than those of persons who had breakfast.

Boys report eating breakfast more frequently and eating breakfasts that provide more nutrients than do girls. Many rationalizations are presented for failure to eat breakfast, including lack of time, lack of appetite, preference for sleep, spending time over personal appearance, or fear of becoming fat.

In one study it was observed that the availability of someone with whom to eat breakfast, someone to prepare it for them, the availability of prepared foods, and the acceptance of the breakfast-eating habit in the peer group all influenced the extent to which breakfast was eaten.

It should be pointed out that breakfast need not be the conventional fruit, cereal, toast, and beverage pattern but can be any combination of foods, either liquid or solid, that provides its nutritional equivalent, at least 300 kilocalories, and sufficient protein and fat to provide a sense of satiety until the next meal.

Concern over teen-agers' diets

Nutritionists express concern over the nutritional habits of the 12- to 19-year-old group for many reasons. This is a period marked by a level of physical and emotional growth that often results in stress and anxiety, which in turn influence physiologic, psychological, and social behavior, all of which affect nutritional behavior.

The incidence of dietary inadequacies is higher during adolescence, which is a stage at which the results of nutrient lack are far-reaching, especially for girls, than at any other stage of the life cycle. Second, many relationships between physical abnormalities and dietary practice have been observed.

The incidence of tuberculosis is highest in adolescence, and there is some evidence to suggest a relationship between nutritional status and onset of tuberculosis, speed of recovery, and rate of reinfection.

Emotional instability, noted especially among girls who mature early, influences the utilization of nutrients. Negative nitrogen and calcium balances have been observed among both young girls and older persons who are under extreme emotional stress.

With 53% of girls between 15 and 19 years of age married, the possibility that a girl will bear a child before she is fully matured herself is a reason to focus special attention on her nutritional status. One out of four mothers bearing her first child is less than 20 years old, and 6% of all deaths among 18- to 19-year-old girls result from the complications of pregnancy. If the nutritive intake of a girl has been inadequate prior to conception she is less able to cope with the added physical stress of pregnancy with the demands of the growing fetus and is unable to make up for her own nutritive deficits. As a result, babies of teen-agers are more often born prematurely, have more congenital defects, and have inadequate nutritive stores to carry them through the initial period of extrauterine life. In all respects the malnourished mother is a poor obstetric risk. Whether a concern over the welfare of their yet unconceived children will provide sufficient motivation to teen-aged girls to modify their food habits remains to be tested, but the concern of nutritionists over the present status of the diets of adolescents has prompted a concerted effort to reach this group.

IMPROVING NUTRITIONAL HABITS

It has been well documented that nutrition knowledge and food habits are not necessarily the same. The key to the application of sound nutritional principles to eating patterns appears to be motivation. In adolescence the most effective motivation is the hope for vitality, good looks, and popularity. Concern over long-term effects of malnutrition or undernutrition on health has relatively little impact on the high school student or even the college student. Of the various methods attempted, the use of group sessions where the group accepts certain standards of eating and then helps provide the incentive and backing to implement them have been most effective. In some cases it is necessary to "unlearn" sets of habits, but for others it is merely a case of modifying or improving the current set of habits. A positive approach that builds on the prevailing habits rather than a negative one that involves pulling all the props out from under a person is preferable and more effective. It is important to start with the present habits of the individual, reinforce the good aspects, and replace the poor with new habits and to recognize that good diets do not just happen but are planned.

SELECTED REFERENCES
Children

Breckenbridge, M. E.: Food attitudes of five to twelve-year-old children, J. Am. Dietet. A. **35**:704, 1959.

Bryan, M. S., and Lowenberg, M. E.: The father's influence on young children's food preferences, J. Am. Dietet. A. **34**:30, 1958.

Committee on Nutrition, American Academy of Pediatrics: Factors affecting food intake, Pediatrics **33**:135, 1964.

Committee on Nutrition, American Academy of Pediatrics: Appraisal of the use of vitamins B₁ and B₁₂ or supplements promoted for the stimulation of growth and appetite in children, Pediatrics **21**:860, 1958.

Dierks, E. C., and Morse, L. M.: Food habits and nutrient intakes of preschool children, J. Am. Dietet. A. **47**:292, 1965.

Hathaway, M. L., and Sargent, D. W.: Overweight in children, J. Am. Dietet. A. **40**:511, 1962.

Haughton, J. G.: Nutritional anemia of infancy and childhood, Am. J. Public Health **53**:1121, 1963.

Lantis, M.: The child consumer—cultural factors influencing his food choices, J. Home Economics **54**:370, 1962.

Lowenberg, M. E.: Food preferences of young children, J. Am. Dietet. A. **24**:430, 1948.

Metheny, M. Y., Hunt, F. E., Patton, M. B., and Heye, H.: The diets of preschool children. I. Nutritional sufficiency findings and family marketing practices, J. Home Economic **54**:297, 1962.

Munro, N.: How do snacks affect total caloric intake of preschool children, J. Am. Dietet. A. **33**:601, 1957.

Norman, F. A., and Pratt, E. L.: Feeding of infants and children in hot weather, J.A.M.A. **166**:2168, 1958.

Adolescence

Christakis, G., Sajecki, S., Hillman, R. W., Miller, E., Blumenthal, S., and Archer, M.: Effect of a combined nutrition education program and physical fitness program on the weight status of obese high school boys, Fed. Proc. **25**:15, 1966.

Everson, G. J.: Bases for concern about teenagers' diets, J. Am. Dietet. A. **36**:17, 1960.

Gallagher, J. R.: Weight control in adolescence, J. Am. Dietet. A **40**:519, 1962.

Heald, F. P.: Natural history and physiological bases of adolescent obesity, Fed. Proc. **25**:1, 1966.

Hinton, M. A., Eppright, E. S., Chadderdon, H., and Wolins, L.: Eating behaviour and dietary intake of girls 12-14 years old. Psychologic, sociologic and physiologic factors, J. Am. Dietet. A. **43**:223, 1963.

Ohlson, M. A., and Hort, B. P.: Influence of breakfast on total day's food intake, J. Am. Dietet. A. **47**:282, 1965.

Peckos, P. S., and Heald, F. P.: Nutrition of adolescents, Children **11**:27, 1964.

Roth, A.: The teenage clinic, J. Am. Dietet. A. **36**:27, 1960.

Steele, B. F., Clayton, U. U., and Tucker, R. E.: Role of breakfast and of between-meal foods in adolescents' nutrient intake, J. Am. Dietet. A. **28**:1054, 1952.

Wharton, M. A.: Nutritive intake of adolescents, J. Am. Dietet. A. **42**:306, 1963.

19

Nutritional considerations in aging

Geriatrics, the branch of medicine concerned with the care of the aging as well as the aged, is concerned with prolonging the prime of life, delaying the onset of the severely degenerative aspects of aging, and treating the diseases of the aged. Gerontology is the broader branch of science dealing with the psychological, sociologic, economic, and physiologic as well as the medical aspects of aging. Both fields of study have witnessed a surge of activity in the last two decades. This increasing concern over the problems of the aging population has been motivated by the increase in both the total numbers and proportion of the population who are living beyond retirement age. Advances in medical technology, environmental hygiene, and nutrition have meant that more people are living longer with greater freedom from disease and in many cases with better health for a longer period of time. The extension of life has meant also that more of the complications of aging, both physiologic and psychological, have become evident and has called **360** for more thorough studies of the problem.

As has been frequently stated, both medical and social scientists are concerned with adding years to life as well as life to years. There are over twice as many people living to 65 years of age in 1960 than in 1900, representing 10% instead of 4% of the population. There has been a similar change in the life expectancy at the time of birth, as shown in Table 19-1.

NATURE OF AGING PROCESS

The human being is the product of his genetic heritage as well as his past and present environment, including the injuries, infections, stresses, fatigues, nutritional imbalances, and emotional trauma associated with them. It therefore stands to reason that the longer a person lives the more complex he becomes and that the physical and physiologic variations found in 70-year-old persons, each of whom have been subjected to widely different environments, make them a very heterogeneous group. Thus it is much more dangerous to generalize about all older people from studies on a few than it is for newborn infants, whose

Table 19-1. Life expectancy at birth

Year of birth	Life expectancy
1850	40 years
1900	47 years
1940	63 years
1950	68 years
1960	73 years

environments by comparison have been relatively homogeneous.

Since the nutritional status of an individual at any age is a reflection of his previous as well as his present dietary habits, Shock has suggested that the best preparation for a healthy old age begins in the office of the pediatrician. As with any biological process, aging occurs at different rates in different individuals even under similar environmental conditions. A person with a chronological age of 80 may have a biological age of 50 and vice versa. One factor believed to be responsible for delaying the onset of the senile process is a high but not excessive level of nutritive adequacy in the presenile years in the presence of adequate but not excessive caloric intake.

In aging, as at any other time, the state of nutrition of the body is determined by the state of nutrition of the individual cells. Cells will be less than adequately nourished under conditions of dietary deficiencies or excesses, impaired digestion, incomplete absorption, inefficient distribution and utilization of nutrients, and accumulation of waste products. Many of these situations are likely to occur as the body ages.

The stresses that affect aging may be subtle and insidious, but when allowed to accumulate over a period of years they become cumulative and detrimental. This can be most vividly illustrated by a caloric imbalance of as little as 10 kilocalories per day, which at the end of a year amounts to a gain or loss of one pound of weight. When accumulated over a 40-year period this represents an appreciable increase in body size. Similarly, rather small stresses in individual cells or organs which accumulate over the years may become sufficiently great to cause impaired cellular functioning. Physiologists have been seeking an answer to the question of the nature of the degenerative changes that occur with aging. Aging, in theory, begins with conception, but during the period of growth, the anabolic or building-up processes exceed the catabolic or degenerative changes so that the net result is one of growth and increased functional capabilities of the organs and tissues of the body. Once the body has reached physiologic maturity the process is reversed, slowly at first, and the rate of degenerative changes outweighs the growth changes. Along with this comes impaired function of many organs of the body. The difficulties of studying one person through the 50 or 60 years of aging are obvious. It is a question as to whether the subject or the investigator is lost first. So far we have relied on data from many different people at different ages, but now there is at least one longitudinal study designed to assess the biochemical and physiologic changes that occur in a group of men to be studied for 20 years. Such an investigation should shed considerable light on the biochemistry and physiology of the aging process.

The concensus of opinion now maintains that decrease in the efficiency of any organ is caused more by a loss of cells than by a change in the functioning level of the remaining cells. It is postulated that with aging the cells form defective RNA from the DNA, which appears to be damaged with age and which contains the genetic code for cellular reproduction and enzyme synthesis. The defective RNA then calls for the synthesis of defective enzymes, which are not capable of performing nor-

Table 19-2. Percentage of functions or tissues remaining in a 75-year-old man compared to a 30-year-old man*

Tissue	Percent remaining in 75-year-old man
Brain weight	56
Number of glomeruli in kidney	69
Number of nerve trunk fibers	63
Number of taste buds	36
Body water content	82

*Adapted from Shock, N. W.: Physiology of aging, Scient. Am. **206**:100, 1962.

mal cellular functions. This, of course, leads to death of the cell. When many cells fail to reproduce effectively or to function, the number of cells of an organ and hence its size and functional capacity are reduced, although each remaining cell is quite functional. The percentage of various tissues remaining in a 75-year-old man compared to those in a 30- year-old man is shown in Table 19-2. A decrement of 10% to 15% in cellular function was found to lead to decrements of 40% to 60% in organ function. Thus, the changes caused by aging are believed to be due to loss of cells rather than to a depressed level of functioning. Some workers, however, have reported a 15% decrease in the number of mitochondria, the site of energy metabolism, in cells from heart and liver tissue, with age suggesting that the capacity of a cell to release energy may be diminished.

The rate of decline in the functioning capacity differs in various systems of the body. Shock has studied and measured the change in 50- and 70-year-old men compared to a 30-year-old man. Some of his results are summarized in Fig. 19-1.

In addition to the decrease in the number of cells of the body in aging there are structural changes associated with collagen, the noncellular protein substance that binds the cells together and through which nutrients must pass from the intercellular fluids into the cells. Collagen, in which the rate of protein turnover is very slow, becomes less elastic and more fibrous as the cell ages. There is some evidence that the connective tissue or collagen replaces some of the more active cells lost from an organ so that the decline in functional capacity of an organ may be greater than that represented by the decrease in organ weight. In muscle tissue, muscle fibers may be replaced by connective tissue. The accumulation of collagen in the skin is believed to contribute to the aging appearance of the skin. Although there is not complete agreement on the cause of aging there is agreement that, generally speaking, the changes are irreversible. It is sometimes difficult to distinguish between physiologic symptoms and pathologic conditions.

NUTRIENT INTAKE

The factors that influence the nutritional habits and intake of older people can be classified as those that affect the intake, the digestion, the metabolism of nutrients, and the elimination of waste products.

Factors affecting the ingestion of nutrients

Long-standing dietary habits. Patterns of eating are established early in life, and there is evidence that people tend to prefer the type of foods they learned to eat when young. Nutrition education has had relatively little impact on the food habits of an individual; thus we find an older person is likely to choose and enjoy the foods he has eaten throughout his life that have become part of this cultural heritage. To him they may represent a certain form of se-

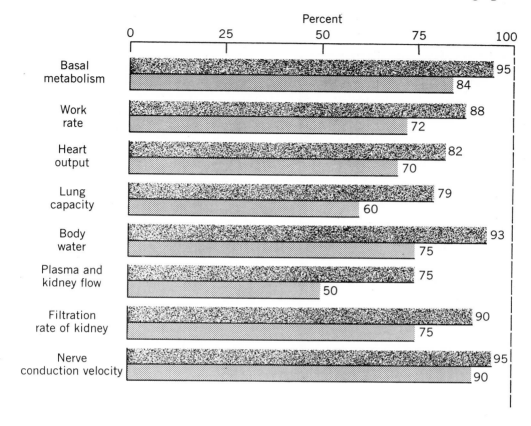

Fig. 19-1

Percentage of certain physiologic functions remaining at ages 50 and 70 compared to age 30. (Adapted from data from Shock, N. W.: Physiology of aging, Scient. Am. **206**:100, 1962.)

curity. Since many experiences with food are pleasant ones, the use of a specific food may conjure up very pleasant memories. Many individuals now in their later years were forming their food habits in an era when the kinds and variety of foods available the year round were much different and fewer than those available in the markets 50 years later. As a result they do not readily make use of the new marketing techniques that increase the variety of food

available and may eat in the same way they learned to eat when the selection was more limited. An examination of dietary intakes of older people reveals that vitamin A and ascorbic acid are the nutrients most likely to be lacking. These, it will be recognized, are provided through ample use of fresh fruits and vegetables that were available only seasonally, unless home-preserved, 60 to 70 years ago.

In old age, as in other stages of life, one

of the major deterrents to optimal nutrition is the established eating habits of the individual. Because the many meanings food has for older people may be more deeply ingrained and more intense, it is likely very unwise to insist on any abrupt change in dietary habits without a thorough knowledge of the individual's reactions to food. A slower, more subtle approach in which modifications are made within the framework of individual's food preferences is more likely to be successful. Where abnormal metabolic conditions such as diabetes, ulcer, or obstruction of the bile duct dictate regulated dietary patterns, the medical necessities of the changes are of primary concern and leave no alternative but a sudden modification of eating habits.

Loss of teeth. The longer one lives the more likely he is to lose his teeth, and the lower his socioeconomic status the less likely he is to replace them with satisfactory dentures. The American Dental Association estimates that of every 100 70-year-olds, 28 men and 38 women have lost all their teeth and that 80% of these either fail to replace them or replace them with ill-fitting dentures. In either case, the absence of a satisfactory method of chewing food leads to many modifications in eating patterns. Food that is inadequately chewed is difficult to swallow. Thus there is a tendency to substitute foods requiring little chewing such as ground meat for those requiring more such as steaks and roast. When foods high in cellulose such as fruits and vegetables, which are difficult to handle, are eliminated from the diet the bulk of the diet is reduced with the resultant decrease in gastric motility and problems of elimination. If fluoridation of the water supply by reducing dental caries decreases the number of edentulous senior citizens, its benefits may be even greater in later years than in childhood.

Diminished sense of taste and smell. The noted decline in the number of taste buds at age 70 to 36% of those at age 30 may explain the observation that there is often a decreased interest in food with increase in age. With a diminished number and sensitivity of taste buds it is understandable that much of the pleasure of eating is removed.

Loss of neuromuscular coordination. The ability to maintain fine neuromuscular coordination declines with the aging process, frequently manifesting itself as an inability to manipulate eating utensils. Rather than risk the embarrassment that would come with spilled food or inability to cut meat or eat soup, a person will avoid all such foods. This may lead to marked dietary changes and often nutritional inadequacies.

Physical discomfort. The discomfort that often accompanies ingestion of certain foods is more pronounced in older people. Some may cause heartburn, others cause gastric distention, and still others are incompletely digested. Efforts to avoid the offending foods may lead to the elimination of nutritious foods.

Economic considerations. The economic pressures to which many older people are subjected plays an important role in determining their dietary adequacy. When it is recognized that 75% of persons over 65 years of age have an income of less than 1000 dollars per year and 15% have less than 500 dollars it is not surprising that they have restricted amounts for food expenditures. The necessity of living on a meager income in order to remain financially independent forces many older people to choose the least expensive foods that provide them with the energy for which they recognize a need. This frequently means substituting the relatively inexpensive carbohydrate foods, bread and cereal products, which are low in the protective nutrients, for the more expensive meat, milk, fresh fruits, and vegetables, which are normally dependable sources of protein, minerals, and most vitamins. The ease with which carbohydrates are obtained and stored enhances their appeal.

A study of the food consumption of older persons in Rochester, New York who were beneficiaries of the Social Security program's old age survivors and disability insurance showed that while less than half the households had diets that furnished full amounts of NRC recommended dietary allowances for all nutrients, one fourth had diets that failed to meet two thirds of this standard for one or more nutrient. When the nutritive adequacy was related to the amount spent for food it was found that 80% of those who spent more than the cost of the USDA liberal cost food plan met the recommended allowances in full while those who spent less than the USDA estimate for the cost of a low-cost food plan failed to meet two thirds of the recommended allowance for one or more nutrients. Those with low incomes of less than 1000 dollars per person per year had diets considered poor two and one half times as often as those with high incomes (2000 dollars for one person or 3000 dollars for two). The relationship between income and dietary adequacy in this study is shown in Fig. 19-2.

The disappearance of the corner groceries from the older residential and downtown areas and their replacement with large supermarkets in suburban shopping plazas have compounded the problem of the older citizen, who characteristically chooses to live in the more familiar, central, less expensive part of town. To take advantage of the lower prices at the larger market he must either pay for public transportation to and from the store or become dependent on friends with cars. Once in the store he may become overwhelmed and confused by the choices with which he is confronted and in the end shop rather in-

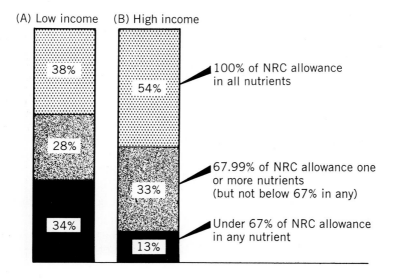

(A) Under $1,000 for one and $2,000 for two members
(B) $2,000 and over for one, $3,000 and over for two members

Fig. 19-2

Diet quality as related to income among older households in Rochester, New York. (From LeBovit, C., and Baker, D. A.: Food consumption and dietary levels of older households in Rochester, New York, Washington, D. C., 1965, U. S. Department of Agriculture Home Economics Research Report No. 25.)

effectively or return to the smaller delicatessen or service store at which prices are higher but which offer the familiar personalized service.

The pervading fear that they may become ill and be unable to look after themselves renders elderly people ready prey for the food faddist or purveyor of natural food and food supplements who promises them excellent health, eternal youth, increased vitality, and assurance that they will avoid the debilitating diseases so feared in old age. All too frequently they are persuaded by door-to-door salesmen to invest a significant part of their income in all-but-worthless products, greatly overpriced, which cannot provide the protection they seek against conditions for which there is no known cure.

Social factors. A person who preserves his independence by living alone may find that this in itself modifies his eating pattern. Lack of motivation to cook regular meals leads to the use of snack-type foods at irregular times with the result of a poorly balanced meal nutritionally. Inexpensive living quarters may lack adequate cooking and refrigeration facilities. Swanson has observed that it not unusual to find an older person showing a very erratic eating pattern—a day of nibbling followed by a day of overeating. In one woman she found daily intakes varying from 800 to 3700 kilocalories accompanied by loss of nitrogen except on days when the intake was above 3000 kilocalories and 100 gm. of protein.

Psychological factors. Conditions of emotional stress or deprivation often lead to modifications in attitudes toward food and in food habits. Persons who are anxious may experience loss of appetite and resultant undernutrition or on the other hand may indulge in compulsive nibbling which leads to overnutrition. Their interest in food may represent emotional poverty or lack of other interests. Some older people who find their living situation quite intolerable escape it by relying on the sedative effect which occurs following a large meal. In spite of this tendency to overeat obesity is rarely a problem in old age, although LeBovit found about one third of her subjects overweight. Others use food as an attention-getting device. The older person who is completely self-sufficient is often neglected by his relatives and friends. On the other hand, the person who does not eat adequate meals becomes a cause of concern and is often the recipient of attention and invitations. The same diet consumed under the emotionally unhappy condition of living alone compared to the pleasant atmosphere of companionship leads to a loss of nitrogen over a period as short as 30 days.

Factors affecting digestion

Changes in digestive secretions. With the degeneration in the size of the salivary glands that occurs after age 60, there is a decrease in the secretion of saliva. The effect of this on carbohydrate digestion is minimal since other enzymes are capable of complete carbohydrate digestion. However, the loss of saliva as a lubricant for food may have a more profound effect. With the decline in saliva there is a trend toward the use of softer, more moist foods such as creamed dishes, mashed potatoes rather than baked potatoes, and thinner starch-thickened products, possibly a means of compensating for the natural lubricants in the saliva.

The secretion of most digestive enzymes shows a decline with aging, but the extent of the decrease and the age at which it occurs has not been fully established. Depending on the extent of the decrease food may be less completely digested or will require a longer time for complete digestion. Impaired liver function with a loss of bile secretion has been shown to influence fat digestion. Evidence reported earlier that a decline in hydrochloric acid secretion of 9% to 35% occurred in aging has been disclaimed in more recent work.

Factors affecting metabolism and excretion

Decline in physiologic function. Many of the changes associated with aging occur in functions that require a coordination among various organ systems that decline at varying rates. The rate at which nerve impulses are conducted does not vary, but the amount of blood the heart can pump and the capacity of the lungs declines with age. Thus there is marked impairment in the amount of physical exercise an older person can tolerate.

The rate of blood flowing through the kidney is decreased to 50% of normal adult capacity. This means that less blood is presented to the filtering system of the kidney through which the waste products of metabolism are eliminated and the nutrients are returned to the general circulation. Thus there is an increase with aging in the time required to excrete waste products.

The normal functioning of individual cells requires a definite chemical composition of the fluids bathing them. This chemical composition varies directly with the composition of the blood, so a measure of blood composition reflects composition of cell environment. There is no measurable difference between the composition of the blood of older and younger subjects, but if the composition is deliberately altered, as it could be by the ingestion of sodium bicarbonate, a person 70 years old requires from four to eight times as long as a person 30 years of age to reestablish normal blood composition. With aging there are other changes in the rate at which the body can adjust to stress.

Hormonal secretions. Changes in hormonal secretions that exert a regulatory effect of a wide range of physiologic processes have a direct or indirect effect on the nutrition of the cells and hence of the whole organism. By regulating the diameter of blood vessels the endocrine glands regulate the amount of blood and hence the nutrients reaching the tissues. In aging persons there is a greater restriction in the size of the blood vessels leading to the kidney than in the size of those leading to the brain, thus assuring more adequate blood supply to the more vital centers.

The adrenal gland, which normally responds to the stimulation by the pituitary hormone during stress, does not respond as rapidly in older people, indicating a reduced capacity to respond to stress. In contrast, the thyroid gland retains its ability to manufacture and secrete thyroxine although there is a slight reduction in the amount of protein-bound iodine, which indicates the level of the circulating thyroid hormone.

Alterations in the blood vessels, such as the narrowing of the lumen, the loss of elasticity, thickening of the wall, and the replacement of elastic muscle fibers with nonelastic material, reduce the capacity of the blood vessels to effectively nourish all parts of the body.

Nutritive needs

The information available on the nutritive needs of persons over 40 years old is very scanty and is based primarily on studies of the intake of healthy persons rather than on experimental balance studies designed to determine the need. In general it is suggested that the nutritive intakes proposed for early adulthood be maintained throughout life. Except for calories there is no evidence that needs either diminish or increase. The extent of information available on each nutrient will be discussed.

Energy. The National Research Council has recognized the change in activity patterns and energy needs that occurs with aging. The trend from active sports to spectator sports, the decline in activity accompanying retirement, the decrease in the amount of housework for women, and the decline in basal metabolic needs as the number of cells in the body decreases with the loss of tissue mass all contribute to this. They suggest that the average reduction in total energy needs with increasing age is 3% per decade for ages 25 to 45, 7.5% per decade for ages 45 to 65, and 10% for the decade from 65 to 75 years, with no further decrements thereafter. The rather small decrease between 30 and 60 recognizes that the decrease in activity is accompanied by a decrease in efficiency of muscular effort that minimizes the caloric reduction.

Studies on nutritive intake of older persons have shown intakes below 1400 kilocalories, representing either efforts to reduce weight, inability to buy or eat more, failure to eat regularly, or an inability to chew food. In addition to failing to meet the individual needs for energy, such diets invariably are inadequate in several other nutrients such as calcium, iron, and several vitamins. Even though the suggested amount of protein might be provided, much which should go into the synthesis of body proteins is diverted to be used as a source of energy leading to negative nitrogen balance. This situation occurred experimentally in diets of less than 1800 kilocalories. The emotional state of the individual influences nitrogen balance with emotional instability depressing nitrogen retention.

Failure to consume adequate calories and with it adequate levels of other nutrients may account for the fatigue, lassitude and lack of interest in life so often experienced by elderly people. The lassitude and fatigue may depress activity to the extent that the need for calories is reduced, leading to weight gain even on a very low energy intake. It is conceivable that the use of nutritionally suboptimal low-calorie meals may be related to the premature signs of aging.

One study of 100 women aged 40 to 70 established a relationship between caloric intake and general level of health. Those whose health was rated good consumed 1650 to 1825 kilocalories while those whose health was rated as poor were consuming 1125 to 1475 kilocalories. They confirmed that the number of symptoms and the likelihood of other nutrient deficiencies increased when the energy value of the diet was lower. It is difficult to separate cause and effect in such a situation, however.

Protein. The National Research Council recommends that an intake of 1 gm. of protein per kilogram of body weight be maintained throughout adulthood. Studies show that average intakes of elderly people are in the neighborhood of 45 gm. daily. This may occur for many reasons. A low protein intake almost always occurs with a low calorie intake. Inability to chew properly reduces the intake of protein-rich meat, and the rejection of milk as a food suitable only for infants eliminates another potentially good source of protein. Protein-rich foods are the most expensive group and may well be reduced for considerations of economy.

In the adult, protein is used primarily for replacing those cells that are constantly breaking down in the wear-and-tear processes of the body and for the synthesis of enzymes needed for digestion and cellular metabolism. If cellular enzymes are not produced the cell cannot function properly and ultimately dies, leading to a loss of cell mass reflected in decreased organ size and reduced organ function. This may account for the observation that as the amount of protein decreased, the number of symptoms reported went up.

Since iron, thiamine, riboflavin, and niacin occur together in many foods high in protein a deficiency of protein will lead to a deficiency of these other nutrients as well. A reduction in thiamine to critically low levels depresses appetite, which further reduces total food intake and compounds the problem of dietary inadequacy.

Calcium. Early in the study of bone and tooth metabolism it was felt that these tissues were metabolically inert and that once they were formed the need for a dietary source of calcium was drastically reduced. Although subsequent research has clearly established that bones are metabolically dynamic tissues calling for a constant source of dietary calcium it has been very difficult to convince older people that they do not outgrow their need for calcium. A failure to provide a dietary source of calcium and the absence of conditions favoring its absorption will lead to loss of calcium from the reserves in the bone shaft with resulting porous, fragile bones very susceptible to fracture and slower to heal than adequately calcified bones.

Until recently, osteoporosis, a bone disease common in older people in which a decreased bone mass was reflected in a shorter stature, was believed to be a disease of endocrine origin. Evidence is now accumulating to suggest that osteoporosis can result from low dietary intakes of calcium that have prevailed over a long period of time, and there is much information to show that osteoporosis can be prevented and possibly cured by a diet high in calcium throughout adult life.

Evidence from dietary studies shows that calcium is the nutrient most likely to be consumed at levels below two thirds of the NRC recommended dietary allowances. We do know that people adapt to low intakes by increasing their level of absorption, but it is equally well established that emotional instability, a frequent accompaniment to old age, leads to increased excretion and decreased absorption with a net loss of calcium or a negative calcium balance.

Ascorbic acid. The intake of vitamin C among older persons is frequently reported to be extremely low. Long-standing food habits have not established the practice of using fresh fruits and vegetables. The relatively high cost of these foods and the bulk that many provide may be some of the factors contributing to a restriction in their use. The beneficial effects that ascorbic acid exerts on the absorption of calcium and iron are reason to encourage a more adequate intake.

Iron. The need for iron does not change for men, but for postmenopausal women who no longer suffer iron losses in monthly menstrual flow the recommended allowances drop back to 10 mg. from 15 mg. The ability to absorb iron does not diminish but with a decrease in caloric intake the iron intake frequently drops. This is especially true if there is a decrease in protein content of the diet.

Fat. Because of possible relationship between high fat intake and the development of atherosclerosis and heart disease, it is suggested that older persons, especially those who may be overweight, restrict their fat intake to a level providing 30% to 35% of the calories. Age per se does not affect tolerance for fat.

ADEQUACY OF DIETS

The assessment of adequacy of diets of aging people is complicated by the difficulty in obtaining subjects. In one study only 13% of the people contacted agreed to participate, raising the question as to how representative they were of the original group. In spite of the difficulties of obtaining the cooperation of a sufficiently large group of aging people, several studies have been successfully completed to give some picture of prevailing dietary patterns. Although the majority have been confined to institutions to facilitate data collection some have been carried out on groups of individuals living in their own homes.

Swanson, comparing the nutrient intake of Iowa women at ages 30 to 39 with those of women over 70, reported a decrease in intake of calories, protein, ascorbic acid, and calcium. The relative and absolute amounts of meat, fish and poultry, and milk products accounted for this decrease. The relationship between the calories contributed by these groups in the two age groups is shown in Fig. 19-3. The amount of cereal products in the diet remained constant but constituted a higher proportion of the total calories as aging people reduced their total caloric content.

Kelly, in a study of food selection of 114 Michigan women, also reported low intakes of calcium, vitamin A, and ascorbic acid,

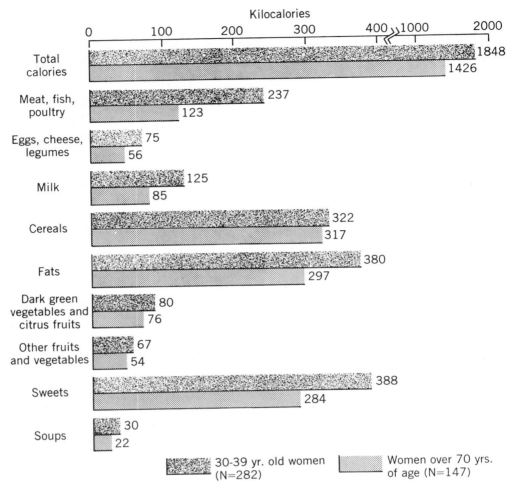

Fig. 19-3

Caloric contribution of various food groups in 30- to 39-year-old women and women over 70. (Based on data from Swanson, P.: Adequacy in old age. Part II. Nutrition education programs for the aging, J. Home Economics **56:**728, 1964.)

with a higher mortality rate among those getting less than 40% of the recommended allowances of one or more nutrients. A large number of her subjects complained of tiredness, pains in joints, shortness of breath, constipation, and other signs of general malaise.

Fry, in a smaller study of 32 women over 65, found their diets to be reasonably adequate, with iron, calcium, and vitamin A the most likely limiting factors. But only

12%, 16%, and 9% of the women showed these specific deficiencies.

A study of 283 households in which the homemaker was over 60 and who were dependent on Old Age Survivors Insurance showed 44% with diets evaluated as good and 25% with poor diets, defined as those containing less than two thirds of the recommended allowances for one or more nutrients. It was observed that diets low in protein were low in at least four other nutrients. Thiamine, lacking in the diets of 40% of the households, calcium, and ascorbic acid, low in 30% of the cases, were the nutrients most often low.

Steinkamp was able to follow a group of 577 aging persons in California over a 14-year period. She found that the mean intake met the standards for all nutrients except calories for men and calcium for women. However, one fourth of the men and one half of the women had less than two thirds of the recommended calcium allowances, and one fourth of both sexes had equally low intakes of ascorbic acid. There was a slight downward trend for all nutrients with age and a sharp downward trend after 75 years. She found that the decrease in calories was associated with a general decrease in the amount of food consumed rather than a decrease in a particular food or food group.

DIETARY SUPPLEMENTS

The fact that older persons are concerned about their health and are highly motivated to take any steps which they believe will help maintain a sufficient level of health that they can maintain their independence means that the use of dietary supplements—especially multivitamin and mineral capsules—is quite widespread. In Rochester, New York it was found that 37% of the households of people 55 or older were using supplements. Of these 104, 48 were consuming diets adequate in all nutrients and needed no supplements, and 56 with fair or poor diets would have benefited from the correct supplement. However, only 12 of this group used supplements that provided all the nutrients lacking in their diets, 31 used products providing some but not all of the nutrients they needed, and 13 supplemented their diets with nutrients they were already getting in adequate amounts in their regular diet but not with the nutrients they needed. A similar situation was noted in a study of men and women over 50 years of age in California where Stein-

kamp found that 35% were using mineral, vitamin, or other food supplements. Of those taking vitamin supplements 37% had diets already adequate in the vitamins taken. Of the 63 diets found low in vitamin A, 12 diets were supplemented; of 43 low in ascorbic acid, 11; for niacin 8 of 45; for riboflavin 4 of 29; and for thiamine 3 of 11. In the case of minerals only three of 89 persons with suboptimal intakes of calcium took supplements including calcium, and none of the 23 needing iron received it. Since the amount spent on supplements may represent an appreciable proportion of the money available for food one would hope that more guidance could be available to help those who would profit from supplements to choose the correct ones and to counsel those whose diets are already adequate against wasting their money.

SELECTED REFERENCES

Batchelder, E. L.: Nutritional status and dietary habits of older people, J. Am. Dietet. A. **33**:471, 1957.

Beeuwkes, A. M.: Studying the food habits of the elderly, J. Am. Dietet. A. **37**:215, 1960.

Brin, M., Dibble, M. U., Peel, A., McMullen, E., Bourquin, A., and Chen, N.: Some preliminary findings on the nutritional status of the aged in Onondoga County, New York, Am. J. Clin. Nutrition **17**:240, 1965.

Caniggia, A.: Medical problems in senile osteoporosis, Geriatrics **20**:330, 1965.

Curtis, H. J.: Biological mechanisms underlying aging process, Science **141**:686, 1963.

Davidson, C. S., Livermore, J., Anderson, P., and Kaufman, S.: Nutrition of a group of apparently healthy aging persons, Am. J. Clin. Nutrition **10**:181, 1962.

Fry, P. C., Fox, H. M., and Linkswiler, H.: Nutrient intakes of healthy older women, J. Am. Dietet. A. **42**:218, 1963.

Garry, R. C.: Symposium. Nutrition and the elderly, Proc. Nutrition Soc. **19**:107, 1960.

Henry, C. E.: Feeding elderly people in their homes, J. Am. Dietet. A. **35**:149, 1959.

Kelly, L., Ohlson, M. A., and Harper, L. J.: Food selection and well-being of aging women, J. Am. Dietet. A. **33**:466, 1957.

LeBovit, C.: The food of older persons living at home, J. Am. Dietet. A. **46**:285, 1965.

Mayer, J.: Nutrition in the aged, Postgrad. Med. **32**:394, 1962.

Shock, N.: Physiology of aging, Scient. Am. **206:** 100, 1962.

Steinkamp, R. C., Cohen, N. L., and Walsh, H. E.: Resurvey of an aging population—fourteen-year followup, J. Am. Dietet. A. **46:**103, 1965.

Swanson, P.: Adequacy in old age. I. Role of nutrition, J. Home Economics **56:**651, 1964.

Watkins, D. M.: New findings in nutrition of older people, Am. J. Pub. Health **55:**548, 1965.

Williams, I., and Smith, C. E.: Home-delivered meals for the aged and handicapped, J. Am. Dietet. A. **35:**146, 1959.

20

Weight control

Weight control is a term generally applied to efforts to maintain body weight within the limits compatible with maximum level of health or to adjust body weight to conform to these established standards. For the vast majority of adults this control is readily achieved with little or no conscious effort on the part of the individual. This is quite impressive when one considers that daily error of 10 kilocalories or 0.5% in caloric intake of a sedentary adult female will accumulate to represent a change in body weight of 1 pound per year, and a 5% error a change of 10 pounds. For a relatively small group of people the problem is one of keeping weight up to desired levels and for a somewhat larger group, estimated as high as 25% of the population, the problem is one of restricting weight gain. Although the health hazards of being underweight may be equally as great as those of being overweight, persons in the latter group are more receptive to advice and more motivated to seek it. They are also the subject of vastly more research and are more ready targets for promoters of food supplements ready to capitalize on their desire for a panacea for weight problems than are the underweight individuals who are, comparatively speaking, totally ignored. As if to accept this as desirable we will reflect the situation by drawing on the vast literature available to discuss obesity rather extensively and conform to established patterns by disposing of the problems of the underweight individual in a few paragraphs. This must not be interpreted to imply that the underweight individual does not warrant attention.

OBESITY

Obesity is generally defined as a condition in which there is an abnormal accumulation of fat in body tissue. When 20% of body weight of a man and 28% to 30% of the weight of a woman is composed of fat compared to normal values of 12% to 18% and 18% to 24% respectively the amount of fat is judged to be abnormally high and the individual is described as obese. An increase in fat above these levels means that the body cells that normally contain some **373** fat have become saturated with fat. In addition, in order to accomodate the fat that must be formed in order to store energy intake in excess of expenditures which the body cannot excrete, new fat or adipose cells capable of holding as much as 62% fat form or connective tissues cells are converted into fat cells. When these new adipose cells accumulate a person is described as being obese. It usually corresponds with a weight at least 15% above ideal or desirable weights. This accumulation of fat is frequently evidenced by a increase in the bulk or size of the body and may be either localized or distributed throughout the body. Formerly described as simple obesity, the condition is now recognized as a symptom of one or more disturbing influences—either physiologic, psychological, or pathological. It is indeed a condition of multiple origins.

In addition to the segment of the population who can be theoretically described as obese there is another group designated as merely overweight whose body weight is above the level believed to be compatible with the optimal level of health but not sufficiently high to represent an excess accumulation of fat. Overweight individuals, of course, are very likely to become obese unless preventive measures are taken when the increments in weight begin.

Bruch suggests that the body may have a preferred weight that bears no relation to an accepted standard but one which the individual tends to maintain or revert to after an attempt at weight adjustment.

Diagnosis

The absence of any single, effective technique for measuring body fat on which to base a diagnosis of obesity has led to the use of many methods.

Appearance. Diagnosis of severe obesity can be made quite reliably on the basis of physical appearance, but this criterion is useless in identifying cases of borderline obesity since it does not distinguish between body size caused by an accumulation of fat and that caused by an accumulation of water or muscle. On the basis of appearance, some persons may be judged to be obese at a body weight that cannot be considered unhealthy.

Skinfold measurements. Efforts to measure subcutaneous fat by measuring the thickness of a skinfold have been only moderately successful. Mayer feels that a single skinfold measurement on the triceps, located at the back of the right upper arm midway between the elbow and the shoulder, is adequate for diagnostic purposes. Others, however, maintain that they must be made in several parts of the body, such as the subscapular area just below the angle of the left scapula, the thigh, hip, abdomen, calf, and pectoral areas. Measurements must be made with a constant pressure caliper (usually 10 gm. per square millimeter). These measurements must then be compared to an established standard for obesity. Generally, the relation of skinfold thickness to body fat is independent of height. The major drawback to this method is the difficulty of getting reliable measurements not only from different technicians but also from the same technicians on separate occasions. The wide variations noted under normal conditions is another complicating factor. For instance in 12-year-old boys the median measurement of triceps skinfold was 9 mm., with a range of 4.5 to 22 mm.

X-ray measurement of body fat. A relatively new technique in which the thickness of fat is measured in various parts of the body as it shows up on an x-ray plate is useful in clinical studies but is of limited value for routine diagnostic purposes because of its high cost and the relative hazard of widespread use of x-ray technique.

Comparison of body weight to an established standard. In spite of the limitations of a comparison of the weight of an individual to established standards of weight for specific age and height it remains the most widely used criterion available. Practically all standards are based on figures made available by insurance companies and are the ones associated with the lowest mortality rates. The current standards which they described as "ideal weights" at age 25 released by the Society of Actuaries are reproduced in Appendix E. It will be noted that these weights are made with normal clothing and heights are taken with 2-inch heels for women and 1-inch heels for men. Moreover, the individual using these tables must arbitrarily classify himself in one of three body frame types—small, medium, or large. This makes it possible for an individual to place himself in the category that best suits his needs as he perceives them and is frequently the one that presents his present status in the most favorable light.

The use of standard height-weight tables to determine presence or absence of obesity, considered 15% to 20% above ideal weight, can be very misleading when the individual is edematous (suffering from an excess accumulation of fluid in the tissues), when he is very muscular, or when his weight is composed of a low proportion of muscle and a high proportion of fat or vice versa.

Determination of lean body mass. There are three major techniques available to determine the relative amounts of fat and lean body mass comprising body weight, but all require trained workers and expensive equipment. The measurement of specific gravity involves comparing the weight under water (corrected for residual air in the lungs) to the weight in air. When the proportion of fat is normal, the ratio of weight in water to weight in air, or specific gravity, will be approximately 1, indicating a normal distribution of musculature and fat. Adipose tissue has a specific gravity of 0.92, compared to 1.1 for the rest of the body. As the proportion of fat increases, the specific gravity decreases since fat is lighter per unit of volume than lean body

mass. The lower the specific gravity, the greater the amount of fat in the body.

Since the amount of water in the body is known to be approximately 72% of lean body mass knowledge of the amount of water in the body can be used to compute the amount of lean body mass. This in turn could be subtracted from the total body weight to determine the amount of body fat. Another technique for measuring body water involves injecting a known amount of either of the chemicals, antipyrine or deuterium oxide, into the blood and removing a sample of blood after a prescribed period to determine the extent to which body water had diluted the chemical. From this determination total body water, then lean body mass, and finally body fat can be calculated.

A technique known as the *whole body counter* is based on the theory that potassium represents a fixed percentage of lean body mass or protoplasm and that potassium[40], a radioactive form of potassium, is a fixed percentage of the potassium in food consumed and hence of the potassium in body tissue. By measuring the radioactivity of potassium[40] in the whole body by subjecting an individual to a short period in front of a Geiger counter, it is possible to measure the amount of this substance in the body, and from this to calculate the total amount of potassium and then the lean body mass. Subtracting this from total body weight, one then calculates the amount of body fat present. Although the equipment is initially expensive and requires a skilled operator, the test subjects the individual to no discomfort or hazards and may have potential as a diagnostic tool.

Other techniques. The search for a simple method of recognizing obesity has led to the development of many gimmicks. For instance, Joliffe suggested the "ruler test," in which a ruler laid from the chest to the abdomen of a subject lying on his back will rise at the end toward the feet in an obese person and be flat or slanted downward in a person of normal weight. Another criterion, the "perfect 36" index, involves subtracting a person's waist measurement in inches from his height in inches. Values of 36 to 40 are considered characteristic of persons of normal body weight while a value less than 25 represents obesity. The limitations of such methods are obvious.

Prevalence

The difficulty of arriving at a suitable criterion for diagnosing obesity has led to confusing reports in the incidence of obesity even when one recognizes that there may be marked differences in various segments of the population. For instance, public health statistics suggest an incidence of 10% to 13%, insurance statistics based on a selected population 6% to 7%, and statistics from a study of Iowa women 25%, if a weight of 15% above that in standard tables of ideal weights is used as the basis for diagnosing obesity. A weight at least 20% above these standards, which represents a doubling of fat reserves, is found in millions of Americans representing 3% of the population over 30 years of age according to MacByrde. Duncan in Philadelphia, basing his figures on the Body Build and Blood Pressure study, reports that 5% of the males (one in twenty) and 11% of women (one in nine) are at least 20% over the desirable weights suggested by life insurance statistics as most conducive to longevity while Pollack in New York placed the figures at 30% for males and 40% for females over 40. One study of 12 thousand schoolchildren showed 30% of them more than 20% overweight based on standard height-weight charts while another reported that 12.5% of adolescent girls and 9.5% of adolescent boys were overweight.

Many of the discrepancies in the reported incidence of obesity can be attributed to differences in the social, cultural, and economic background of the sample with a higher incidence of obesity found in the middle than either the high or low socioeconomic groups in adolescents.

Practically all studies agree that obesity becomes a progressively greater public health problem as the ability to regulate exercise and intake is lost from ages 20 to 60 with the gradual decline in energy requirements. At birth the infant requires 50 kilocalories per kilogram of body weight for basal metabolism, at five years a child needs 45 kilocalories, and at 15 an adolescent needs 40 kilocalories, after which needs decline steadily at a rate approximating 1% per year. After age 60 to 70 incidence of obesity declines, reflecting the higher mortality rates prevailing among younger obese people in the population so that the obese do not live to become a statistic at age 60.

Disadvantages

Before a person is motivated to correct a condition such as obesity, which calls for considerable willpower and perseverance over a long period, he must be convinced that the disadvantages of the condition are sufficiently great to warrant the self-discipline involved. In obesity there are many disadvantages from a health standpoint as well as physically, physiologically, economically, and socially.

Health hazards. It is well established that chronic illness is more prevalent among obese than nonobese and that even for people only 10% to 15% overweight mortality rates are higher. Table 20-1 shows the increase in mortality rates that occurs with progressively higher body weights and the concomitant decrease in life expectancy that occurs. For each pound of weight above ideal weights, the death rate increases by approximately 1%. Table 20-2 shows the effect of obesity on mortality rates from specific diseases. It is evident that the risk of cardiovascular disease, cerebral hemorrhage, and nephritis is much higher among obese than nonobese persons. Even with greatly improved surgical techniques the obese person subjected to

Table 20-1. Increase in mortality rates with severity of obesity

Percent overweight	Percent increase in death rate
10	10–15
20	20–25
30	40–45
40	70

Table 20-2. Mortality rates from various causes among overweight men and women—percent actual of expected deaths*

Causes of death	Men	Women
Cardiovascular-renal diseases	149	177
Diabetes	383	372
Cirrhosis of the liver	249	147
Appendicitis	223	195
Ulcers	67	—
Suicide	78	73
Tuberculosis	21	35
Pneumonia	102	129

*From Marks, H. H.: Influence of obesity on morbidity and mortality, Bull. New York Acad. Med. **36:**15, 1960.

surgery is still in considerable hazard. The relationship between heart disease and obesity can be appreciated when one recognizes that for every pound of added fat the heart must pump blood through an additional two thirds mile of blood vessels.

The relationship between obesity and diabetes may not be one of cause and effect, since current theories suggest that obesity may be an early sign of adult-onset diabetes and may be caused by essentially the same metabolic defect. Obesity may be a stress factor in diabetes when it overtaxes the homeostatic mechanisms involved in carbohydrate metabolism to the point that diabetes is precipitated in susceptible individuals.

While the presence of some fat surrounding vital organs such as the kidney, heart and lungs is desirable, excessive fat accumulation interferes with their mechanical efficiency.

Seltzer has found that in men a decrease in the ponderal index (height in inches/cube root of weight in pounds) below 12.5 is closely related to an increase in mortality. This index represents body shape rather than body size with a curvilinear relationship between variables, as shown in Fig. 20-1, in which there is a precipitous rise in mortality at the lower end of the ponderal index range. The lower end of the index represents extreme endomorphs who have long been characterized by obesity.

Social disadvantages. The obese person frequently finds himself caught in a vicious circle from a social point of view. Often the initial weight gain is a reflection of an unhappy social adjustment. The resultant obesity leads to social rejection, which in turn leads to more overeating, to increased weight, and to continued or more profound rejection. Adolescents in particular are victims in this chain of events. Excessive weight precludes their effective participation in many active sports, such as tennis, badminton, or swimming, and in social activities, such as dancing. The reduced activity often accompanied by a nibbling pattern of eating makes weight gain easier, again setting up a vicious circle.

Economic disadvantages. The obese individual finds that certain occupations, such as airline stewardess, nursing, selling, receptionist, or other jobs where public impressions are important or mobility essential, are closed to him. Some employers are

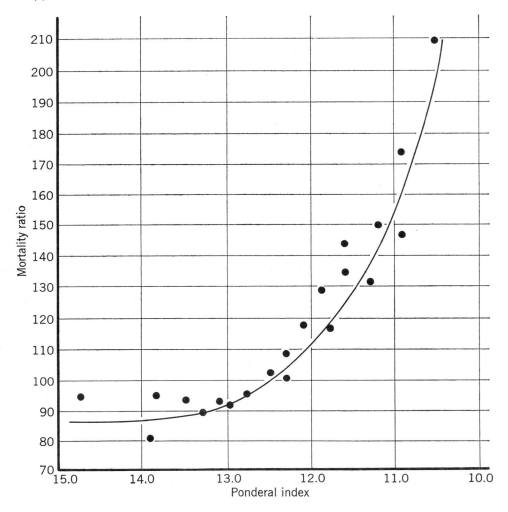

Fig. 20-1

Association of mortality ratio with ponderal index for men, issue ages 40 to 49. Data derived from Build and blood pressure study, 1959. Ponderal index = height in inches divided by cubic root of weight in pounds. (From Seltzer, C. C.: Some reevaluations of build and blood pressure study 1959 as related to ponderal index, somatotype, and mortality, New England J. Med. **274**:254, 1966.)

reluctant to train persons who are obviously health risks. This not only limits the vocational choices open but also curtails advancement in many occupations. In addition this person may find that the cost of special clothes, furniture, or transportation will increase his cost of living well above normal. In considering economic factors

one might also consider the amount which may well be spent in potential cures or weight-reducing panaceas or the cost of his excessive food intake.

Psychological factors. Although it has been impossible to associate any particular personality traits with obese individuals there have been several studies that have revealed some interesting relationships. It is difficult to determine if psychological factors are a cause or effect of obesity, but it is easy to underestimate the psychological effects of obesity on an obese individual, especially an adolescent girl. For instance, Mayer observed that obese girls had personality characteristics similar to those of racial and ethnic minority groups—self-blame, withdrawal, passivity, inferiority feelings, and sensitivity about one's status. Lack of family support exposed obese adolescents to greater tension. Obese persons have been found to have "distorted body images," a preoccupation with weight, and a tendency to blame all failures and disappointments on their weight. It is possible that social pressures on obese juveniles affect their personalities permanently.

Causes

The development of the concept that obesity is a disease of multiple origins or a syndrome rather than a single disease entity does not represent any rejection of the long-established concept that fat will accumulate only when the intake or consumption of energy (measured in kilocalories) exceeds the output or expenditure of energy. It does, however, propose that the cause of a failure to make a successful adjustment in caloric intake may be found in diverse areas and even suggests that perhaps not all persons should reduce. It still holds true that when calorie intake exceeds calorie expenditure the excess cannot be excreted and will be stored as body fat once the limited glycogen reserves of liver and muscle have been saturated. Nor is there any reason to believe that body fat arises spontaneously. It arises only as a storage form of energy. In the growing individual, however, energy will also be used in the increase in body musculature and bone. In short, the law of conservation of energy still holds. In general, the factors that influence the individual's ability to ad-

just calorie intake to expenditure will be classified as environmental, psychological, genetic, cultural, and physiologic.

Environmental factors

Availability of food. Obesity is a significant problem for large segments of the population only in countries where the food supply exceeds the demand. It is, in essence, a disease of plenty. The middle and upper socioeconomic classes in most countries have always had plenty of food and hence have been the ones who have tended to become obese. This is depicted in medieval paintings where the corpulent rich man is shown being waited on by lean servants. In many societies today one evidence of a successful man is a plump, well-fed wife.

Advertisers are constantly inducing us, especially our children, to buy more food; at the same time another segment of the industry is promoting weight-reducing aids for those who have bought and consumed too much food.

Comfort of environment. Well-heated houses and warm, lightweight clothing have reduced the amount of energy needed to maintain normal body temperature in temperate climates, and the energy costs of procuring food have been decreasing constantly with the mechanization of the food and agriculture industries.

Food and hospitality. The use of food as an expression of hospitality does much to increase the energy intake of the population by having food more constantly available. People are offered food and drink in almost all social situations from the early-morning coffee klatsch to the late-evening buffet supper and midnight snack. Failure to offer food in a social situation may be interpreted as a lack of hospitality, and failure to accept food on the part of the guest may be interpreted as a rejection of hospitality. The more important the occasion, the greater the amount of food and drink offered. In many cultures, even the very poor feel compelled to save or borrow for a special festive occasion such as a wedding or baptism in order to save face by providing a feast.

Family food habits. Long-standing family food habits, many of which were established when existence involved more strenuous physical activity and everyone worked harder with less protection against extremes of weather, have been retained in the current push-button, air-conditioned era. The daughter serves the same kind of meal to her family that her mother served several decades earlier in spite of marked changes that have occurred in family energy needs.

The pattern of food intake is a significant factor among overweight persons, with 75% of one group found to consume most of their food between four o'clock in the afternoon and midnight. Only 17% of the subjects reported eating only three meals a day.

Decreased activity. A decrease in the amount and intensity of physical activity tends to occur with increasing age with the transition from active to spectator sports. In addition, for the woman there is often a decrease in the activity associated with homemaking. Not only does she exercise less in looking after the needs of her children and home but expects them to take over some of the household tasks she formerly did herself. The increased availability of labor-saving devices and more readily available transportation has resulted in lower energy expenditures among succeeding generations. For instance, power steering in a tractor reduces the energy expenditure by 20% compared to regular steering. A secretary working six hours a day on an electric typewriter expends 450 kilocalories less per week than her counterpart using a standard typewriter. Similarly, it has been estimated that the average man expends 210 kilocalaries in walking one mile, 171 kilocalories in cycling the same distance, and 17 kilocalories in driving an automobile. If traditional meal patterns are not adjusted accordingly, the likelihood of an undesirable weight gain is increased.

Mayer, in studying the activity patterns of obese and nonobese children, found that the obese exercised significantly less each day with less enthusiasm than did the nonobese. Even when they reportedly participated in an activity for a comparable period of time their actual time of activity was as little as one third that of nonobese. They also ate less, but the adjustment was not sufficiently large to compensate for the decreased caloric requirements. Because of their larger weight load, obese individuals are often less skilled in sports and may limit their participation even more. Mayer also observed that adolescent obesity usually began in the winter, traditionally a period of reduced activity in the temperate climate. For some persons, periods of forced immobility coupled with admonitions to eat to keep up strength may initiate an excessive weight gain. The widespread use of school buses, often for reasons of safety, in transporting children to and from school further deprives young people of a mild but consistent form of exercise. To compensate for such things these people must make a conscious effort to increase their activity since prescribed physical education programs in schools are much too short to substitute for this. It has been shown similarly that obese women walked only half as much as controls or twenty miles less during a week. In many cases they sought ways of reducing activity, such as use of elevators, efficient schedule planning to reduce activity, or choosing a mode of living that called for a minimum energy expenditure.

Decreased basal energy needs. The need for energy to carry on the vital body functions known as basal metabolism declines very gradually with age. While the difference in needs between one year and the next may be imperceptible and call for no conscious adjustment in energy intake, failure to make a satisfactory adjustment of intake to needs over a period of years can lead to an appreciable positive calorie balance in old age.

Patterns of infant feeding. The tendency of mothers to consider large weight gains in early infancy as highly desirable and to compare the eating habits of their infants to those of other infants leads them to introduce solid foods at an early age and to force large quantities of food. Bakwin attributes some of the problems of obesity in adolescence to a pattern of eating in which the individual is trained to eat beyond the point where he experiences normal satiety signals to the point where he is overeating. He feels that such a situation can be conditioned by patterns of feeding in early infancy. The developmental pattern of some infants has centered around eating as much as he wants as frequently as he wants while minimizing physical activity.

Psychological factors

Investigations as to whether psychological factors are causative or perpetuating in obese persons were begun in the late 1940's and have not yet identified any personality factors common to persons who experience difficulty in making a satisfactory weight adjustment. The psychological makeup of the individual influences not only the intake of food but also the level of activity and hence the energy expenditure.

An extensive review of the relationship between specific psychological factors and the incidence of obesity is well beyond the scope of the discussion, but some of the more established relationships will be discussed. While obesity is compatible with normal personality factors, some characteristics occur more frequently in obese than nonobese subjects. According to Bruch, overeating may be a balancing factor in adjustment to life. If overeating is to be stopped, the individual must be helped to find some other form of emotional support.

Failure to do so may result not only in unsuccessful weight reducing but may produce trauma far worse than the obesity it was designed to cure. The threat of earlier mortality from many diseases is not a motivating factor for many. To them, the prospect of dying early and happy is much less threatening than is the prospect of an unhappy life adjustment that comes with an inability to reduce in face of continuing efforts. Indeed, without his pattern of overeating he may be in danger of developing a form of mental illness. The need for individual therapy is evident. From a psychological point of view, overeating may be a response to nonspecific emotional tensions or a symptom of underlying emotional tensions, or it may represent an addiction to food.

Anxiety. An anxious person deprived for one reason or another of an outlet in physical activity may seek solace in food, the consumption of which represents a pleasureful pastime. The greater the level of anxiety, the less likely weight loss is to occur.

Substitute for love and security. To at least some obese individuals, overeating, a pleasant experience, is used as a substitute for love and affection or as an expression of self-pity. An overprotective mother may overfeed her child in order to reinforce her love for him. For others the strength symbolized by a large body is apparently a source of security representing a bulwark against an unfriendly world.

Tenseness or frustration. In some persons food is a response to, compensation for, or defense against tension and frustration.

Genetic factors

Characteristics of an individual that determine his level of intake and pattern of utilization of food may be determined by heredity. Such factors may explain the different responses in different individuals in common environments or similar responses among identical twins in markedly different environments.

Somatotype. The anthropologic classification of somatic body types as endomorphic (plump and round), mesomorphic (muscular), and ectomorphic (linear and fragile) is based on genetically determined traits. The endomorph is quite likely to become obese while the individual with few of the endomorphic characteristics tends to remain slim, as does the individual with a high ectomorphic component in his body build. The mesomorph will become obese if his build includes more of an endomorphic than ectomorphic component. In a study of obese girls it was shown that none of them had an elevated ectomorphic component while 40% of endomorphs of normal weight had a high ectomorphic component in their body structure. The endomorph tends to gain weight easily while the ectomorph seldom does. Obese girls have been demonstrated to have broader, shorter hands than nonobese, which further points to a relationship between the fragile bony structure of the ectomorph and the absence of obesity. In Britain, Withers showed that mesomorph-endomorphs had a ratio of 2.4:1 as many relatives in the same somatotype as ectomorphs.

Level of enzyme activity. Recent evidence has suggested that the rate of production of enzymes involved in either fat storage or fat mobilization can affect the formation of fat and the ease with which it can be used as a source of energy. An efficient or active enzyme system involved is fat formation (lipogenesis) may remove glucose from the bloodstream so rapidly that the normal satiety signals to reduce food intake do not operate quickly enough to regulate food intake, leading to an increased food intake and hence fat formation. This rate of lipogenesis in obese persons may be as much as five times greater than normal. Once fat has been deposited in adipose tissue primarily as triglycerides, it must be broken down into fatty acids and

glycerol (lipolysis) before the fat can be released from the storage site to be transported in the bloodstream for use as a source of energy in tissues requiring energy. This lipolysis depends on the presence of a fat-splitting enzyme—a lipase. In obese people the level of activity of this enzyme may be low or inhibited so that they do not mobilize or release stored fat rapidly enough to meet the body's demand for a source of energy. In order to meet the need the individual is forced to consume more food. It has also been established that once fat has been deposited in adipose tissue that the cell will store fat more readily again following its removal. Thus it is easier for a person who has been obese to become obese again than for one who has never been overweight.

While each gram of carbohydrate or protein has the potential of yielding 4 kilocalories in the body and each gram of fat 9 kilocalories, there are many enzymes involved in the many steps in their conversion to carbon dioxide, water, and energy in the form of ATP. Since we have much evidence of biochemical individuality in many enzyme reactions in the body, it is logical to assume that there are wide individual differences in the degree of efficiency with which energy will be released from these potential sources and with which it will be converted to mechanical, chemical, osmotic, or electrical energy for vital body functions. Such differences are undoubtedly genetically determined and are encoded in the DNA of the cell nucleus. An individual with a low lipase activity or a very efficient enzyme system for the release of energy may have more difficulty regulating this weight. Conversely, a person with an adequate lipase activity and a low efficiency rate in the release of energy will make a much more adequate weight adjustment. Aerobic metabolism is more efficient than anaerobic metabolism, in which it is necessary to expend energy to resynthesize glycogen. It is possible that the tendency toward aerobic metabolism, the more efficient type, may be genetically determined, leaving more energy to be stored. Such differences are well known to animal breeders, who choose animals whose genetic characteristics allow them to gain the most weight on the smallest amount of food, which facilitates the production of wool, milk, or eggs.

Genetically determined characteristics also influence a person's athletic aptitude and hence his participation in active sports. The sensitivity of the appetite-regulating center of the brain, the hypothalamus, appears to be genetically determined. A sensitive hypothalamus responds quickly to an elevated level of arterial blood glucose relative to venous blood glucose and depresses appetite. A less sensitive hypothalamus will respond more slowly and allow the individual to eat more before a feeling of satiety is reached.

Studies to determine the incidence of obesity in children of obese parents have shown that if both parents are obese there is a 73% chance that the children will be. If one parent is obese, the chances are 50%, while if neither parent is obese, there is only a 9% chance that the children will be. Where the children are reared in the same environment as the parents, the relationship is undoubtedly partially environmental and partially hereditary. However, Mayer, in studying the effect of environment on the incidence of obesity, found that infants adopted into families with one or more obese parents did not become obese while those born into similar families did become obese.

Once genetic factors are recognized as determinants, it would be reasonable from a public health standpoint to encourage persons with an hereditary predisposition to obesity to participate in a preventative program based on a regime of activity and a regulation of food intake begun at an early age. Genetically determined differences between individuals may be impos-

sible to detect with the sensitivity of present analytical methods, but if even small differences cumulate they become appreciable.

Cultural factors

The meaning of body size varies from one cultural group to another and influences attitudes towards obesity. To many groups a large body represents success; the man with the large wife is one who is sufficiently successful to provide her with adequate food. The sterotype of the plump, successful nineteenth century businessman, an object of envy by his less successful contemporaries, is gradually being replaced by that of the sleek, well-dressed, efficient young man. In certain primitive tribes young girls will be kept in, fed, and fattened into attractive young women. In many royal courts the women carried about on litters vie with one another to be the most attractive to royalty.

Food assumes special meanings in various life situations; it is frequently offered in times of sickness or death; it is basic to the feasts used to celebrate births, marriages, and deaths in many cultures, in which the provision of adequate food may involve incurring large debts.

The kind of food served and the manner in which it is served are often a basis of distinction among social classes, ranging from the use of relatively inexpensive high-starch diets among the poor to the conspicuous consumption of food by the higher socioeconomic groups.

Physiologic factors

Secretion of endocrine glands. The basal metabolic rate is determined by the level of secretion of the thyroid gland, thyroxine. In most individuals this is maintained within a normal range, but a very small segment of the population may find their energy needs depressed because of a depressed secretion of thyroxine. Some persons experience a very easy accumulation of fat and may find it easier to achieve calorie balance if either thyroxine or the closely related compound, thyronine, is administered. Because of the hazards from unsupervised use of the hormone it is available only on prescription.

Insulin, the secretion of the pancreas that is necessary for the conversion of carbohydrate to fat as well as for the utilization of carbohydrate as a primary source of energy, can influence the rate at which adipose tissue is formed.

Some endocrine secretions influence the distribution of fat in various parts of the body, and abnormal distributions represent an abnormal endocrine balance.

Adaptation. A severe calorie restriction for a period of time activates an adaptive mechanism that leads to a lowered basal metabolic rate and a greater efficiency in energy expenditure, thus conserving the energy available.

Decrease in basal metabolism. The basal energy needs of the body gradually decrease with age, necessitating an adjustment in energy intake if fat is not to be stored.

Regulation of food intake. The mechanisms by which the amount of food a person eats is regulated are still subject to much study, but it now appears that there is both a short-term and long-term regulation.

Short-term regulation. The meal-to-meal or short-term regulation of intake is controlled by the appetite-regulating center of the brain, the hypothalamus. The glucostatic theory suggests that the medial part of the hypothalamus is sensitive to the level of glucose but not amino acids or lipids in the bloodstream. When the difference in glucose content of arterial and venous blood (the A-V difference) is large, indicating that the tissues have more glucose available than they are removing, the hypothalamus stimulates a satiety response that depresses the appetite and feelings of hunger. When the A-V difference is small, the hypothalamus responds by stimulating

the hunger sensation and producing an increased intake of food. While it is generally agreed that the hypothalamus regulates food intake there is not complete agreement that it responds to blood glucose levels since there is some evidence that it may respond to the heat produced by the specific dynamic action of food.

Long-term regulation. The long-term regulation of food intake is governed by the reserves of fat in the adipose tissue cells of the body. It is hypothesized that a type of feedback mechanism operates whereby the food intake of one day reflects the intake of the previous days, being stimulated when low intakes have led to a depletion of fat reserves.

Persons who have difficulties in reducing weight have low, free-fatty acid levels in the blood after fasting compared to those in persons whose obesity responds to reduced caloric intake. This suggests a difference in their ability to mobilize fat reserves to supply energy during calorie restriction. These same persons respond slowly to the presence of a fat-mobilizing substance such as epinephrine. It may be the result of a metabolic defect that limits the breakdown of body fat stores or one that hastens the reformation of fatty acids and glycerol into fat depots or the presence of a lipase inhibitor.

CLASSIFICATION

Obesity can be classified on several bases. One classification chooses to differentiate between *juvenile onset obesity,* which usually develops before the child is ten years old, and *adult onset obesity,* which develops with increased age. The former is generally more severe than the latter, is more difficult to treat, has a poor response to therapy, and occurs twice as frequently in girls as boys. Frequently it is associated with a low intelligence and occurs among those with relatively little schooling. In some respects it may be an inherited condition caused by either more efficient use of energy or greater efficiency in energy expenditure. In contrast, adult onset obesity is characterized by a constant food intake in conjunction with a slowly declining energy expenditure both for basal metabolism and for activity. It is the result of the slow insidious weight gain of as little as a half pound to one pound per year, which may occur with aging but go unrecognized until it is well advanced. Sometimes the reduction in cell mass that occurs with reduced activity masks the accumulation of fat, which signals the onset of obesity.

In another classification based on pathogenesis, Van Itallie, Bates, and Mayer have identified obesity as either *regulatory,* in which there is either psychological or physiologic defect in the regulation of food intake in relation to energy expenditure or *metabolic,* where there is an underlying metabolic defect in the handling of either carbohydrate or lipid, which can be enzymatic, hormonal, or neurologic in nature. There is some suggestion that juvenile onset obesity and metabolic obesity are the same and that adult onset and regulatory obesity are the same. Bruch, whose experience is primarily with persons seeking psychological help, has suggested that *constitutional obesity* due primarily to physiologic causes, in which the person has a healthier personality adjustment to obesity and may suffer some form of maladjustment if forced to reduce, can be distinguished from *reactive obesity,* most common in adults in which overeating as a response to tension or frustration is often accompanied by decreased physical activity. Episodes of grief or depression frequently correspond to weight gains. Persons with reactive obesity often experience a night-eating syndrome, a higher rate of eating corresponding with periods of depression. These two forms in turn, she believes, are different from developmental obesity, which is common in children whose emotional development centers around eating

as much as they want while avoiding physical activity and social contacts.

In general, the basis on which the classification is made reflects the perspective of the investigator. It may be that physiologic factors mediate the psychological trauma that leads to overeating.

Treatment

The treatment of obesity involves the successful reversal of the positive caloric balance that caused the condition, i.e., a calorie intake less than calorie expenditure. Because of the multiple origins of obesity and the many meanings of food to individuals it is often difficult to find the cause of obesity. Until the cause is known, efforts to cure the conditions are discouraging. While the effectiveness of treatment depends on many factors, the motivation of the patient and the establishment of a realistic goal are of prime importance. In most cases the obesity is the result of a very slow calorie surplus over a long period of time. A very small error in intake when accumulated over a period of years is reflected in a sizeable weight gain. Conversely, a constant intake of 100 calories less than daily expenditure will result in a ten-pound weight loss in one year.

The patient launching a weight-reducing regime should be aware that for some persons there will be no drop in body weight for perhaps two or three weeks regardless of strict adherence to a diet known to be deficient in calories. The explanation is that as fat is withdrawn from storage sites water may enter the cells to replace fat and remain there for a period of time, after which it may be released very rapidly. Unfortunately, this phenomenon occurs at the stage in weight reducing when a person is most in need of some evidence of success. Usually when weight loss is looked at over a longer period of two to three months the predicted weight loss will be observed. It is quite common for a person to experience spurts of weight loss followed by a plateau, even with constant caloric intake and expenditure.

Studies on the prognosis of treatment have shown that success is more likely in adult onset than in juvenile onset obesity, in males than in females, in younger people than in older people, in married persons than in widowed, separated, or divorced persons, in single persons, especially women under 30, in the higher socioeconomic groups, in those making their first attempt than those making subsequent attempts, among those less than 60% overweight, among emotionally mature and well-adjusted rather than anxious or depressed persons, and among those with a medical problem that is complicated by obesity. It should also be emphasized that success will be greater if attempts are made in early stages and if done under supervision of a physician who concerns himself with the underlying causes than with a quack, charlatan, faddist, pseudoscientist, or well-meaning but misguided friends.

The reversal of the caloric balance involves setting the total calorie intake at a level less than that required to meet energy needs. This may be accomplished by either decreasing the intake or increasing activity. The level of caloric intake that will accomplish this varies greatly from one person to another because of the many individual factors that contributed to the situation.

Decreased caloric intake. Decreased caloric intake may be achieved by a very strict diet that prescribes a specific number of calories from specific foods or by a prudent diet in which an individual maintains his customary eating patterns but selects smaller portions and avoids foods of high caloric value. While popular literature abounds in diets designed to lead to a painless loss of weight, very few have stood the test of time, and the search for the panacea continues.

One currently popular theory is that weight loss is more effective if calories are derived from fat and protein rather than carbohydrates. Experimental evidence, however, shows that weight loss is a function of calorie intake regardless of the source of calories. The distribution of total calories throughout the day can influence the relative amount of muscle and fat deposited. If a large number of calories is consumed at one time in a condition described as *nutrient overload,* some calories that might have been used in muscle growth or in tissue repair are diverted to fat depots because of the demand suddenly placed on one metabolic pathway. The same number of calories distributed in smaller, more frequent feedings leads to decreased fat and increased muscle increments. Thus there appears to be some evidence in support of the nibbling habit in weight reduction, provided, of course, the amount of food nibbled does not exceed the needs of the individuals.

In addition to a restriction in the total caloric intake, there are certain other considerations that may be important in dieting success. Understanding guidance and support from physician or friends or family is crucial. A very rigid diet may be anxiety-producing. Eating slowly, tasting food thoroughly, using a smaller than average plate, and including such carbohydrates as potatoes because of their satiety value may contribute to a successful weight-reducing program. Even more important is the necessity of developing a set of eating patterns in which the calorie intake is restricted and which can be maintained to replace the eating pattern that led to the weight gain. For some persons this may involve a reeducation of their concept of serving size. Some research shows that the overweight person's concept of an average serving of food is a much larger quantity than that of a person of normal weight.

Complete starvation diets and those completely devoid of carbohydrates are effective because they lead to the accumulation of ketone bodies in the bloodstream, which in turn depress the appetite. The hazards involved in overtaxing the body's capacity to counteract excess ketones dictate that such regimes be employed only in extreme obesity that has been refractory to all other conventional methods and that they be undertaken under strict medical supervision. Such persons are usually hospitalized and kept in bed because of the extreme weakness accompanying the loss of sodium that occurs. The short-term results of such programs have given dramatic results, but on the long term the results have been very discouraging, with very few patients maintaining, let alone continuing, their weight loss. Part of the rapid initial weight loss can be attributed to an initial loss of sodium with the concurrent loss of water and the fact that protein has been deaminated to provide sufficient glucogenic amino acids to obtain the glucose needed to maintain the energy supply for the central nervous system and erythrocytes. This is reflected in negative nitrogen balance. Since protein is a less concentrated storage form of calories than fat tissue, much more must be catabolized to provide the same number of calories. The extensive loss of protein in starvation diets is manifest by a negative nitrogen balance and loss of body potassium. The catabolism of a pound of muscle tissue yields about one sixth as many calories as a pound of fat tissue.

Intermittent fasts of one to twelve days' duration following an initial fast of one to fifteen days have given promising results initially, giving the patient a feeling of well-being and cheerfulness, but have proven no more satisfactory than a continuous reduction in calorie intake in the long run. Persons who have been on a fasting regime usually eat less immediately afterwards and experience satiety with less food. This has led to the hypothesis that during fasting the satiety center in the hypothalamus may become more sensitive to satiety signals. Criteria for evaluating diets designed for caloric restriction are discussed in Chapter 5.

Increased activity. The effectiveness of an increased level of activity in establish-

ing caloric equilibrium has been alternately overrated and underrated. As illustrated in Chapter 5, the 3000 to 3500 kilocalories represented by one pound of stored body fat represents sufficient energy for many hours of such vigorous activity as tennis. However, a few minutes of the same activity every day for a longer period will help maintain the fine daily calorie balance necessary for weight control without undue stimulation of the appetite. Thus, while a 60-kg. (132-pound) woman will have to walk for 30 hours at an energy cost of 2 kilocalories per kilogram per hour to use the energy stored in one pound of body fat, if she walks half a mile a day at this rate of 3 miles per hour, after 180 days she will have used the equivalent amount of energy. Such a mild degree of exercise can represent two pounds per year. Sometimes the initiation of a program of moderate exercise not only increases caloric expenditures sufficiently that a weight loss will occur on a diet that previously maintained weight but also improves muscle tonus, stimulates circulation, and creates a general sense of well-being. Strenuous exercise, on the other hand, may stimulate the appetite to counterbalance any advantages of the regime.

A study to determine the effectiveness of a program of nutrition education and exercise on the course of obesity in 13- to 14-year-old boys more than 30% overweight in the beginning of the program showed that obese boys in the experimental group gained 5.8 pounds during the 18-month study period while those in the control group who did not receive nutrition education and who did not participate in a program of physical activity gained 13.5 pounds. These results suggest that a program of nutrition education coupled with one of prescribed physical activity can be an effective method of controlling adolescent obesity.

Dietary aids

A discussion of weight control would not be complete without some mention of the types of dietary aids, representing a 100 million dollar business, with which the adult public is constantly confronted. The magnitude of this enterprise likely reflects the observation that many obese persons cannot adhere to a diet without supportive measures. It also represents the constant search of the overweight for some easy, painless, and quick road to weight loss. Since very few of these aids stand the test of time and remain on the market for more than a brief period, this discussion will be confined to the general types of dietary aids.

Agents reducing food intake. Appetite depressants or anorexigenic drugs are the basis of many dietary aids. Pills containing sugar, milk solids, or gelatin taken about half an hour before meals act as an appetite depressant by raising blood glucose levels, increasing the difference between arterial and venous glucose levels, hence depressing the appetite at mealtime. These are relatively harmless but generally greatly overpriced even when the cost of minerals and vitamins that are often added to them is considered. The same effect could be achieved with caramels from the corner grocery store if only one were taken. Fruit juices high in carbohydrate, such as grape juice or prune juice, would have a similar effect.

Stimulants. Products containing amphetamines, which are stimulants for the central nervous system, are useful in overcoming depression and its attendant nibbling. They are the basis of other products but must be used with caution since they result in an elevated blood pressure, dryness of the mouth, and a rapid heartbeat, effects that cannot be divorced from its effect on the appetite. Dexedrine and Benzedrine, common appetite depressants, are also cardiac stimulants, as are epinephrine or ephedrine-like compounds. These anorexigenic drugs may be an essential crutch in the initial period of caloric restriction for the person who has become ad-dicted to food and who eats compulsively.

Tranquilizers as weight-reducing aids function by decreasing activity but at the same time reducing nibbling, which may have been the cause of weight gain.

Loss of body water. Diuretics lead to a loss of body water but no loss of body fat. If extra weight is caused by an accumulation of water in the tissues, diuretics will lead to permanent weight loss, but under normal conditions such water must be quickly replaced to maintain normal electrolyte balance. Steam baths, special plastic clothing, and bath salts—also designed to reduce weight by reduction in body water—will effect only transient weight loss.

Bulk-producing substances. Noncaloric substances such as methyl cellulose are advocated as appetite depressants because of their affinity for water and their tendency to increase in volume on the theory that bulk in the stomach will depress appetite. It has been experimentally demonstrated that the swelling of methyl cellulose takes place in the small intestine rather than in the stomach, thus limiting its supposed effectiveness.

Psychological aids. Testimony of individuals who have thought or prayed their way to slimness is evidence of the use being made of psychologically oriented devices in weight control. Other devices with strong powers of suggestion such as records played during sleep or pictures of the individual in slimming clothes are some of the current psychological gimmicks.

Transition diet

Once a desired weight adjustment is achieved it is important that the individual be given guidance in the transition from a reducing diet to a maintenance diet. It is especially important that one recognize the level of intake that will maintain the desired weight and that is sufficiently different from the regular diet that led to the initial weight gain to prevent a recurrence. Any maintenance diet must be sufficiently individualized to conform to the cultural, environmental, and social situation in which the individual lives.

Prevention

From a public health point of view the most feasible attacks on the problem of obesity are through prevention. By learning to identify those individuals who, because of genetic makeup, personality characteristics, or environmental factors, are most likely to become obese it should be possible to develop an educational program designed to control weight gain in the incipient stage. Such an approach could embrace a program of exercise coupled with education and training in the choice of foods and patterns of eating to minimize caloric intake. Christakis introduced an 18-month program of nutrition education and supervised exercise among 13- to 14-year-old obese high school boys in New York City that resulted in significantly lower weight gains in the experimental group than in the control group. Pediatricians, with access to weight grids, which help identify deviations in growth patterns in the early stages, have an opportunity to alert parents and encourage them to help the child acquire a set of eating patterns that will help forestall weight gain. Obstetricians and gynecologists working with women during pregnancy and menopause, two periods when weight gain is very easy, are in a position to help the women to cope with such an eventuality. Similarly, physicians dealing with middle-aged males working under any form of emotional stress who have a family history of heart disease have a unique opportunity to offer preventive therapy before weight reaches the stage where it enhances the possibility of coronary or arteriosclerotic heart disease. Persons with deviant activity patterns are just as prone to caloric imbalances as are those with deviant eating habits; thus it is important to work on both sides of the energy equation, promoting a habit of moderate but consistent exercise along with moderation in food intake.

UNDERWEIGHT

A person whose weight is more than 15% below desirable weight, while not subjected to the same social pressures as his overweight counterpart to adjust, is more susceptible to certain health hazards. He is almost twice as likely to succumb to respiratory diseases such as tuberculosis and has greater difficulty maintaining body temperature as environmental temperature drops.

Treatment

The treatment of underweight individuals involves creating a positive energy balance by increasing energy consumption beyond energy expenditure regardless of the level of the latter. Just as in obesity, it is important to recognize the cause of the undernutrition if it is to be adequately treated. If a depressed appetite is involved, various techniques can be used. Thiamine-deficiency anorexia may be reversed by the use of thiamine supplements. Handling of anorexia nervosa is considerably more complex and should involve determining the underlying cause. The use of smaller, more frequent meals of lower calorie value rather than fewer larger meals may help promote an increased energy intake. The addition of highly concentrated sources of energy such as sugar, jellies, butter, mayonnaise, sauces, or dried milk solids to regular foods is a fairly successful way of increasing the energy value of a diet without an increase in bulk. Just as in weight reduction the adjustment in weight needs to be made gradually, and it may be even more difficult, albeit more pleasant, for an underweight person to try to gain one pound per week than for an obese person to lose it.

SELECTED REFERENCES
Obesity
Ayers, W.: Changing attitudes toward overweight and reducing, J. Am. Dietet. A. 34:23-28, 1958.

Bortz, W. M., Wroldsen, A., Issekietz, B., and Rodahl, K.: Weight loss and frequency of feeding, New England J. Med. 274:376, 1966.

Drenick, E. J., and Smith, R.: Weight reduction by prolonged starvation, Postgrad. Med. 36:A95, 1964.

Darling, C. D., and Summerskill, J.: Emotional factors in obesity and weight reduction, J. Am. Dietet. A. 29:1204, 1953.

Fellner, C. H., and Levitt, H.: A new approach to overweight, Am. J. Clin. Nutrition 15:50, 1964.

Forbes, G.: Lean body mass and fat in obese children, Pediatrics 34:308, 1964.

Goldberg, M., and Gordon, E. S.: Energy metabolism in human obesity, J.A.M.A. 189:616, 1964.

Gordon, E. S.: New concepts of the biochemistry and physiology of obesity, M. Clin. North America 48:1285, 1964.

Halpern, S. L.: Methodology of effective weight reduction, M. Clin. North America 48:1335, 1964.

Hamburger, W. W.: The psychology of weight reduction, J. Am. Dietet. A. 34:17, 1958.

Hashim, S. A., and Van Itallie, T. B.: Clinical and physiologic aspects of obesity, J. Am. Dietet. A. 46:15, 1965.

Jacobs, D., Heald, F. P., White, P. L., and McGanity, W. J.: Obesity prevention, J.A.M.A. (supplement 1) 186:27, 1963.

MacBryde, C. M.: The diagnosis of obesity, M. Clin. North America 48:1307, 1964.

McCracken, B. H.: Etiological aspects of obesity, Am. J. M. Sc. 243:99, 1962.

Mayer, J.: Some aspects of the problem of the regulation of food intake and obesity, New England J. Med. 274:610, 662, 722, 1966.

Mayer, J.: Physical activity and anthropometric measurements of obese adolescents, Fed. Proc. 25:11, 1966.

Mendelson, M.: Psychological aspects of obesity, M. Clin. North America 48:1373, 1964.

Mendelson, M.: Deviant patterns of feeding behavior in man, Fed. Proc. (part 1) 23:69, 1964.

Moore, M. E., Stunkard, A., and Strole, L.: Obesity, social class and mental illness, J.A.M.A. 181:962, 1962.

Pollack, H., Conzllazio, C. F., and Issac, G. J.: Metabolic demands as a factor in weight control, J. Am. Dietet. A. 167:217, 1958.

Pollack, H.: Prophylaxis of obesity in the adult, Bull. New York Acad. Med. 36:87, 1960.

Prugh, D. E.: Some psychological considerations concerned with the problem of over nutrition, Am. J. Clin. Nutrition 9:538, 1961.

Rosenberg, B. A., Bloom, W., and Spencer, H.: Obesity—treatment and hazards, J.A.M.A. 186:43 (supplement), 1963.

Sebrell, W. H.: Weight control through prevention of obesity, J. Am. Dietet. A. 34:919, 1958.

Seltzer, C. C., and Mayer, J.: Body build and obesity. Who are the obese?, J.A.M.A. 189:677, 1964.

Seltzer, C. C.: Some re-evaluations of the build and blood pressure study 1959 as related to ponderal index, somatotype and mortality, New England J. Med. 274:254, 1966.

Seltzer, C. C., Goldman, R. F., and Mayer, J.: The triceps skinfold as a predictive measure of body density and body fat in obese adolescent girls, Pediatrics 36:212, 1965.

Shank, R.: Weight reduction and its significance, Nutr. Rev. 19:289, 1961.

Shipman, W. G., and Plesset, M. R.: Predicting the outcome for obese dieters, J. Am. Dietet. A. 42:383, 1963.

Swendseid, M. E., Mulcare, D. B., and Drenick, E. J.: Nitrogen and weight losses during starvation and realimentation in obesity, J. Am. Dietet. A. 46:276, 1965.

Wright, F. H.: Preventing obesity in childhood, J. Am. Dietet. A. 40:516, 1962.

Young, C.: The prevention of obesity, M. Clin. North America 48:1317, 1964.

Young, C. M.: Some comments on the obesities, J. Am. Dietet. A. 45:134, 1963.

21

Food faddism and quackery

Food faddism and quackery are aspects of nutrition that are receiving an increasing amount of attention from nutritionists because of the health, economic, and social problems they create. Nutritionists are recognizing that the food quack, with his strongly emotional appeal, his exaggerated claims, and his powers of persuasion, is commanding attention from a significant segment of the population and rapidly undermining the teaching of the legitimate nutritionists, who cannot compete with the faddist because of their unwillingness to misrepresent the knowledge in the field by making unrealistic claims. Faddism is not confined to the superstitious, the uninformed, and the poor. Although they are easily influenced, faddism frequently attracts persons with the easiest access to sound scientific information in the field. The forces that operate to keep food faddism alive are a complex of economic, ethical, sociocultural, and educational factors.

Food fads, which can be defined as favored or popular fashions in food consumption that prevail for a period of time, are constantly changing. Although some basic beliefs of the food faddist keep recurring and have gained wider acceptance, the form in which they are manifest is constantly changing and they can usually be destroyed if adequately and persistently attacked. A person who follows a food fad, usually with exaggerated zeal, becomes known as a food faddist, and the whole subject of fashions in food in which special properties are attributed to it is known as food faddism. Some of the food fads such as coffee drinking are merely fashions that cannot be considered harmful in any way, but others, such as the use of food grown only on organically fertilized soil, may lead to bizarre eating habits at greatly inflated costs. In addition to attacking the problem of food fads, the legitimate nutritionist is constantly combatting food misinformation, which is often more difficult to fight since it involves scientific half-truths, distortions, or misrepresentations of scientific information as well as outright fallacies and fancies. The food quack pretends to have information he does not possess, perpetrates his ideas or products on large groups of people, and is usually motivated by personal financial gain.

EXTENT OF FOOD FADDISM AND QUACKERY

The Food and Drug Administration believes that 10 million Americans are being bilked of at least half a billion dollars per year by food quacks, purveyors of nutritional supplements, and vendors of books and special devices reputed to solve the nutritional ills of the country. If a comparable amount were spent on improved food intakes both the consumer and the food industry would benefit. Such a large expenditure of money on unnecessary supplementation or modification of the diet could occur only in an affluent society and reflects the health-consciousness of the nation and our eternal quest for longer and healthier lives. Thus, we find food quackery only in the technically developed countries that enjoy a high standard of living. It has been suggested that if the amount of money spent in the United States on dietary supplements is any indication of the nutritional status of the population, it could only be classed as the most poorly nourished nation in the world. In reality it takes more effort to be malnourished than well nourished with prevailing food patterns in the United States.

Jalso, in a study of nutritional beliefs and practices in New York state, found that food faddists had less formal education and less nutrition education than nonfaddists and were concentrated in the older age and lower socioeconomic groups. On the basis of a personality test, food faddists were found to have more rigid personalities than nonfaddists.

Nature of food fads

Food fads, in addition to representing mere fashions in food or the persistence of folk beliefs, follow several prescribed patterns, usually stressing a food concept rather than a nutrient concept.

Exaggeration of the virtues of a particular food. Many food fads revolve around the belief that specific foods have almost magical medicinal properties, usually in the cure of conditions over which medical science has produced no effective control or cure. Among the more common beliefs are that fruits cure cancer, carrot juice relieves leukemia, garlic reduces high blood pressure, and royal jelly extends the prime of life and leads to sexual rejuvenation. It is interesting to note that different cultures ascribe different properties to the same food. For instance, the tomato is considered poisonous by some, an aphrodisiac by others, and a cancer cure in still other situations.

Food quacks constantly refer to the "secret formula" of a product, to which they attribute its special merits. In one case the secret formula was alfalfa, ground bones, and the germ from cereal products and in another garlic, lecithin, and wheat germ.

Omission of foods because of harmful properties. The omission of certain foods is as much a food fad as is the exaggerated use of them in the diet. The notion that any food enriched with nutrients (called chemicals by the faddists) is poisonous has led to the rejection of such staples in the diet as enriched white bread or milk fortified with vitamin D. The proposed relationship between fruit and fever has led to the exclusion of fruit from the diet.

Foods high in cholesterol are avoided by many persons in the fear that their use will lead to heart disease. In place of cholesterol-containing foods, it is not unusual to find a person substituting high intakes of liquid oils without the benefit of medical guidance.

Emphasis on "natural" foods. A whole segment of the food faddist cult supports the notion that only "natural" foods are safe for human consumption. To qualify as a natural food, it must have been grown on soil fertilized by natural or organic fertilizers rather than chemical fertilizers, it must have not been subjected to herbicides or pesticides, and it must be unprocessed. Stores devoted entirely to sale of foods reportedly grown on naturally fertilized soil do a thriving business with customers who have lost all faith in the adequacy of food bought in normal food outlets. These persons travel long distances and pay exorbitant prices to avoid these "contaminants" in the food supply. A list of the foods available in such an outlet includes carrot juice, stone-milled buckwheat flour, unsulfured fruit, wheat germ, fertile eggs, and Irish sea moss as well as more conventional food items. All of these, the customer is led to believe, have been grown on soil that has not been treated with chemical fertilizers and are sold in their natural, unprocessed form. The use of such terms as "counterfeited," "prefabricated," "worthless," "national scandal," and "devitalized" to describe processed foods and "natural" and "vital" for unprocessed foods is designed to heighten the effect. Natural foods are for the most part wholesome foods that are rich in nutrients and flavor and certainly should never be condemned from a nutritional standpoint, but neither are they *essential* for health. Most processed foods are equally as good and should not be excluded.

Many natural food organizations with very impressive and authoritative-sounding names propound the basic philosophy that all mental and metabolic diseases are caused by commercially processed foods. In several cases it has been established that the president of the organization or editor of its publication is the owner of a natural food store. Their propaganda war against all foods other than natural foods is continuous and knows no bounds.

Special devices. Food faddists may also direct their attention to the types of equipment in which or on which food is prepared. Great merit has been attributed to devices for grating or shredding vegetables, to blenders often selling at twice the price of conventional blenders, or to cooking utensils (available only in large sets) that are said to be capable of conserving nutrients.

Dangers of food faddism

The major concern of the government and other agencies involved in protecting the consumer against the fraudulent claims and ineffectual products of the food quack stems not only from a fear that the product he sells is in itself harmful but also from a concern over the economic and ethical aspects of his operation. The government is concerned that millions of people are spending money for products that cannot possibly do what they are reported to do and more specifically that among the victims are many who can ill afford to divert their food money to nutritional supplements or overrated food products. The vitamins in many products are useless unless they have some substrate on which to act, so that the supplements are useless without food. Older people in whom the fear of becoming ill or dependent is ever present are particularly susceptible. In addition to spending money on a product that is worthless for the purpose for which it was bought, people, in the belief that it may be effective, often delay the time when competent medical advice is sought until the damage is irreparable.

Mode of operation of the quack

The food quack capitalizes on people's desire for information and creates a market for his product or ideas through a variety of highly emotional appeals. He capitalizes on the overriding fear of many that they will become incapacitated through illness. For others he provides a crutch for their organic and psychic ailments. Quacks undermine the public's faith in the adequacy of the nation's food supply to provide them with the essentials for good health. Not only do they suggest that it may be incapable of providing the essentials, they also suggest that certain products used to increase our food production, such as herbicides, pesticides, and the chemicals used in processing, are toxic substances undermining health and leading to all kinds of dire consequences.

By his contentions that all disease is caused by faulty diet, that the population suffers from widespread malnutrition, that food-processing destroys the nutritive value of foods, and that soil depletion is an underlying cause of faulty diets, the quack is able to create such a fear of sickness in his victim that he has little trouble selling his panacea. The imaginary illnesses he conjures up are often created by the use of vague, meaningless terms such as "roundness of corpuscles," "tired blood," and "vitagenic," all of which have scientific overtones to the gullible.

Food quacks frequently pose as members of legitimate-sounding professional organizations. It is virtually impossible for a lay person to recognize the names of the official organs of the profession let alone discriminate them from others with equally impressive names. To expect that the general public will recognize that the American Institute of Nutrition, the official organization of nutritionists, is different from the American Academy of Applied Nutrition or the American Nutrition Society, both of which are nonscientific organizations, is to assume a level of interest that does not exist. In at least one case the telephone number listed on the letterhead of one of these pseudoscientific societies is answered by a health food store. Many of these organizations publish their own monthly journal with "scientific" articles by their own members, most of which support the use of the type of product sold in their outlets. Even reputable scientific groups have been temporarily deceived into accepting them as scientific. Besides mentioning specific organizations quacks also promote themselves by the use of self-conferred titles such as "world-renowned nutrition-

ist," "dietician," "international authority," and other convincing accolades. Indeed, several individuals who have earned degrees that qualify them to use the title of doctor have been diverted into the lucrative food faddism business. By quoting scientific data out of context or in an incomplete form or by applying findings of animal studies to humans they are able to create an illusion of scientific know-how.

The faddist is quick to capitalize on new developments in science by taking an observation from scientific literature and by smart and timely merchandising parlaying it into a neat profit. The promoters of safflower oil as an aid to reducing blood cholesterol levels were able for a short time to convince the public to buy it at the drugstore in 1100-mg. capsules at six cents each or approximately 25 dollars per pint while the same product was available across the street in the grocery store at 80 cents a pint. Similarly, people with the unfounded belief that gelatin will improve the condition of their fingernails eagerly pay two dollars per ounce for gelatin in capsule form that the grocer offers at ten cents for the same amount. The ingredients in one widely distributed pill selling for 12 cents each were found to be the same as those in half a cent's worth of dried nonfat milk solids. The discovery of vitamin K, naturally present in alfalfa, as necessary for blood coagulation gave food supplement promoters another product in which the margin of profit was very high. Vitamin E, for which a human deficiency has never been demonstrated, is a favorite promotion of the quack, who attributes to the human being all of the most severe deficiency symptoms ever observed in animals.

Characteristics of a quack

One can be suspicious of food quackery when a person operates under one of several conditions:

1. The promoter claims that his food has miraculous powers, usually in the cure of

conditions that are still baffling medical men, such as arthritis, leukemia, and arteriosclerosis. He usually claims to have information not available through regular medical channels.

2. He claims that he is being persecuted by medical "trusts and cartels" whose livelihood is threatened by him and his product.

3. He maintains that the soil is depleted and no longer capable of producing a food supply capable of meeting the nutritional needs of the population. His only solutions to this are the use of food supplements or the exclusive use of the nutritious foods grown in soil fertilized with organic fertilizers.

4. He maintains that practically everyone is suffering from some degree of malnutrition that cannot possibly be corrected by foods readily available. He attributes this to the following dietary habits:

1. Use of pasteurized rather than raw milk.
2. Use of nonfertile rather than fertile eggs.
3. Ingestion of mixed meals.
4. Use of canned fruits and vegetables.
5. Use of white flour rather than freshly milled whole grains or sprouted grains.
6. Use of refined sugars.
7. Use of plant foods of all types grown on impoverished soils.
8. Use of chemically pure or synthetic vitamins.
9. Use of chemically-contaminated foodstuffs resulting from pesticides, etc. (addition of fluorides to water supplies is opposed).

Methods of merchandising

Food quacks can be found in almost any aspect of the food-marketing business, but they have tended to rely on the less conventional merchandising procedures. High-pressure advertising in their own publications, Sunday supplements, and some maga-zines in which an introductory offer with refund privileges for dissatisfied customers is offered are very common. They are sufficiently astute psychologists to realize that very few disillusioned buyers are going to bother to seek a refund.

Door-to-door salesmen or "doorbell doctors" are very successful in convincing the housewife that the only way she can protect her own health and her family's health is through the use of whatever product he is promoting, be it special saucepans, a recipe book, vitamins, food supplements, or a potential cure for asthma. Usually these products are available at a "special low price" for quantity purchases on a cash basis. In many cases a victim realizes too late that in order to safeguard the health of her whole family she has committed an unreasonable part of the family income. In some door-to-door selling situations the parent company protects itself against responsibility for the claims of its salesmen, making it difficult to take effective legal action to stop the sales.

Public lectures, often "by invitation only," are used to lure people. After an initial period in which some fairly plausible nutritional information is given, the lecturer launches into a train of thought designed to lead the audience to only one conclusion—that their only hope of salvation is to rely on the product for which he will be glad to take orders. Radio and television time are also purchased and used in much the same way.

Health food stores thrive in the densely populated areas of large cities, especially when they offer food grown on organically grown soil. Their inventory includes several hundred items such as carrot powder, papaya tablets, alfalfa concentrates, rose hips, miracle wafers, amino acid tablets, royal jelly, millet, special-formula tablets of natural vitamins and minerals, bone meal, wheat germ, brewer's yeast, dessicated liver, alfalfa, fish-liver oil, kelp, parsley, and iron. At the other end of the merchandising continuum are the health food farms located in a pastoral setting uncontaminated by herbicides, pesticides, and chemical fertilizers to which the devotee may travel for the privilege of paying two to three times regular grocery prices for the same products. Practically all these outlets also offer mail order service.

The labelling on a product may also purposefully be misleading. For instance, 10-gm. capsules of gelatin bore a listing of the percentage of the total protein represented by seventeen different amino acids, the names of which would give the average consumer the impression that the product was highly nutritious. The fact that the whole capsule provided about 0.0014% of the day's protein requirement was not mentioned.

Books on nutrition have been a source of much misinformation and half-truths for the consumer and a source of tremendous income for the successful writer. Since the food quack is not limited in his claims by established findings he is able to make a much stronger, more emotional appeal than the legitimate scientist who often tends to be overly cautious in his attempts to avoid violating the limits of knowledge. A perusal of the titles of the chapters in some of the more popular publications such as *"Are poisons making you old?" "Help for prostates," "Learn to live without an ulcer," "Skin problems are more than skin deep,"* and *"Arthritis can often be relieved!"* gives the reader some notion of the approach used. Again much of the information is based on sound basic principles of nutrition, but in their zeal to sell books the authors couch everything in terms of a strong emotional appeal. The sale of half a million copies of a book can earn the author a quarter of a million dollars and the publisher half a million, so the motivation to appeal to a wide audience is great.

Special equipment for food preparation has been another lucrative approach of the food quack. This is often demonstrated at fairs, summer resorts, arcades, department stores, or invitational parties in private homes where the promoter relies heavily on impulse buying. He attributes a wide range of merits to the equipment, such as increasing the consumption of fruits and vegetables, eliminating poisons from foods, conserving vitamins, or incorporating oxygen in food.

Types of products

"Shotgun" formula. Products characterized by "shotgun" formulas may list as many as fifty different nutrients on the label and are designed to impress the gullible consumer who is awed by the range of items included. Some of these are nutrients for which recommended daily allowances and minimum daily requirements have been established; others are those known to be essential but for which no requirements have been established; and others are substances of no known nutritional significance but harmless. Of those known to be required some will be present at many times the recommended level while others will be present in insignificant amounts. For instance, one product in the recommended daily dose contains 400% of the minimum daily requirement of vitamins A, D, C, B, and B_2 and about 2% of the daily requirement of potassium. This same product lists 10 mg. of unsaturated fatty acids, which represents about 0.1% of the 1% of the calories from linoleic acid recommended in the adult diet. The mixture is obviously irrational from a nutritional and physiologic point of view but completely rational from the point of view of the uninformed consumer.

"Loaded" formula. The term *"loaded" formula* is applied to the high-potency product that competes by providing more of a nutrient than its competitor. Thus, we find a spiraling in trade competition, with one company adding more of a nutrient for a very insignificant difference in price than his competitor. The average consumer does

not realize that he merely excretes the excess amounts of the water-soluble vitamins and may develop toxic reactions from excessive levels of the fat-soluble vitamins. Recent rulings (1965) of the Food and Drug Administration limiting the levels of the fat-soluble vitamins A and D that can be included without a prescription should help rectify this situation.

Natural organic products. Natural organic foods are reportedly grown in organically fertilized soil without the benefit of insecticides and herbicides or chemical fertilizers.

Miracle products. Miracle products include such products as garlic pills to relieve high blood pressure, honey and vinegar for arthritis, wheat germ for sterility, and lecithin for coronary disease.

Unnecessary supplements. The sale of protein supplements to the American population may well be questioned, especially at suggested prices. One firm created doubts as to the adequacy of protein in the American diet to soften the market for its protein pills, each of which contained 728 mg. of protein. In order to obtain the equivalent of the 20 gm. of protein in one serving of meat, a person would need to take 28 pills at a cost of 25 cents.

Useless products. Sea water, which enterprising persons living in coastal areas were shipping all over the country, would be placed in the category of useless products. When the cost of shipping used up some of the profit they reverted to dehydrated sea water to further enhance their earnings. Many products that might be beneficial in significant amount are useless at the levels at which they are sold.

COMBATTING MISINFORMATION AND FOOD FADDISTS

Efforts to protect the public against unscrupulous purveyors of misinformation and nutritional supplements in the name of nutritional science and to prevent exaggerated claims of the efficiency of food products are the concern of several government and community agencies.

Better Business Bureaus in many communities attempt to police, restrict, or regulate the activities of peddlers of health foods, special cooking devices, or nutrition supplements within their regions. They also require the registration of all persons giving public lectures, and on the basis of information available from one community to another are able to deny lecture privileges to those with a reputation for abusing them. They describe their efforts to combat food misinformation as preventive, corrective, and educational.

The Food and Drug Administration is constantly concerned with protecting the consumer against mislabelling and harmful, contaminated, and worthless products. When personnel and funds are limited, it is frequently necessary to restrict their activities to those aspects that present immediate dangers to the population. It takes time to prove that labelling is misleading or may lead to injury. After the FDA feels it has sufficient evidence to press charges, court proceedings are extremely slow and costly to both parties. In some instances, by the time enforcement agencies have been prepared to take action, the defendant has already realized sufficient profit that he does not contest the action. Regulations enacted in 1963 which require that a company present evidence that the product it proposes to sell is safe for human consumption have done much to lighten the load of this agency, which previously had to prove that a product was harmful before its sale could be restricted. A reluctance on the part of the public to initiate charges against a firm by which they have been victimized also hampers the operation of enforcement agencies. To admit that one has been "taken" is to admit a human frailty that many persons prefer not to publicize.

The Food and Drug Administration is responsible for formulating and enforcing regulations regarding the processing and sale of food products. On their recommendation the amount of folic acid that can be included in nutritional supplements was restricted to 0.1 mg. in a daily dose; the addition of vitamin D was limited to milk and infant formula at a level to provide no more than 400 I.U. in the recommended daily dose, and the use of the term *low-calorie* is allowed only for foods providing less than 20 kilocalories in an average serving. It has suggested that the quantities of vitamins and minerals in nutritional supplements be limited to amounts that are nutritionally useful to reduce the wild claims of manufacturers and also that only nutrients for which a deficiency is likely to occur be allowed. It has suggested that for only eight vitamins—thiamine, riboflavin, niacin, pyridoxine, vitamin A, vitamin D, vitamin K, and ascorbic acid—and four minerals—calcium, phosphorus, iron, and iodine—is there any justification for their inclusion in dietary supplements, that the use of artificial sweeteners should be restricted, and that a more meaningful term than minimum daily requirement be used in labelling foods. It is also concerned with artificial and natural contaminants in food.

Many of the efforts of the Food and Drug Administration to have more effective legislation enacted have been actively opposed by natural food organizations, which have launched an organized mail campaign to the members of Congress and the Department of Health, Education, and Welfare opposing the proposed legislation.

The American Medical Association has recognized the threat that quackery and faddism poses for the health of the nation and have launched a counterattack in the form of an exposé of the tactics and claims of the quack and faddist. They have developed films for use in nutrition education programs with supporting literature; they prepare periodical statements of their stand on prevailing practices and products; and they publish a popular magazine that frequently includes articles pertaining to the use of nutritional supplements and special health foods or devices. In spite of the efforts of this professional group to promote sound information, occasionally one of their own members, under the protection and aura associated with his degree, has published books on nutrition-related topics about which he was not adequately informed or qualified to speak. The American Medical Association also maintains a Bureau of Investigation that answers inquiries about specific persons or products and promotes an active campaign against quackery.

Other professional groups such as the American Public Health Association, The American Dietetics Association, and the American Home Economics Association all have active programs designed to combat food faddism and misinformation and are constantly attempting to inform the public in an effort to help them separate the foibles from the facts.

The Federal Trade Commission is involved in the fight against food quackery in its responsibility to protect the American public against false and misleading advertising. Cases involving charges of false advertising may take several years to try and will involve hundreds of hours of testimony. Some of their cases have revolved around such claims as the superiority of vitamins from natural sources over synthetic vitamins, the need for delivery of garden-fresh vitamins, the need for time-released vitamin-mineral capsules, and claims that juices prepared in special blenders have miraculous curative powers.

The Post Office department, which regulates the use of the mails to defraud, also performs a watchdog function to protect the public against nutritional hoaxes.

On the theory that an informed public is a less gullible public, nutrition education should be one of the most effective ways of combatting food fads and quackery, especially with the potential of all the media available to disseminate sound information. When even the well-educated and scientifically enlightened are prey to the wiles of the faddist and the quack, one wonders what level of education is necessary to protect people from becoming victims of the promoter who claims his product will cure everything from corns to sterility to leukemia. To combat faddism it is necessary to recognize the emotional and psychological influences which perpetuate it. Thus an educational campaign aimed at combatting it must be multifaceted, attacking as many of the forces that support it as possible.

Only through a constant flow of legitimate nutrition information can progress be made in combatting the high pressure salesmanship of the quack. It appears that for every one person involved in merchandising sound nutritional information there are several hundred merchandising their own pet schemes. Several nutritionists who write regular syndicated columns for daily or weekly newspapers utilize this opportunity to fight faddism and help enlighten the public. Dietitians in some larger cities operate a service known as Dial-a-titian in which people with questions related to nutrition may call the service and have their query referred to the person most qualified to answer it.

The difficulties in combatting misinformation in the press are much more formidable than those on labels or ads for products. Only when a book containing untenable claims for a certain food or product is displayed in a store along with the product it recommends can the book be confiscated along with the product on the grounds that it constitutes labelling. Even then it must involve interstate trade.

The final chapter in the saga of food faddism is far from written. One can only hope that it can be brought under reasonable control before the health of too many persons is jeopardized by the use of products promoted by unscrupulous salesmen.

SELECTED REFERENCES

Beeuwkes, A. M.: Food faddism and consumer, Fed. Proc. **13**:785, 1954.

Bernard, V. W.: Why people become the victims of medical quackery, Am. J. Pub. Health **55**:1142, 1965.

Darby, W. J.: The rational use of vitamins in medical practice, M. Clin. North America **48**:1203, 1964.

Council on Foods and Nutrition: Vitamin preparations as dietary supplements and as therapeutic agents, J.A.M.A. **169**:41, 1959.

Council on Foods and Nutrition: Problems of antibiotics in food, J.A.M.A. **170**:139, 1959.

Council on Foods and Nutrition: Safe use of chemicals in food, J.A.M.A. **178**:749, 1961.

Council on Foods and Nutrition: General policy on addition of specific nutrients to foods, J.A.M.A. **178**:1024, 1961.

Larrick, G. P.: The nutritive adequacy of our food supply, J. Am. Dietet. A. **39**:117, 1961.

Jalso, S. B., Burns, M. M., and Rivers, J. M.: Nutritional beliefs and practices, J. Am. Dietet. A. **47**:263, 1965.

Kulp, K., Golosinec, O. C., Shank, C. W., and Bradley, W. B.: Current practices in bread enrichment, J. Am. Diet. A. **32**:331, 1956.

Milstead, K. L.: Science works through law to protect consumers, J. Am. Dietet. A. **48**:187, 1966.

Mitchell, H. S.: Food fads—what protection have we?, J. Home Economics **53**:100, 1961.

Mott, M. A.: Better business bureaus fight food faddism, J. Am. Diet. A. **39**:122, 1961.

Nutrition Foundation: The role of nutrition education in combating food fads, New York, 1959, Nutrition Foundation.

Olson, R. E.: Food faddism—why?, Nutr. Rev. **16**:97, 1958.

Sebrell, W. H.: Food faddism and public health, Fed. Proc. **13**:780, 1954.

Sipple, H. L.: Opportunities in nutrition education, J. Am. Dietet. A. **42**:140, 1963.

Todhunter, E. N.: The foods we eat, J. Home Economics **50**:510, 1958.

Walker, A. R. P.: Problems in nutritional supplementation and enrichment. Am. J. Clin. Nutrition **12**:157-60, 1963.

Appendices

Appendix A

Glossary

absorption Process by which the products of digestion are transferred from the intestinal tract into the blood and lymph or by which substances in the interstitial fluid are taken up by the cells.

acid-base balance Relationship of acid-forming and base-forming elements in the body.

aerobic Living or functioning in air or free oxygen.

active transport An energy-requiring process by which a substance crosses a biological membrane.

alopecia Loss of hair.

amino acid Organic compounds of carbon, hydrogen, oxygen, and nitrogen. Each amino acid molecule contains one or more amino group ($-NH_2$) and at least one carboxyl group ($-COOH$). In addition, some amino acids (cystine and methionine) contain sulfur. Many amino acids are linked together in some definite pattern to form a molecule of protein.

anabolism The process by which substances are formed or built up. It includes all the chemical reactions that nutrients undergo in the construction of body compounds, such as blood, enzymes, muscle tissue, and fat.

anaerobic Living or functioning in the absence of air or free oxygen. The opposite of aerobic.

antibody One of many specific substances produced in the body to react against disease-producing or other foreign materials in the bloodstream.

Some antibodies remain available for many years and help to give a person permanent immunity.

antioxidant A substance capable of chemically protecting other substances against oxidation.

antivitamin or vitamin antagonist Substance chemically similar to a vitamin that is able to replace the vitamin in an essential compound but not capable of performing its role.

anorexia Pathologic absence of appetite or hunger in spite of a need for food.

apatite The crystals of calcium phosphate that give strength to bone or tooth matrix.

appetite Complex sensations by which organism is aware of desire for and anticipation of ingestion of palatable food.

atrophy Wasting away or degeneration.

basal metabolism The irreducible minimum of energy needed to carry on the body processes vital to life.

biosynthesis The coming together of chemical building units to form new materials in the living plant or animal.

blood serum Whole blood from which cells and clotting factor have been removed. It is the colorless fluid portion of the blood that separates when blood clots.

buffer A substance that can help a solution resist or counteract changes in free acid or alkali concentration. There are many buffers in the body, which help maintain the acid-base balance compatible with life.

calcification Process by which organic tissue becomes hardened by a deposit of calcium salts.

calorimeter An instrument for measuring heat changes in any system.

calorimetry The science of measuring heat.

carbon The chemical element present in all substances designated as organic. These include proteins, carbohydrates, and fats. When a compound containing carbon combines with oxygen in the body, energy is liberated and carbon dioxide is formed. Compounds that do not contain carbon are classed as inorganic.

cartilage A special form of white connective tissue that is attached to the ends of bones that are either divided into joints or united by joints. It is more flexible but not as strong as bone. Cartilage is the first substance to form in growing bone; then calcium and phosphorus are deposited in the cartilage to change it to bone.

carbon dioxide A compound that is formed when carbon combines with oxygen. It leaves the body chiefly when air is exhaled from the lungs.

catalyst A substance that speeds up the rate of a chemical reaction but is not itself used up in the reaction.

catabolism The breaking down in the body of chemical compounds into simpler ones, usually accompanied by the production of heat.

cell Smallest structural unit of living material.

cheilosis A condition characterized by lesions of the lips and corners of the mouth.

coenzmes An enzyme usually containing a vitamin that activates or combines with another enzyme to give a substance with enzyme activity.

chlorophyll The magnesium-containing green coloring matter present in growing plants, which under stimulus of light is active in the manufacture of carbohydrates from carbon dioxide and water in a process known as photosynthesis.

chylomicrons Very small (micro-) globules of fat of varying sizes in transport in the blood.

collagen A protein that forms the chief constituent of the connective tissue, cartilage, tendon, bone, and skin. Collagen is changed to gelatin by the action of water and heat.

colostrum A thin watery yellowish fluid secreted during the first few days of lactation.

combustion The combination of substances with oxygen accompanied by the liberation of energy.

decalcification The withdrawal of calcium from the bones on teeth where it has been deposited.

edema Swelling of a part of or the entire body caused by the accumulation of excess of water.

endemic Occurring infrequently but more or less constantly in a particular region or population.

endocrine Secreting internally or into the blood-stream, as in endocrine glands or glands of internal secretion.

endogenous Originating within or inside the cells or tissues.

enrichment Addition of nutrients, usually thiamine, riboflavin, niacin, and iron, to cereal products.

element Any one of the fundamental atoms of which all matter is composed.

enzymatic Related to that class of complex organic substances called enzymes, such as amylase and pepsin, that accelerate (catalyze) specific chemical reactions in plants and animals, as in digestion of foods.

epithelial Those cells that form the outer layer of the skin or those that line all the portions of the body that have contact with the external air, such as the eyes, ears, nose, throat, and lungs.

erythropoiesis The process by which red blood cells are produced.

exudation The abnormal outpouring of a substance that becomes deposited in or on tissues.

etiology Theory or study of the causes of a disease or a disorder.

Food and Agriculture Organization (FAO) A branch of the United Nations concerned with problems of food supply and distribution on a worldwide basis to help provide an adequate level of nutrition for all people.

Food and Nutrition Board A group of scientists in foods and nutrition or related fields who act in an advisory capacity to the National Research Council of the National Academy of Sciences.

fetus The unborn young or embryo of animals in the later stages of their development before birth (adjective, fetal).

flora (intestinal) The bacteria and other small organisms that are found in the intestinal contents.

gluconeogenesis Formation of glucose from noncarbohydrate substances such as amino acids or glycerol.

homeostatis Steady biochemical states in the body maintained by physiologic processes.

hormone A chemical substance that is produced in an organ called an endocrine gland and is transported by the blood or other body fluids to other cells. A hormone greatly influences the functions of some specific organs and of the body as a whole.

hunger The complex of unpleasant sensations felt after prolonged deprivation that will impel an animal or man to seek, work, or fight for immediate relief by ingestion of food.

hydrogenation The addition of hydrogen to any unsaturated compounds. Oils are changed to solid fats by hydrogenation.

hydrolysis The splitting of a substance into the smaller units of which it is composed by the addition of the elements of water. For example, when starch is heated in water containing a small amount of acid or subjected to the action of digestive enzymes, the simpler sugar glucose is released.

hypervitaminosis A condition in which the level of a vitamin in the blood or tissues is high enough to cause undesirable symptoms.

ingest To eat or take in through the mouth.

isocaloric Having the same energy value.

labile Unstable; easily decomposed.

lactation The secretion of milk or the period during which milk is formed.

lipids A broad term for fats and fatlike substances; characterized by the presence of one or more fatty acids. Lipids include fats, cholesterol, lecithins, phospholipids, and similar substances that do not mix readily with water.

lysosome (perinuclear dense body) The organelle of the cell that contains enzymes capable of destroying the cell.

matrix The intercellular framework of a tissue.

metabolism All the chemical changes that occur from the time nutrients are absorbed until they are built into body substances or are excreted.

microorganisms Very small living cells such as bacteria, yeasts, and molds.

mitochondrion Organelle of the cell in which most of the transformation of energy occurs.

mucosa The mucous membrane in an epithelial tissue that lines the passages and cavities of the body, such as the gastrointestinal tract and the respiratory tract. It usually has the ability to secrete.

National Research Council A group of leading scientists appointed by the National Academy of Sciences to coordinate the efforts of major scientific and technical societies of this country to serve science and government.

organelle Part or division of a cell that has a definite structure and function within the cells.

osmosis The transfer of materials that takes place through a semipermeable membrane that separates two solutions or between a solvent and a solution that tends to equalize their concentrations. The walls of living cells are semipermeable membranes, and much of the activity of the cells depends on osmosis.

organic acids Acids containing only carbon, hydrogen, and oxygen. Among the best known are citric acid (in citrus fruits) and acetic acid (in vinegar).

oxidation The removal of electrons in the most general sense; may also mean the combining with oxygen or the removal of hydrogen.

phagocyte A cell that can engulf particles or cells that are foreign or harmful to the body. Phagocytes are present in the blood and lymph and also in the lungs, liver, and spleen.

phosphorylate A chemical term that applies to the introduction of a phosphorus and oxygen group into a complex chemical compound.

physiologic Refers to the science of physiology, which deals with functions of living organisms or their parts.

placenta An organ on the wall of the uterus (womb), to which the developing young animal is attached by means of the umbilical cord. Nourishment is transferred from the maternal organism to the fetus and fetal waste products returned to the maternal circulation through it.

plasma The colorless fluid portion of the blood from which the cells have been removed.

protoplasm Living matter possessing capability for growth, repair, and reproduction. It is composed of water, inorganic salts, and organic compounds.

ossification The process of forming bone. Cartilage is made into bone by the process of ossification. The minerals, calcium, and phosphorus are deposited in the cartilage, changing it into bone.

portal vein Blood vessel leading from the wall of the intestine to the liver.

passive transport Process by which a substance crosses a biological membrane by diffusion or without the use of energy.

pituitary gland A gland in the lower part of the brain that produces a number of hormones that regulate the growth of all body tissues and regulate the development and action of other endocrine glands such as the thyroid, pancreas, and adrenal glands.

radical In chemistry, a group of elements joined in a set formation, which appears as a unit in a series of compounds or behaves as one piece without decomposition in chemical reactions. Examples are the glycerol radical in fats, the carboxyl group in organic acids, and the phenol radical (benzene ring) in certain amino acids. The amino acids themselves act as larger radicals in making up proteins.

reticuloendothelial system The liver, spleen, and bone marrow.

ribosome Organelle of a cell responsible for protein synthesis. Frequently occurs in groupings of known as polyribosomes, polysomes, or ergosomes.

satiety Cessation of desire for further nourishment at the end of the meal.

syndrome A medical term meaning a group of symptoms that occur together.

synthesis Process by which a new substance is formed from its individual parts.

toxicity The quality of a substance that makes it poisonous or toxic; sometimes refers to the degree of severity of the poison or the possibility of being poisonous.

trimester Three months or one third of the nine months of pregnancy. The nine months of pregnancy are divided into the first, second, and third trimesters.

urinary Occurring in the urine.

Meaning of prefixes and suffixes used in nutrition terms

Prefix	Meaning	Example
a-	lack of	avitaminosis
ab-	away from	abnormal
ad-	toward	addiction
amyl-	starch	amylose
an-	negative, lack of	anemia
ante-	before, preceding	antenatal
anti-	against	antibiotic
bi-	two, double	bilateral
calori-	heat	calorimetry
co-	with	coenzymes
di-	in two parts	disaccharides
dys-	bad	dysentery
endo-	within	endogenous
epi-	upon, on, over, above	epithelium
ex-	out	exogenous
hepato-	pertaining to the liver	hepatitis
hyper-	excessive, above	hyperactive
iso-	the same	isocaloric
hypo-	under	hypothyroidism
lacto-	pertaining to milk	lactose
lip-	fat	lipid
leuko-	white	leukocyte
mono-	one	monosaccharide
neo-	new	neonatal
os-	bone	osteoblast
pan-	all, entire	panacea
peri-	around, on all sides	pericardium
poly-	many	polyneuritis

Prefix	Meaning	Example
post-	after, behind	postnatal
ren-	kidney	renal
syn-	with, together	synthesis
tachy-	rapid	tachycardia
thio-	containing sulphur	thiamine
tox-	poison	toxemia

Suffix	Meaning	Example
-algia	suffering, pain	neuralgia
-ase	enzyme	protease
-blast	cell that builds	osteoblast
-cide	causing death	pesticide
-clast	cell that destroys	osteoclast
-cyte	mature cell	erythrocyte
-emia	blood	anemia
-ectomy	removal	thyroidectomy
-gen	get or produce	antigen
-genesis	produce	glucogenesis
-gram	tracing or mark	cardiogram
-graph	instrument	cardiograph
-heme	iron-containing	hemoglobin
-ie, iasis	disease of	cholelithiasis
-itis	inflammation of	hepatitis
-logy	study of	biology
-lysis	solution, breakdown	hydrolysis
-meter	instrument for measuring	calorimeter
-oid	like	lipoid
-oma	tumor, swelling	adenoma

Suffix	Meaning	Example	Suffix	Meaning	Example
-osis	disease of, state or condition	fluorosis	-phobia	fear of, antagonism	hydrophobia
-pathy	suffering, disease	osteopathy	-plasty	repair of	rhinoplasty
-phagia	swallowing, eating	hyperphagia	-rhea	to flow, discharge	steatorrhea
			-tomy	cut into	appendectomy

Appendix C

National Research Council recommended allowances

National Research Council recommended allowances

Recommended daily dietary allowances designed for the maintenance of good nutrition of practically all healthy persons in the U.S.A.

(Allowances are intended for persons normally active in a temperate climate.)*

	Persons			Food energy†	Protein	Calcium	Iron	Vitamin A	Thiamine	Riboflavin	Niacin equivalent	Ascorbic acid	Vitamin D
	Age in years§ From up to	Weight in pounds	Height in inches	Calories	Grams	Grams	Milligrams	International units	Milligrams	Milligrams	Milligrams	Milligrams	International units
Men	18 35	154	69	2,900	70	0.8	10	5,000	1.2	1.7	19	70	
	35 55	154	69	2,600	70	.8	10	5,000	1.0	1.6	17	70	
	55 75	154	69	2,200	70	.8	10	5,000	.9	1.3	15	70	

Women	18	35	128	64	2,100	58	.8	15	5,000	.8	1.3	14	70	400
	35	55	128	64	1,900	58	.8	15	5,000	.8	1.2	13	70	400
	55	75	128	64	1,600	58	.8	10	5,000	.8	1.2	13	70	400
Pregnant (second and third trimester)					+200	+20	+.5	+5	+1,000	+.2	+.3	+3	+30	+400
Lactating‖					+1,000	+40	+.5	+5	+3,000	+.4	+.6	+7	+30	+400
Infants‖	0		18		lb. x 52 ± 7	lb. x 1.1 ± 0.2	.7	lb. x 0.45	1,500	.4	.6	6	30	400
Children	1	3	29	34	1,300	32	.8	8	2,000	.5	.8	9	40	400
	3	6	40	42	1,600	40	.8	10	2,500	.6	1.0	11	50	400
	6	9	53	49	2,100	52	.8	12	3,500	.8	1.3	14	60	400
Boys	9	12	72	55	2,400	60	1.1	15	4,500	1.0	1.4	16	70	400
	12	15	98	61	3,000	75	1.4	15	5,000	1.2	1.8	20	80	400
	15	18	134	68	3,400	85	1.4	15	5,000	1.4	2.0	22	80	400
Girls	9	12	72	55	2,200	55	1.1	15	4,500	.9	1.3	15	80	400
	12	15	103	62	2,500	62	1.3	15	5,000	1.0	1.5	17	80	400
	15	18	117	64	2,300	58	1.3	15	5,000	.9	1.3	15	70	400

*Adapted from Recommended Dietary Allowances, Publication 1146, 59 pp., revised 1964. Published by National Academy of Sciences—National Research Council, Washington, D.C., 20418. Price $1.00. Also available in libraries. The allowance levels are intended to cover individual variations among most normal persons as they live in the United States under usual environmental stresses.

†Tables 1 and 2 and figures 1 and 2 in Publication 1146 show calorie adjustments for weight and age.

‡Niacin equivalents include dietary sources of the preformed vitamin and the precursor, tryptophan (60 milligrams tryptophan represents 1 milligram niacin).

§Entries on lines for age range 18 to 35 years represent the 25-year age. All other entries represent allowances for the midpoint of the specified age periods, i.e., line for children 1 to 3 is for age 2 years (24 months); 3 to 6 is for age 4½ years (54 months), etc.

‖The calorie and protein allowances per pound for infants are considered to decrease progressively from birth. Allowances for calcium, thiamine, riboflavin, and niacin increase proportionately with calories to the maximum values shown.

Note. The Recommended Daily Dietary Allowances should not be confused with Minimum Daily Requirements. The Recommended Dietary Allowances are amounts of nutrients recommended by the Food and Nutrition Board of National Research Council, and are considered adequate for maintenance of good nutrition in healthy persons in the United States. The allowances are revised from time to time in accordance with newer knowledge of nutritional needs. The Minimum Daily Requirements are the amounts of various nutrients that have been established by the Food and Drug Administration as standards for labeling purposes of foods and pharmaceutical preparations for special dietary uses. These are the amounts regarded as necessary in the diet for the prevention of deficiency diseases and generally are less than the Recommended Dietary Allowances. The Minimum Daily Requirements are set forth in the Federal Register, vol. 6, No. 227 (Nov. 22, 1941), beginning on p. 5921, and amended as stated in the Federal Register (June 1, 1957), vol. 22, No. 106, p. 3841.

Growth standards for children*

Height and weight of children aged 4-18 years

Ages (years)	Height (in inches)			Weight (in pounds)		
	5th P	50th P	95th P	5th P	50th P	95th P
		Boys 4-18 years				
4	38.3	40.8	43.3	30.0	36.1	42.2
5	40.3	43.4	46.4	33.0	40.3	47.6
6	42.8	45.9	49.0	36.0	44.7	53.4
7	44.8	48.1	51.4	40.3	50.9	61.5
8	46.9	50.5	54.1	44.4	57.4	70.4
9	48.8	52.8	56.8	48.0	64.4	80.4
10	50.6	54.9	59.2	51.4	71.4	91.4
11	51.9	56.4	60.9	53.3	78.9	102.5
12	53.5	58.6	63.7	60.0	86.0	113.5
13	55.2	61.3	67.4	65.3	98.6	131.9
14	57.5	64.1	70.7	75.5	111.8	148.1
15	61.0	66.9	72.8	88.0	124.3	160.6
16	63.8	68.9	74.0	97.8	133.8	169.8
17	65.2	69.8	74.4	106.5	139.8	174.0
18	65.9	70.2	74.5	110.3	144.8	179.3

*From Falkner, F.: Some physical growth standards for white North American children, Pediatrics **29**:448, 1962.
†P=percentile.

Height and weight of children aged 4-18 years—cont'd

Ages (years)	Height (in inches)			Weight (in pounds)		
	5th P	50th P	95th P	5th P	50th P	95th P
			Girls 4-18 years			
4	38.1	40.7	43.3	28.8	36.1	43.4
5	40.6	43.4	46.2	32.2	40.9	49.6
6	42.8	45.9	49.0	35.5	45.7	55.9
7	44.5	47.8	51.1	38.3	51.0	63.7
8	46.4	50.0	53.6	42.0	57.2	72.4
9	48.2	52.2	56.2	45.1	63.6	82.1
10	49.9	54.5	59.1	48.2	71.0	95.0
11	51.9	57.0	62.1	55.4	82.0	108.6
12	54.1	59.5	64.9	63.9	94.4	124.9
13	57.1	62.2	66.8	72.8	105.5	138.2
14	58.5	63.1	67.7	83.0	113.0	144.0
15	59.5	63.8	68.1	89.5	120.0	150.5
16	59.8	64.1	68.4	95.1	123.0	150.1
17	60.1	64.2	68.3	97.9	125.8	153.7
18	60.1	64.4	68.7	96.0	126.2	156.4

Annual height gains (in inches)			*Annual weight gains (in pounds)*		
Boys	Age (years)	Girls	Boys	Age (years)	Girls
2.8	4	2.8	4.4	4	4.4
2.6	5	2.7	4.5	5	4.4
2.5	6	2.5	4.8	6	4.4
2.4	7	2.25	5.5	7	5.3
2.4	8	2.3	6.4	8	6.4
2.3	9	2.3	7.0	9	7.6
2.1	10	2.4	7.0	10	9.4
1.7	11	2.5	6.8	11	10.6
1.6	11½	—	7.4	11½	—
1.9	12	3.1	8.4	12	12.6
2.6	13	2.3	—	12½	13.3
3.0	13½	—	11.8	13	13.2
3.2	14	1.4	—	13½	—
3.4	14½	—	15.0	14	8.6
3.1	15	0.6	15.4	14½	—
2.0	16	0.3	10.8	15	4.4
0.9	17	0.1	8.8	16	2.8
0.4	18	0.0	6.6	17	0.7
			4.4	18	0.0

Ideal weights for height for adults

Desirable weights for men of 25 and over*

Height with shoes on (1-inch heels)		Small frame	Medium frame	Large frame
Feet	Inches			
5	2	112–120	118–129	126–141
5	3	115–123	121–133	129–144
5	4	118–126	124–136	132–148
5	5	121–129	127–139	135–152
5	6	124–133	130–143	138–156
5	7	128–137	134–147	142–161
5	8	132–141	138–152	147–166
5	9	136–145	142–156	151–170
5	10	140–150	146–160	155–174
5	11	144–154	150–165	159–179
6	0	148–158	154–170	164–184
6	1	152–162	158–175	168–189
6	2	156–167	162–180	173–194
6	3	160–171	167–185	178–199
6	4	164–175	172–190	182–204

*Weight in pounds, according to frame (in indoor clothing).
(Courtesy Metropolitan Life Insurance Company, How to Control Your Weight, New York, 1960, supplement. Based on 1959 Body Build and Blood Pressure Study.)

Desirable weights for women of 25 and over*

Height with shoes on (2-inch heels)		Small frame	Medium frame	Large frame
Feet	Inches			
4	10	92–98	96–107	104–119
4	11	94–101	98–110	106–122
5	0	96–104	101–113	109–125
5	1	99–107	104–116	112–128
5	2	102–110	107–119	115–131
5	3	105–113	110–122	118–134
5	4	108–116	113–126	121–138
5	5	111–119	116–130	125–142
5	6	114–123	120–135	129–146
5	7	118–127	124–139	133–150
5	8	122–131	128–143	137–154
5	9	126–135	132–147	141–158
5	10	130–140	136–151	145–163
5	11	134–144	140–155	149–168
6	0	138–148	144–159	153–173

*Weight in pounds, according to frame (in indoor clothing).
(Courtesy Metropolitan Life Insurance Company, How to Control Your Weight, New York, 1960, supplement. Based on 1959 Body Build and Blood Pressure Study.)

Appendix F

Table of food composition

Table of food composition*†

Milk, cream, cheese; related products

Milk, cow's:

Food, approximate measure, and weight (in grams)		Water (%)	Food energy (cal.)‡	Pro-tein (gm.)	Fat (total lipid) (gm.)	Fatty acids			Carbo-hydrate (gm.)	Cal-cium (mg.)	Iron (mg.)	Vita-min A value (I.V.)	Thia-mine (mg.)	Ribo-flavin (mg.)	Niacin (mg.)	Ascor-bic acid (mg.)
						Satu-rated (total) (gm.)	Unsaturated									
							Oleic (gm.)	Linoleic (gm.)								
Fluid, whole (3.5% fat).	1 cup	87	160	9	9	5	3	Trace	12	288	0.1	350	0.08	0.42	0.1	2
Fluid, nonfat (skim)	1 cup	90	90	9	Trace	—	—	—	13	298	0.1	10	0.10	0.44	0.2	2
Buttermilk, cultured, from skim milk.	1 cup	90	90	9	Trace	—	—	—	13	298	0.1	10	0.09	0.44	0.2	2
Evaporated, un-sweetened, undiluted.	1 cup	74	345	18	20	11	7	1	24	635	0.3	820	0.10	0.84	0.5	3

Food	Measure	Weight (g)	Water (%)	Food energy (Cal.)	Protein (g)	Fat (g)	Saturated fat (g)	Oleic (g)	Linoleic (g)	Carbohydrate (g)	Calcium (mg)	Iron (mg)	Vitamin A (I.U.)	Thiamine (mg)	Riboflavin (mg)	Niacin (mg)	Ascorbic acid (mg)
Condensed, sweetened, undiluted.	1 cup	306	27	980	25	27	15	9	1	166	802	0.3	1,090	0.23	1.17	0.5	3
Dry, whole	1 cup	103	2	515	27	28	16	9	1	39	936	0.5	1,160	0.30	1.50	0.7	6
Dry, nonfat, instant	1 cup	70	3	250	25	Trace	—	—	—	36	905	0.4	20	0.24	1.25	0.6	5
Milk, goat's:																	
Fluid, whole	1 cup	244	88	165	8	10	6	2	Trace	11	315	0.2	390	0.10	0.27	0.7	2
Cream:																	
Half-and-half (cream and milk).	1 cup	242	80	325	8	28	16	9	1	11	261	0.1	1,160	0.08	0.38	0.1	2
	1 tablespoon	15	80	20	Trace	2	1	1	Trace	1	16	Trace	70	Trace	0.02	Trace	Trace
Light, coffee or table	1 cup	240	72	505	7	49	27	16	1	10	245	0.1	2,030	0.07	0.36	0.1	2
	1 tablespoon	15	72	30	Trace	3	2	1	Trace	1	15	Trace	130	Trace	0.02	Trace	Trace
Whipping, unwhipped (volume about double when whipped):																	
Light	1 cup	239	62	715	6	75	41	25	2	9	203	0.1	3,070	0.06	0.30	0.1	2
	1 tablespoon	15	62	45	Trace	5	3	2	Trace	1	13	Trace	190	Trace	0.02	Trace	Trace
Heavy	1 cup	238	57	840	5	89	49	29	3	7	178	0.1	3,670	0.05	0.26	0.1	2
	1 tablespoon	15	57	55	Trace	6	3	2	Trace	Trace	11	Trace	230	Trace	0.02	Trace	Trace
Cheese:																	
Blue or Roquefort type	1 ounce	28	40	105	6	9	5	3	Trace	1	89	0.1	350	0.01	0.17	0.1	0
Cheddar or American:																	
Ungrated	1 inch cube	17	37	70	4	5	3	2	Trace	Trace	128	0.2	220	Trace	0.08	Trace	0
Grated	1 cup	112	37	445	28	36	20	12	1	2	840	1.1	1,470	0.03	0.51	0.1	0
	1 tablespoon	7	37	30	2	2	1	1	Trace	Trace	52	0.1	90	Trace	0.03	Trace	0
Cheddar, process	1 ounce	28	40	105	7	9	5	3	Trace	1	219	0.3	350	Trace	0.12	Trace	0
Cheese foods, Cheddar	1 ounce	28	43	90	6	7	4	2	Trace	2	162	0.2	280	0.01	0.16	Trace	0
Cottage cheese, from skim milk:																	
Creamed	1 cup	225	78	240	31	9	5	3	Trace	7	212	0.7	380	0.07	0.56	0.2	0
	1 ounce	28	78	30	4	1	1	Trace	Trace	1	27	0.1	50	0.01	0.07	Trace	0
Uncreamed	1 cup	225	79	195	38	1	Trace	Trace	—	6	202	0.9	20	0.07	0.63	0.2	0
	1 ounce	28	79	25	5	Trace	Trace	Trace	—	1	26	0.1	Trace	0.01	0.08	Trace	0
Cream cheese	1 ounce	28	51	105	2	11	6	4	Trace	1	18	0.1	440	Trace	0.07	Trace	0
	1 tablespoon	15	51	55	1	6	3	2	Trace	Trace	9	Trace	230	Trace	0.04	Trace	0
Swiss (domestic)	1 ounce	28	39	105	8	8	4	3	Trace	1	262	0.3	320	Trace	0.11	Trace	0
Milk beverages:																	
Cocoa	1 cup	242	79	235	9	11	6	4	Trace	26	286	0.9	390	0.09	0.45	0.4	2
Chocolate-flavored milk drink (made with skim milk).	1 cup	250	83	190	8	6	3	2	Trace	27	270	0.4	210	0.09	0.41	0.2	2

*From Nutritive values of the edible part of foods, Home and Garden Bulletin No. 72, Washington, D. C., 1960, U. S. Department of Agriculture.

†Dashes show that no basis could be found for imputing a value although there was some reason to believe that a measurable amount of the constituent might be present.

‡Cal. = K calories

Table of food composition—cont'd

Food, approximate measure, and weight (in grams)		Water (%)	Food energy (cal.)	Protein (gm.)	Fat (total lipid) (gm.)	Fatty acids			Carbohydrate (gm.)	Calcium (mg.)	Iron (mg.)	Vitamin A value (I.V.)	Thiamine (mg.)	Riboflavin (mg.)	Niacin (mg.)	Ascorbic acid (mg.)
						Saturated (total) (gm.)	Unsaturated Oleic (gm.)	Unsaturated Linoleic (gm.)								
Malted milk	1 cup	78	280	13	12	—	—	—	32	364	0.8	670	0.17	0.56	0.2	2
Milk desserts:																
Cornstarch pudding, plain (blanc mange).	1 cup	76	275	9	10	5	3	Trace	39	290	0.1	390	0.07	0.40	0.1	2
Custard, baked	1 cup	77	285	13	14	6	5	1	28	278	1.0	870	0.10	0.47	0.2	1
Ice cream, plain, factory packed:																
Slice or cut brick, 1/8 of quart brick.	1 slice or cut brick.	62	145	3	9	5	3	Trace	15	87	0.1	370	0.03	0.13	0.1	1
Container	3½ fluid ounces.	62	130	2	8	4	3	Trace	13	76	0.1	320	0.03	0.12	0.1	1
Container	8 fluid ounces.	62	295	6	18	10	6	1	29	175	0.1	740	0.06	0.27	0.1	1
Ice milk	1 cup	67	285	9	10	6	3	Trace	42	292	0.2	390	0.09	0.41	0.2	2
Yoghurt, from partially skimmed milk.	1 cup	89	120	8	4	2	1	Trace	13	295	0.1	170	0.09	0.43	0.2	2
Eggs																
Eggs, large, 24 ounces per dozen:																
Raw:																
Whole, without shell	1 egg	74	80	6	6	2	3	Trace	Trace	27	1.1	590	0.05	0.15	Trace	0
White of egg	1 white	88	15	4	Trace	—	—	—	Trace	3	Trace	0	Trace	0.09	Trace	0
Yolk of egg	1 yolk	51	60	3	5	2	2	Trace	Trace	24	0.9	580	0.04	0.07	Trace	0
Cooked:																
Boiled, shell removed	2 eggs	74	160	13	12	4	5	1	1	54	2.3	1,180	0.09	0.28	0.1	0
Scrambled, with milk and fat.	1 egg	72	110	7	8	3	3	Trace	1	51	1.1	690	0.05	0.18	Trace	0
Meat, poultry, fish, shellfish; related products																
Bacon, broiled or fried, crisp.	2 slices	8	100	5	8	3	4	1	1	2	0.5	0	0.08	0.05	0.8	—

Note: the "weight (in grams)" column values are: Malted milk 270; Cornstarch pudding 248; Custard 248; Slice/cut brick 71; Container 3½ fl oz 62; Container 8 fl oz 142; Ice milk 187; Yoghurt 246; Whole egg 50; White of egg 33; Yolk of egg 17; Boiled eggs 100; Scrambled egg 64; Bacon 16.

Food	Measure															
Beef, trimmed to retail basis,* cooked:																	
Cuts braised, simmered, or pot-roasted:																	
Lean and fat	3 ounces	85	53	245	23	16	8	7	Trace	0	10	2.9	30	0.04	0.18	3.5	—
Lean only	2.5 ounces	72	62	140	22	5	2	2	Trace	0	10	2.7	10	0.04	0.16	3.3	—
Hamburger (ground beef), broiled:																	
Lean	3 ounces	85	60	185	23	10	5	4	Trace	0	10	3.0	20	0.08	0.20	5.1	—
Regular	3 ounces	85	54	245	21	17	8	8	Trace	0	9	2.7	30	0.07	0.18	4.6	—
Roast, oven-cooked, no liquid added:																	
Relatively fat, such as rib:																	
Lean and fat	3 ounces	85	40	375	17	34	16	15	1	0	8	2.2	70	0.05	0.13	3.1	—
Lean only	1.8 ounces	51	57	125	14	7	3	3	Trace	0	6	1.8	10	0.04	0.11	2.6	—
Relatively lean, such as heel of round:																	
Lean and fat	3 ounces	85	62	165	25	7	3	3	Trace	0	11	3.2	10	0.06	0.19	4.5	—
Lean only	2.7 ounces	78	65	125	24	3	1	1	Trace	0	10	3.0	Trace	0.06	0.18	4.3	—
Steak, broiled:																	
Relatively fat, such as sirloin:																	
Lean and fat	3 ounces	85	44	330	20	27	13	12	1	0	9	2.5	50	0.05	0.16	4.0	—
Lean only	2 ounces	56	59	115	18	4	2	2	Trace	0	7	2.2	10	0.05	0.14	3.6	—
Relatively lean, such as round:																	
Lean and fat	3 ounces	85	55	220	24	13	6	6	Trace	0	10	3.0	20	0.07	0.19	4.8	—
Lean only	2.4 ounces	68	61	130	21	4	2	2	Trace	0	9	2.5	10	0.06	0.16	4.1	—
Beef, canned:																	
Corned beef	3 ounces	85	59	185	22	10	5	4	Trace	0	17	3.7	20	0.01	0.20	2.9	—
Corned beef hash	3 ounces	85	67	155	7	10	5	4	Trace	9	11	1.7	—	0.01	0.08	1.8	—
Beef, dried or chipped	2 ounces	57	48	115	19	4	2	2	Trace	0	11	2.9	—	0.04	0.18	2.2	—
Beef and vegetable stew	1 cup	235	82	210	15	10	5	5	Trace	15	28	2.8	2,310	0.13	0.17	4.4	15
Beef potpie, baked: Individual pie, 4¾-inch diameter, weight before baking about 8 ounces.	1 pie	227	55	560	23	33	9	20	2	43	32	4.1	1,860	0.25	0.27	4.5	7
Chicken, cooked:																	
Flesh only, broiled	3 ounces	85	71	115	20	3	1	1	1	0	8	1.4	80	0.05	0.16	7.4	—
Breast, fried, ½ breast:																	
With bone	3.3 ounces	94	58	155	25	5	1	2	1	1	9	1.3	70	0.04	0.17	11.2	—
Flesh and skin only	2.7 ounces	76	58	155	25	5	1	2	1	1	9	1.3	70	0.04	0.17	11.2	—

*Outer layer of fat on the cut was removed to within approximately ½ inch of the lean. Deposits of fat within the cut were not removed.

Table of food composition—cont'd

Food, approximate measure, and weight (in grams)		Water (%)	Food energy (cal.)	Protein (gm.)	Fat (total lipid) (gm.)	Fatty acids Saturated (total) (gm.)	Unsaturated Oleic (gm.)	Unsaturated Linoleic (gm.)	Carbohydrate (gm.)	Calcium (mg.)	Iron (mg.)	Vitamin A value (I.V.)	Thiamine (mg.)	Riboflavin (mg.)	Niacin (mg.)	Ascorbic acid (mg.)
Drumstick, fried:																
With bone	2.1 ounces — 59	55	90	12	4	1	2	1	Trace	6	0.9	50	0.03	0.15	2.7	—
Flesh and skin only	1.3 ounces — 38	55	90	12	4	1	2	1	Trace	6	0.9	50	0.03	0.15	2.7	—
Chicken, canned, boneless	3 ounces — 85	65	170	18	10	3	4	2	0	18	1.3	200	0.03	0.11	3.7	3
Chicken potpie. See Poultry potpie.																
Chile con carne, canned:																
With beans	1 cup — 250	72	335	19	15	7	7	Trace	30	80	4.2	150	0.08	0.18	3.2	—
Without beans	1 cup — 255	67	510	26	38	18	17	1	15	97	3.6	380	0.05	0.31	5.6	—
Heart, beef, lean, braised	3 ounces — 85	61	160	27	5	—	—	—	1	5	5.0	20	0.21	1.04	6.5	1
Lamb, trimmed to retail basis,* cooked:																
Chop, thick, with bone, broiled.	1 chop, 4.8 ounces. — 137	47	400	25	33	18	12	1	0	10	1.5	—	0.14	0.25	5.6	—
Lean and fat	4.0 ounces[c] — 112	47	400	25	33	18	12	1	0	10	1.5	—	0.14	0.25	5.6	—
Lean only	2.6 ounces — 74	62	140	21	6	3	2	Trace	0	9	1.5	—	0.11	0.20	4.5	—
Leg, roasted:																
Lean and fat	3 ounces — 85	54	235	22	16	9	6	Trace	0	9	1.4	—	0.13	0.23	4.7	—
Lean only	2.5 ounces — 71	62	130	20	5	3	2	Trace	0	9	1.4	—	0.12	0.21	4.4	—
Shoulder, roasted:																
Lean and fat	3 ounces — 85	50	285	18	23	13	8	1	0	9	1.0	—	0.11	0.20	4.0	—
Lean only	2.3 ounces — 64	61	130	17	6	3	2	Trace	0	8	1.0	—	0.10	0.18	3.7	—
Liver, beef, fried	2 ounces — 57	57	130	15	6	—	—	—	3	6	5.0	30,280	0.15	2.37	9.4	15
Pork, cured, cooked:																
Ham, light cure, lean and fat, roasted.	3 ounces — 85	54	245	18	19	7	8	2	0	8	2.2	0	.40	.16	3.1	—
Luncheon meat:																
Boiled ham, sliced	2 ounces — 57	59	135	11	10	4	4	1	0	6	1.6	0	0.25	0.09	1.5	—
Canned, spiced or unspiced.	2 ounces — 57	55	165	8	14	5	6	1	1	5	1.2	0	0.18	0.12	1.6	—

Food	Measure																
Pork, fresh, trimmed to retail basis,* cooked:																	
Chop, thick, with bone	1 chop, 3.5 ounces	98	42	260	16	21	8	9	2	0	8	2.2	0	0.63	0.18	3.8	—
Lean and fat	2.3 ounces	66	42	260	16	21	8	9	2	0	8	2.2	0	0.63	0.18	3.8	—
Lean only	1.7 ounces	48	53	130	15	7	2	3	1	0	7	1.9	0	0.54	0.16	3.3	—
Roast, oven-cooked, no liquid added:																	
Lean and fat	3 ounces	85	46	310	21	24	9	10	2	0	9	2.7	0	0.78	0.22	4.7	—
Lean only	2.4 ounces	68	55	175	20	10	3	4	1	0	9	2.6	0	0.73	0.21	4.4	—
Cuts, simmered:																	
Lean and fat	3 ounces	85	46	320	20	26	9	11	2	0	8	2.5	0	0.46	0.21	4.1	—
Lean only	2.2 ounces	63	60	135	18	6	2	3	1	0	8	2.3	0	0.42	0.19	3.7	—
Poultry potpie (based on chicken potpie).	1 pie	227	57	535	23	31	10	15	3	42	68	3.0	3,020	0.25	0.26	4.1	5
Individual pie, 4¼-inch diameter, weight before baking about 8 ounces.																	
Sausage:																	
Bologna, slice, 4.1 by 0.1 inch.	8 slices	227	56	690	27	62	—	—	—	2	16	4.1	—	0.36	0.49	6.0	—
Frankfurter, cooked	1 frankfurter	51	58	155	6	14	—	—	—	1	3	0.8	—	0.08	0.10	1.3	—
Pork, links or patty, cooked.	4 ounces	113	35	540	21	50	18	21	5	Trace	8	2.7	0	0.89	0.39	4.2	—
Tongue, beef, braised	3 ounces	85	61	210	18	14	—	—	—	Trace	6	1.9	—	0.04	0.25	3.0	—
Turkey potpie. See Poultry potpie.																	
Veal, cooked:																	
Cutlet, without bone, broiled.	3 ounces	85	60	185	23	9	5	4	Trace	—	9	2.7	—	0.06	0.21	4.6	—
Roast, medium fat, medium done; lean and fat.	3 ounces	85	55	230	23	14	7	6	Trace	0	10	2.9	—	0.11	0.26	6.6	—
Fish and shellfish:																	
Bluefish, baked or broiled.	3 ounces	85	68	135	22	4	—	—	—	0	25	0.6	40	0.09	0.08	1.6	—
Clams:																	
Raw, meat only	3 ounces	85	82	65	11	1	—	—	—	2	59	5.2	90	0.08	0.15	1.1	—
Canned, solids and liquid.	3 ounces	85	86	45	7	1	—	—	—	2	47	3.5	—	0.01	0.09	0.9	8

*Outer layer of fat on the cut was removed to within approximately ½ inch of the lean. Deposits of fat within the cut were not removed.

Table of food composition—cont'd

Food, approximate measure, and weight (in grams)		Water (%)	Food energy (cal.)	Protein (gm.)	Fat (total lipid) (gm.)	Fatty acids			Carbohydrate (gm.)	Calcium (mg.)	Iron (mg.)	Vitamin A value (I.V.)	Thiamine (mg.)	Riboflavin (mg.)	Niacin (mg.)	Ascorbic acid (mg.)
						Saturated (total) (gm.)	Unsaturated Oleic (gm.)	Unsaturated Linoleic (gm.)								
Crabmeat, canned	3 ounces	85	77	85	15	2	—	—	—	1	38	0.7	—	0.07	0.07	1.6	—
Fish sticks, breaded, cooked, frozen; stick, 3.8 by 1.0 by 0.5 inch	10 sticks or 8-ounce package	227	66	400	38	20	5	4	10	15	25	0.9	—	0.09	0.16	3.6	—
Haddock, fried	3 ounces	85	66	140	17	5	1	3	Trace	5	34	1.0	—	0.03	0.06	2.7	2
Mackerel:																	
Broiled, Atlantic	3 ounces	85	62	200	19	13	—	—	—	0	5	1.0	450	0.13	0.23	6.5	—
Canned, Pacific, solids and liquid.*	3 ounces	85	66	155	18	9	—	—	—	0	221	1.9	20	0.02	0.28	7.4	—
Ocean perch, breaded (egg and bread-crumbs), fried.	3 ounces	85	59	195	16	11	—	—	—	6	28	1.1	—	0.08	0.09	1.5	—
Oysters, meat only: Raw, 13–19 medium selects.	1 cup	240	85	160	20	4	—	—	—	8	226	13.2	740	0.33	0.43	6.0	—
Oyster stew, 1 part oysters to 3 parts milk by volume, 3–4 oysters.	1 cup	230	84	200	11	12	—	—	—	11	269	3.3	640	0.13	0.41	1.6	—
Salmon, pink, canned	3 ounces	85	71	120	17	5	1	1	Trace	0	†167	0.7	60	0.03	0.16	6.8	—
Sardines, Atlantic, canned in oil, drained solids.	3 ounces	85	62	175	20	9	—	—	—	0	372	2.5	190	0.02	0.17	4.6	—
Shad, baked	3 ounces	85	64	170	20	10	—	—	—	0	20	0.5	20	0.11	0.22	7.3	—
Shrimp, canned, meat only.	3 ounces	85	70	100	21	1	—	—	—	1	98	2.6	50	0.01	0.03	1.5	—
Swordfish, broiled with butter or margarine.	3 ounces	85	65	150	24	5	—	—	—	0	23	1.1	1,750	0.03	0.04	9.3	—
Tuna, canned in oil, drained solids.	3 ounces	85	61	170	24	7	—	—	—	0	7	1.6	70	0.04	0.10	10.1	—

Mature dry beans and peas, nuts, peanuts; related products

Food	Measure																
Almonds, shelled	1 cup	142	5	850	26	77	6	52	15	28	332	6.7	0	0.34	1.31	5.0	Trace
Beans, dry:																	
Common varieties, such as Great Northern, navy, and others, canned:																	
Red	1 cup	256	76	230	15	1	—	—	—	42	74	4.6	Trace	0.13	0.10	1.5	—
White, with tomato sauce:																	
With pork	1 cup	261	71	320	16	7	3	3	1	50	141	4.7	340	0.20	0.08	1.5	5
Without pork	1 cup	261	68	310	16	1	—	—	—	60	177	5.2	160	0.18	0.09	1.5	5
Lima, cooked	1 cup	192	64	260	16	1	—	—	—	48	56	5.6	Trace	0.26	0.12	1.3	Trace
Brazil nuts	1 cup	140	5	915	20	94	19	45	24	15	260	4.8	Trace	1.34	0.17	2.2	—
Cashew nuts, roasted	1 cup	135	5	760	23	62	10	43	4	40	51	5.1	140	0.58	0.33	2.4	—
Coconut:																	
Fresh, shredded	1 cup	97	51	335	3	34	29	2	Trace	9	13	1.6	0	0.05	0.02	0.5	3
Dried, shredded, sweetened	1 cup	62	3	340	2	24	21	2	Trace	33	10	1.2	0	0.02	0.02	0.2	0
Cowpeas or black-eyed peas, dry, cooked	1 cup	248	80	190	13	1	—	—	—	34	42	3.2	20	0.41	0.11	1.1	Trace
Peanuts, roasted, salted:																	
Halves	1 cup	144	2	840	37	72	16	31	21	27	107	3.0	—	0.46	0.19	24.7	0
Chopped	1 tablespoon	9	2	55	2	4	1	2	1	2	7	0.2	—	0.03	0.01	1.5	0
Peanut butter	1 tablespoon	16	2	95	4	8	2	4	2	3	9	0.3	—	0.02	0.02	2.4	0
Peas, split, dry, cooked	1 cup	250	70	290	20	1	—	—	—	52	28	4.2	100	0.37	0.22	2.2	—
Pecans:																	
Halves	1 cup	108	3	740	10	77	5	48	15	16	79	2.6	140	0.93	0.14	1.0	2
Chopped	1 tablespoon	7.5	3	50	1	5	Trace	3	1	1	5	0.2	10	0.06	0.01	0.1	Trace
Walnuts, shelled:																	
Black or native, chopped.	1 cup	126	3	790	26	75	4	26	36	19	Trace	7.6	380	0.28	0.14	0.9	—
English or Persian:																	
Halves	1 cup	100	4	650	15	64	4	10	40	16	99	3.1	30	0.33	0.13	0.9	3
Chopped	1 tablespoon	8	4	50	1	5	Trace	1	3	1	8	0.2	Trace	0.03	0.01	0.1	Trace

*Vitamin values based on drained solids.

†Based on total contents of can. If bones are discarded, value will be greatly reduced.

Table of food composition—cont'd

Food, approximate measure, and weight (in grams)		Water (%)	Food energy (cal.)	Protein (gm.)	Fat (total lipid) (gm.)	Fatty acids			Carbohydrate (gm.)	Calcium (mg.)	Iron (mg.)	Vitamin A value (I.V.)	Thiamine (mg.)	Riboflavin (mg.)	Niacin (mg.)	Ascorbic acid (mg.)
						Saturated (total) (gm.)	Unsaturated Oleic (gm.)	Unsaturated Linoleic (gm.)								
Vegetables and vegetable products																
Asparagus:																
Cooked, cut spears	1 cup	175	94	35	4	Trace	—	—	—	6	37	1.0	1,580	0.27	0.32	2.4	46
Canned spears, medium:																
Green	6 spears	96	92	20	2	Trace	—	—	—	3	18	1.8	770	0.06	0.10	0.8	14
Bleached	6 spears	96	92	20	2	Trace	—	—	—	4	15	1.0	80	0.05	0.06	0.7	14
Beans:																
Lima, immature, cooked	1 cup	160	71	180	12	1	—	—	—	32	75	4.0	450	0.29	0.16	2.0	28
Snap, green:																
Cooked:																
In small amount of water, short time.	1 cup	125	92	30	2	Trace	—	—	—	7	62	0.8	680	0.08	0.11	0.6	16
In large amount of water, long time.	1 cup	125	92	30	2	Trace	—	—	—	7	62	0.8	680	0.07	0.10	0.4	13
Canned:																
Solids and liquid	1 cup	239	94	45	2	Trace	—	—	—	10	81	2.9	690	0.08	0.10	0.7	9
Strained or chopped (baby food).	1 ounce	28	92	5	Trace	Trace	—	—	—	1	9	0.3	110	0.01	0.02	0.1	Trace
Bean sprouts. *See* Sprouts.																
Beets, cooked, diced	1 cup	165	91	50	2	Trace	—	—	—	12	23	0.8	40	0.04	0.07	0.5	11
Broccoli spears, cooked	1 cup	150	91	40	5	Trace	—	—	—	7	132	1.2	3,750	0.14	0.29	1.2	135
Brussels sprouts, cooked	1 cup	130	88	45	5	1	—	—	—	8	42	1.4	680	0.10	0.18	1.1	113
Cabbage:																
Raw:																
Finely shredded	1 cup	100	92	25	1	Trace	—	—	—	5	49	0.4	130	0.05	0.05	0.3	47
Coleslaw	1 cup	120	83	120	1	9	2	2	5	9	52	0.5	180	0.06	0.06	0.3	35
Cooked:																
In small amount of water, short time.	1 cup	170	94	35	2	Trace	—	—	—	7	75	0.5	220	0.07	0.07	0.5	56

Food	Measure	Weight (g)	Water (%)	Food energy	Protein	Fat				Carbohydrate	Calcium	Iron	Vitamin A	Thiamine	Riboflavin	Niacin	Ascorbic acid
In large amount of water, long time.	1 cup	170	94	30	2	Trace	—	—	—	7	71	0.5	200	0.04	0.04	0.2	40
Cabbage, celery or Chinese: Raw, leaves and stalk, 1-inch pieces.	1 cup	100	95	15	1	Trace	—	—	—	3	43	0.6	150	0.05	0.04	0.6	25
Cabbage, spoon (or pakchoi), cooked.	1 cup	150	95	20	2	Trace	—	—	—	4	222	0.9	4,650	0.07	0.12	1.1	23
Carrots: Raw: Whole, 5½ by 1 inch, (25 thin strips).	1 carrot	50	88	20	1	Trace	—	—	—	5	18	0.4	5,500	0.03	0.03	0.3	4
Grated	1 cup	110	88	45	1	Trace	—	—	—	11	41	0.8	12,100	0.06	0.06	0.7	9
Cooked, diced	1 cup	145	91	45	1	Trace	—	—	—	10	48	0.9	15,220	0.08	0.07	0.7	9
Canned, strained or chopped (baby food).	1 ounce	28	92	10	Trace	Trace	—	—	—	2	7	0.1	3,690	0.01	0.01	0.1	1
Cauliflower, cooked, flowerbuds.	1 cup	120	93	25	3	Trace	—	—	—	5	25	0.8	70	0.11	0.10	0.7	66
Celery, raw: Stalk, large outer, 8 by about 1½ inches at root end.	1 stalk	40	94	5	Trace	Trace	—	—	—	2	16	0.1	100	0.01	0.01	0.1	4
Pieces, diced	1 cup	100	94	15	1	Trace	—	—	—	4	39	0.3	240	0.03	0.03	0.3	9
Collards, cooked	1 cup	190	91	55	5	1	—	—	—	9	289	1.1	10,260	0.27	0.37	2.4	87
Corn, sweet: Cooked, ear 5 by 1¾ inches.*	1 ear	140	74	70	3	1	—	—	—	16	2	0.5	310†	0.09	0.08	1.0	7
Canned, solids and liquid.	1 cup	256	81	170	5	2	—	—	—	40	10	1.0	690†	0.07	0.12	2.3	13
Cowpeas, cooked, immature seeds.	1 cup	160	72	175	13	1	—	—	—	29	38	3.4	560	0.49	0.18	2.3	28
Cucumbers, 10-ounce; 7½ by about 2 inches: Raw, pared	1 cucumber	207	96	30	1	Trace	—	—	—	7	35	0.6	Trace	0.07	0.09	0.4	23
Raw, pared, center slice ⅛-inch thick.	6 slices	50	96	5	Trace	Trace	—	—	—	2	8	0.2	Trace	0.02	0.02	0.1	6

*Measure and weight apply to entire vegetable or fruit, including parts not usually eaten.

†Based on yellow varieties; white varieties contain only a trace of cryptoxanthin and carotenes, the pigments in corn that have biological activity.

Table of food composition—cont'd

Food, approximate measure, and weight (in grams)	Water (%)	Food energy (cal.)	Protein (gm.)	Fat (total lipid) (gm.)	Fatty acids Saturated (total) (gm.)	Unsaturated Oleic (gm.)	Unsaturated Linoleic (gm.)	Carbohydrate (gm.)	Calcium (mg.)	Iron (mg.)	Vitamin A value (I.V.)	Thiamine (mg.)	Riboflavin (mg.)	Niacin (mg.)	Ascorbic acid (mg.)
Dandelion greens, cooked. 1 cup	180	90	60	4	1	—	—	—	12	252	3.2	21,060	0.24	0.29	—	32
Endive, curly (including escarole). 2 ounces	57	93	10	1	Trace	—	—	—	2	46	1.0	1,870	0.04	0.08	0.3	6
Kale, leaves including stems, cooked. 1 cup	110	91	30	4	1	—	—	—	4	147	1.3	8,140	—	—	—	68
Lettuce, raw:																
Butterhead, as Boston types; head, 4-inch diameter. 1 head	220	95	30	3	Trace	—	—	—	6	77	4.4	2,130	0.14	0.13	0.6	18
Crisphead, as iceberg; head, 4¾-inch diameter. 1 head	454	96	60	4	Trace	—	—	—	13	91	2.3	1,500	0.29	0.27	1.3	29
Looseleaf, or bunching varieties, leaves. 2 large	50	94	10	1	Trace	—	—	—	2	34	0.7	950	0.03	0.04	0.2	9
Mushrooms, canned, solids and liquid. 1 cup	244	93	40	5	Trace	—	—	—	6	15	1.2	Trace	0.04	0.60	4.8	4
Mustard greens, cooked 1 cup	140	93	35	3	1	—	—	—	6	193	2.5	8,120	0.11	0.19	0.9	68
Okra, cooked, pod 3 by ⅝ inch. 8 pods	85	91	25	2	Trace	—	—	—	5	78	0.4	420	0.11	0.15	0.8	17
Onions:																
Mature:																
Raw, onion 2½-inch diameter. 1 onion	110	89	40	2	Trace	—	—	—	10	30	0.6	40	0.04	0.04	0.2	11
Cooked 1 cup	210	92	60	3	Trace	—	—	—	14	50	0.8	80	0.06	0.06	0.4	14
Young green, small, without tops. 6 onions	50	88	20	1	Trace	—	—	—	5	20	0.3	Trace	0.02	0.02	0.2	12
Parsley, raw, chopped 1 tablespoon	3.5	85	1	Trace	Trace	—	—	—	Trace	7	0.2	300	Trace	0.01	Trace	6
Parsnips, cooked 1 cup	155	82	100	2	1	—	—	—	23	70	0.9	50	0.11	0.13	0.2	16
Peas, green:																
Cooked 1 cup	160	82	115	9	1	—	—	—	19	37	2.9	860	0.44	0.17	3.7	33
Canned, solids and liquid. 1 cup	249	83	165	9	1	—	—	—	31	50	4.2	1,120	0.23	0.13	2.2	22

Food	Measure																
Peppers, hot, red, without seeds, dried (ground chili powder, added seasonings).	1 tablespoon	15	8	50	2	2	—	—	—	8	40	2.3	9,750	0.03	0.17	1.3	2
Peppers, sweet: Raw, medium, about 6 per pound: Green pod without stem and seeds.	1 pod	62	93	15	1	Trace	—	—	—	3	6	0.4	260	0.05	0.05	0.3	79
Red pod without stem and seeds.	1 pod	60	91	20	1	Trace	—	—	—	4	8	0.4	2,670	0.05	0.05	0.3	122
Canned, pimientos, medium.	1 pod	38	92	10	Trace	Trace	—	—	—	2	3	0.6	870	0.01	0.02	0.1	36
Potatoes, medium (about 3 per pound raw): Baked, peeled after baking.	1 potato	99	75	90	3	Trace	—	—	—	21	9	0.7	Trace	0.10	0.04	1.7	20
Boiled: Peeled after boiling	1 potato	136	80	105	3	Trace	—	—	—	23	10	0.8	Trace	0.13	0.05	2.0	22
Peeled before boiling	1 potato	122	83	80	2	Trace	—	—	—	18	7	0.6	Trace	0.11	0.04	1.4	20
French-fried, piece 2 by ½ by ½ inch: Cooked in deep fat	10 pieces	57	45	155	2	7	2	2	4	20	9	0.7	Trace	0.07	0.04	1.8	12
Frozen, heated	10 pieces	57	53	125	2	5	1	1	2	19	5	1.0	Trace	0.08	0.01	1.5	12
Mashed: Milk added	1 cup	195	83	125	4	1	—	—	—	25	47	0.8	50	0.16	0.10	2.0	19
Milk and butter added.	1 cup	195	80	185	4	8	4	3	Trace	24	47	0.8	330	0.16	0.10	1.9	18
Potato chips, medium, 2-inch diameter.	10 chips	20	2	115	1	8	2	2	4	10	8	0.4	Trace	0.04	0.01	1.0	3
Pumpkin, canned	1 cup	228	90	75	2	1	—	—	—	18	57	0.9	14,590	0.07	0.12	1.3	12
Radishes, raw, small, without tops.	4 radishes	40	94	5	Trace	Trace	—	—	—	1	12.	0.4	Trace	0.01	0.01	0.1	10
Sauerkraut, canned, solids and liquid.	1 cup	235	93	45	2	Trace	—	—	—	9	85	1.2	120	0.07	0.09	0.4	33
Spinach: Cooked	1 cup	180	92	40	5	1	—	—	—	6	167	4.0	14,580	0.13	0.25	1.0	50
Canned, drained solids	1 cup	180	91	45	5	1	—	—	—	6	212	4.7	14,400	0.03	0.21	0.6	24
Canned, strained or chopped (baby food).	1 ounce	28	88	10	1	Trace	—	—	—	2	18	0.2	1,420	0.01	0.04	0.1	2

Table of food composition—cont'd

Food, approximate measure, and weight (in grams)	Water (%)	Food energy (cal.)	Protein (gm.)	Fat (total lipid) (gm.)	Fatty acids Saturated (total) (gm.)	Fatty acids Unsaturated Oleic (gm.)	Fatty acids Unsaturated Linoleic (gm.)	Carbohydrate (gm.)	Calcium (mg.)	Iron (mg.)	Vitamin A value (I.V.)	Thiamine (mg.)	Riboflavin (mg.)	Niacin (mg.)	Ascorbic acid (mg.)
Sprouts, raw:															
Mung bean 1 cup 90	89	30	3	Trace	—	—	—	6	17	1.2	20	0.12	0.12	0.7	17
Soybean 1 cup 107	89	40	6	2	—	—	—	4	46	0.7	90	0.17	0.16	0.8	4
Squash:															
Cooked:															
Summer, diced 1 cup 210	96	30	2	Trace	—	—	—	7	52	0.8	820	0.10	0.16	1.6	21
Winter, baked, mashed 1 cup 205	81	130	4	1	—	—	—	32	57	1.6	8,610	0.10	0.27	1.4	27
Canned, winter, strained and chopped (baby food). 1 ounce 28	92	10	Trace	Trace	—	—	—	2	7	0.1	510	0.01	0.01	0.1	1
Sweet potatoes:															
Cooked, medium, 5 by 2 inches, weight raw about 6 ounces:															
Baked, peeled after baking. 1 sweet potato 110	64	155	2	1	—	—	—	36	44	1.0	8,910	0.10	0.07	0.7	24
Boiled, peeled after boiling. 1 sweet potato 147	71	170	2	1	—	—	—	39	47	1.0	11,610	0.13	0.09	0.9	25
Candied, 3½ by 2¼ inches. 1 sweet potato 175	60	295	2	6	2	3	1	60	65	1.6	11,030	0.10	0.08	0.8	17
Canned, vacuum or solid pack. 1 cup 218	72	235	4	Trace	—	—	—	54	54	1.7	17,000	0.10	0.10	1.4	30
Tomatoes:															
Raw, medium, 2 by 2½ inches, about 3 per pound. 1 tomato 150	94	35	2	Trace	—	—	—	7	20	0.8	1,350	0.10	0.06	1.0	34*
Canned 1 cup 242	94	50	2	Trace	—	—	—	10	15	1.2	2,180	0.13	0.07	1.7	40
Tomato juice, canned 1 cup 242	94	45	2	Trace	—	—	—	10	17	2.2	1,940	0.13	0.07	1.8	39
Tomato catsup 1 tablespoon 17	69	15	Trace	Trace	—	—	—	4	4	0.1	240	0.02	0.01	0.3	3
Turnips, cooked, diced 1 cup 155	94	35	1	Trace	—	—	—	8	54	0.6	Trace	0.06	0.08	0.5	33

Turnip greens:																	
Cooked:																	
In small amount of water, short time.	1 cup	145	93	30	3	Trace	—	—	—	5	267	1.6	9,140	0.21	0.36	0.8	100
In large amount of water, long time.	1 cup	145	94	25	3	Trace	—	—	—	5	252	1.4	8,260	0.14	0.33	0.8	68
Canned, solids and liquid	1 cup	232	94	40	3	1	—	—	—	7	232	3.7	10,900	0.04	0.21	1.4	44
Fruits and fruit products																	
Apples, raw, medium, 2½-inch diameter, about 3 per pound.†	1 apple	150	85	70	Trace	Trace	—	—	—	18	8	0.4	50	0.04	0.02	0.1	3
Apple brown betty	1 cup	230	64	345	4	8	4	3	—	68	41	1.4	230	0.13	0.10	0.9	3
Apple juice, bottled or canned.	1 cup	249	88	120	Trace	Trace	—	—	Trace	30	15	1.5	—	0.01	0.04	0.2	2
Applesauce, canned:																	
Sweetened	1 cup	254	76	230	1	Trace	—	—	—	60	10	1.3	100	0.05	0.03	0.1	3
Unsweetened or artificially sweetened.	1 cup	239	88	100	Trace	Trace	—	—	—	26	10	1.2	100	0.04	0.02	0.1	2
Applesauce and apricots, canned, strained or junior (baby food).	1 ounce	28	77	25	Trace	Trace	—	—	—	6	1	0.1	170	Trace	Trace	Trace	1
Apricots:																	
Raw, about 12 per pound.†	3 apricots	114	85	55	1	Trace	—	—	—	14	18	0.5	2,890	0.03	0.04	0.7	10
Canned in heavy syrup:																	
Halves and syrup	1 cup	259	77	220	2	Trace	—	—	—	57	28	0.8	4,510	0.05	0.06	0.9	10
Halves (medium) and syrup.	4 halves; 2 tablespoons syrup.	122	77	105	1	Trace	—	—	—	27	13	0.4	2,120	0.02	0.03	0.4	5
Dried:																	
Uncooked, 40 halves, small.	1 cup	150	25	390	8	1	—	—	—	100	100	8.2	16,350	0.02	0.23	4.9	19
Cooked, unsweetened, fruit and liquid.	1 cup	285	76	240	5	1	—	—	—	62	63	5.1	8,550	0.01	0.13	2.8	8
Apricot nectar, canned	1 cup	250	85	140	1	Trace	—	—	—	36	22	0.5	2,380	0.02	0.02	0.5	7

*Year-round average. Samples marketed from November through May average around 15 milligrams per 150-gram tomato; from June through October, around 39 milligrams.

†Measure and weight apply to entire vegetable or fruit including parts not usually eaten.

Table of food composition—cont'd

Food, approximate measure, and weight (in grams)		weight (in grams)	Water (%)	Food energy (cal.)	Protein (gm.)	Fat (total lipid) (gm.)	Fatty acids			Carbohydrate (gm.)	Calcium (mg.)	Iron (mg.)	Vitamin A value (I.V.)	Thiamine (mg.)	Riboflavin (mg.)	Niacin (mg.)	Ascorbic acid (mg.)
							Saturated (total) (gm.)	Unsaturated Oleic (gm.)	Linoleic (gm.)								
Avocados, raw:																	
California varieties, mainly Fuerte:																	
10-ounce avocado, about 3⅓ by 4¼ inches, peeled, pitted.	½ avocado	108	74	185	2	18	4	8	2	6	11	0.6	310	0.12	0.21	1.7	15
½-inch cubes	1 cup	152	74	260	3	26	5	12	3	9	15	0.9	440	0.16	0.30	2.4	21
Florida varieties:																	
13-ounce avocado, about 4 by 3 inches, peeled, pitted.	½ avocado	123	78	160	2	14	3	6	2	11	12	0.7	360	0.13	0.24	2.0	17
½-inch cubes	1 cup	152	78	195	2	17	3	8	2	13	15	0.9	440	0.16	0.30	2.4	21
Bananas, raw, 6 by 1½ inches, about 3 per pound.*	1 banana	150	76	85	1	Trace	—	—	—	23	8	0.7	190	0.05	0.06	0.7	10
Blackberries, raw	1 cup	144	84	85	2	1	—	—	—	19	46	1.3	290	0.05	0.06	0.5	30
Blueberries, raw	1 cup	140	83	85	1	1	—	—	—	21	21	1.4	140	0.04	0.08	0.6	20
Cantaloupes, raw; medium, 5-inch diameter, about 1⅔ pounds.*	½ melon	385	91	60	1	Trace	—	—	—	14	27	0.8†	6,540	0.08	0.06	1.2	63
Cherries:																	
Raw, sweet, with stems*	1 cup	130	80	80	2	Trace	—	—	—	20	26	0.5	130	0.06	0.07	0.5	12
Canned, red, sour, pitted, heavy syrup.	1 cup	260	76	230	2	1	—	—	—	59	36	0.8	1,680	0.07	0.06	0.4	13
Cranberry juice cocktail, canned.	1 cup	250	83	160	Trace	Trace	—	—	—	41	12	0.8	Trace	0.02	0.02	0.1	‡
Cranberry sauce, sweetened, canned, strained.	1 cup	277	62	405	Trace	1	—	—	—	104	17	0.6	40	0.03	0.03	0.1	5
Dates, domestic, natural and dry, pitted, cut.	1 cup	178	22	490	4	1	—	—	—	130	105	5.3	90	0.16	0.17	3.9	0
Figs:																	
Raw, small, 1½-inch diameter, about 12 per pound.	3 figs	114	78	90	1	Trace	—	—	—	23	40	0.7	90	0.07	0.06	0.5	2

Food	Measure	Weight (g)	Water (%)	Food energy	Protein	Fat				Carbohydrate	Calcium	Iron	Vitamin A	Thiamine	Riboflavin	Niacin	Ascorbic acid
Fruit cocktail, canned in heavy syrup, solids and liquid.	1 cup	256	80	195	1	1	—	—	—	50	23	1.0	360	0.04	0.03	1.1	5
Grapefruit:																	
Raw, medium, 4¼-inch diameter, size 64:																	
White*	½ grapefruit	285	89	55	1	Trace	—	—	—	14	22	0.6	10	0.05	0.02	0.2	52
Pink or red*	½ grapefruit	285	89	60	1	Trace	—	—	—	15	23	0.6	640	0.05	0.02	0.3	52
Raw sections, white	1 cup	194	89	75	1	Trace	—	—	—	20	31	0.8	20	0.07	0.03	0.3	72
Canned, white:																	
Syrup pack, solids and liquid.	1 cup	249	81	175	1	Trace	—	—	—	44	32	0.7	20	0.07	0.04	0.5	75
Water pack, solids and liquid.	1 cup	240	91	70	1	Trace	—	—	—	18	31	0.7	20	0.07	0.04	0.5	72
Grapefruit juice:																	
Fresh	1 cup	246	90	95	1	Trace	—	—	—	23	22	0.5	§	.09	0.04	0.4	92
Canned, white:																	
Unsweetened	1 cup	247	89	100	1	Trace	—	—	—	24	20	1.0	20	0.07	0.04	0.4	84
Sweetened	1 cup	250	86	130	1	Trace	—	—	—	32	20	1.0	20	0.07	0.04	0.4	78
Frozen, concentrate, unsweetened:																	
Undiluted, can, 6 fluid ounces.	1 can	207	62	300	4	1	—	—	—	72	70	0.8	60	0.29	0.12	1.4	236
Diluted with 3 parts water, by volume.	1 cup	247	89	100	1	Trace	—	—	—	24	25	0.2	20	0.10	0.04	0.5	96
Frozen, concentrate, sweetened:																	
Undiluted, can, 6 fluid ounces.	1 can	211	57	350	3	1	—	—	—	85	59	0.6	50	0.24	0.11	1.2	245
Diluted with 3 parts water, by volume.	1 cup	249	88	115	1	Trace	—	—	—	28	20	0.2	20	0.08	0.03	0.4	82
Dehydrated:																	
Crystals, can, net weight 4 ounces.	1 can	114	1	430	5	1	—	—	—	103	99	1.1	90	0.41	0.18	2.0	399
Prepared with water (1 pound yields about 1 gallon).	1 cup	247	90	100	1	Trace	—	—	—	24	22	0.2	20	0.10	0.05	0.5	92

*Measure and weight apply to entire vegetable or fruit including parts not usually eaten.

†Value based on varieties with orange-colored flesh; for green-fleshed varieties value is about 540 I.U. per ½ melon.

‡About 5 milligrams per 8 fluid ounces is from cranberries. Ascorbic acid is usually added to approximately 100 milligrams per 8 fluid ounces.

§For white-fleshed varieties value is about 20 I.U. per cup; for red-fleshed varieties, 1,080 I.U. per cup.

Table of food composition—cont'd

Food, approximate measure, and weight (in grams)	Water (%)	Food energy (cal.)	Protein (gm.)	Fat (total lipid) (gm.)	Fatty acids Saturated (total) (gm.)	Unsaturated Oleic (gm.)	Unsaturated Linoleic (gm.)	Carbohydrate (gm.)	Calcium (mg.)	Iron (mg.)	Vitamin A value (I.V.)	Thiamine (mg.)	Riboflavin (mg.)	Niacin (mg.)	Ascorbic acid (mg.)
Grapes, raw:															
American type (slip skin), such as Concord, Delaware, Niagara, Catawba, and Scuppernong.* 1 cup	82	65	1	1	—	—	—	15	15	0.4	100	0.05	0.03	0.2	3
European type (adherent skin), such as Malaga, Muscat, Thompson Seedless, Emperor, and Flame Tokay.* 1 cup	81	95	1	Trace	—	—	—	25	17	0.6	140	0.07	0.04	0.4	6
Grape juice, bottled or canned. 1 cup	83	165	1	Trace	—	—	—	42	28	0.8	—	0.10	0.05	0.6	Trace
Lemons, raw, medium, 2½-inch diameter, size 150.* 1 lemon	90	20	1	Trace	—	—	—	6	18	0.4	10	0.03	0.01	0.1	38
Lemon juice:															
Fresh 1 cup	91	60	1	Trace	—	—	—	20	17	0.5	40	0.08	0.03	0.2	113
1 tablespoon	91	5	Trace	Trace	—	—	—	1	1	Trace	Trace	Trace	Trace	Trace	7
Canned, unsweetened 1 cup	92	55	1	Trace	—	—	—	19	17	0.5	40	0.07	0.03	0.2	102
Lemonade concentrate, frozen, sweetened:															
Undiluted, can, 6 fluid ounces. 1 can	48	430	Trace	Trace	—	—	—	112	9	0.4	40	0.05	0.06	0.7	66
Diluted with 4⅓ parts water, by volume. 1 cup	88	110	Trace	Trace	—	—	—	28	2	0.1	10	0.01	0.01	0.2	17
Lime juice:															
Fresh 1 cup	90	65	1	Trace	—	—	—	22	22	0.5	30	0.05	0.03	0.3	80
Canned 1 cup	90	65	1	Trace	—	—	—	22	22	0.5	30	0.05	0.03	0.3	52

Food	Measure	Weight (g)	Water (%)	Food energy	Protein	Fat			Carbohydrate	Calcium	Iron	Vitamin A	Thiamine	Riboflavin	Niacin	Ascorbic acid
Limeade concentrate, frozen, sweetened:																
Undiluted, can, 6 fluid ounces.	1 can	218	50	410	Trace	Trace	—	—	108	11	0.2	Trace	0.02	0.02	0.2	26
Diluted with 4⅓ parts water, by volume.	1 cup	248	90	105	Trace	Trace	—	—	27	2	Trace	Trace	Trace	Trace	Trace	6
Oranges, raw:																
California, navel (winter), 2⅘-inch diameter, size 88.*	1 orange	180	85	60	2	Trace	—	—	16	49	0.5	240	0.12	0.05	0.5	75
Florida, all varieties, 3-inch diameter.*	1 orange	210	86	75	1	Trace	—	—	19	67	0.3	310	0.16	0.06	0.6	70
Orange juice:																
Fresh:																
California, Valencia (summer).	1 cup	249	88	115	2	1	—	—	26	27	0.7	500	0.22	0.06	0.9	122
Florida varieties:																
Early and mid-season.	1 cup	247	90	100	1	Trace	—	—	23	25	0.5	490	0.22	0.06	0.9	127
Late season, Valencia.	1 cup	248	88	110	1	Trace	—	—	26	25	0.5	500	0.22	0.06	0.9	92
Canned, unsweetened	1 cup	249	87	120	2	Trace	—	—	28	25	1.0	500	0.17	0.05	0.6	100
Frozen concentrate:																
Undiluted, can, 6 fluid ounces.	1 can	210	58	330	5	Trace	—	—	80	69	0.8	1,490	0.63	0.10	2.4	332
Diluted with 3 parts water, by volume.	1 cup	248	88	110	2	Trace	—	—	27	22	0.2	500	0.21	0.03	0.8	112
Dehydrated:																
Crystals, can, net weight 4 ounces.	1 can	113	1	430	6	2	—	—	100	95	1.9	1,900	0.76	0.24	3.3	406
Prepared with water, 1 pound yields about 1 gallon.	1 cup	248	88	115	1	Trace	—	—	27	25	0.5	500	0.20	0.06	0.9	108
Orange and grapefruit juice:																
Frozen concentrate:																
Undiluted, can, 6 fluid ounces.	1 can	209	59	235	4	1	—	—	78	61	0.8	790	0.47	0.06	2.3	301
Diluted with 3 parts water, by volume.	1 cup	248	88	110	1	Trace	—	—	26	20	0.2	270	0.16	0.02	0.8	102

*Measure and weight apply to entire vegetable or fruit including parts not usually eaten.

Table of food composition—cont'd

Food, approximate measure, and weight (in grams)		Water (%)	Food energy (cal.)	Protein (gm.)	Fat (total lipid) (gm.)	Fatty acids			Carbohydrate (gm.)	Calcium (mg.)	Iron (mg.)	Vitamin A value (I.V.)	Thiamine (mg.)	Riboflavin (mg.)	Niacin (mg.)	Ascorbic acid (mg.)
						Saturated (total) (gm.)	Unsaturated Oleic (gm.)	Unsaturated Linoleic (gm.)								
Papayas, raw, ½-inch cubes.	1 cup	89	70	1	Trace	—	—	—	18	36	0.5	3,190	0.07	0.08	0.5	102
Peaches:																
Raw:																
Whole, medium, 2-inch diameter, about 4 per pound.*	1 peach	89	35	1	Trace	—	—	—	10	9	0.5	1,320†	0.02	0.05	1.0	7
Sliced	1 cup	89	65	1	Trace	—	—	—	16	15	0.8	2,230†	0.03	0.08	1.6	12
Canned, yellow-fleshed, solids and liquid:																
Syrup pack, heavy:																
Halves or slices	1 cup	79	200	1	Trace	—	—	—	52	10	0.8	1,100	.02	0.06	1.4	7
Halves (medium) and syrup.	2 halves and 2 tablespoons syrup.	79	90	Trace	Trace	—	—	—	24	5	0.4	500	.01	0.03	0.7	3
Water pack	1 cup	91	75	1	Trace	—	—	—	20	10	0.7	1,100	0.02	0.06	1.4	7
Strained or chopped (baby food).	1 ounce	78	25	Trace	Trace	—	—	—	6	2	0.1	140	Trace	0.01	0.2	1
Dried:																
Uncooked	1 cup	25	420	5	1	—	—	—	109	77	9.6	6,240	0.02	0.31	8.5	28
Cooked, unsweetened, 10-12 halves and 6 tablespoons liquid.	1 cup	77	220	3	1	—	—	—	58	41	5.1	3,290	0.01	0.15	4.2	6
Frozen:																
Carton, 12 ounces, not thawed.	1 carton	76	300	1	Trace	—	—	—	77	14	1.7	2,210	0.03	0.14	2.4	135‡
Can, 16 ounces, not thawed.	1 can	76	400	2	Trace	—	—	—	103	18	2.3	2,950	0.05	0.18	3.2	181‡
Peach nectar, canned	1 cup	87	120	Trace	Trace	—	—	—	31	10	0.5	1,080	0.02	0.05	1.0	1

Food	Measure																
Pears:																	
Raw, 3 by 2½-inch diameter.*	1 pear	182	83	100	1	1	—	—	—	25	13	0.5	30	0.04	0.07	0.2	7
Canned, solids and liquid: Syrup pack, heavy:																	
Halves or slices	1 cup	255	80	195	1	1	—	—	—	50	13	0.5	Trace	0.03	0.05	0.3	4
Halves (medium) and syrup.	2 halves and 2 tablespoons syrup.	117	80	90	Trace	Trace	—	—	—	23	6	0.2	Trace	0.01	0.02	0.2	2
Water pack	1 cup	243	91	80	Trace	Trace	—	—	—	20	12	0.5	Trace	0.02	0.05	0.3	4
Strained or chopped (baby food).	1 ounce	28	82	20	Trace	Trace	—	—	—	5	2	0.1	10	Trace	0.01	0.1	1
Pear nectar, canned	1 cup	250	86	130	1	Trace	—	—	—	33	8	0.2	Trace	0.01	0.05	Trace	1
Persimmons, Japanese or kaki, raw, seedless, 2½-inch diameter.*	1 persimmon	125	79	75	1	Trace	—	—	—	20	6	0.4	2,740	0.03	0.02	0.1	11
Pineapple:																	
Raw, diced	1 cup	140	85	75	1	Trace	—	—	—	19	24	0.7	100	0.12	0.04	0.3	24
Canned, heavy syrup pack, solids and liquid:																	
Crushed	1 cup	260	80	195	1	Trace	—	—	—	50	29	0.8	120	0.20	0.06	0.5	17
Sliced, slices and juice.	2 small or 1 large and 2 tablespoons juice.	122	80	90	Trace	Trace	—	—	—	24	13	0.4	50	0.09	0.03	0.2	8
Pineapple juice, canned	1 cup	249	86	135	1	Trace	—	—	—	34	37	0.7	120	0.12	0.04	0.5	22
Plums, all except prunes:																	
Raw, 2-inch diameter, about 2 ounces.*	1 plum	60	87	25	Trace	Trace	—	—	—	7	7	0.3	140	0.02	0.02	0.3	3
Canned, syrup pack (Italian prunes):																	
Plums (with pits) and juice.*	1 cup	256	77	205	1	Trace	—	—	—	53	22	2.2	2,970	0.05	0.05	0.9	4
Plums (without pits) and juice.	3 plums and 2 tablespoons juice.	122	77	100	Trace	Trace	—	—	—	26	11	1.1	1,470	0.03	0.02	0.5	2

*Measure and weight apply to entire vegetable or fruit including parts not usually eaten.

†Based on yellow-fleshed varieties; for white-fleshed varieties value is about 50 I.U. per 114-gram peach and 80 I.U. per cup of sliced peaches.

‡Average weighted in accordance with commercial freezing practices. For products without added ascorbic acid, value is about 37 milligrams per 12-ounce carton and 50 milligrams per 16-ounce can; for those with added ascorbic acid, 139 milligrams per 12 ounces and 186 milligrams per 16 ounces.

Table of food composition—cont'd

| Food, approximate measure, and weight (in grams) | | Water (%) | Food energy (cal.) | Protein (gm.) | Fat (total lipid) (gm.) | Fatty acids | | | Carbohydrate (gm.) | Calcium (mg.) | Iron (mg.) | Vitamin A value (I.V.) | Thiamine (mg.) | Riboflavin (mg.) | Niacin (mg.) | Ascorbic acid (mg.) |
| | | | | | | Saturated (total) (gm.) | Unsaturated | | | | | | | | | |
							Oleic (gm.)	Linoleic (gm.)								
Prunes, dried, "softened", medium:																
Uncooked*	4 prunes	28	70	1	Trace	—	—	—	18	14	1.1	440	0.02	0.04	0.4	1
Cooked, unsweetened, 17-18 prunes and ⅓ cup liquid.*	1 cup	66	295	2	1	—	—	—	78	60	4.5	1,860	0.08	0.18	1.7	2
Prunes with tapioca, canned, strained or junior (baby food).	1 ounce	77	25	Trace	Trace	—	—	—	6	2	0.3	110	0.01	0.02	0.1	1
Prune juice, canned	1 cup	80	200	1	Trace	—	—	—	49	36	10.5	—	0.02	0.03	1.1	4
Raisins, dried	1 cup	18	460	4	Trace	—	—	—	124	99	5.6	30	0.18	0.13	0.9	2
Raspberries, red:																
Raw	1 cup	84	70	1	1	—	—	—	17	27	1.1	160	0.04	0.11	1.1	31
Frozen, 10-ounce carton, not thawed.	1 carton	74	275	2	1	—	—	—	70	37	1.7	200	0.06	0.17	1.7	59
Rhubarb, cooked, sugar added.	1 cup	63	385	1	Trace	—	—	—	98	212	1.6	220	0.06	0.15	0.7	17
Strawberries:																
Raw, capped	1 cup	90	55	1	1	—	—	—	13	31	1.5	90	0.04	0.10	1.0	88
Frozen, 10-ounce carton, not thawed.	1 carton	71	310	1	1	—	—	—	79	40	2.0	90	0.06	0.17	1.5	150
Frozen, 16-ounce can, not thawed.	1 can	71	495	2	1	—	—	—	126	64	3.2	150	0.09	0.27	2.4	240
Tangerines, raw, medium, 2½-inch diameter, about 4 per pound.*	1 tangerine	87	40	1	Trace	—	—	—	10	34	0.3	350	0.05	0.02	0.1	26
Tangerine juice:																
Canned, unsweetened	1 cup	89	105	1	Trace	—	—	—	25	45	0.5	1,040	0.14	0.04	0.3	56
Frozen concentrate:																
Undiluted, can, 6 fluid ounces.	1 can	58	340	4	1	—	—	—	80	130	1.5	3,070	0.43	0.12	0.9	202
Diluted with 3 parts water, by volume.	1 cup	88	115	1	Trace	—	—	—	27	45	0.5	1,020	0.14	0.04	0.3	67
Watermelon, raw, wedge, 4 by 8 inch (1/16 of 10	1 wedge	93	115	2	1	—	—	—	27	30	2.1	2,510	0.13	0.13	0.7	30

Weight (in grams) values: Uncooked* 32; Cooked 270; Prunes with tapioca 28; Prune juice 256; Raisins 160; Raspberries Raw 123; Frozen 284; Rhubarb 272; Strawberries Raw 149; Frozen carton 284; Frozen can 454; Tangerines 114; Tangerine juice canned 248; Undiluted 210; Diluted 248; Watermelon 925.

Grain products

Food	Measure																
Barley, pearled, light, uncooked.	1 cup	203	11	710	17	2	Trace	1	2	160	32	4.1	0	0.25	0.17	6.3	0
Biscuits, baking powder with enriched flour, 2½-inch diameter.	1 biscuit	38	27	140	3	6	2	3	1	17	46	0.6	Trace	0.08	0.08	0.7	Trace
Bran flakes (40% bran) added thiamine.	1 ounce	28	3	85	3	1	—	—	—	23	20	1.2	0	0.11	0.05	1.7	0
Breads:																	
Boston brown bread, slice, 3 by ¾ inch.	1 slice	48	45	100	3	1	—	—	—	22	43	0.9	0	0.05	0.03	0.6	0
Cracked-wheat bread:																	
Loaf, 1-pound, 20 slices.	1 loaf	454	35	1,190	39	10	2	5	2	236	399	5.0	Trace	0.53	0.42	5.8	Trace
Slice	1 slice	23	35	60	2	1	—	—	—	12	20	0.3	Trace	0.03	0.02	0.3	Trace
French or vienna bread:																	
Enriched, 1-pound loaf.	1 loaf	454	31	1,315	41	14	3	8	2	251	195	10.0	Trace	1.26	0.98	11.3	Trace
Unenriched, 1-pound loaf.	1 loaf	454	31	1,315	41	11	3	8	2	251	195	3.2	Trace	0.39	0.39	3.6	Trace
Italian bread:																	
Enriched, 1-pound loaf.	1 loaf	454	32	1,250	41	4	Trace	1	2	256	77	10.0	0	1.31	0.93	11.7	0
Unenriched, 1-pound loaf.	1 loaf	454	32	1,250	41	4	Trace	1	2	256	77	3.2	0	0.39	0.27	3.6	0
Raisin bread:																	
Loaf, 1-pound, 20 slices.	1 loaf	454	35	1,190	30	13	3	8	2	243	322	5.9	Trace	0.24	0.42	3.0	Trace
Slice	1 slice	23	35	60	2	1	—	—	—	12	16	0.3	Trace	0.01	0.02	0.2	Trace
Rye bread:																	
American, light (⅓ rye, ⅔ wheat):																	
Loaf, 1-pound, 20 slices.	1 loaf	454	36	1,100	41	5	—	—	—	236	340	7.3	0	0.81	0.33	6.4	0
Slice	1 slice	23	36	55	2	Trace	—	—	—	12	17	0.4	0	0.04	0.02	0.3	0
Pumpernickel, loaf, 1 pound.	1 loaf	454	34	1,115	41	5	—	—	—	241	381	10.9	0	1.05	0.63	5.4	0

*Measure and weight apply to entire vegetable or fruit including parts not usually eaten.

Table of food composition—cont'd

Food, approximate measure, and weight (in grams)		Water (%)	Food energy (cal.)	Protein (gm.)	Fat (total lipid) (gm.)	Fatty acids			Carbohydrate (gm.)	Calcium (mg.)	Iron (mg.)	Vitamin A value (I.V.)	Thiamine (mg.)	Riboflavin (mg.)	Niacin (mg.)	Ascorbic acid (mg.)
						Saturated (total) (gm.)	Unsaturated Oleic (gm.)	Unsaturated Linoleic (gm.)								
White bread, enriched:																
1% to 2% nonfat dry milk:																
Loaf, 1-pound, 20 slices.	1 loaf	454	36	1,225	39	15	3	8	2	229	318	10.9	Trace	1.13	0.77	10.4	Trace
Slice	1 slice	23	36	60	2	1	Trace	Trace	Trace	12	16	0.6	Trace	0.06	0.04	0.5	Trace
3% to 4% nonfat dry milk:*																
Loaf, 1-pound	1 loaf	454	36	1,225	39	15	3	8	2	229	381	11.3	Trace	1.13	0.95	10.8	Trace
Slice, 20 per loaf	1 slice	23	36	60	2	1	Trace	Trace	Trace	12	19	0.6	Trace	0.06	0.05	0.6	Trace
Slice, toasted	1 slice	20	25	60	2	1	Trace	Trace	Trace	12	19	0.6	Trace	0.05	0.05	0.6	Trace
Slice, 26 per loaf	1 slice	17	36	45	1	1	Trace	Trace	Trace	9	14	0.4	Trace	0.04	0.04	0.4	Trace
5% to 6% nonfat dry milk:																
Loaf, 1-pound, 20 slices.	1 loaf	454	35	1,245	41	17	4	10	2	228	435	11.3	Trace	1.22	0.91	11.0	Trace
Slice	1 slice	23	35	65	2	1	Trace	Trace	Trace	12	22	0.6	Trace	0.06	0.05	0.6	Trace
White bread, unenriched:																
1% to 2% nonfat dry milk:																
Loaf, 1-pound, 20 slices.	1 loaf	454	36	1,225	39	15	3	8	2	229	318	3.2	Trace	0.40	0.36	5.6	Trace
Slice	1 slice	23	36	60	2	1	Trace	Trace	Trace	12	16	0.2	Trace	0.02	0.02	0.3	Trace
3% to 4% nonfat dry milk:*																
Loaf, 1-pound	1 loaf	454	36	1,225	39	15	3	8	2	229	381	3.2	Trace	0.31	0.39	5.0	Trace
Slice, 20 per loaf	1 slice	23	36	60	2	1	Trace	Trace	Trace	12	19	0.2	Trace	0.02	0.02	0.3	Trace
Slice, toasted	1 slice	20	25	60	2	1	Trace	Trace	Trace	12	19	0.2	Trace	0.01	0.02	0.3	Trace
Slice, 26 per loaf	1 slice	17	36	45	1	1	Trace	Trace	Trace	9	14	0.1	Trace	0.01	0.01	0.2	Trace
5% to 6% nonfat dry milk:																
Loaf, 1 pound, 20 slices.	1 loaf	454	35	1,245	41	17	4	10	2	228	435	3.2	Trace	0.32	0.59	4.1	Trace
Slice	1 slice	23	35	65	2	1	Trace	Trace	Trace	12	22	0.2	Trace	0.02	0.03	0.2	Trace

Food	Measure															
Whole-wheat bread, made with 2% nonfat dry milk:																
Loaf, 1-pound, 20 slices	1 loaf	454	36	1,105	48	14	3	6	3	216	449	10.4	Trace	1.17	0.56	12.9	Trace
Slice	1 slice	23	36	55	2	1	Trace	Trace	Trace	11	23	0.5	Trace	0.06	0.03	0.7	Trace
Slice, toasted	1 slice	19	24	55	2	1	Trace	Trace	Trace	11	22	0.5	Trace	0.05	0.03	0.6	Trace
Breadcrumbs, dry, grated	1 cup	88	6	345	11	4	1	2	1	65	107	3.2	Trace	0.19	0.26	3.1	Trace
Cakes:†																
Angelfood cake; sector, 2-inch (1/12 of 8-inch-diameter cake).	1 sector	40	32	110	3	Trace	—	—	—	24	4	0.1	0	Trace	0.06	0.1	0
Chocolate cake, chocolate icing; sector, 2-inch (1/16 of 10-inch-diameter layer cake).	1 sector	120	22	445	5	20	8	10	1	67	84	1.2	190*	0.03	0.12	0.3	Trace
Fruitcake, dark (made with enriched flour); piece, 2 by 2 by 1/2 inch.	1 piece	30	18	115	1	5	1	3	1	18	22	0.8	40‡	0.04	0.04	0.2	Trace
Gingerbread (made with enriched flour); piece, 2 by 2 by 2 inches.	1 piece	55	31	175	2	6	1	4	Trace	29	37	1.3	50	0.06	0.06	0.5	0
Plain cake and cupcakes, without icing:																
Piece, 3 by 2 by 1 1/2 inches.	1 piece	55	24	200	2	8	2	5	1	31	35	0.2	90‡	0.01	0.05	0.1	Trace
Cupcake, 2 3/4-inch diameter.	1 cupcake	40	24	145	2	6	1	3	Trace	22	26	0.2	70‡	0.01	0.03	0.1	Trace
Plain cake and cupcakes, with chocolate icing:																
Sector, 2-inch (1/16 of 10-inch-layer cake).	1 sector	100	21	370	4	14	5	7	1	59	63	0.6	180‡	0.02	0.09	0.2	Trace
Cupcake, 2 3/4-inch diameter.	1 cupcake	50	21	185	2	7	2	4	Trace	30	32	0.3	90‡	0.01	0.04	0.1	Trace

*When the amount of nonfat dry milk in commercial white bread is unknown, values for bread with 2% to 4% nonfat dry milk are suggested.

†Unenriched cake flour and vegetable cooking fat used unless otherwise specified.

‡If the fat used in the recipe is butter or fortified margarine, the vitamin A value for chocolate cake with icing will be 490 I. U. per 2-inch sector; 100 I. U. for fruitcake; for plain cake without icing, 300 I. U. per piece; 220 I. U. per cupcake; for plain cake with icing, 440 I. U. per 2-inch sector; 220 I. U. per cupcake; and 300 I. U. for pound cake.

Table of food composition—cont'd

Food, approximate measure, and weight (in grams)		Water (%)	Food energy (cal.)	Protein (gm.)	Fat (total lipid) (gm.)	Fatty acids			Carbo-hydrate (gm.)	Cal-cium (mg.)	Iron (mg.)	Vita-min A value (I.V.)	Thia-mine (mg.)	Ribo-flavin (mg.)	Niacin (mg.)	Ascor-bic acid (mg.)
						Satu-rated (total) (gm.)	Unsaturated Oleic (gm.)	Unsaturated Linoleic (gm.)								
Pound cake, old-fashioned (equal weights flour, sugar, fat, eggs); slice, 2¾ by 3 by ⅝ inch.	1 slice	30	17	140	2	9	2	5	1	14	6	0.2	80*	0.01	0.03	0.1	0
Sponge cake; sector, 2-inch (1/12 of 8-inch-diameter cake).	1 sector	40	32	120	3	2	1	1	Trace	22	12	0.5	180	0.02	0.06	0.1	Trace
Cookies:																	
Plain and assorted, 3-inch diameter.	1 cooky	25	3	120	1	5	—	—	—	18	9	0.2	20	0.01	0.01	0.1	Trace
Fig bars, small	1 fig bar	16	14	55	1	1	—	—	—	12	12	0.2	20	0.01	0.01	0.1	Trace
Corn, rice and wheat flakes, mixed, added nutrients.	1 ounce	28	3	110	2	Trace	—	—	—	24	11	0.5	0	0.11	—	0.9	0
Corn flakes, added nutrients:																	
Plain	1 ounce	28	4	110	2	Trace	—	—	—	24	5	0.4	0	0.12	0.02	0.6	0
Sugar-covered	1 ounce	28	2	110	1	Trace	—	—	—	26	3	0.3	0	0.12	0.01	0.5	0
Corn grits, degermed, cooked:																	
Enriched	1 cup	242	87	120	3	Trace	—	—	—	27	2	0.7†	150‡	0.10	0.07†	1.0†	0
Unenriched	1 cup	242	87	120	3	Trace	—	—	—	27	2	0.2	150‡	0.05	0.02	0.5	0
Cornmeal, white or yellow, dry:																	
Whole ground, unbolted	1 cup	118	12	420	11	5	1	2	2	87	24	2.8	600‡	0.45	0.13	2.4	0
Degermed, enriched	1 cup	145	12	525	11	2	Trace	1	1	114	9	4.2†	640‡	.64	0.38†	5.1†	0
Corn muffins, made with enriched degermed cornmeal and enriched flour; muffin, 2¾-inch diameter.	1 muffin	48	33	150	3	5	2	2	Trace	23	50	0.8	80§	.09	0.11	0.8	Trace

Food	Measure														
Corn, puffed, pre-sweetened, added nutrients.	1 ounce	28	5	110	1	Trace	—	—	26	3	0.5	0	0.12	0.05	0.6	0
Corn, shredded, added nutrients.	1 ounce	28	3	110	2	Trace	—	—	25	1	0.7	0	0.12	0.05	0.6	0
Crackers: Graham, plain	4 small or 2 medium.	14	6	55	1	1	—	—	10	6	0.2	0	0.01	0.03	0.2	0
Saltines, 2 inches square.	2 crackers	8	4	35	1	1	—	—	6	2	0.1	0	Trace	Trace	0.1	0
Soda: Cracker, 2½ inches square.	2 crackers	11	4	50	1	1	Trace	Trace	8	2	0.2	0	Trace	Trace	0.1	0
Oyster crackers	10 crackers	10	4	45	1	1	Trace	Trace	7	2	0.2	0	Trace	Trace	0.1	0
Cracker meal	1 tablespoon	10	6	45	1	1	Trace	Trace	7	2	0.1	0	0.01	0.01	0.1	0
Doughnuts, cake type	1 doughnut	32	24	125	1	6	6	1	16	13	0.4‖	30	0.05‖	0.05‖	0.4‖	Trace
Farina, regular, enriched, cooked.	1 cup	238	90	100	3	Trace	Trace	—	21	10	0.7†	0	0.11	0.07‡	1.0†	0
Macaroni, cooked: Enriched: Cooked, firm stage (8 to 10 minutes; undergoes additional cooking in a food mixture).	1 cup	130	64	190	6	1	1	—	39	14	1.4*	0	0.23*	0.14*	1.9*	0
Cooked until tender	1 cup	140	72	155	5	1	1	—	32	11	1.3*	0	0.19*	0.11*	1.5*	0
Unenriched: Cooked, firm stage (8 to 10 minutes; undergoes additional cooking in a food mixture).	1 cup	130	64	190	6	1	1	—	39	14	0.6	0	0.02	0.02	0.5	0
Cooked until tender	1 cup	140	72	155	5	1	1	—	32	11	0.6	0	0.02	0.02	0.4	0

*If the fat used in the recipe is butter or fortified margarine, the vitamin A value for chocolate cake with chocolate icing will be 490 I.U. per 2-inch sector; 100 I.U. for fruitcake; for plain cake without icing, 300 I.U. per piece; 220 I.U. per cupcake; for plain cake with icing, 440 I.U. per 2-inch sector; 220 I.U. per cupcake; and 300 I.U. for pound cake.

†Iron, thiamine, riboflavin, and niacin are based on the minimum levels of enrichment specified in standards of identity promulgated under the Federal Food, Drug, and Cosmetic Act.

‡Vitamin A value based on yellow product. White product contains only a trace.

§Based on recipe using white cornmeal; if yellow cornmeal is used, the vitamin A value is 140 I.U. per muffin.

‖Based on product made with enriched flour. With unenriched flour, approximate values per doughnut are: Iron, 0.2 milligram; thiamine, 0.01 milligram; riboflavin, 0.03 milligram; niacin, 0.2 milligram.

Table of food composition—cont'd

Food, approximate measure, and weight (in grams)			*Water (%)*	*Food energy (cal.)*	*Protein (gm.)*	*Fat (total lipid) (gm.)*	*Fatty acids: Saturated (total) (gm.)*	*Fatty acids: Unsaturated: Oleic (gm.)*	*Fatty acids: Unsaturated: Linoleic (gm.)*	*Carbohydrate (gm.)*	*Calcium (mg.)*	*Iron (mg.)*	*Vitamin A value (I.V.)*	*Thiamine (mg.)*	*Riboflavin (mg.)*	*Niacin (mg.)*	*Ascorbic acid (mg.)*
Marcaroni (enriched) and cheese, baked.	1 cup	220	58	470	18	24	11	10	1	44	398	2.0	950	0.22	0.44	2.0	Trace
Muffins, with enriched white flour; muffin, 2¾-inch diameter.	1 muffin	48	38	140	4	5	1	3	Trace	20	50	0.8	50	0.08	0.11	0.7	Trace
Noodles (egg noodles), cooked:																	
Enriched	1 cup	160	70	200	7	2	1	1	Trace	37	16	1.4*	110	0.23*	0.14*	1.8*	0
Unenriched	1 cup	160	70	200	7	2	1	1	Trace	37	16	1.0	110	0.04	0.03	0.7	0
Oats (with or without corn) puffed, added nutrients.	1 ounce	28	3	115	3	2	Trace	1	1	21	50	1.3	0	0.28	0.05	0.5	0
Oatmeal or rolled oats, regular or quick-cooking, cooked.	1 cup	236	86	130	5	2	Trace	1	1	23	21	1.4	0	0.19	0.05	0.3	0
Pancakes (griddlecakes), 4-inch diameter:																	
Wheat, enriched flour (home recipe).	1 cake	27	50	60	2	2	Trace	1	Trace	9	27	0.4	30	0.05	0.06	0.3	Trace
Buckwheat (buckwheat pancake mix, made with egg and milk).	1 cake	27	58	55	2	2	1	1	Trace	6	59	0.4	60	0.03	.04	0.2	Trace
Piecrust, plain, baked:																	
Enriched flour:																	
Lower crust, 9-inch shell.	1 crust	135	15	675	8	45	10	29	3	59	19	2.3	0	0.27	.19	2.4	0
Double crust, 9-inch pie.	1 double crust	270	15	1,350	16	90	21	58	7	118	38	4.6	0	0.55	.39	4.9	0
Unenriched flour:																	
Lower crust, 9-inch shell.	1 crust	135	15	675	8	45	10	29	3	59	19	0.7	0	0.04	.04	0.6	0

Food	Measure																
Double crust, 9-inch pie.	1 double crust	270	15	1,350	16	90	21	58	7	118	38	1.4	0	0.08	.07	1.3	0
Pies (piecrust made with unenriched flour); sector, 4-inch, 1/7 of 9-inch-diameter pie:																	
Apple	1 sector	135	48	345	3	15	4	9	1	51	11	0.4	40	0.03	.02	0.5	1
Cherry	1 sector	135	47	355	4	15	4	10	1	52	19	0.4	590	0.03	.03	0.6	1
Custard	1 sector	130	58	280	8	14	5	8	1	30	125	0.8	300	0.07	.21	0.4	0
Lemon meringue	1 sector	120	47	305	4	12	4	7	1	45	17	0.6	200	0.04	.10	0.2	4
Mince	1 sector	135	43	365	3	16	4	10	1	56	38	1.4	Trace	0.09	.05	0.5	1
Pumpkin	1 sector	130	59	275	5	15	5	7	1	32	66	0.6	3,210	0.0004	.13	0.6	Trace
Pizza (cheese); 5½-inch sector; 1/8 of 14-inch-diameter pie.	1 sector	75	45	185	7	6	2	3	Trace	27	107	0.7	290	0.04	.12	0.7	Trace
Popcorn, popped, with added oil and salt.	1 cup	14	3	65	1	3	2	Trace	Trace	8	1	0.3	—	—	.01	0.2	0
Pretzels, small stick	5 sticks	5	8	20	Trace	Trace	—	—	—	4	1	0	0	Trace	Trace	Trace	0
Rice, white (fully milled or polished), enriched, cooked:																	
Common commercial varieties, all types.	1 cup	168	73	185	3	Trace	—	—	—	41	17	1.5†	0	0.19†	0.01†	1.6†	0
Long grain, parboiled	1 cup	176	73	185	4	Trace	—	—	—	41	33	1.4†	0	0.19†	0.02†	2.0†	0
Rice, puffed, added nutrients (without salt).	1 cup	14	4	55	1	Trace	—	—	—	13	3	0.3	0	0.06	0.01	0.6	0
Rice flakes, added nutrients.	1 cup	30	3	115	2	Trace	—	—	—	26	9	0.5	0	0.10	0.02	1.6	0
Rolls:																	
Plain, pan; 12 per 16 ounces:																	
Enriched	1 roll	38	31	115	3	2	1	1	Trace	20	28	0.7	Trace	0.11	0.07	0.8	Trace
Unenriched	1 roll	38	31	115	3	2	1	1	Trace	20	28	0.3	Trace	0.02	0.03	0.3	Trace
Hard, round; 12 per 22 ounces.	1 roll	52	25	160	5	2	1	1	Trace	31	24	0.4	Trace	0.03	0.05	0.4	Trace
Sweet, pan; 12 per 18 ounces.	1 roll	43	32	135	4	4	1	2	Trace	21	37	0.3	30	0.03	0.06	0.4	Trace
Rye wafers, whole-grain, 1⅞ by 3½ inches.	2 wafers	13	6	45	2	Trace	—	—	—	10	7	0.5	0	0.04	0.03	0.2	0

*Iron, thiamine, riboflavin, and niacin are based on the minimum levels of enrichment specified in standards of identity promulgated under the Federal Food, Drug, and Cosmetic Act.
†Iron, thiamine, and niacin are based on the minimum levels of enrichment specified in standards of identity promulgated under the Federal Food, Drug, and Cosmetic Act. Riboflavin is based on unenriched rice. When the minimum level of enrichment for riboflavin specified in the standards of identity becomes effective the value will be 0.12 milligram per cup of parboiled rice and of white rice.

Table of food composition—cont'd

| Food, approximate measure, and weight (in grams) | | Water (%) | Food energy (cal.) | Protein (gm.) | Fat (total lipid) (gm.) | Fatty acids | | | Carbohydrate (gm.) | Calcium (mg.) | Iron (mg.) | Vitamin A value (I.V.) | Thiamine (mg.) | Riboflavin (mg.) | Niacin (mg.) | Ascorbic acid (mg.) |
						Saturated (total) (gm.)	Unsaturated Oleic (gm.)	Unsaturated Linoleic (gm.)								
Spaghetti:																
Cooked, tender stage (14 to 20 minutes):																
Enriched	1 cup	72	155	5	1	—	—	—	32	11	1.3*	0	0.19*	0.11*	1.5*	0
Unenriched	1 cup	72	155	5	1	—	—	—	32	11	.6	0	0.02	0.02	0.4	0
Spaghetti with meat balls in tomato sauce (home recipe)	1 cup	70	335	19	12	4	6	1	39	125	3.8	1,600	0.26	0.30	4.0	22
Spaghetti in tomato sauce with cheese (home recipe)	1 cup	77	260	9	9	2	5	1	37	80	2.2	1,080	0.24	0.18	2.4	14
Waffles, with enriched flour, ½ by 4½ by 5½ inches	1 waffle	41	210	7	7	2	4	1	28	85	1.3	250	0.13	0.19	1.0	Trace
Wheat, puffed:																
With added nutrients (without salt)	1 ounce	3	105	4	Trace	—	—	—	22	8	1.2	0	0.15	0.07	2.2	0
With added nutrients, with sugar and honey	1 ounce	3	105	2	1	—	—	—	25	7	0.9	0	0.14	0.05	1.8	0
Wheat, rolled; cooked	1 cup	80	175	5	1	—	—	—	40	19	1.7	0	0.17	0.06	2.1	0
Wheat, shredded, plain (long, round, or bite-size)	1 ounce	7	100	3	1	—	—	—	23	12	1.0	0	0.06	0.03	1.2	0
Wheat and malted barley flakes, with added nutrients	1 ounce	3	110	2	Trace	—	—	—	24	14	0.7	0	0.13	0.03	1.1	0
Wheat flakes, with added nutrients	1 ounce	4	100	3	Trace	—	—	—	23	12	1.2	0	0.18	0.04	1.4	0
Wheat flours:																
Whole-wheat, from hard wheats, stirred	1 cup	12	400	16	2	Trace	1	1	85	49	4.0	0	0.66	0.14	5.2	0

Food	Measure																
All-purpose or family flour:																	
Enriched, sifted	1 cup	110	12	400	12	1	Trace	Trace	Trace	84	18	3.2*	0	0.48	0.29*	3.8*	0
Unenriched, sifted	1 cup	110	12	400	12	1	Trace	Trace	Trace	84	18	0.9	0	0.07	0.05	1.0	0
Self-rising, enriched	1 cup	110	11	385	10	1	Trace	Trace	Trace	82	292	3.2*	0	0.49*	0.29*	3.9*	0
Cake or pastry flour, sifted.	1 cup	100	12	365	8	1	Trace	Trace	Trace	79	17	0.5	0	0.03	0.03	0.7	0
Wheat germ, crude, commercially milled.	1 cup	68	11	245	18	7	1	2	4	32	49	6.4	0	1.36	.46	2.9	0
Fats, oils																	
Butter, 4 sticks per pound:																	
Sticks, 2	1 cup	227	16	1,625	1	184	101	61	6	1	45	0	7,500†	—	—	—	0
Stick, ⅛	1 tablespoon	14	16	100	Trace	11	6	4	Trace	Trace	3	0	460†	—	—	—	0
Pat or square (64 per pound).	1 pat	7	16	50	Trace	6	3	2	Trace	Trace	1	0	230†	—	—	—	0
Fats, cooking:																	
Lard	1 cup	220	0	1,985	0	220	84	101	22	0	0	0	0	0	0	0	0
Lard	1 tablespoon	14	0	125	0	14	5	6	1	0	0	0	0	0	0	0	0
Vegetable fats	1 cup	200	0	1,770	0	200	46	130	14	0	0	0	—	0	0	0	0
Vegetable fats	1 tablespoon	12.5	0	110	0	12	3	8	1	0	0	0	—	0	0	0	0
Margarine, 4 sticks per pound:																	
Sticks, 2	1 cup	227	16	1,635	1	184	37	105	33	1	45	0	7,500‡	0	0	0	0
Sticks, ⅛	1 tablespoon	14	16	100	Trace	11	2	6	2	Trace	3	0	460‡	0	0	0	0
Pat or square (64 per pound).	1 pat	7	16	50	Trace	6	1	3	1	Trace	1	0	230‡	0	0	0	0
Oils, salad or cooking:																	
Corn	1 tablespoon	14	0	125	0	14	1	4	7	0	0	0	—	0	0	0	0
Cottonseed	1 tablespoon	14	0	125	0	14	4	3	7	0	0	0	—	0	0	0	0
Olive	1 tablespoon	14	0	125	0	14	2	11	1	0	0	0	—	0	0	0	0
Soybean	1 tablespoon	14	0	125	0	14	2	3	7	0	0	0	—	0	0	0	0
Salad dressings:																	
Blue cheese	1 tablespoon	16	32	80	1	8	2	2	4	1	13	Trace	30	Trace	0.02	Trace	Trace
Commercial, mayonnaise type.	1 tablespoon	15	41	65	Trace	6	1	1	3	2	2	Trace	30	Trace	Trace	Trace	—

*Iron, thiamine, riboflavin, and niacin are based on the minimum levels of enrichment specified in standards of identity promulgated under the Federal Food, Drug, and Cosmetic Act.

†Year-round average.

‡Based on the average vitamin A content of fortified margarine. Federal specifications for fortified margarine require a minimum of 15,000 I.U. of vitamin A per pound.

Table of food composition—cont'd

Food, approximate measure, and weight (in grams)		Water (%)	Food energy (cal.)	Protein (gm.)	Fat (total lipid) (gm.)	Fatty acids Saturated (total) (gm.)	Fatty acids Unsaturated Oleic (gm.)	Fatty acids Unsaturated Linoleic (gm.)	Carbohydrate (gm.)	Calcium (mg.)	Iron (mg.)	Vitamin A value (I.V.)	Thiamine (mg.)	Riboflavin (mg.)	Niacin (mg.)	Ascorbic acid (mg.)
French	1 tablespoon	15	39	60	Trace	6	1	1	3	3	2	0.1	—	—	—	—	—
Home cooked, boiled	1 tablespoon	17	68	30	1	2	1	1	Trace	3	15	0.1	80	0.01	0.03	Trace	Trace
Mayonnaise	1 tablespoon	15	15	110	Trace	12	2	3	6	Trace	3	0.1	40	Trace	0.01	Trace	—
Thousand island	1 tablespoon	15	32	75	Trace	8	1	2	4	2	2	0.1	50	Trace	Trace	Trace	Trace
Sugars, sweets																
Candy:																
Carmels	1 ounce	28	8	115	1	3	2	1	Trace	22	42	0.4	Trace	0.01	0.05	Trace	Trace
Chocolate, milk, plain	1 ounce	28	1	150	2	9	5	3	Trace	16	65	0.3	80	0.02	0.09	0.1	Trace
Fudge, plain	1 ounce	28	8	115	1	3	2	1	Trace	21	22	0.3	Trace	0.01	0.03	0.1	Trace
Hard candy	1 ounce	28	1	110	0	Trace	—	—	—	28	6	0.5	0	0	0	0	0
Marshmallows	1 ounce	28	17	90	1	Trace	—	Trace	—	23	5	0.5	0	0	Trace	Trace	0
Chocolate syrup, thin type	1 tablespoon	20	32	50	Trace	Trace	Trace	Trace	Trace	13	3	0.3	—	Trace	0.01	0.1	0
Honey, strained or extracted.	1 tablespoon	21	17	65	Trace	0	—	—	—	17	1	0.1	0	Trace	0.01	0.1	Trace
Jams and preserves	1 tablespoon	20	29	55	Trace	Trace	—	—	—	14	4	0.2	Trace	Trace	0.01	Trace	Trace
Jellies	1 tablespoon	20	29	55	Trace	Trace	—	—	—	14	4	0.3	Trace	Trace	0.01	Trace	1
Molasses, cane:																
Light (first extraction)	1 tablespoon	20	24	50	—	—	—	—	—	13	33	0.9	—	0.01	0.01	Trace	—
Blackstrap (third extraction).	1 tablespoon	20	24	45	—	—	—	—	—	11	137	3.2	—	0.02	0.04	0.4	—
Syrup, table blends (chiefly corn, light and dark).	1 tablespoon	20	24	60	0	0	—	—	—	15	9	0.8	0	0	0	0	0
Sugars (cane or beet):																
Granulated	1 cup	200	Trace	770	0	0	—	—	—	199	0	0.2	0	0	0	0	0
	1 tablespoon	12	Trace	45	0	0	—	—	—	12	0	Trace	0	0	0	0	0
Lump, 1⅛ by ¾ by ⅜	1 lump	6	Trace	25	0	0	—	—	—	6	0	Trace	0	0	0	0	0

Food	Measure	Grams	Water (%)	Food energy (cal.)	Protein (g)	Fat (g)	Saturated (total) (g)	Unsat. Oleic (g)	Unsat. Linoleic (g)	Carbohydrate (g)	Calcium (mg)	Iron (mg)	Vitamin A (I.U.)	Thiamine (mg)	Riboflavin (mg)	Niacin (mg)	Ascorbic acid (mg)
Powdered, stirred before measuring.	1 cup	128	Trace	495	0	0	—	—	—	127	0	0	0	0	0	0	0
	1 tablespoon	8	Trace	30	0	0	—	—	—	8	0	Trace	0	0	0	0	0
Brown, firm-packed	1 cup	220	2	820	0	0	—	—	—	212	187	7.5	0	0.02	0.07	0.4	0
	1 tablespoon	14	2	50	0	0	—	—	—	13	12	0.5	0	Trace	Trace	Trace	0
Miscellaneous items																	
Beer (average 3.6 percent alcohol by weight).	1 cup	240	92	100	1	0	—	—	—	9	12	Trace	—	0.01	0.07	1.6	—
Beverages, carbonated:																	
Cola type	1 cup	240	90	95	0	0	—	—	—	24	—	—	0	0	0	0	0
Ginger ale	1 cup	230	92	70	0	0	—	—	—	18	—	—	0	0	0	0	0
Bouillon cube, ⅝ inch	1 cube	4	4	5	1	Trace	—	—	—	Trace	—	—	—	—	—	—	—
Chili powder. *See* Vegetables, peppers.																	
Chili sauce (mainly tomatoes).	1 tablespoon	17	68	20	Trace	Trace	—	—	—	4	3	0.1	240	0.02	0.01	0.3	3
Chocolate:																	
Bitter or baking	1 ounce	28	2	145	3	15	8	6	Trace	8	22	1.9	20	0.01	0.07	0.4	0
Sweet	1 ounce	28	1	150	1	10	6	4	Trace	16	27	0.4	Trace	0.01	0.04	0.1	Trace
Cider. *See* Fruits, apple juice.																	
Gelatin, dry:																	
Plain	1 tablespoon	10	13	35	9	Trace	—	—	—	0	—	—	—	—	—	—	—
Dessert powder, 3-ounce package.	½ cup	85	2	315	8	0	—	—	—	75	—	—	—	—	—	—	—
Gelatin dessert, ready-to-eat:																	
Plain	1 cup	239	84	140	4	0	—	—	—	34	—	—	—	—	—	—	—
With fruit	1 cup	241	82	160	3	Trace	—	—	—	40	—	—	—	—	—	—	—
Olives, pickled:																	
Green	4 medium or 3 extra large or 2 giant.	16	78	15	Trace	2	Trace	2	Trace	Trace	8	0.2	40	—	—	—	—
Ripe: Mission	3 small or 2 large.	10	73	15	Trace	2	Trace	2	Trace	Trace	9	0.1	10	Trace	Trace	—	—
Pickles, cucumber:																	
Dill, large, 4 by 1¾ inches	1 pickle	135	93	15	1	Trace	—	—	—	3	35	1.4	140	Trace	0.03	Trace	8
Sweet, 2¾ by ¾ inches	1 pickle	20	61	30	Trace	Trace	—	—	—	7	2	0.2	20	Trace	Trace	Trace	1
Popcorn. *See* Grain products.																	
Sherbet, orange	1 cup	193	67	260	2	2	2	Trace	Trace	59	31	Trace	110	0.02	0.06	Trace	4

Table of food composition—cont'd

Food, approximate measure, and weight (in grams)	Water (%)	Food energy (cal.)	Protein (gm.)	Fat (total lipid) (gm.)	Saturated (total) (gm.)	Unsaturated Oleic (gm.)	Unsaturated Linoleic (gm.)	Carbohydrate (gm.)	Calcium (mg.)	Iron (mg.)	Vitamin A value (I.V.)	Thiamine (mg.)	Riboflavin (mg.)	Niacin (mg.)	Ascorbic acid (mg.)
Soups, canned; ready-to-serve (prepared with equal volume of water):															
Bean with pork 1 cup 250	84	170	8	6	1	2	2	22	62	2.2	650	0.14	0.07	1.0	2
Beef noodle 1 cup 250	93	70	4	3	1	1	1	7	8	1.0	50	0.05	0.06	1.1	Trace
Beef bouillon, broth, consomme. 1 cup 240	96	30	5	0	0	0	0	3	Trace	0.5	Trace	Trace	0.02	1.2	—
Chicken noodle 1 cup 250	93	65	4	2	Trace	1	1	8	10	0.5	50	0.02	0.02	0.8	Trace
Clam chowder 1 cup 255	92	85	2	3				13	36	1.0	920	0.03	0.03	1.0	—
Cream soup (mushroom) 1 cup 240	90	135	2	10	1	3	5	10	41	0.5	70	0.02	0.12	0.7	Trace
Minestrone 1 cup 245	90	105	5	3				14	37	1.0	2,350	0.07	0.05	1.0	—
Pea, green 1 cup 245	86	130	6	2	1	1	Trace	23	44	1.0	340	0.05	0.05	1.0	7
Tomato 1 cup 245	90	90	2	2	Trace	1		16	15	0.7	1,000	0.06	0.05	1.1	12
Vegetable with beef broth. 1 cup 250	92	80	3	2				14	20	0.8	3,250	0.05	0.02	1.2	—
Starch (cornstarch) 1 cup 128	12	465	Trace	Trace				112	0	0	0	0	0	0	0
1 tablespoon 8	12	30	Trace	Trace				7	0	0	0	0	0	0	0
Tapioca, quick-cooking granulated, dry, stirred before measuring. 1 cup 152	13	535	1	Trace				131	15	0.6	0	0	0	0	0
1 tablespoon 10	13	35	Trace	Trace				9	1	Trace	0	0	0	0	0
Vinegar 1 tablespoon 15	—	2	0	—				1	1	0.1	—	—	—	—	—
White sauce, medium 1 cup 265	73	430	10	33	18	11	1	23	305	0.5	1,220	0.12	0.44	0.6	Trace
Yeast:															
Baker's:															
Compressed 1 ounce 28	71	25	3	Trace				3	4	1.4	Trace	0.20	0.47	3.2	Trace
Dry active 1 ounce 28	5	80	10	Trace				11	12	4.6	Trace	0.66	1.53	10.4	Trace
Brewer's, dry, debittered. 1 tablespoon 8	5	25	3	Trace				3	17	1.4	Trace	1.25	0.34	3.0	Trace
Yoghurt. *See* Milk, cream, cheese; related products.															

Selected sources of reliable nutrition information

American Dental Association
222 E. Superior Street
Chicago, Illinois 60611

American Dietetic Association
620 N. Michigan Avenue
Chicago, Illinois 60611

American Institute of Baking
400 E. Ontario Street
Chicago, Illinois 60611

American Medical Association
535 N. Dearborn Street
Chicago, Illinois 60610

Borden Company
350 Madison Avenue
New York, N. Y. 10017

National Academy of Sciences
National Research Council
2101 Constitution Avenue
Washington, D. C. 20418

National Dairy Council
111 N. Canal Street
Chicago, Illinois 60606

National Meat and Livestock Board
33 S. Wabash Avenue
Chicago, Illinois 60603

Nutrition Foundation, Inc.
99 Park Avenue
New York, N. Y. 10016

Superintendent of Documents
U. S. Government Printing Office
Washington, D. C. 20402

U. S. Department of Agriculture
Washington, D. C. 20250

Index

A